AAOS
AMERICAN ACADEMY OF ORTHOPAEDIC SURGEONS

ECSI
EMERGENCY CARE & SAFETY INSTITUTE

First Aid, CPR, and AED ADVANCED

Meets CPR and ECC Guidelines

EIGHTH EDITION

American College of Emergency Physicians®
ADVANCING EMERGENCY CARE

Authors

Alton L. Thygerson, EdD, FAWM

Steven M. Thygerson, PhD, MSPH, CIH

Justin S. Thygerson, PhD, CSP

Medical Editors

Alfonso Mejia, MD, MPH, FAAOS

Bob Elling, MPA, EMT-P

JONES & BARTLETT LEARNING

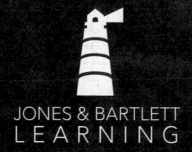

World Headquarters
Jones & Bartlett Learning
5 Wall Street
Burlington, MA 01803
978-443-5000
info@jblearning.com
www.jblearning.com
www.psglearning.com

Substantial discounts on bulk quantities of Jones & Bartlett Learning publications are available to corporations, professional associations, and other qualified organizations. For details and specific discount information, contact the special sales department at Jones & Bartlett Learning via the above contact information or send an email to specialsales@jblearning.com.

Jones & Bartlett Learning books and products are available through most bookstores and online booksellers. To contact the Jones & Bartlett Learning Public Safety Group directly, call 800-832-0034, fax 978-443-8000, or visit our website, www.psglearning.com.

The material presented in *Advanced First Aid, CPR, and AED, Eighth Edition* has been made available by the American Academy of Orthopaedic Surgeons (AAOS) for educational purposes only. This material is not intended to present the only, or necessarily best, methods or procedures for the medical situations discussed, but rather is intended to represent an approach, view, statement, or opinion of the author(s) or producer(s), which may be helpful to others who face similar situations. Medical providers should use their own, independent medical judgment, in addition to open discussion with patients, when developing patient care recommendations and treatment plans. Medical care should always be based on a medical provider's expertise that is individually tailored to a patient's circumstances, preferences and rights. Some drugs or medical devices demonstrated in AAOS courses or described in AAOS print or electronic publications have not been cleared by the Food and Drug Administration (FDA) or have been cleared for specific uses only. The FDA has stated that it is the responsibility of the physician to determine the FDA clearance status of each drug or device he or she wishes to use in clinical practice and to use the products with appropriate patient consent and in compliance with applicable law. Furthermore, any statements about commercial products are solely the opinion(s) of the author(s) and do not represent an AAOS endorsement or evaluation of these products. These statements may not be used in advertising or for any commercial purpose.

There may be images in this book that feature models; these models do not necessarily endorse, represent, or participate in the activities represented in the images. Any screenshots in this product are for educational and instructive purposes only. Any individuals and scenarios featured in the case studies throughout this product may be real or fictitious but are used for instructional purposes only.

The procedures and protocols in this book are based on the most current recommendations of responsible medical sources. AAOS and the publisher, however, make no guarantee as to, and assume no responsibility for, the correctness, sufficiency, or completeness of such information or recommendations. Other or additional safety measures may be required under particular circumstances.

This textbook is intended solely as a guide to the appropriate procedures to be employed when rendering emergency care to the sick and injured. It is not intended as a statement of the standards of care required in any particular situation, because circumstances and the patient's physical condition can vary widely from one emergency to another. Nor is it intended that this textbook shall in any way advise emergency personnel concerning legal authority to perform the activities or procedures discussed. Such local determination should be made only with the aid of legal counsel.

23142-7

Production Credits
VP, Product Development: Christine Emerton
Director of Product Management: Cathy Esperti
Product Manager: Carly Mahoney
Content Strategist: Ashley Procum
Project Manager: Kristen Rogers
Project Specialist: John Fuller
Senior Digital Project Specialist: Angela Dooley
Director of Marketing Operations: Brian Rooney
Content Services Manager: Colleen Lamy
VP, Manufacturing and Inventory Control: Therese Connell
Composition: S4Carlisle Publishing Services
Cover and Text Design: Scott Moden
Senior Media Development Editor: Troy Liston
Rights & Permissions Manager: John Rusk
Rights Specialist: Rebecca Damon
Cover and title page image: © Microgen/Shutterstock
Printing and Binding: LSC Communications

Library of Congress Cataloging-in-Publication Data
Names: Thygerson, Alton L. First aid, CPR, and AED. Advanced. | American Academy of Orthopaedic Surgeons, issuing body.
Title: First aid, CPR, and AED. Advanced / American Academy of Orthopaedic Surgeons.
Description: Eighth edition. | Burlington, MA : Jones & Bartlett Learning, [2022] | Preceded by First aid, CPR, and AED. Advanced / Alton L. Thygerson, Steven M. Thygerson. Seventh edition. [2017]. | Includes bibliographical references and index.
Identifiers: LCCN 2021010019 | ISBN 9781284231427 (paperback)
Subjects: MESH: First Aid | Emergencies | Cardiopulmonary Resuscitation | Electric Countershock
Classification: LCC RC86.7 | NLM WA 292 | DDC 616.02/52--dc23
LC record available at https://lccn.loc.gov/2021010019

6048

Printed in the United States of America
25 24 23 22 10 9 8 7 6 5 4 3

Brief Contents

Contents

Skill Sheets

Flowcharts

Welcome to the Emergency Care & Safety Institute

Welcome to the Emergency Care and Safety Institute (ECSI), brought to you by the American Academy of Orthopaedic Surgeons (AAOS) and the American College of Emergency Physicians (ACEP).

ECSI is an internationally renowned organization that provides training and certifications that meet job-related requirements as defined by regulatory authorities such as the Occupational Safety and Health Administration (OSHA), the Joint Commission, and state offices of Emergency Medical Services (EMS), Education, Transportation, and Health. Our courses are delivered throughout a range of industries and markets worldwide, including colleges and universities, business and industry, governments, public safety agencies, hospitals, private training companies, and secondary school systems.

ECSI programs are offered in association with the AAOS and ACEP. AAOS, the world's largest medical association of musculoskeletal specialists, is known as the original name in EMS publishing, putting out the first EMS textbook ever in 1971, and ACEP is widely recognized as the leading name in all of emergency medicine.

ECSI Course Catalog

Individuals seeking training from ECSI can choose from among various traditional classroom-based courses or alternative online courses, such as:

- Advanced Cardiac Life Support (ACLS)
- Basic Life Support (BLS) for Health Care Providers
- Bloodborne and Airborne Pathogens
- CPR and AED
- First Aid (standard, advanced, pediatric, pet, sports, wilderness)

ECSI
EMERGENCY CARE
& SAFETY INSTITUTE

ECSI offers a wide range of textbooks, instructor and student support materials, and interactive technology, including online courses. ECSI student manuals are the center of an integrated teaching and learning system that offers resources to better support instructors and train students. The instructor supplements provide practical, hands-on, time-saving tools such as slides in PowerPoint format, skills demonstration videos, and Web-based, distance learning resources. Technology resources provide interactive exercises and simulations to help students become prepared for any emergency.

Documents attesting to ECSI's recognitions of satisfactory course completion will be issued to those who successfully meet the course requirements. Written acknowledgment of a participant's successful course completion is provided in the form of a Course Completion Card, issued by the ECSI.

Visit **www.ECSInstitute.org** today!

Preface

2020 Guideline Updates and the COVID-19 Pandemic

This book exceeds the requirements of the 2020 American Heart Association (AHA) Emergency Cardiovascular Care (ECC) Guidelines and the 2020 International Liaison Committee on Resuscitation (ILCOR) Consensus on Science with Treatment Recommendations (CoSTR). At this time, we find ourselves in the middle of a 100-year event: the COVID-19 pandemic. These updates were made with the pandemic in mind.

Although we are perhaps more mindful than ever of the importance of personal protective equipment (PPE) during first aid treatment, readers will still notice some variability throughout this textbook with regard to PPE worn by first aid providers as they care for those who are injured or ill. They may also question the inclusion of skills and techniques that are discouraged in the context of COVID-19.

We have tried throughout the text to apply the best current knowledge and practices available. However, that science is developing rapidly, and we will make every attempt to make supplemental material available that reflects the most updated knowledge.

Face Masks

Prior to 2020, the level of PPE commonly worn by all first aid providers during first aid treatment typically included disposable gloves when possible. Face masks are now standard equipment for all interpersonal encounters, not just during first aid treatment. Social distancing guidelines mandate the use of masks in public. People without symptoms can still be infected with the virus and thus transmit it to others. Asking everyone to wear a mask during first aid treatment can make those encounters safer.

Art and Photos

Revising the illustrations and images throughout the book has been a challenge. Organizing photo shoots has been dramatically hindered by necessary social distancing restrictions. For this reason, we ensured that first aid providers and other relevant parties were wearing face masks and appropriate eye protection in any new images that were shot for this textbook. However, we were not able to update all the photos to reflect new practice guidelines. It is certainly our hope that by the time the next edition is published, our knowledge of best practices with regard to PPE will be more static and there will be more consistency in the appearance of PPE in images throughout the text.

Cardiopulmonary Resuscitation

This revised text includes coverage of mouth-to-mouth cardiopulmonary resuscitation (CPR) and mouth-to-barrier CPR. These techniques are still key competencies for the first aid provider whose partner or family member has, for example, experienced cardiac arrest. This text also includes coverage of hands-only CPR for instances where the first aid provider is unable or unwilling to provide rescue breaths. In the midst of the COVID-19 pandemic, ILCOR recommends that layperson first aid providers consider hands-only CPR and defibrillation for treating those who are not members of the provider's household and consider rescue breaths and chest compressions for infants and children.

Acknowledgments

The authors, medical editors, Jones & Bartlett Learning Public Safety Group, American Academy of Orthopaedic Surgeons, and American College of Emergency Physicians would like to thank all of the reviewers who generously offered their time, expertise, and talent to the making of this eighth edition.

Reviewers

Erwin J. Banola, MS
CAHPERD
SHAPE America
Santa Clarita, California

Gwen Barnett, BS, MT (ASCP)
Southern Indiana Career and Technical Center
Evansville, Indiana

Gabriel Beecham, MD, MRCEM, MCAI, DipIMC (RCSEd)
Specialist Registrar
Children's Health Ireland
Crumlin, Dublin, Ireland

Mark A. Boisclair, MPA, NRP
EMS Programs
Chattahoochee Valley Community College
Phenix City, Alabama

Isabel Jeannette Brea, MD, MPH, FACEP, FAAEM
Herbert Wertheim College of Medicine Florida International University
Miami, Florida

Scott C. Bryan II, MA, DA
American Heart Association BLS Instructor
Emmanuel College
Franklin Springs, Georgia

Thomas E. Charlton, MD, MHSA, FACEP, FAEMS
Assistant Program Director
CMU College of Medicine
Department of Emergency Medicine, Division of EMS
Saginaw-Tuscola MCA
Mount Pleasant, Michigan

Alexander R. Chiu, MD, MBA, FACEP
Chief Executive Officer
Air Visits, Inc
Faculty, Health + Hospitals/Coney Island Hospital
Assistant Professor
State University of New York Downstate College of Medicine
Chairman
Technology SIG, American Telemedicine Association
New York, New York

Kent Courtney
Paramedic, Fire Fighter, Rescue Technician, Educator
Essential Safety Training and Consulting
Rimrock, Arizona

Chance Cummings, Lieutenant, Paramedic
EMS Liaison Officer
Starkville Fire Department
Starkville, Mississippi

Kathleen E. Curran, MSHA/Ed, MSP
Kean University
Union, New Jersey

Daniel Du Pont, MD, MBE
Resident Physician
Emergency Medicine
Hospital of the University of Pennsylvania
Philadelphia, Pennsylvania

Alyson G. Dykes, MS, BSN-RN
Lindenwood University
Saint Charles, Missouri

Frank Fannin, MD, EMT-P, FACEP, EMS
Prospect, Kentucky

Jeffrey D. Ferguson, MD, NRP, FACEP
Department of Emergency Medicine
Virginia Commonwealth University
Richmond, Virginia

James W. Fogal, MA, NRP
Auburn University
Auburn, Alabama

Emerson Franke, MD
Rutgers/RWJBarnabas Health
New Jersey

Scott B. Fredericks, NRAEMT
EMS Instructor
Harrisburg Area Community College
Shumaker Public Safety Center
Harrisburg, Pennsylvania

Fidel O. Garcia, Paramedic
Professional EMS Education
Grand Junction, Colorado

Gary D. Harmon, MS, BS, AAS, NRP
Lees-McRae College
Banner Elk, North Carolina

Joe Holley, MD, FACEP, FAEMS
University of Tennessee Memphis
Emergency Medicine
Memphis, Tennessee

Nate Hunt, MD, PGY-5
EMS Fellow
Department of Emergency Medicine
University of Michigan
Ann Arbor, Michigan

Charna Klein
Adjunct Lecturer
ARC Instructor Trainer
Brooklyn College
Brooklyn, New York

Ellen Komosinski, BPS, NYS EMT, CIC
Adjunct Professor
Suffolk County Community College
Selden, New York

Peri L. Krichbaum, MS, ATC
Columbia State Community College
Columbia, Tennessee

David S. Kugler, MD, MPH, MA, EMT-P, FACEP, FAEMS
Medical Director
SkyHealth
Assistant Professor of Emergency Medicine
Northwell Health
Department of Emergency Medicine
Attending Physician
Associate Medical Director
Center for Emergency Medical Services Hofstra Northwell Health School of Medicine
Chief Division of Aeromedical and Tactical Medicine
New York

David B. Latham, EMT-P
Adjunct Faculty
Oxnard Community College
Camarillo, California

Stu Mavros, EMT, OEC I-T, ECSI I-T
Patrol Rep, Director of High Point Nordic Ski Patrol
Chief and K9 Unit Lead of Search, Rescue, Response & Recovery of New Jersey
Ramsey, New Jersey

Tyler McCardell, BS, NRAEMT
Wakefield EMS
Peach Bottom, Pennsylvania

Gregory S. Neiman, MS, NRP, NCEE
EMS Community Liaison
VCU Health
Richmond, Virginia

Glad Nwaozo, MS, MS4
Drexel University College of Medicine
Philadelphia, Pennsylvania

Brian Oakes, MS, LAT
Assistant Professor
Mansfield University
Mansfield, Pennsylvania

Monty Putman, MD
Orange County EMS System
Orlando, Florida

Jason Quick, Maj., NRP, LP, CAP
Commander
388th CS, Texas Wing, Civil Air Patrol
Fort Worth, Texas

Craig Ramsay, BS, BA, ACP, EMSI
Central Ohio Technical College
Newark, Ohio
Ohio University
Athens, Ohio

Robert Root, DO
Associate Professor of Emergency Medicine
Texas Tech University Health Science Center El Paso
El Paso, Texas

Jared L. Ross, DO, NRP, TCCC, FAAEM
President
EMSEC, LLC
Emergency Medicine Physician
BJC Christian Hospital Northeast
St. Louis, Missouri

Eli Schned, MD, FAWM, DiMM
Monadnock Community Hospital
Peterborough, New Hampshire

Jeremy H. Smith, NRP
Training Officer
Joint Special Operations Medical Training Center
Fort Bragg, North Carolina

Cara L. Stewart
Carl Albert State College
Poteau, Oklahoma

Briana Tully, DO, PHP
Charlottesville, Virginia

William H. Turner, NRP, Paramedic
Assistant Professor, Program Director
Shawnee State University
Portsmouth, Ohio

Scott Webb, NRP
Columbia Safety
Kennewick, Washington

Josh Weiner, NRP, FP-C
Regions Hospital EMS
St. Paul, Minnesota

Deitra E. Wengert, PhD, MCHES
Towson University
Towson, Maryland

Christopher C. Williams, PhD, NRP
Guilford County EMS
Greensboro, North Carolina

Kenneth A. Williams, MD, FACEP, FAEMS
Brown Emergency Medicine
Providence, Rhode Island

Leland "Lee" Yarger, MSEd
Coordinator of Aquatic Degrees, Senior Lecturer of Aquatics
Ball State University School of Kinesiology
Muncie, Indiana

Christian C. Zuver, MD, FACEP
Orange County EMS System
Orlando, Florida

1

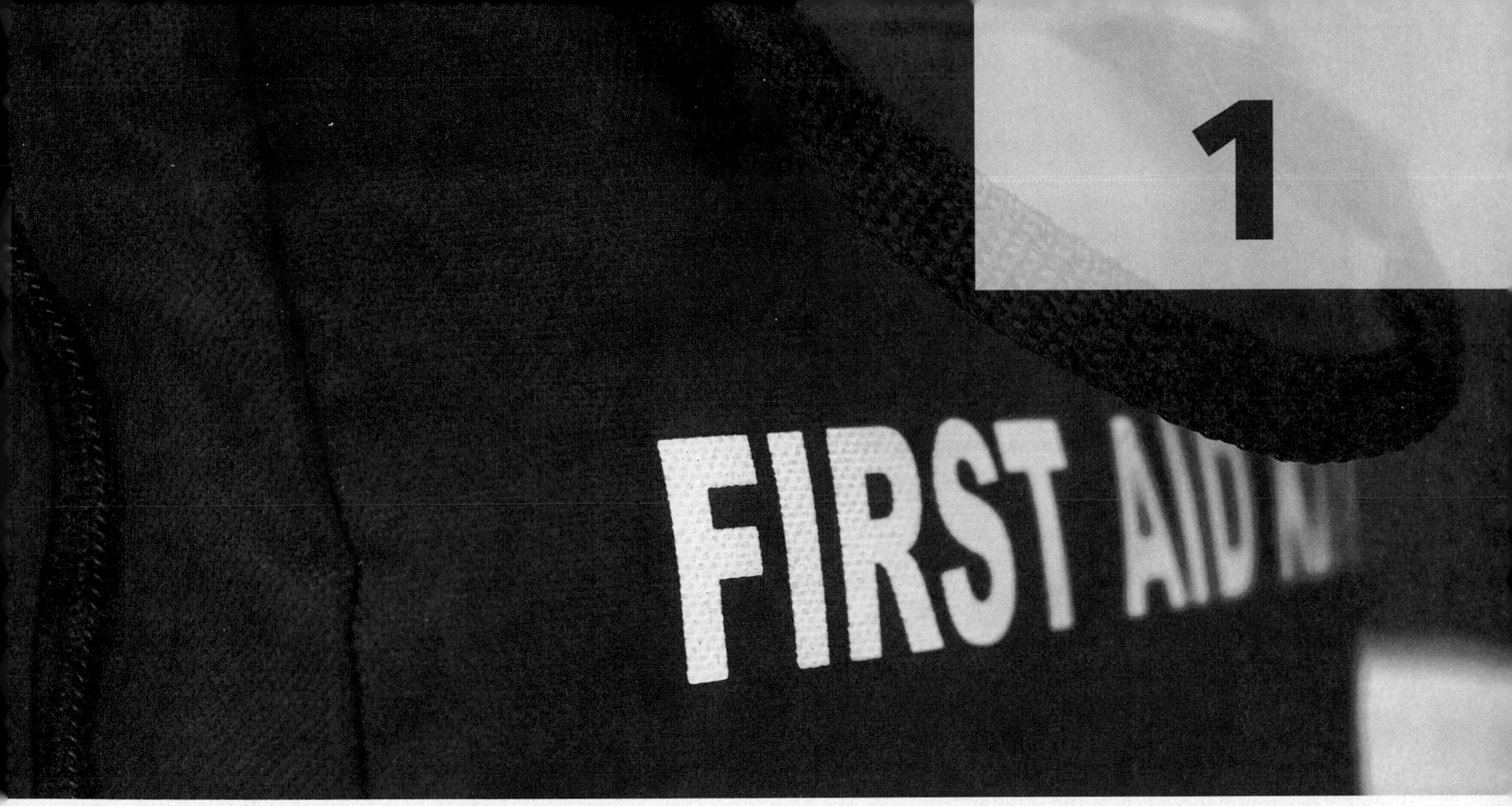

Introduction

CHAPTER AT A GLANCE

Why Is First Aid Important?

A large truck swings around a corner, crashes into an automobile, and pushes it over an embankment. Bystanders rush to the rescue. They pull the injured driver from the car, lift him to his feet, stop a passing car, and send the injured man to a nearby hospital in a sitting position. Because of the lack of knowledge and unskilled handling, the man's spinal cord is injured by the sharp edge of a broken vertebra, and he will remain paralyzed for the rest of his life. This tragic outcome could have been avoided if someone had known what to do in an emergency.

A backcountry hiker is bitten by a rattlesnake. Her frantic companion cuts and sucks the bitten area, not realizing that this is an outdated and harmful procedure. They have now unnecessarily been exposed to her blood. By the time the woman seeks appropriate professional medical care, she has suffered extensive tissue damage. A trained first aid provider would have known the proper procedures to care for this person.

A group of beachgoers removes an unresponsive swimmer from the water. No one helps because no one knows cardiopulmonary resuscitation (CPR). The emergency medical services (EMS) ambulance arrives, and because nothing has been done so far, they are unable to revive the swimmer. CPR would have served as an interim action and preserved life for the few minutes needed until the ambulance arrived, potentially giving the EMS providers a chance of reviving the swimmer.

Late at night, a man who had earlier smashed a finger in a car door can no longer stand the excruciating pain caused by the pressure of blood accumulating underneath the fingernail. He drives himself to a hospital emergency department where a physician relieves a blood clot. The man later receives an expensive hospital bill. If he had known the proper first aid procedure, he could have potentially relieved the pain sooner and saved money.

These cases clearly point out the need for first aid training. *It is better to know it and not need it than to need it and not know it.* Everyone should be able to perform first aid, because most people will eventually find themselves in a situation requiring it for another person or for themselves. First aid providers do not diagnose (this is what physicians do); however they can suspect what the problem is and then provide first aid.

Who Needs First Aid?

Just as heart disease and cancer demand public attention because of the critical health risks they pose in the United States, injury—both unintentional and intentional—must be recognized as a major threat to public health. This threat has been called the neglected epidemic. **TABLE 1-1** shows the role of injury as a cause of death by age group and ranking compared with other causes of death.

Death statistics do not always reflect the extent or severity of the injury problem. Most injuries and sudden illnesses do not result in death, but rather result in hospitalization; treatment in an emergency department, urgent care center, or physician office; or treatment from a first aid provider. According to the World Health Organization, in the world's high-income countries, for every person killed by injury, 30 people are hospitalized and 300 people are treated in emergency departments; even more are treated in other health care facilities and by first aid providers.

> **FYI**
>
> **OSHA (Occupational Safety and Health Administration) Regulations**
>
> Standard 29 CFR 1910.151: Medical Services and First Aid—General Industry:
> "In the absence of an infirmary, clinic, or hospital in near proximity to workplace which is used for the treatment of all injured employees, a person or persons shall be adequately trained to render first aid. Adequate first aid supplies shall be readily available."

The injury pyramid, as shown in **FIGURE 1-1**, helps illustrate the distribution of injury severity. The top of the pyramid is composed of deaths caused by injury. Although deaths from injury are fewer in number than other types of injuries, they are more visible because they are considered newsworthy and often appear on radio and television, in the print newspapers, social media, and online news resources. The second category is composed of severe injuries that result in hospitalization and disability. Severe injuries are followed on the pyramid by less-severe injuries, those that require emergency department care or urgent care centers, and those that are treated in basic health care facilities. Finally, at the bottom of the pyramid are injuries that do not require professional medical care and that are instead treated by a first aid provider.

TABLE 1-2 shows the leading causes of nonfatal injuries treated at hospital emergency departments by age group in the United States. Each year, one in four people experiences a nonfatal injury serious enough to need professional medical care or to restrict activity for at least 1 day. More sports-related nonfatal injuries are treated in hospital emergency departments than any other type of unintentional injury.

Death occurs when a person's heart stops. Therefore, what a bystander does can mean the difference between life and death. Fortunately, most injuries and sudden illnesses do not require life-saving efforts. During their entire lifetimes, most people will rarely, if ever, see a life-threatening condition outside of a medical facility. Saving lives is important, but first aid providers are more frequently called upon to provide initial care for less-severe conditions. If not properly treated, these less-severe injuries can evolve into something more serious. As such, these skills demand attention during first aid training.

Each year, the injuries of millions of Americans go unreported. For many of these people, the injury causes temporary pain and inconvenience; for others, however, the injury leads to disability, chronic pain, and a profound change in lifestyle. Given the size of the injury and sudden illness problem, everyone should be prepared to deal with an emergency.

Value of First Aid to Self

Although many people learn first aid to help others, the training primarily helps oneself. It enables first aid providers to give proper immediate care to their own injuries and sudden illnesses. If people are too seriously injured to help themselves, they could be able to direct others in proper care. First aid training also helps develop safety awareness. Discussing injuries teaches people how injuries occur and thus promotes injury prevention.

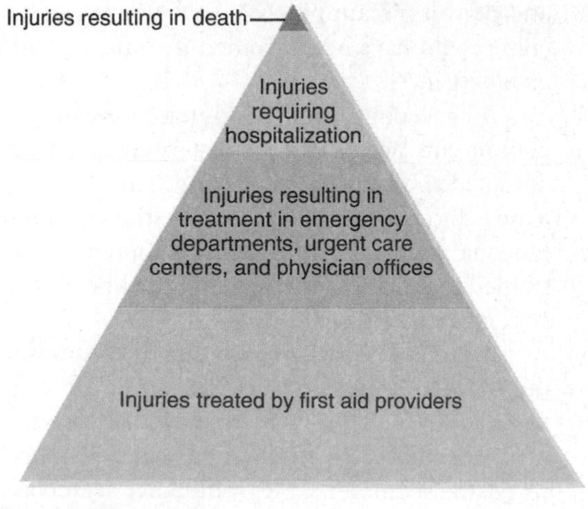

FIGURE 1-1 Injury pyramid.

TABLE 1-1 Ten Leading Causes of Death by Age Group, United States, 2018

Age Groups (Years)										
<1	1–4	5–9	10–14	15–24	25–34	35–44	45–54	55–64	65+	Total
Congenital anomalies 4,473	Unintentional injury 1,226	Unintentional injury 734	Unintentional injury 692	Unintentional injury 12,044	Unintentional injury 24,614	Unintentional injury 22,677	Malignant neoplasms 37,301	Malignant neoplasms 113,957	Heart disease 526,509	Heart disease 655,381
Short gestation 3,679	Congenital anomalies 384	Malignant neoplasms 393	Suicide 596	Suicide 6,211	Suicide 8,020	Malignant neoplasms 10,640	Heart disease 32,220	Heart disease 81,042	Malignant neoplasms 431,102	Malignant neoplasms 599,274
Maternal pregnancy complications 1,358	Homicide 353	Congenital anomalies 201	Malignant neoplasms 450	Homicide 4,607	Homicide 5,234	Heart disease 10,532	Unintentional injury 23,056	Unintentional injury 23,693	Chronic lower respiratory disease 135,560	Unintentional injury 167,127
SIDS 1,334	Malignant neoplasms 326	Homicide 121	Congenital anomalies 172	Malignant neoplasms 1,371	Malignant neoplasms 3,684	Suicide 7,521	Suicide 8,345	Chronic lower respiratory disease 18,804	Cerebrovascular causes 127,244	Chronic lower respiratory disease 159,486
Unintentional injury 1,168	Influenza and pneumonia 122	Influenza and pneumonia 71	Homicide 168	Heart disease 905	Heart disease 3,3561	Homicide 3,304	Liver disease 8,157	Diabetes mellitus 14,941	Alzheimer disease 120,658	Cerebrovascular causes 147,810
Placenta cord membranes 724	Heart disease 115	Chronic lower respiratory disease 68	Heart disease 101	Congenital anomalies 354	Liver disease 1,088	Liver disease 3,108	Diabetes mellitus 6,414	Liver disease 13,945	Diabetes mellitus 60,182	Alzheimer disease 122,019
Bacterial sepsis 579	Perinatal period 62	Heart disease 68	Chronic lower respiratory disease 64	Diabetes mellitus 246	Diabetes mellitus 837	Diabetes mellitus 2,282	Cerebrovascular causes 5,128	Cerebrovascular causes 12,789	Unintentional injury 57,213	Diabetes mellitus 84,946
Circulatory system disease 428	Septicemia 54	Cerebrovascular causes 34	Cerebrovascular causes 54	Influenza and pneumonia 200	Cerebrovascular causes 567	Cerebrovascular causes 1,704	Chronic lower respiratory disease 3,807	Suicide 8,540	Influenza and pneumonia 48,888	Influenza and pneumonia 59,120
Respiratory distress 390	Chronic lower respiratory disease 50	Septicemia 34	Influenza and pneumonia 51	Chronic lower respiratory disease 165	HIV 482	Influenza and pneumonia 956	Septicemia 2,380	Septicemia 5,956	Nephritis 42,232	Nephritis 51,386
Neonatal hemorrhage 375	Cerebrovascular 43	Benign neoplasms 19	Benign neoplasms 30	Complicated Pregnancy 151	Influenza and pneumonia 457	Septicemia 829	Influenza and pneumonia 2,339	Influenza and pneumonia 5,858	Parkinson disease 32,988	Suicide 48,344

Data from National Vital Statistics System, National Center for Health Statistics, CDC.

TABLE 1-2 Ten Leading Causes of Nonfatal Injuries Treated in Hospital Emergency Departments in the United States, 2017

Age Groups (Years)										
<1	1–4	5–9	10–14	15–24	25–34	35–44	45–54	55–64	65+	Total
Fall 120,007	Fall 699,107	Fall 530,390	Struck by/against 451,267	Struck by/against 755,114	Fall 647,408	Fall 623,997	Fall 828,731	Fall 1,047,959	Fall 2,970,720	Fall 8,591,683
Struck by/against 23,356	Struck by/against 254,793	Struck by/against 323,525	Fall 451,183	Fall 671,408	MV-occupant 579,446	Other specified 436,726	Other specified 473,726	Other specified 356,187	Struck by/against 312,954	Struck by/against 3,685,012
Other bite/sting 13,505	Other bite/sting 139,941	Other bite/sting 107,577	Overexertion 222,433	MV-occupant 595,092	Struck by/against 528,104	Struck by/against 396,695	Overexertion 362,246	Struck by/against 278,211	Overexertion 227,817	Overexertion 2,569,850
Other specified 9,737	Foreign body 121,422	Cut/pierce 88,488	Cut/pierce 99,249	Overexertion 493,072	Other specified 517,628	Overexertion 395,791	Struck by/against 360,767	Overexertion 258,488	MV-occupant 215,666	MV-occupant 2,500,353
Foreign body 8,618	Cut/pierce 60,421	Overexertion 65,413	Unknown/unspecified 67,107	Cut/pierce 345,982	Overexertion 482,430	MV-occupant 381,110	Poisoning 337,444	MV-occupant 249,192	Cut/pierce 162,819	Other specified 2,365,891
Inhalation/suffocation 8,518	Overexertion 58,727	MV-occupant 53,791	MV-occupant 64,349	Other specified 331,389	Poisoning 401,819	Poisoning 321,267	MV-occupant 331,388	Poisoning 245,289	Other specified 143,563	Cut/pierce 1,823,358
Fire/burn 7,567	Other specified 47,348	Foreign body 52,756	Other bite/sting 57,014	Other assault, struck by/against 312,205	Cut/pierce 327,787	Cut/pierce 269,865	Cut/pierce 235,597	Cut/pierce 184,284	Poisoning 137,849	Poisoning 1,755,044
Unknown/unspecified 4,618	Fire/burn 41,066	Pedal cyclist 39,388	Other assault, struck by/against 54,366	Poisoning 246,611	Other assault, struck by/against 355,927	Other assault, struck by/against 212,483	Other assault, struck by/against 171,022	Other bite/sting 115,933	Other bite/sting 116,191	Other assault, struck by/against 1,261,580
Cut/pierce 3,844	Unknown/unspecified 38,207	Dog bite 33,586	Pedal cyclist 49,283	Pedal cyclist 147,861	Other bite/sting 176,855	Other bite/sting 131,323	Other bite/sting 135,907	Other assault, struck by/against 95,550	Unknown/unspecified 96,304	Other bite/sting 1,142,130
Poisoning 3,459	Poisoning 37,493	Unknown/unspecified 32,336	Other transport 40,876	Unknown/unspecified 122,980	Unknown/unspecified 120,116	Unknown/unspecified 98,759	Unknown/unspecified 95,913	Unknown/unspecified 78,898	Other transport 79,829	Unknown/unspecified 755,567

* With the exception of the "Other assault" category, all causes of injury in this table are unintentional.

Abbreviation: MV, motor vehicle

Data from Office of Statistics and Programming, National Center for Injury Prevention and Control, CDC.

Value of First Aid to Others

People with first aid training are more likely to give proper assistance to injured family members. Although the main beneficiaries are the trained person and their family, the benefits of knowing appropriate first aid techniques extend further, usually to coworkers, acquaintances, and strangers.

Value of First Aid in Remote Areas

Should an injury or sudden illness require professional medical care, time, distance, and availability are major considerations. EMS can reach most people who are severely injured or suddenly ill within 10 to 20 minutes. However, some people are long distances from professional medical care. Although many people associate long distances and lack of professional medical care with wilderness settings involving outdoor recreational activities (eg, hiking, camping, hunting, and snowmobiling), other settings also demand that people be prepared to give first aid for an extended time. The following are some examples:

- Urban areas after a disaster that destroys or overwhelms EMS
- Remote areas relating to one's occupation (eg, farming, ranching, commercial fishing, and forestry)
- Remote communities
- Developing countries

First aid needed in remote locations is similar to that needed in urban settings, but extra skills are sometimes required. See Chapter 24, *Wilderness First Aid*, for information on delivering first aid in remote locations.

What Is First Aid?

The International Liaison Committee on Resuscitation (ILCOR) guidelines define **first aid** as the helping behaviors and initial care provided for an acute illness or injury. According to the guidelines, the goals of the first aid provider include "preserving life, alleviating suffering, preventing further illness or injury, and promoting recovery." First aid, which includes self-care, can be initiated by anyone in any situation but should be based on medical and scientific evidence or expert consensus. First aid competencies include the following:

- Recognizing, assessing, and prioritizing the need for first aid
- Providing care by using appropriate knowledge, skills, and behaviors
- Recognizing limitations and seeking additional care when needed

First aid does not take the place of professional medical care. In most cases, professional medical care is unnecessary and the ill or injured person will safely recover.

Legal Aspects of First Aid

Legal and ethical issues concern all first aid providers. For example, are you required to stop and give care at an automobile crash? Are you allowed to treat a child with a broken arm even when the parents cannot be contacted for their consent? These and many other legal and ethical questions confront first aid providers.

A first aid provider can be sued. However, do not become overly concerned about being sued; it rarely happens. Ways to minimize the risk of a lawsuit include the following:

- Obtain the person's consent before helping and touching them.
- Follow this text's guidelines, and do not exceed your training level.
- Review the standards of first aid, and stay up to date on best practices.
- Explain any first aid you are about to give.
- Treat everyone with respect.
- Once you have started to care for a person, stay with that person. You are legally bound to remain with the person until care is turned over to an equally or better trained person.

> **Q&A**
>
> **What level of care am I expected to give?**
>
> The level of care required of a provider is referred to as the **standard of care.** A first aid provider cannot provide the same level of care as a physician or an emergency medical technician. When you are providing first aid, you must do the following to meet the standard of care: (1) do what is expected of someone with first aid training and experience working under similar conditions, and (2) treat the person to the best of your ability. If the first aid you provide is not up to the expected standard, you may be held liable for your actions.

Consent

A first aid provider must have the person's **consent** (permission) before giving first aid. Touching another person without their consent (which is known as **battery**) is unlawful and could be grounds for a lawsuit. The lawsuit could also include a charge of **assault**, a threat or attempt to touch another person. Likewise, giving first aid without the person's consent is unlawful.

Informed (Expressed) Consent

Consent must be obtained from every alert, mentally competent (able to make a rational decision) person of legal age. Tell the person that you have first aid training and explain what you will be doing. The person may give permission verbally or with a nod of the head, which would indicate **expressed consent**.

Implied Consent

Implied consent involves an unresponsive person with a life-threatening condition. It is assumed or implied that an unresponsive person would consent to life-saving interventions. An alert person who does not resist the care of a first aid provider is also assumed to have given implied consent.

Children and Incompetent Adults

Consent must be obtained from the parent or guardian of a child, as legally defined by the state. In some states, a minor can give consent to receive medical care, depending on the minor's age and maturity. In many states, minors who are married, are members of the armed services, or are parents are legally considered adults. Consent must also be obtained from the parent or guardian of an adult who is mentally incompetent (unable to make a rational decision). A care giver or health care proxy could provide consent for an adult who has dementia and is unable to consent for themselves.

When life-threatening situations exist and a parent or legal guardian is not available for consent, first aid should be given based on implied consent. Do not withhold first aid just to obtain consent from a parent or guardian.

Psychiatric emergencies present difficult issues of consent. Under most conditions, a police officer is the only person with the authority to restrain and transport a person against that person's will. A first aid provider should not intervene unless directed to do so by a police officer or unless it is obvious that the person is about to do life-threatening harm to themselves or others.

Q&A

How can I avoid a lawsuit resulting from giving first aid?

Before giving first aid, get the person's consent or permission. Then provide quality care, keep within your training level, be nice to the person, and try to ensure that witnesses are on hand. Afterward, write down what you did, who was present (ie, names of witnesses), and who took over the person's care from you.

Refusing Help

Although it seldom happens, a person might refuse assistance for countless reasons, such as religious grounds, avoidance of possible pain, or the desire to be examined by a physician rather than by a first aid provider. Whatever the reason for refusing first aid, or even if no reason is given, an alert and mentally competent adult can reject help.

Generally, the wisest approach is for you to inform the person of their medical condition, what you propose to do, and why the help is necessary. If the person understands the consequences and still refuses treatment, there is little else you can do. Call 9-1-1 and, while awaiting arrival, do the following:

- Try again to persuade the person to accept care, and encourage others at the scene to persuade the person. A person could change their mind after a short time.
- Make certain you have witnesses. A person could refuse consent and then deny having done so.
- Consider calling for law enforcement assistance. In most locations, the police can place a person in protective custody and require them to go to a hospital.

Do not worry about the legal implications if someone denies refusing consent. Unless you have a duty to act (see the "Duty to Act" section below), you are not required to give first aid.

Abandonment

Abandonment means leaving a person after starting to give help without first ensuring that the person will receive continued care at the same level or higher. Once you have responded to an emergency, you must not leave a person who needs continuing first aid until another competent and trained person takes responsibility for the person. This might seem obvious, but cases exist in which critically ill or injured people were left unattended and then died. Thus, a first aid provider must stay with the person until another equally or better trained person takes over.

Negligence

Negligence means not following the accepted standards of care, resulting in further injury to the person. Negligence involves the following:

1. Having a duty to act (ie, an obligation to give first aid)
2. Breaching that duty (either by not giving care or by giving substandard care)
3. Causing injury and damages
4. Exceeding your level of training

Duty to Act

No one is required to give first aid unless a legal **duty to act** exists. Usually, the decision to help in an emergency is an ethical (moral) one. However, a legal duty to act could apply in the following situations:

- *When employment requires it.* If your employer designates you as the person responsible for providing first aid to meet OSHA requirements and you are called to an injury scene, you have a duty to act. Examples of occupations that involve a legal obligation to give first aid include law enforcement officers, park rangers, athletic trainers, lifeguards, flight attendants, and fire fighters.

  A person's employment-related duty to act may extend to off-duty hours. Some states require certain people who are trained by the state to give emergency care regardless of their on- or off-duty status. In other words, these people are considered to be always on duty. Other states require such people to act when on duty but not generally when they are off duty, unless they are in uniform or have other visible insignia and appear to be on duty, in which case these people must respond.
- *When a preexisting responsibility exists.* You might have a preexisting relationship with other people that makes you responsible for them, which means you must give first aid should they need it. For example, a parent has a preexisting responsibility for a child and teachers for their students.

- *When you were involved in the events that led to the person's injuries.* Regardless of who was at fault, if you possess first aid training, you are legally obligated to offer care to any person who has been injured or becomes ill as a result of actions in which you are involved. For example, all drivers are required to provide reasonable assistance, including contacting 9-1-1 if professional medical care is needed.

Duty to act means following guidelines for standards of care. *Standards of care* ensure quality care and protection for injured or suddenly ill people. The elements that make up standards of care include the following:

- *The type of rescuer.* A first aid provider should provide the level and type of care expected of a reasonable person with the same amount of training and in similar circumstances. Different standards of care apply to physicians, nurses, emergency medical technicians (EMTs), and first aid providers.
- *Published guidelines.* Organizations and societies devoted to emergency care publish recommended first aid procedures. For example, the American Heart Association publishes guidelines for giving CPR, and the Wilderness Medical Society publishes guidelines for assisting people who are in remote locations. Once trained, you should stay up to date on the latest first aid practices.

Breach of Duty

A **breach of duty** happens when a first aid provider fails to provide the type of care that would be given by a person having the same or similar training. A breach of duty can occur in two ways: through omission and through commission. An **act of omission** is the failure to do what a reasonably prudent person with the same or similar training would do in the same or similar circumstances. An **act of commission** is doing something that a reasonably prudent person would not do under the same or similar circumstances. Forgetting to apply a dressing is an act of omission; cutting the site of a snakebite is an act of commission.

Injury and Damages Inflicted

The unfortunate outcome of a breach of duty is harm to the person in need of care. The most obvious harm is the physical damage produced at the point of contact. However, injury and damage can include subsequent physical pain and suffering, mental anguish, medical expenses, and sometimes loss of earnings and earning capacity. First aid providers can help prevent such adverse outcomes, and can avoid any liability should they occur, by conforming to the appropriate standard of care.

Level of Training Restrictions

As mentioned in the discussion of duty to act, the standard of care expected of a provider depends on the provider's training level and on organizational recommendations. It may seem that meeting the prescribed standard of care is the bare minimum to which a provider should aspire and that going beyond this standard would be commendable. However, in meeting the standard of care, doing the minimum is enough. Providers should not exceed their skill level. Doing more than what is defined by the standard of care may be dangerous to the injured or ill person and possibly even to the provider. If a provider chooses to exceed the standard of care, they can be held liable for any damage done in the process. For example, watching a professional medical procedure portrayed on a medical drama television show or actual procedures shown on the Internet or social media does not qualify a layperson to perform it.

Confidentiality

First aid providers might learn confidential information. It is important that you be extremely cautious about revealing information you learn while caring for someone. The law recognizes that people have the right to privacy. Do not discuss what you know with anyone other than those who have a medical need to know. The exception to this rule is when state laws require the reporting of certain incidents, such as rape, abuse, and gunshot wounds.

Good Samaritan Laws

Starting in the late 1950s, a number of states (beginning with California in 1959) enacted laws designed to protect physicians and other medical personnel from legal actions that might arise from emergency treatment they provided while not in the line of duty. These laws, known as **Good Samaritan laws**, encourage people to assist others in distress by granting them protection from lawsuits. Although the laws vary from state to state, Good Samaritan protection generally applies only when the rescuer (1) is acting during an emergency; (2) is acting in good faith, which means they have good intentions; (3) is acting without compensation; and (4) is not guilty of malicious misconduct or gross negligence toward the person (deviating from rational first aid guidelines).

Although Good Samaritan laws originally covered physician and other health care providers, all states have expanded them to include laypeople serving as first aid providers. In fact, some states have several Good Samaritan laws that cover different types of people in various situations. These laws will not protect first aid providers who have caused further injury to a person. Good Samaritan laws are not a protection for poorly given first aid, nor do they authorize providers to exceed their scope of training. Fear of lawsuits has made some people hesitant about becoming involved in emergency situations. First aid providers, however, are rarely sued.

Some Good Samaritan laws have been expanded to protect the injured or ill and witnesses calling 9-1-1 to report an illness or injury related to illegal activity. For example, certain immunity is offered to people calling in an opioid overdose. Callers may be protected from arrest, charge, and prosecution. These life-saving laws are aimed at reducing the numbers of unintentional deaths from opioid overdoses.

Q&A

What is the rescue doctrine?

The rescue doctrine is an unfamiliar concept to most first aid providers and emergency personnel. The rescue doctrine says that people who are injured while performing a rescue may, unless they have acted rashly or recklessly, recover damages from the person whose negligence created the peril that necessitated the rescue in the first place. In other words, in some cases, an injured first aid provider has the right to recover for injuries sustained while attempting to assist others from those responsible for causing the dangerous rescue. The following are examples of situations covered by the rescue doctrine:

- A person intervenes to rescue another person who is being attacked by a dog and the rescuer is injured. The owner of the dog will be held responsible for the injury.
- A distracted driver fails to see a stop sign. A bystander on a nearby street curb realizes that the driver is about to hit a pedestrian, runs into the street to push the pedestrian out of the way and is hit by the vehicle instead. The driver will be liable for bystander's injury as well for any injuries to the other pedestrian.

Injury Prevention

"An ounce of prevention is worth a pound of cure" refers to the fact that it is better to prevent an injury or illness than it is to treat one. Effective prevention requires a combination of interventions known as the **3Es**: education, enforcement, and engineering.

Educational interventions are the most well known because they are the easiest to implement. Education attempts to change behavior by informing a target group about potential hazards, explaining risks, and persuading people to adopt safer behavior.

Enforcement tries to reduce dangerous behaviors through enforcing laws and regulations. For most laws to be effective, they should incorporate the following elements:

- A perceived high likelihood of apprehension
- Swift penalty delivery
- Penalties that do not always have to be extreme or severe

Engineering makes changes to the environment or product design to protect everyone automatically. This is called a passive or automatic intervention because it requires no work on the part of the person.

Examples of interventions are listed in **TABLE 1-3**.

TABLE 1-3 Examples of Interventions

Education/ Persuasion	Enforcement/Laws	Engineering/ Technology
■ Swimming lessons ■ Gun safety course ■ Social media clip showing a safety procedure or message ■ Weather and road condition alerts for drivers	■ Laws requiring seat belt and helmet use ■ Prohibition of fireworks ■ Laws requiring that personal flotation devices be worn when boating ■ Building codes and inspections	■ Airbags in cars ■ Helmets ■ Child-resistant packaging on medications and chemicals ■ Smoke and carbon monoxide detectors

Haddon Matrix

The **Haddon Matrix** is a strategy for identifying interventions that can be applied to any type of illness or injury. As seen in **TABLE 1-4**, the three major phases progress horizontally from left to right and can be viewed as time phases:

TABLE 1-4 Sample Haddon Matrix

Injury Type	Pre-event	Event	Post-event
Motor vehicle crash	Passing and enforcing drinking and driving laws	Wearing seat belts	Initiating rapid EMS response
Poisoning	Labeling toxic products	Packaging poisons in small, nonlethal amounts	Calling the National Poison Control telephone number
Drowning	Constructing fences around backyard swimming pools	Wearing personal flotation devices	Performing CPR

- *Pre-event.* In this phase, interventions attempt to stop or hinder an event (eg, drowning) from happening. This phase involves prevention efforts.
- *Event.* This phase attempts to modify the consequences of such events either to prevent or to reduce the severity of an injury (eg, airbag inflating on impact).
- *Post-event.* This phase focuses on returning the person to optimal functioning in society after an injury or illness. This phase involves rescue, first aid, medical treatment, and rehabilitation.

Table 1-4 shows examples of interventions related to crashes, poisoning, and drowning.

PREP KIT

Ready for Review

- Everyone should be able to perform first aid because most people will eventually find themselves in a situation requiring it for another person or for themselves.
- First aid is the immediate care given to an injured or suddenly ill person. First aid does not take the place of professional medical care.
- Legal and ethical issues concern all first aid providers.
- A first aid provider must have the person's consent (permission) before giving first aid.
- First aid providers might learn confidential information. It is important that first aid providers be extremely cautious about revealing information they learn while caring for someone.
- Varying from state to state, Good Samaritan laws encourage people to assist others in distress by granting them protection from lawsuits.

Vital Vocabulary

abandonment Failure to continue first aid until relieved by someone with an equal or higher level of training.

act of commission A breach of duty in which the provider does something that a reasonably prudent person would not do under the same or similar circumstances.

act of omission A breach of duty in which the provider fails to do what a reasonably prudent person with the same or similar training would do in the same or similar circumstances.

assault A threat or attempt to touch another person without consent.

battery Touching a person or providing first aid without consent.

breach of duty Failure of a first aid provider to deliver the type of care that would be given by a person having the same or similar training.

consent An agreement by a person in need of care to accept treatment offered as explained by medical personnel or first aid providers.

duty to act A person's responsibility to provide care.

expressed consent Permission for care that a person gives verbally or with a head nod.

first aid Immediate care given to an injured or suddenly ill person.

Good Samaritan laws Laws that encourage people to voluntarily help an injured or suddenly ill person by minimizing the liability for errors made while rendering emergency care in good faith.

Haddon Matrix A strategy for identifying interventions that can be applied to any type of illness or injury. Interventions proceed through three stages: pre-event, event, and post-event.

implied consent The legally permissible assumption that an unconscious person in need of emergency life-saving treatment would accept treatment, were they alert and able.

negligence Deviation from the accepted standard of care that results in further injury to the person.

standard of care The level of care legally and ethically required of a provider. To meet the standard of care when providing first aid, a provider must (1) do what is expected of someone with first aid training and experience working under similar conditions, and (2) treat the person to the best of their ability.

3Es A strategy to produce effective prevention by combining three types of intervention: education, enforcement, and engineering.

Assessment in Action

Toward the end of the ski season, you hear that a ski resort in a neighboring state is nearly empty of skiers and the resort is offering reduced ticket prices during weekdays. You decide to take advantage of the reduced prices and take a few days off to go skiing. As you ski down the mountain on a run with trees bordering on both sides, you come across a man lying motionless in the snow near a tree that he may have crashed into. No other skiers are in sight and you are alone. As you approach the person, you see no obvious injuries. You have no first aid supplies. Your first aid certification is current.

Directions: Circle Yes if you agree with the statement; circle No if you disagree.

1. You have to stop to help the man.

   YES **NO**

2. You have implied consent to help this man.

   YES **NO**

PREP KIT continued

3. After tapping on the man's shoulder to see if he is okay, he remains unresponsive but is breathing. You can leave and assume that the ski patrol will be coming shortly.

   YES NO

4. You are an off-duty paramedic and you decide to help. Can you expect to be paid for the time spent helping the skier?

   YES NO

Check Your Knowledge

Directions: Circle Yes if you agree with the statement; circle No if you disagree.

1. Because an ambulance can arrive within minutes in most locations, most people do not need to learn first aid.

   YES NO

2. Correct first aid can mean the difference between life and death.

   YES NO

3. During your lifetime, you are likely to encounter many life-threatening emergencies.

   YES NO

4. All injured people require professional medical care.

   YES NO

5. Before giving first aid to an alert, competent adult, you must get consent (permission) from the person.

   YES NO

6. If you ask an injured adult if you can help, and they say, "No," you can ignore them and proceed to provide care.

   YES NO

7. People who are designated as first aid providers by their employers must give first aid to injured employees while on the job.

   YES NO

8. First aid providers who help injured people are rarely sued.

   YES NO

9. Good Samaritan laws provide a degree of protection for first aid providers who act in good faith and without compensation.

   YES NO

10. You are required to provide first aid to any injured or suddenly ill person you encounter.

    YES NO

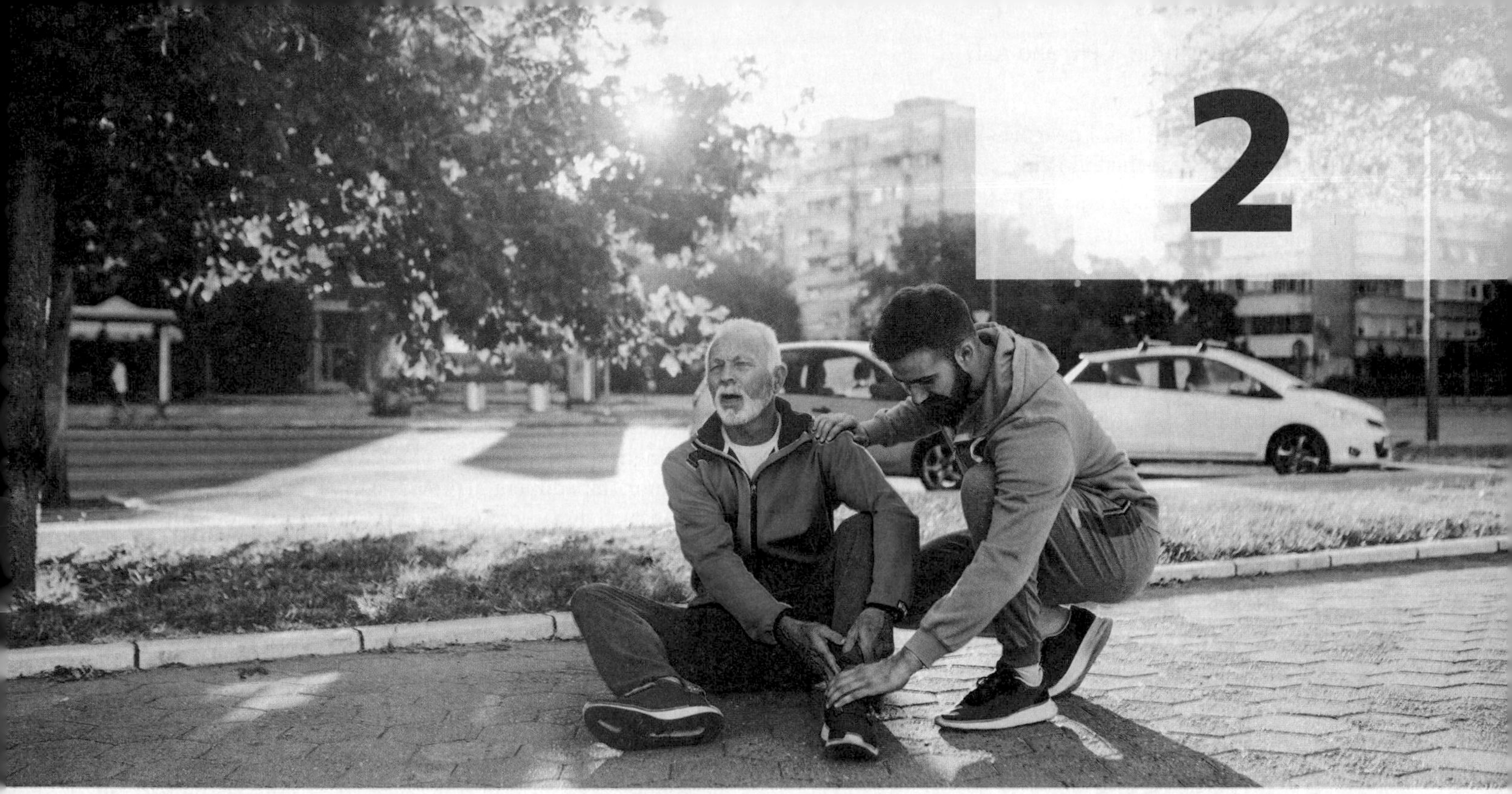

2

Action at an Emergency

CHAPTER AT A GLANCE

Emergencies

Emergencies have the following distinctive characteristics:

- *Dangerous*. People's lives, well-being, or property are threatened.
- *Unusual and rare*. The average person will probably encounter fewer than a half dozen serious emergencies in a lifetime.
- *Different from one another*. Each emergency presents a unique set of issues.
- *Unforeseen*. Emergencies happen suddenly and without warning.
- *Urgent*. If the emergency is not dealt with immediately, the situation will escalate.

Bystander Actions

The bystander is a vital link between **emergency medical services (EMS)** and the injured or suddenly ill person. Typically it is a bystander who recognizes a situation as an emergency and acts to help the person. If a bystander is to intervene in an emergency, they must make not just one but a series of decisions and actions quickly and reliably. These include the following:

1. Recognizing the emergency
2. Deciding to help
3. Calling 9-1-1 if EMS is needed
4. Checking the injured or ill person
5. Giving first aid

Compared with health care providers, ordinary bystanders are significantly less likely to offer help in emergencies that occur in public places. Some reasons for this include the following:

- Lack of knowledge and training
- Confusion about what constitutes an emergency
- Characteristics of the emergency (eg, unpleasant physical appearance of the person, the presence of other bystanders)
- Fear of being infected with a disease
- Concern about legal consequences of helping (see Chapter 1, *Introduction*, Legal Aspects of First Aid)

Lack of Knowledge

The average layperson is unaware of many aspects of emergency care and has difficulty recognizing common medical emergencies and deciding to call 9-1-1 for help. In addition, a person who does not feel competent to deal with an emergency is not likely to offer even minimal help. The person who does not feel competent can escape this uncomfortable feeling by failing to acknowledge the situation as an emergency. The implication is that bystanders who are uncertain of their ability to deal with a seriously injured person are more likely to assume that the person is not seriously injured.

Confusion About What Is an Emergency

Sometimes, laypeople have difficulty deciding when an emergency exists **FIGURE 2-1**. For example, motor vehicle crashes can be easier to recognize as emergencies than heart attacks. Underestimating the severity of an emergency can lead to delays in calling 9-1-1 and to inappropriate decisions, such as transporting people with life-threatening conditions by private vehicles rather than calling 9-1-1.

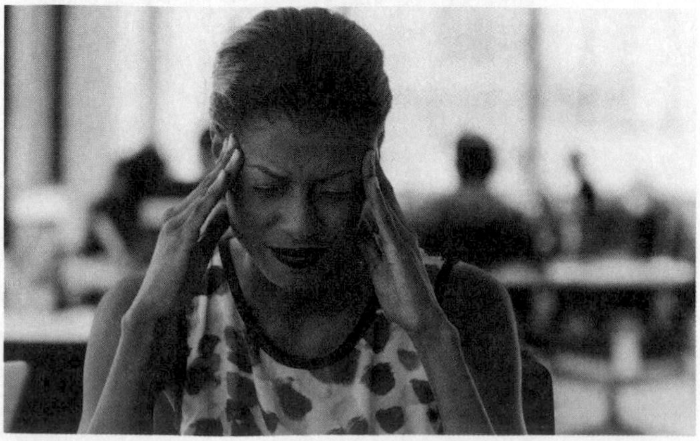

FIGURE 2-1 It is not always clear at first glance whether an emergency exists.

Other Factors That Influence Whether a Bystander Helps

In addition to lack of knowledge and confusion, bystanders encounter other barriers that can slow or prevent action in an emergency. Many people are put off by unpleasant physical characteristics such as blood, vomitus, or alcohol on the breath. An unwillingness to approach or touch a person who is bleeding is a common impediment to providing care. Concerns about contracting such diseases as human immunodeficiency virus (HIV, the virus that can cause acquired immunodeficiency syndrome [AIDS]), coronavirus disease 19 (COVID-19), and tuberculosis (TB) can worsen this issue.

Another factor involved in helping behavior is the bystander's time of arrival. A bystander who sees the emergency happen is more likely to help than a bystander who arrives after the event.

Fear of being sued may also prevent some people from assisting during an emergency. Good Samaritan laws offer first aid providers protection from lawsuits as long as the first aid provider is not guilty of malicious misconduct and gross negligence. These laws are described further in Chapter 1, *Introduction*. The care must also be provided during an emergency, in good faith, and without compensation.

Quality of Help Provided by Bystanders

First aid and other assistance given by bystanders can be inadequate or potentially dangerous. Failure to keep an open airway and the decision to transport the person in a private vehicle rather than by EMS are two examples. Usually, transporting a person in a private vehicle can be dangerous. However, in mass casualty incidents, such as the Las Vegas shooting when the system was overwhelmed, the decision to use private vehicles was seen as correct. Many people, trained decades ago or remembering a home remedy, might use outdated and unproven first aid procedures for various injuries or sudden illnesses. A few examples include the following:

- Putting butter on a burn
- Treating a nosebleed by tilting the head back
- Using hydrogen peroxide to clean a wound
- Sticking an object between the teeth of a person experiencing a seizure to prevent the person from biting their tongue
- Giving syrup of ipecac for a swallowed poison
- Applying suction on a venomous snake bite

What Should Be Done?

As stated at the beginning of this chapter, injured or suddenly ill people would benefit if bystanders could quickly and reliably do the following **FLOWCHART 2-1**:

1. Recognize the emergency.
2. Decide to help.

Flowchart 2-1 Role of the First Aid Provider

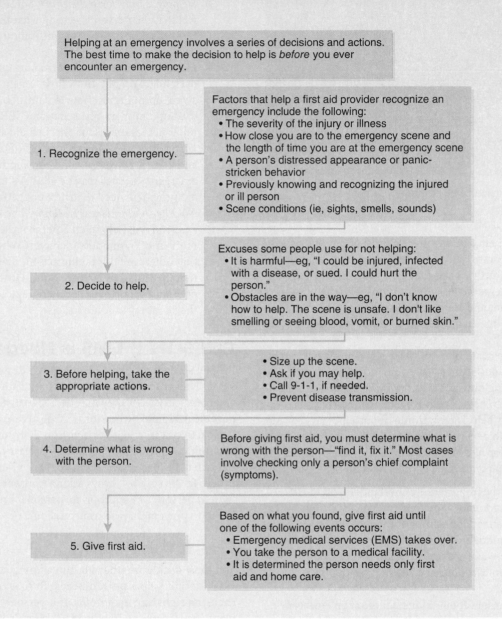

Helping at an emergency involves a series of decisions and actions. The best time to make the decision to help is *before* you ever encounter an emergency.

1. Recognize the emergency.

Factors that help a first aid provider recognize an emergency include the following:

- The severity of the injury or illness
- How close you are to the emergency scene and the length of time you are at the emergency scene
- A person's distressed appearance or panic-stricken behavior
- Previously knowing and recognizing the injured or ill person
- Scene conditions (ie, sights, smells, sounds)

2. Decide to help.

Excuses some people use for not helping:

- It is harmful—eg, "I could be injured, infected with a disease, or sued. I could hurt the person."
- Obstacles are in the way—eg, "I don't know how to help. The scene is unsafe. I don't like smelling or seeing blood, vomit, or burned skin."

3. Before helping, take the appropriate actions.

- Size up the scene.
- Ask if you may help.
- Call 9-1-1, if needed.
- Prevent disease transmission.

4. Determine what is wrong with the person.

Before giving first aid, you must determine what is wrong with the person—"find it, fix it." Most cases involve checking only a person's chief complaint (symptoms).

5. Give first aid.

Based on what you found, give first aid until one of the following events occurs:

- Emergency medical services (EMS) takes over.
- You take the person to a medical facility.
- It is determined the person needs only first aid and home care.

3. Call 9-1-1 if EMS is needed.
4. Check the person.
5. Give first aid.

Recognize the Emergency

To help in an emergency, the bystander first has to notice that something is wrong. Factors that help a first aid provider recognize that something is wrong include the following:

- *Severity*. Severe, catastrophic emergencies such as a motor vehicle crash involving an overturned vehicle or several vehicles attract attention.
- *Physical distance*. The closer a bystander is to an emergency situation, the more likely they are to notice it.
- *Relationship*. Knowing the person increases the likelihood of noticing an emergency. For example, you would notice your child's injuries before you might notice the same injuries on a stranger.
- *Time exposed*. Evidence indicates that the longer a bystander is aware of the situation, the more likely they are to recognize it as an emergency.
- *Scene conditions*. Gory sights, terrible smells, and gruesome sounds repel many people.
- *Person's appearance*. A bystander is likely to notice a person who has a distressed appearance or is exhibiting panic-stricken behavior.

Decide to Help

At some time, everyone will have to decide whether to help another person **FIGURE 2-2**. Unless the decision to act in an emergency is considered well in advance of an actual emergency, the many obstacles that make it difficult or unpleasant

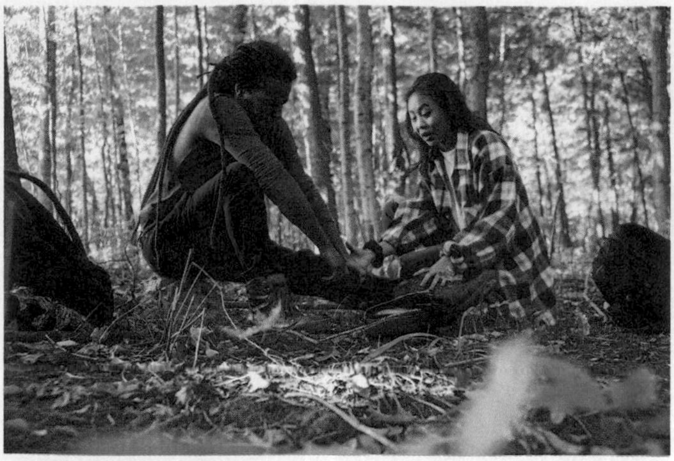

FIGURE 2-2 Be willing to take the time to help.

for a bystander to help a stranger are almost certain to impede action. One important strategy that people use to avoid action is to refuse (consciously or unconsciously) to acknowledge the emergency. Many emergencies do not look like the ones portrayed on television, and the uncertainty of the real event can make it easier for the bystander to avoid acknowledging the emergency.

Bystanders are more likely to promptly get involved at the time of an emergency if they have previously considered the possibility of helping others. Thus, the most important time to make the decision to help is before ever encountering an emergency. Deciding to help is an attitude about emergencies and about one's ability to deal with emergencies. It is an attitude that takes time to develop and is affected by a number of factors. To develop such a helping attitude, people must do the following:

- Appreciate the importance of bystander help to an injured or suddenly ill person.
- Feel confident about helping someone who is seriously injured or suddenly ill, even if someone else is present.
- Be willing to take the time to help.
- Be able to put the potential risks of helping in perspective.
- Feel comfortable about taking charge at an emergency scene. This is accomplished by maintaining skill competency as well as by gaining experience, either actual or simulated.
- Feel comfortable about seeing or touching a person who is bleeding or vomiting or who appears dead.

Deciding Not to Help

A bystander could always find excuses for not helping in emergency situations. The following are reasons, some of them more legitimate than others, that people often give for not aiding others:

- *Helping could be harmful.* Bystanders have lost their lives or been severely injured while attempting to rescue others. Attempting any rescue must be made as safe as possible based on the surrounding hazards and the first aid provider's training. The fear of being sued or contracting a disease such as HIV or tuberculosis can also act as a deterrent. Some would-be first aid providers have been attacked by dogs protecting their disabled owners.
- *Helping is not worth the effort.* Some bystanders might feel that the person is getting what they deserve. Rewards, if any, are not significant for first aid providers.
- *Helping requires advanced training and skills.* Many bystanders do not know how to help. They cannot swim, do not know how to control bleeding or perform cardiopulmonary resuscitation (CPR), or do not have other necessary rescue and first aid skills.
- *Unpleasant conditions.* The sight of blood, vomit, and other unpleasant conditions sometimes found at emergency scenes may be all that some would-be first aid providers need to justify not getting involved.
- *No other bystanders are helping.* The likelihood that a person will help in an emergency decreases as the number of bystanders increases. When bystanders see that others are not taking action, they may conclude that the situation is not serious. Further, the presence of other bystanders may encourage a person to leave the situation to someone else.

Call 9-1-1 if EMS Is Needed

People sometimes make the wrong decision about calling 9-1-1. They may delay calling 9-1-1 until absolutely sure that an emergency exists, or they may decide to bypass EMS and transport the person to professional medical care in a private vehicle. Such actions can endanger a person. Fortunately, most injuries and sudden illnesses do not require professional medical care—only first aid. Size up the scene to determine if EMS or first aid is needed. Be sure to always ask for consent before helping any injured person. Use appropriate personal protective equipment (PPE) to prevent disease transmission.

Check the Person

You must decide whether life-threatening conditions exist and what kind of help a person needs. In most cases, this involves checking signs and symptoms of a person's main (chief) complaint. See Chapter 4, *Finding Out What Is Wrong*, for details.

FYI

Actual Versus Perceived EMS Response Time

People's perceptions of ambulance response times are inaccurate. They tend to overestimate response time while underestimating scene time and time to professional medical care.

Data from Harvey AH, Gerard WC, Rice GF, Finch H. Actual vs. perceived EMS response time. *Prehosp Emerg Care*. 1999;3(1):11–14.

Give First Aid

Often the most critical life support measures are effective only if started immediately by the nearest available person. That person usually will be a layperson—a bystander. Continue to give first aid until EMS takes over or it is determined the person needs only first aid and home care.

Seeking Professional Medical Care

Knowing when to call 9-1-1 for help from EMS is important. To know when to call, you must be able to tell the difference between a minor injury or illness and a life-threatening one. For example, upper abdominal pain may be attributed to something as simple as indigestion or ulcers, but it may also be an early sign of a heart attack. Wheezing could be related to a person's asthma, for which the person can use their prescribed inhaler for quick relief, or it can be as serious as a severe allergic reaction from a bee sting.

Not every cut requires stitches, nor does every burn require professional medical care. It is, however, always best to err on the side of caution. According to the American College of Emergency Physicians (ACEP), if the answer to any of the following questions is "yes," or if you are unsure, call 9-1-1 for professional medical help:

- Is the condition life-threatening?
- Could the condition get worse on the way to the hospital?
- If you move the person, will it cause further injury?
- Does the person need the skills or equipment of EMS?
- Would distance or traffic cause a delay in getting the person to the hospital?

ACEP also recommends immediate transport to the hospital emergency department, by EMS or by private vehicle, for the following conditions that are warning signs of more serious conditions:

- Difficulty breathing, especially if it does not improve with rest
- Chest or upper abdominal pain or pressure lasting 2 minutes or more
- A fast heartbeat (more than 120 to 150 beats per minute) at rest, especially if associated with shortness of breath or feeling faint
- Fainting (passing out) or unresponsiveness
- Difficulty speaking, or numbness or weakness of any part of the body
- Sudden dizziness
- Confusion or changes in mental status, unusual behavior, or difficulty walking
- Sudden blindness or vision changes
- Bleeding from any wound that will not stop with direct pressure
- Broken bones visible through an open wound, or a broken leg
- Drowning (submersion)
- Choking
- Severe burn
- Allergic reaction, especially if there is any difficulty breathing
- Extremely hot or cold body temperature
- Poisoning or drug overdose
- Sudden, severe headache
- Any sudden or severe pain
- Severe or persistent vomiting or diarrhea
- Coughing or vomiting of blood
- Behavioral emergencies (threatening to hurt or kill themselves or someone else)

Wounds requiring immediate professional medical care include the following (see Chapter 9, *Wounds*, for additional information on wounds requiring professional medical care):

- Bleeding from a cut that does not slow during the first 15 minutes of steady direct pressure
- Signs of shock
- Breathing difficulty resulting from a cut to the neck or chest
- All penetrating wounds, especially from a gunshot or a sharp weapon, to the chest or abdomen
- A cut to the eyeball
- A cut that amputates or partially amputates an extremity

When a serious situation occurs, call 9-1-1 *first*. **DO NOT** call your physician, the hospital, a friend, relatives, or neighbors for help before you call 9-1-1. Calling anyone else first only wastes time. Calling 9-1-1 has several advantages over driving to the hospital emergency department by private vehicle:

- Many injured or suddenly ill people should not be moved except by trained personnel.
- The EMS personnel who arrive with the ambulance know what to do. In addition, they are in radio contact with hospital physicians.
- Care provided by EMS personnel at the scene and on the way to the hospital can increase a person's chances of survival and rate of recovery. The condition could get worse and become life threatening on the way to the hospital, in which case, the presence of trained professionals is vital.
- An ambulance usually can get a person to the hospital more quickly.

If the situation is not an emergency, call your physician. However, if you have any doubt about whether the situation is an emergency, call 9-1-1. Later chapters identify when to call 9-1-1 for specific conditions.

Q&A

Should the family be present during resuscitation?

Controversy exists regarding this question. Studies indicate that most family members want to be present. Offering select family members the opportunity to be present is reasonable. If family members are present during resuscitation, be sensitive to them by answering their questions, clarifying information, and providing them comfort.

Data from: Kleinman ME, et al. 2015 American Heart Association guidelines for cardiopulmonary resuscitation and emergency cardiovascular care science. *Circulation.* 2015;132:S424.

How to Call EMS

According to the National Emergency Number Association, over 98% of people in the United States and Canada are covered by some type of 9-1-1 service. Many areas also have Enhanced 9-1-1, which allows the dispatcher to see the caller's phone number and address if the call is placed on a landline. When you call 9-1-1 from a mobile phone, however, Enhanced 9-1-1 cannot identify your exact address, because mobile phone signals only provide a general location **FIGURE 2-3**. Because of this key difference, make sure you know your exact address or location to give the 9-1-1 dispatcher.

When you call 9-1-1, speak slowly and clearly. Be ready to give the dispatcher the following information:

1. *The person's location.* Give the address, names of intersecting roads, and other landmarks, if possible. Location details are the most important information you can provide. Also, tell the specific location of the person. (For example, "in the basement" or "in the backyard.")
2. *The phone number you are calling from and your name.* This information allows dispatchers to detect false reports, thus minimizing their frequency, and it allows a dispatch center without Enhanced 9-1-1 to call back if disconnected or if additional information is needed.
3. *A description of what happened.* State the nature of the emergency. (For example, "My husband fell off a ladder and is not moving.")
4. *The number of people needing help and any special conditions.* (For example, "There was a car crash involving two cars. Three people are trapped.")
5. *A description of the person's condition.* (For example, "My husband's head is bleeding.") List any first aid you have attempted, such as pressing on the site of the bleeding.

DO NOT hang up the phone unless the dispatcher instructs you to do so **FIGURE 2-4**. The EMS dispatcher could tell you how best to care for the person. If you send someone else to call, have the person report back to you so you can be sure the call was made. Other tips include the following:

- Teach children what 9-1-1 is for and how and when to call. Refer to "nine-one-one," not "nine-eleven," because children might expect to find an eleven on the keypad.
- Do not hang up without explanation if you call 9-1-1 by mistake; if you hang up, the dispatcher will have to call back to see if you need help.

Rescuer Reactions

The sight of blood and the cries of people can be upsetting to people attempting to rescue and help an injured person. Seeing a grotesque amputation, being splattered with vomit or blood, or smelling disagreeable odors from urine and feces can be unnerving. More than one first aid provider has felt nauseated and weak, vomited, or fainted when helping injured people. Even the toughest of physicians and emergency medical technicians have difficult moments when exposed to certain situations.

It is essential that first aid providers stay alert and keep working at an injury scene. A first aid provider who collapses while aiding an injured person diverts attention from the original person, whose condition is usually more serious. All the knowledge and skills a first aid provider has are useless if they collapse or have to leave the scene because of weakness or fainting.

Desensitization

Some emergency care providers seem to have ice in their veins. They always appear calm and unaffected by even the worst injuries. These people might seem callous, but the proper psychological term is *desensitized.* A specialty within psychology deals with **desensitization** and suggests ways of overcoming anxieties caused by unpleasant sights and sounds. Desensitization is a deconditioning or a counterconditioning process that can reduce fears and anxieties. The idea is to weaken an undesirable response such as fainting by strengthening an incompatible response. When responses are incompatible (calmness versus anxiety), the occurrence of either one prevents the

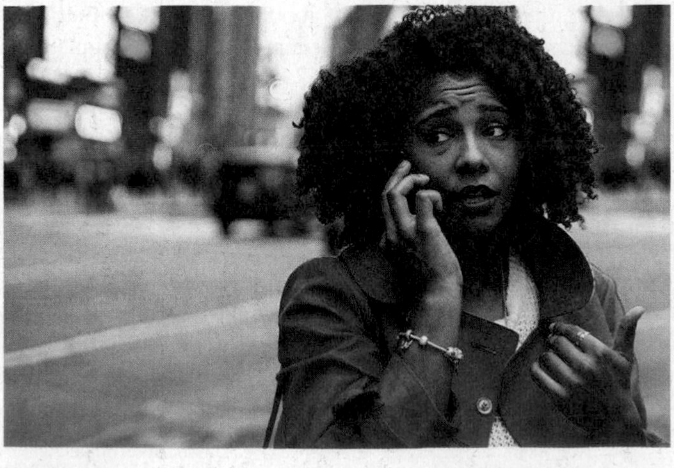

FIGURE 2-3 For help, call 9-1-1 or the local emergency number.

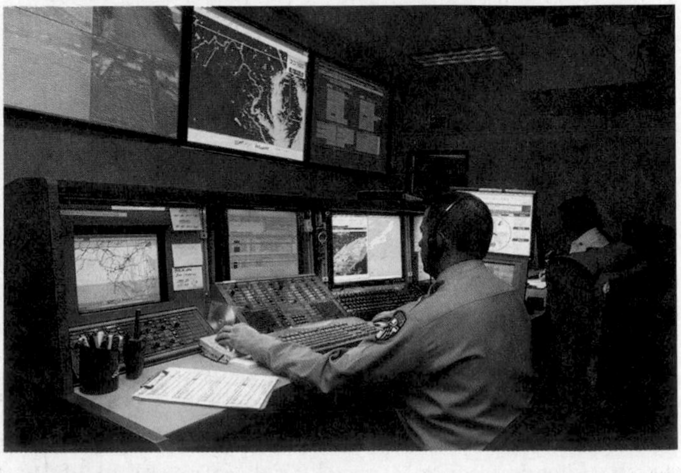

FIGURE 2-4 9-1-1 dispatch center.

occurrence of the other. By desensitizing, you learn to associate relaxation with situations that elicit anxiety so that eventually you do not experience anxiety. But you first need to learn how to invoke relaxation before gradually exposing yourself to anxiety-producing situations such as the sight of blood.

A simple way to desensitize (calm) yourself while helping another person is to change your thought patterns from the unpleasant to the pleasant by singing a favorite song to yourself (not out loud, of course, for the obvious reason of how you might appear to the person or observers). You can begin a process of gradual exposure to unpleasant scenes by viewing television programs, movies, or pictures of injuries in medical journals. You might eventually consider volunteering at a hospital emergency department where you can see injuries.

Physical–Emotional Intersect

A provider's ability to withstand emotional strains can be directly affected by their physical condition. In a number of cases, a first aid provider who fainted had failed to eat breakfast. It is strongly recommended that everyone maintain an adequate blood glucose level through proper eating habits. Eating breakfast is especially important.

Postcare Reactions

After giving first aid for severe injuries, a person might feel an emotional letdown, which is frequently overlooked. A stressful event can be psychologically overwhelming and can result in a condition known as **posttraumatic stress disorder (PTSD)**. Its symptoms include depression and flashbacks of the event.

Discussing your feelings, fears, and reactions within 24 to 72 hours of helping at an emergency helps prevent later emotional conditions. You could discuss your feelings with a trusted friend, a mental health professional, or a member of the clergy. Bringing out your feelings quickly can relieve personal anxieties and stress.

Scene Size-up

If you are at the scene of an emergency situation, do a quick **scene size-up** **FLOWCHART 2-2**, trying to answer the following questions:

- Are hazards present that could be dangerous to you, the injured or suddenly ill person or people, or bystanders?
- How many people are involved?
- What is wrong?
- What happened?
- Are bystanders available to help?

Are Hazards Present?

As you approach an emergency scene, scan the area for immediate dangers to yourself or to the person **FIGURE 2-5**. For example, if a car crash is obstructing traffic, you have to consider whether you can safely approach the vehicle of the person requiring help. Or you might notice that gasoline is dripping from the gas tank and that the battery has shorted out and is sparking. Other conditions include hazardous conditions such as chemical spills, toxic fumes, explosives, gas leaks, or live electric wires. In some locations, dangers such as an avalanche, landslides, fires, flash floods, or attack dogs might exist. If the scene is dangerous, stay away and call 9-1-1. You are not being cowardly, merely realistic. Never attempt a rescue that you have not been specifically trained to do. You cannot help another person if you also become injured or ill.

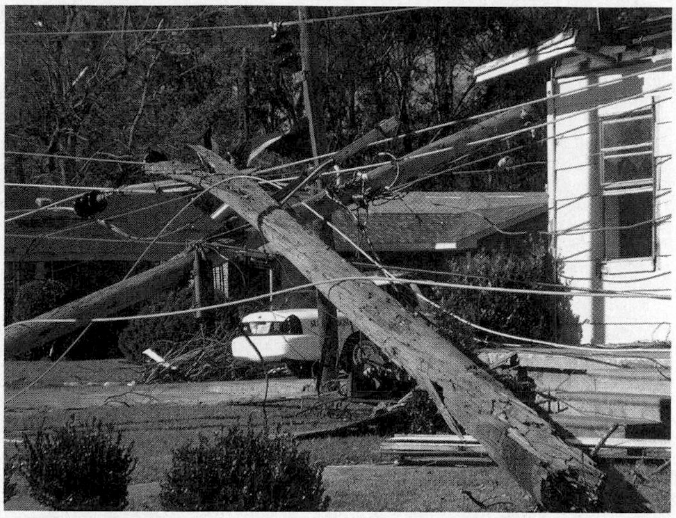

FIGURE 2-5 The scene size-up includes evaluating the scene for hazardous conditions.
Courtesy of Lara Shane/FEMA.

How Many People Are Involved?

The second step is to determine how many people are involved. There could be more than one person in need of help, so look around and ask about others involved.

What Is Wrong? What Happened?

Next, to try to determine what is wrong and what happened. For example, if the emergency department physician knows that a person's abdomen hurts and they were thrown against a steering wheel, they will check for liver, spleen, and cardiac injuries. Be sure to tell EMS personnel about your findings so they can identify the extent of any injuries.

Are Bystanders Available to Help?

Finally, see if there are other bystanders available to help. They can tell you what happened, call 9-1-1, or help calm the injured person.

Q&A

Should I leave my vehicle headlights on at a crash scene?

Always turn your hazard lights on at a scene. Unless your headlights are needed to light up the scene, turn off your headlights when parked. Your headlights can blind approaching vehicles, making it difficult for the drivers to see rescue personnel walking around the scene.

Flowchart 2-2 Scene Size-up

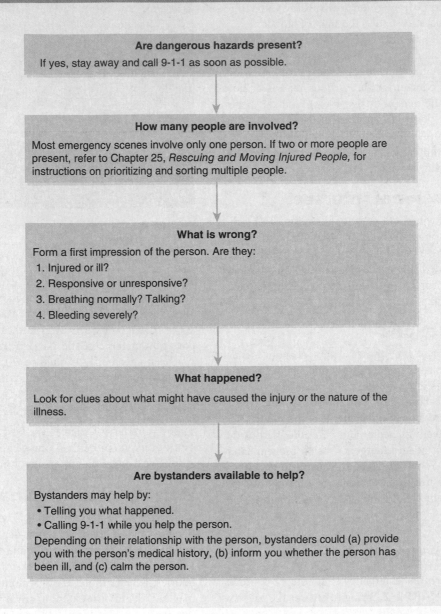

Are dangerous hazards present?

If yes, stay away and call 9-1-1 as soon as possible.

↓

How many people are involved?

Most emergency scenes involve only one person. If two or more people are present, refer to Chapter 25, *Rescuing and Moving Injured People*, for instructions on prioritizing and sorting multiple people.

↓

What is wrong?

Form a first impression of the person. Are they:

1. Injured or ill?
2. Responsive or unresponsive?
3. Breathing normally? Talking?
4. Bleeding severely?

↓

What happened?

Look for clues about what might have caused the injury or the nature of the illness.

↓

Are bystanders available to help?

Bystanders may help by:

- Telling you what happened.
- Calling 9-1-1 while you help the person.

Depending on their relationship with the person, bystanders could (a) provide you with the person's medical history, (b) inform you whether the person has been ill, and (c) calm the person.

Disease Precautions

First aid providers must understand the risks from infectious diseases, which can range in severity from mild to life threatening. First aid providers should know how to reduce the risk of contamination to themselves and to others.

An **infectious disease** is a medical condition caused by the growth and spread of small, harmful organisms within the body. A **communicable disease** is a disease that can spread from one person to another. Immunizations, protective techniques, and handwashing can minimize the risk of infection. Because there are so many different infectious diseases to be concerned about, the Centers for Disease Control and Prevention (CDC) developed a set of **standard precautions**, which advise you to assume that all people are infected and can spread an organism that poses a risk for transmission of infectious diseases. These protective measures are designed to prevent first aid providers from coming into direct contact with infectious agents.

Handwashing

Handwashing is one of the simplest, yet most effective ways to control disease transmission **FIGURE 2-6**. Even if you are wearing medical exam gloves, you should wash your hands before, if possible, and definitely after every contact with an ill or injured person. The longer the germs remain with you, the greater their chance of infecting you.

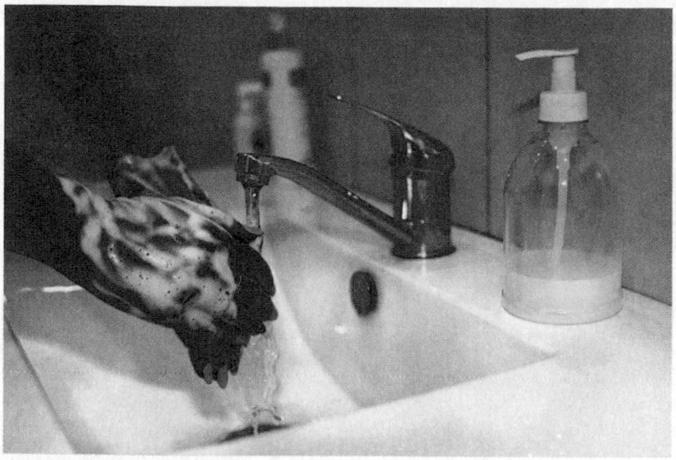

FIGURE 2-6 Handwashing.

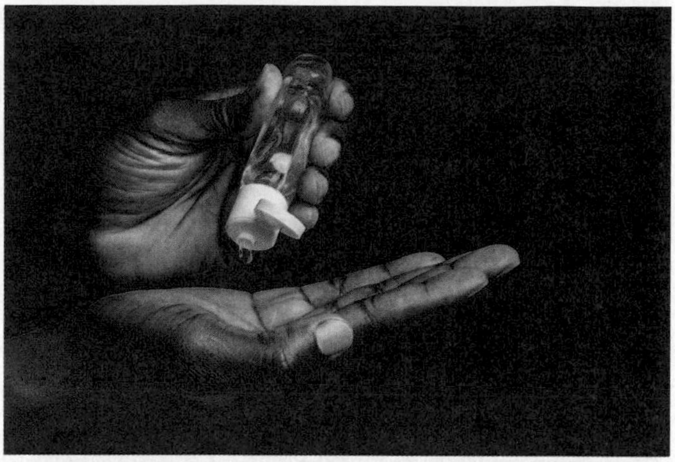

FIGURE 2-7 Use a 60% alcohol hand sanitizer if there is no running water available.

The proper procedure for washing your hands is as follows:

1. Use soap and warm water, if possible. All types of soap are acceptable when washing with water.
2. Rub your hands together for 20 seconds (Sing "Happy Birthday" to yourself two times) to work up a lather. Wash all surfaces well, including wrists, palms, backs of hands, and fingers. Clean the dirt from under your fingernails.
3. Rinse the soap from your hands.
4. Dry your hands completely with a clean cloth or paper towel if possible (this helps remove the germs). If towels are not available, however, it is okay to allow your hands to air dry.

If soap and water are not available, use a hand sanitizer that contains at least 60% alcohol to clean your hands **FIGURE 2-7**. Apply the gel to one hand and rub your hands together, covering all surfaces of your hands and fingers, until the hands are dry. If your mucous membranes (eg, your eyes, nose, or mouth) are splashed by blood or body fluid, immediately flush the area with clean water.

Personal Protective Equipment

Personal protective equipment (PPE) for first aid providers includes such items as medical exam gloves, mouth-to-barrier devices, face masks, and eye protection. PPE provides a barrier between the first aid provider and infectious diseases.

Medical Exam Gloves

Medical exam gloves are the most common type of PPE and should always be worn when there is any possibility of exposure to blood or body fluids. All first aid kits should contain several pairs of gloves **FIGURE 2-8**. Because some people may have allergic reactions to latex, use latex-free gloves when giving first aid. When handling blood or other potentially infectious body fluids, use nitrile gloves, which are latex-free. Although vinyl gloves are latex-free, they are not recommended for first aid. Store medical exam gloves in their original packaging away from direct heat and sunlight. Gloves should not be used past their expiration date or if they are cracked, torn, or discolored.

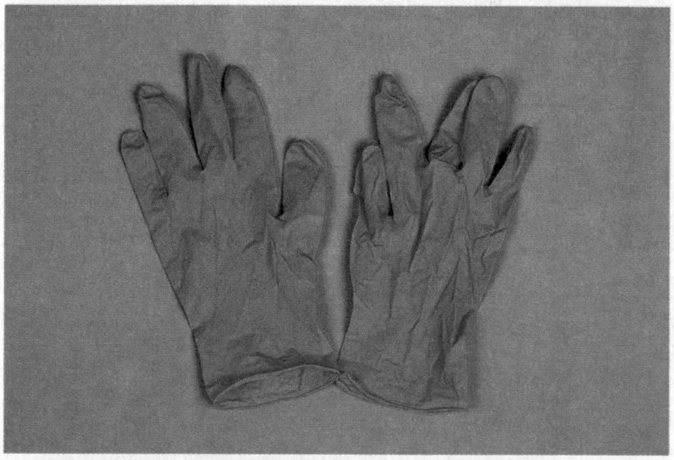

FIGURE 2-8 Disposable gloves.

It is important to use the proper technique when removing used gloves so you do not contaminate yourself. When removing used gloves, do not touch their outer surface **SKILL SHEET 2-1**.

You might consider putting on a second pair of gloves over the first if there is major, significant external bleeding or body fluid. If the gloves are cut or torn, replace them.

Q&A

Why is the use of latex gloves a concern?

Natural latex, which is used in latex gloves, contains natural proteins that have been shown to sensitize and cause allergic reactions in some people over time with repeated use. People who are sensitive or allergic to latex may experience a wide variety of symptoms, including rash, asthma, moderate or life-threatening food allergies, anaphylaxis, and death. A large amount of literature is available regarding concerns over the use of latex gloves. Alternative materials used in making gloves are nitrile, neoprene, and vinyl.

SKILL SHEET 2-1 Removing Gloves

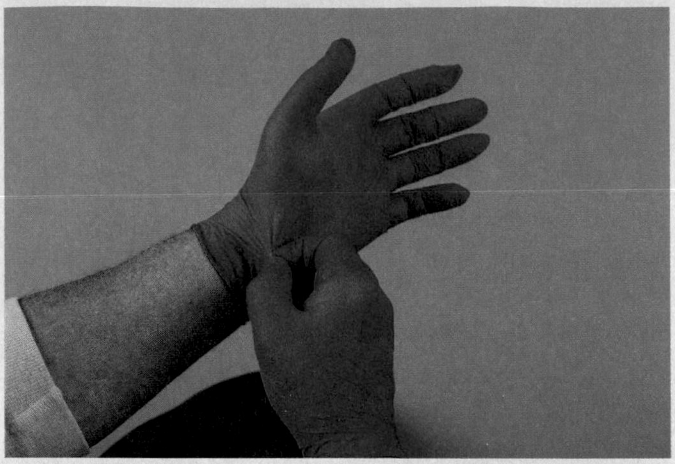

1 Begin by removing one glove. Pinch one glove on the outside near the wrist.

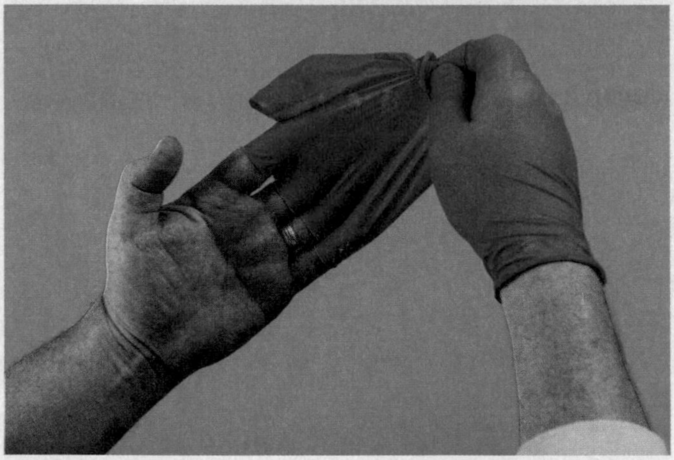

2 Gently pull the glove off, turning it inside out as you pull it off with the hand that is still gloved.

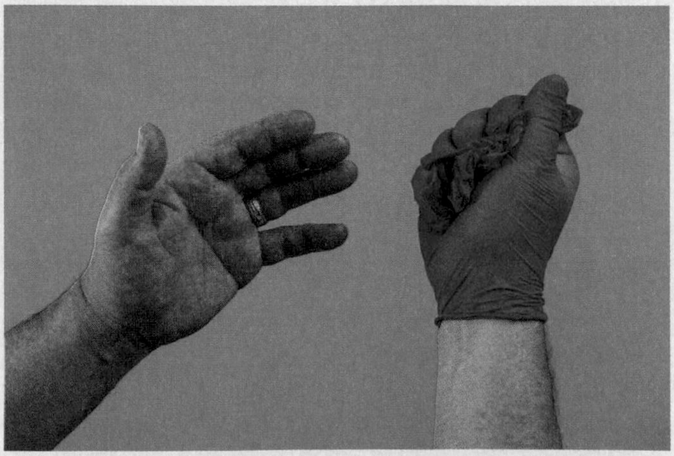

3 When removed, hold it in your gloved hand.

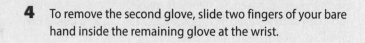

SKILL SHEET 2-1 Removing Gloves (*Continued*)

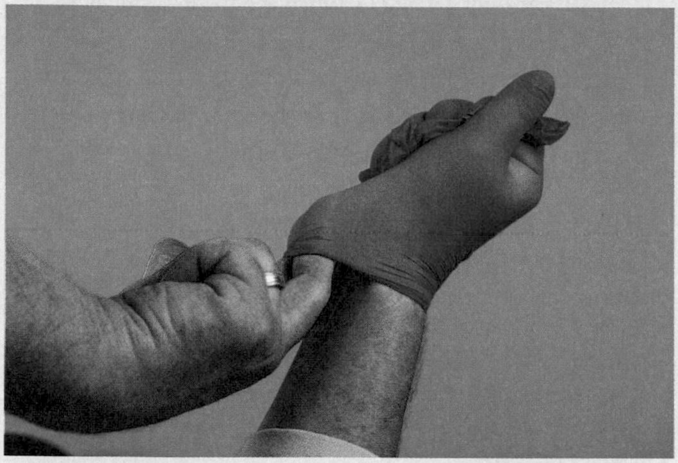

©Jones & Bartlett Learning.

4 To remove the second glove, slide two fingers of your bare hand inside the remaining glove at the wrist.

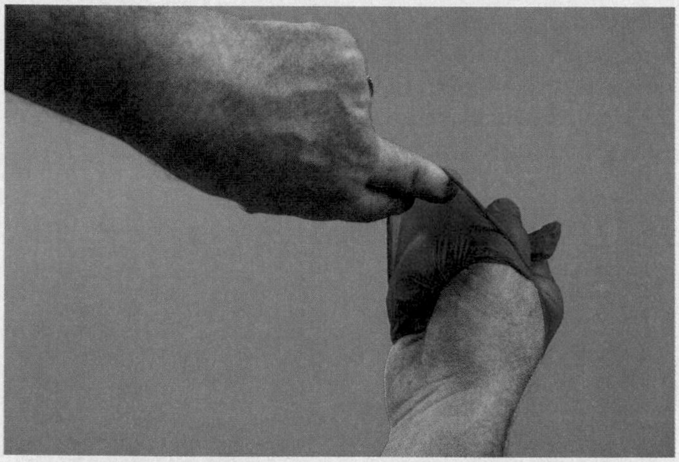

©Jones & Bartlett Learning.

5 Gently stretch the glove away from the hand and gently pull the glove off, keeping the inside out. The first glove remains inside the second glove.

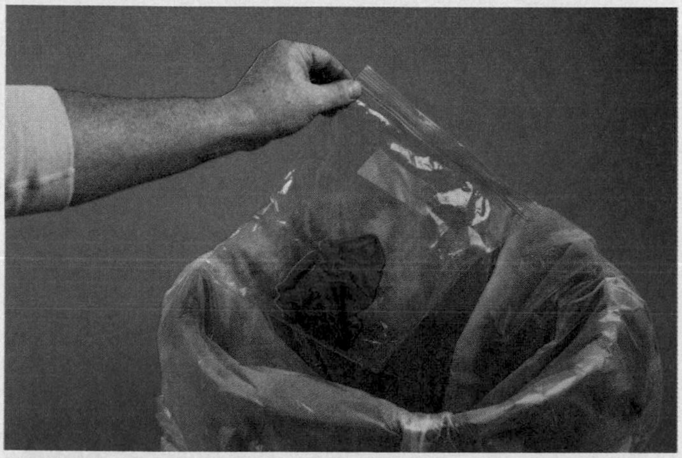

©Jones & Bartlett Learning.

6 If possible, dispose of the gloves in a biohazard container or a sealed plastic bag. If one is not available, dispose in a trash can. Wash your hands with soap and running water. If they are not available, use an alcohol-based hand sanitizer.

Masks

For years the terms "face mask" and "face shield" were used to refer to mouth-to-barrier devices used when giving rescue breaths during CPR. Currently, "face mask" is more commonly used to refer to coverings worn in public for disease prevention, such as those used during the COVID-19 pandemic. "Face shield" is used to refer to a clear plastic mask that covers the eyes, nose, and mouth **FIGURE 2-9**.

Wearing a face mask is new for first aid providers because in years past, only health care providers wore them. Wearing a mask that covers your nose and mouth helps protect you from being infected by others. Mask wearing also keeps you from spreading infection to others. As directed by local or state health officials, it is important to wear a mask even if you have no symptoms. This is especially true when helping people who are not members of your household. When putting on a mask, handle it only by the ear loops or around-the-head strings. **DO NOT** touch the portion of the mask that will cover your face. If you touch any part other than the loops or strings, wash your hands or use hand sanitizer with 60% alcohol.

Wearing a proper face mask is strongly recommended during first aid care. **DO NOT** put the mask under your nose, around your neck, or up on your forehead. To put on a face mask, take the following steps **FIGURE 2-10**. When possible and appropriate, the person receiving first aid care should also wear a face mask or face covering over their mouth and nose.

1. Wash your hands.
2. Pick up the mask by the ear loops or around-the-head strings only. **DO NOT** touch the front of the mask.
3. Using the ear loops or strings, pull the mask to your face, covering your nose and mouth.
4. Fit the mask snugly against the sides of your face and under your chin, and secure the ear loops or around-the-head strings.

Mouth-to-Barrier Devices For CPR

Mouth-to-barrier devices are recommended **FIGURE 2-11**. Although there are few documented cases of disease transmission to first aid providers as a result of performing unprotected mouth-to-mouth resuscitation on a person with an infection, use a barrier device such as a pocket mask when providing CPR whenever possible.

Other Personal Protective Equipment

Other PPE includes eye protection, gowns, and aprons. The Occupational Safety and Health Administration (OSHA) requires these items to be available in some workplaces, especially for health care workers. They are not required for first aid providers and usually will not be available.

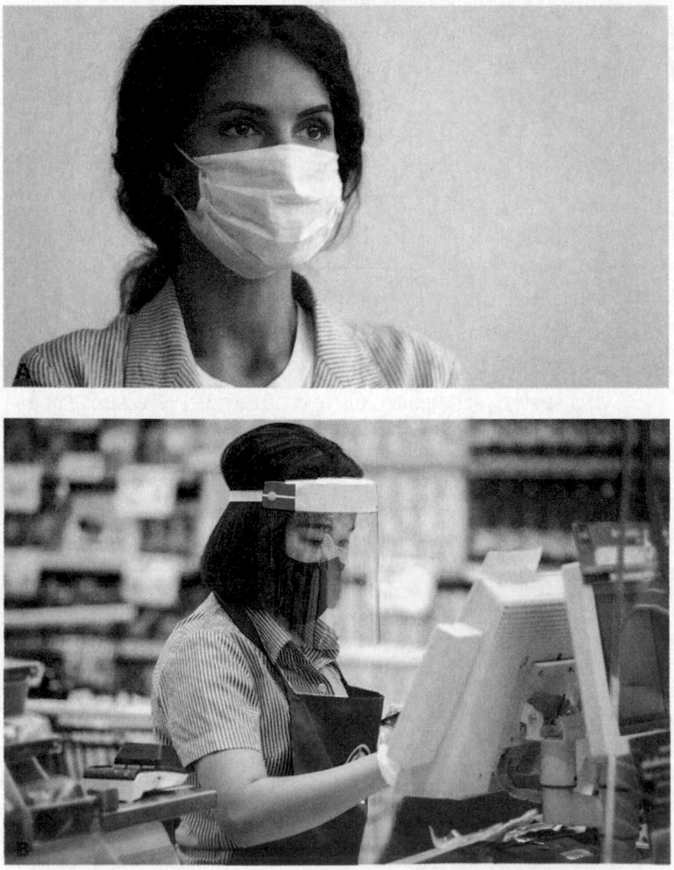

FIGURE 2-9 A. Face mask for public health. **B**. Face shield for public health.

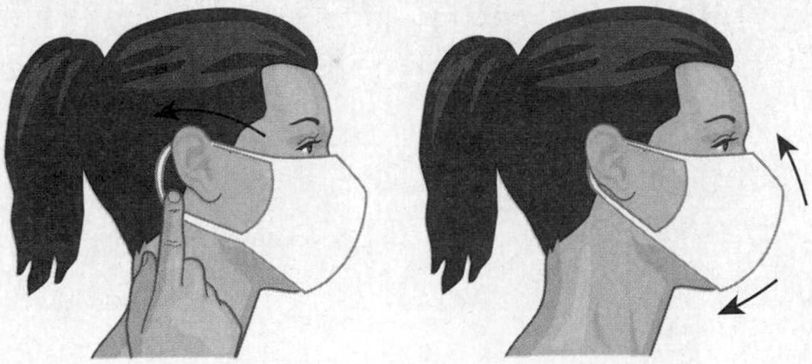

FIGURE 2-10 A correctly fitting face mask should cover your nose and mouth and be secured around your ears or head.

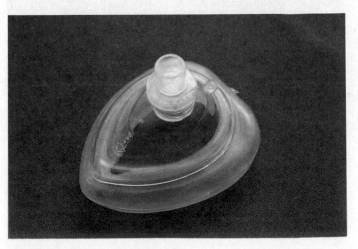

FIGURE 2-11 Pocket face mask with a one-way valve for CPR.

Cleaning Up After an Emergency

When cleaning up blood or other body fluids, protect yourself and others against disease transmission by following these steps:

1. Wear thicker gloves over disposable medical exam gloves.
2. If you have been trained in the correct procedures, use absorbent barriers to soak up blood or other infectious materials.
3. Clean the spill area using soap and water. After cleaning, disinfect with a solution of 1 part bleach and 10 parts water. Isopropyl alcohol can also be used to disinfect. At stronger concentrations these solutions can corrode or discolor certain fabrics, leathers, plexiglass, vinyl, or other synthetic materials.
4. Discard contaminated materials in an appropriate waste disposal container.

If you have been exposed to blood or body fluids, follow these steps:

1. Use soap and water to wash the parts of your body that have been contaminated.
2. If the exposure happened at work, report the incident to your supervisor. Otherwise, contact your personal physician. If the exposure was significant, seek professional medical care. Early action can prevent the development of certain infections.

The best protection against disease is using the safeguards described here. By following these guidelines, first aid providers can decrease their chances of contracting bloodborne illnesses.

FYI

On-the-Job Protection

People infected with hepatitis B virus (HBV) or HIV might not show symptoms and might not even know they are infected. For that reason, consider all human blood and body fluids potentially infectious, and take precautions to avoid contact. Standard precautions recommend that you assume that all body fluids are a possible risk. EMS personnel routinely follow standard precautions, even if blood or body fluids are not visible.

OSHA requires any company with employees who are expected to give first aid in an emergency to follow standard precautions. OSHA applies the Good Samaritan definition to an employee who assists another with a nosebleed or a cut. Such acts, however, are not considered occupational exposure unless the employee who provides the assistance is a member of a first aid team or is designated or expected to provide first aid as part of their job. In essence, OSHA's requirement excludes unassigned employees who perform unanticipated first aid.

Whenever there is a chance that you could be exposed to bloodborne pathogens, your employer must provide appropriate PPE, which might include eye protection, gloves, gowns, and masks. The PPE must be accessible, and your employer must provide training to help you choose the right PPE for your work.

EMS personnel follow standard precautions, and OSHA requires designated worksite first aid providers to follow standard precautions. But what procedures should a typical first aid provider follow? It makes sense for first aid providers to follow standard precautions and assume that all blood and body fluids are infectious.

Some Diseases of Special Concern

Bloodborne Diseases

Some diseases are carried in the blood of a person with an infection (**bloodborne diseases**). **Human immunodeficiency virus (HIV)** is the virus that can cause AIDS. The virus is transmitted by direct contact with infected blood, semen, or vaginal secretions; there is no scientific documentation that the virus is transmitted by contact with sweat, saliva, tears, sputum, urine,

FYI

Emergency Medical Services

If you or someone you know is ever sick or injured and needs emergency help, remember, there are a lot of people who are specially trained to help you!

- *Emergency medical technicians*. Emergency medical technicians (EMTs) have different amounts of training, depending on their jobs. Sometimes EMTs are dispatchers who answer calls for help and send ambulances and rescue vehicles to the scene of the emergency. Other EMTs drive the ambulance, assist with rescues, and perform basic emergency medical care.
- *Paramedics*. Paramedics have a high level of training. They are able to perform many medical procedures at the scene of the emergency or in the ambulance on the way to the hospital. Using a radio to communicate, paramedics often get instructions from a physician at the emergency department or at the base station (the paramedic's headquarters).
- *Emergency nurses*. If you were a patient in the emergency department, an emergency nurse would probably be the first person you would see. One of the nurse's jobs is to ask you questions about your medical condition and help decide when you can see the physician. Emergency nurses are specially trained to help treat emergency patients.
- *Emergency physicians*. Emergency physicians are specially trained to take care of a certain type of patient: emergency patients. Physicians who are specially trained are often called specialists. Emergency physicians specialize in helping people who are injured or who suddenly become sick, such as someone who is having a heart attack or has a very high fever.
- *Emergency medical responders*. Police officers and firefighters are some of the other people who might help you, especially if you have to be rescued.

Data from American College of Emergency Physicians.

feces, vomitus, or nasal secretions, unless these fluids contain visible signs of blood. No vaccine is currently available to prevent HIV infection, however, postexposure prophylaxis is one way to help prevent the transmission of HIV in a person who may have recently been exposed to the virus.

Hepatitis B virus (HBV) is also spread by direct contact with infected blood. The term *hepatitis* refers to an inflammation (and often infection) of the liver. A vaccine is available for HBV and is recommended for all infants and for adults who might have contact with carriers of the disease or with blood. **Hepatitis C virus (HCV)** can cause liver disease or cancer. It cannot be cured, and no vaccine currently exists.

Airborne Diseases

Airborne diseases are transmitted through the air by coughing or sneezing. **Tuberculosis (TB)**, a chronic bacterial disease that usually affects the lungs, is becoming a common condition and is hard to distinguish from other diseases. People who present the highest risk often have a cough. TB is more common in people who have lived in a homeless shelter or in a developing country.

New and reemerging diseases such as **severe acute respiratory syndrome coronavirus 2 (SARS-CoV-2)**, which causes an infection called coronavirus disease 2019 (COVID-19) can be potentially life threatening. Currently, coronavirus disease is a major concern for first aid providers and the people they are helping. The virus is thought to spread mainly from person-to-person through respiratory droplets produced when an infected person coughs, sneezes, or talks. These droplets can land in the mouths or noses of people who are nearby or possibly be inhaled into the lungs. COVID-19 can be spread by people who are not showing symptoms. Several vaccines are now available. For the most up-to-date information on the COVID-19 pandemic, check your county or state health departments or the CDC website.

Death and Dying

Few incidents are as emotionally stressful as a life-and-death situation. Witnessing death and dying is an unfortunate possibility accepted by those who provide emergency care.

The Dying Person

Assisting a person who is dying presents a difficult situation. The following guidelines can help you provide compassionate, effective care:

- Avoid negative statements about the person's condition. Even an unresponsive person can hear what is being said.
- Assure the person that you will locate and inform their family of what has happened. Attempt to have family members present; they can provide great comfort to the person.
- Allow some hope. Do not tell the person that they are dying. Instead, say something like, "I will not give up on you, so do not give up on yourself."
- Do not volunteer information about the person or others who might also be injured. However, if the person asks a question about a family member, tell the truth. Provide simple, honest, clear information if it is requested, and repeat it as often as necessary.
- Use a gentle tone of voice.
- Use a reassuring touch, if appropriate.
- Let the person know that everything that can be done to help will be done.
- Give realistic answers to the person's questions, but try to be positive. Do not make a promise you cannot keep.

The Stages of Grieving

People who lose a loved one go through a **grieving process**. This process generally involves five stages, but not all people move through the process in the same way or at the same pace.

1. *Denial* ("Not me."). The person cannot believe what is happening. This stage serves as a buffer for the person experiencing the situation. This reaction is normal.
2. *Anger* ("Why me?"). First aid providers and bystanders could be the target of the anger. Do not take the anger or insults personally. Be tolerant, use good listening skills, and be empathetic.
3. *Bargaining* ("OK, but first let me . . ."). In the person's mind, an agreement will postpone an unpleasant event, such as death.
4. *Depression* ("But I have not . . ."). This stage is characterized by sadness and despair. The person is usually silent and retreats into their own world.
5. *Acceptance* ("OK, I am not afraid."). Acceptance does not mean a person is happy about the situation. The family often requires more support during this stage than the person does.

With an understanding of these five stages, you can better understand the reactions of those who are grieving as well as your own reactions to stressful situations.

Interacting With Survivors

Interact with the family members of a dead or dying person as follows:

- Do not pronounce death; leave the confirmation of death to a physician.
- Allow survivors to grieve in whatever way seems right to them (eg, anger, rage, crying).
- Provide simple, honest, clear information as it is requested, and repeat it as often as necessary.
- Offer as much support and comfort as possible by your presence and by your words. Do not leave an individual survivor alone, but respect that person's right to privacy.
- Use a gentle tone of voice.
- Use a reassuring touch, if appropriate.

PREP KIT

Ready for Review

- Emergencies are dangerous, unusual, rare, and unforeseen, and they must be dealt with before the situation becomes worse.
- A bystander is a vital link between the EMS system and the person in need of care.
- Injured or suddenly ill people would benefit if bystanders could quickly and reliably do the following:
  - Recognize the emergency.
  - Decide to help.
  - Call 9-1-1 if EMS is needed.
  - Check the person.
  - Give first aid.
- Knowing when to call 9-1-1 is important. To do so, you must be able to tell the difference between a minor injury or illness and a life-threatening one.
- In most communities, call 9-1-1 to receive emergency assistance.
- The sight of blood and the cries of people at an emergency scene can be upsetting, but it is essential that first aid providers remain alert and keep working at an injury scene.
- If you are at the scene of an emergency situation, do a quick scene size-up looking for hazards, the cause of the injury or illness, and the number of people involved.
- First aid providers should take precautions to protect against infectious diseases.
- Few incidents are as emotionally stressful as the life-and-death situations that you might face when providing emergency care.

Vital Vocabulary

airborne disease An infection transmitted through the air, such as tuberculosis (TB).

bloodborne disease An infection transmitted through the blood, such as human immunodeficiency virus (HIV) or hepatitis B virus (HBV).

communicable disease A disease that can spread from person to person or from animal to person.

desensitization A process of deconditioning or counterconditioning designed reduce a person's fears and anxieties. The idea is to weaken an undesirable response such as fainting by strengthening an incompatible response.

emergency medical services (EMS) A system that represents the combined efforts of several professionals and agencies to provide emergency medical care.

grieving process The emotional process that a person works through after a stressful situation that causes personal pain. People go through several stages of grieving.

hepatitis B virus (HBV) A viral infection of the liver for which a vaccine is available.

hepatitis C virus (HCV) A viral infection of the liver for which no vaccine is currently available.

human immunodeficiency virus (HIV) The virus that can cause acquired immunodeficiency syndrome (AIDS).

infectious disease A medical condition caused by the growth of small, harmful organisms within the body.

personal protective equipment (PPE) Equipment, such as exam gloves, used to block the entry of an organism into the body.

posttraumatic stress disorder (PTSD) A delayed stress reaction to a prior emergency event.

scene size-up A quick assessment of the scene and the surroundings for safety issues, the cause of injury or nature of illness, and the number of people; it is completed before starting first aid.

severe acute respiratory syndrome coronavirus 2 (SARS-CoV-2) The virus that causes an infection called coronavirus 2019 (COVID-19), which primarily affects the lungs and can lead to respiratory failure and death.

standard precautions Protective measures that have traditionally been developed by the Centers for Disease Control and Prevention (CDC) for use in dealing with objects, blood, body fluids, or other potential exposure risks of communicable disease.

tuberculosis (TB) A bacterial disease usually affecting the lungs.

PREP KIT continued

Assessment in Action

You are walking from house to house in an unfamiliar neighborhood collecting donated clothing for a local charitable organization. You find no one home at a particular house but hear a loud explosion in the garage. You decide to see what happened. On entering the garage, you find a teenage boy lying on the ground. There is a strong gasoline odor. You have a mobile phone with you.

Directions: Circle Yes if you agree with the statement; circle No if you disagree.

1. This scene could be dangerous.
   YES **NO**
2. You should not be concerned about other people.
   YES **NO**
3. In most communities, 9-1-1 can be used to contact EMS.
   YES **NO**
4. If you do not know the exact address of the emergency, be prepared to give a description of the location as best as you can.
   YES **NO**

Check Your Knowledge

Directions: Circle Yes if you agree with the statement; circle No if you disagree.

1. A quick scene survey should be done before giving first aid to an injured person.
   YES **NO**
2. For a severely injured person, call the person's physician before calling for an ambulance.
   YES **NO**
3. Nitrile are the recommended gloves for first aid providers.
   YES **NO**
4. First aid providers should assume that blood and all body fluids are infectious.
   YES **NO**
5. If you are exposed to blood while on the job, report it to your supervisor, and if off the job, to your personal physician.
   YES **NO**
6. First aid kits should contain exam gloves.
   YES **NO**
7. Wash your hands with soap and water after giving first aid.
   YES **NO**
8. Protective eyewear, medical exam gloves, and face shields are examples of PPE.
   YES **NO**
9. Exam gloves can be made of almost any material as long as they fit the hand well.
   YES **NO**
10. TB is a bloodborne disease.
    YES **NO**

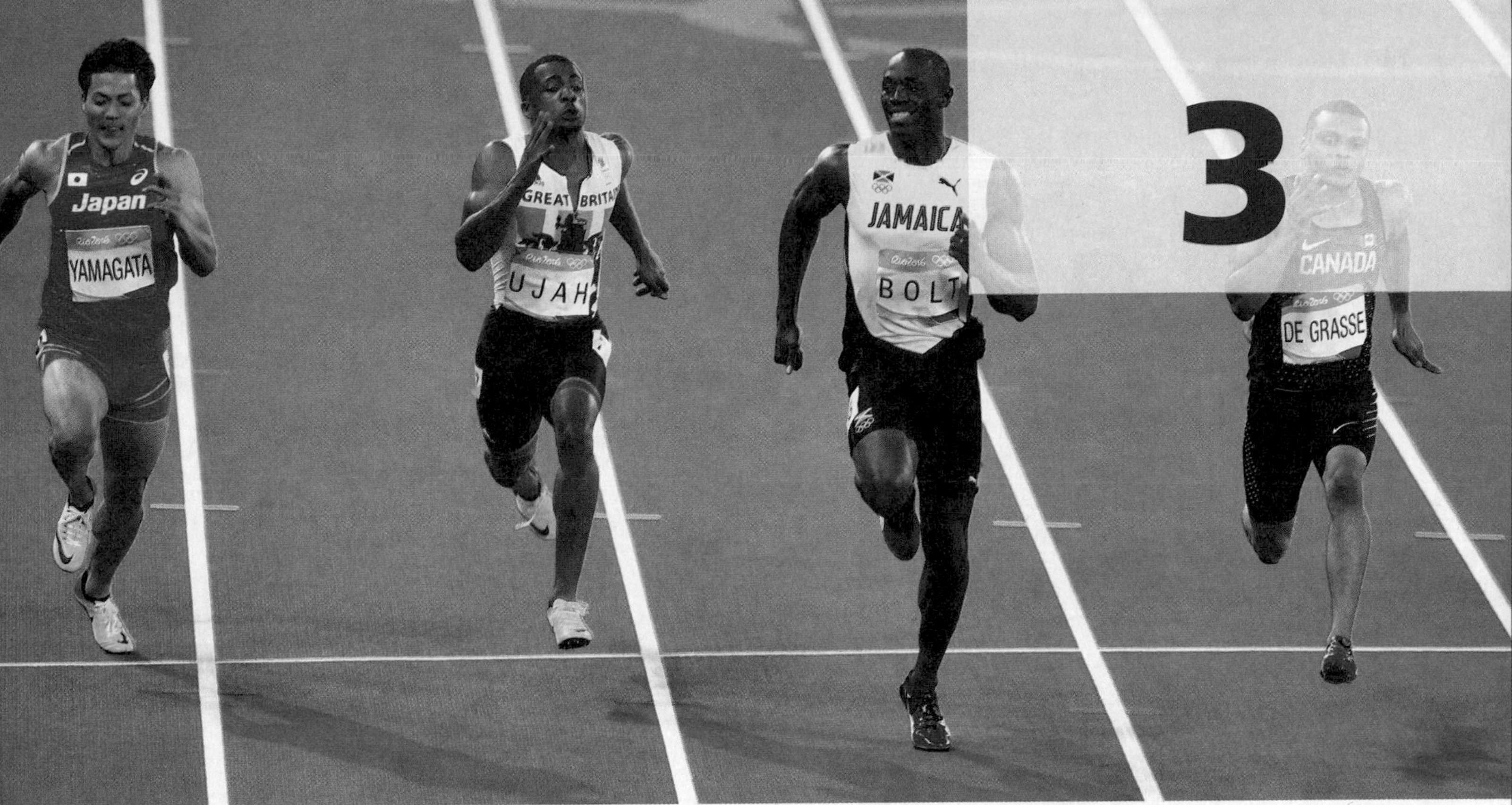

3

The Human Body

CHAPTER AT A GLANCE

- The Human Body
- Directional Terms
- The Body Systems
- The Respiratory System
- The Cardiovascular System
- The Nervous System
- The Skeletal System
- The Muscular System
- The Skin

The Human Body

To assess a person's condition adequately and to give effective first aid, a first aid provider must be familiar with the basic structure and functions of the human body. This knowledge provides a solid cornerstone for building the essentials of quality assessment and emergency first aid. By using the proper medical terms, you will be able to communicate more effectively with the person you are assessing and with professional medical care providers.

Directional Terms

When you are discussing where an injury is located or how a pain moves throughout the body, you need to know the correct directional terms **FIGURE 3-1**. The terms right and left refer to the person's right and left sides, not to your right and left sides. **Anterior** refers to the front of the body and **posterior** refers to the back of the body. **Superior** parts of the body are closer to the head; the parts closer to the feet are called **inferior**. **Lateral** (outer) parts of the body are farther from the middle of the body; the parts closer to the middle of the body are called **medial** (inner).

The terms *proximal* and *distal* are used when discussing an arm or leg. **Proximal** (close) refers to areas that are close to the center of

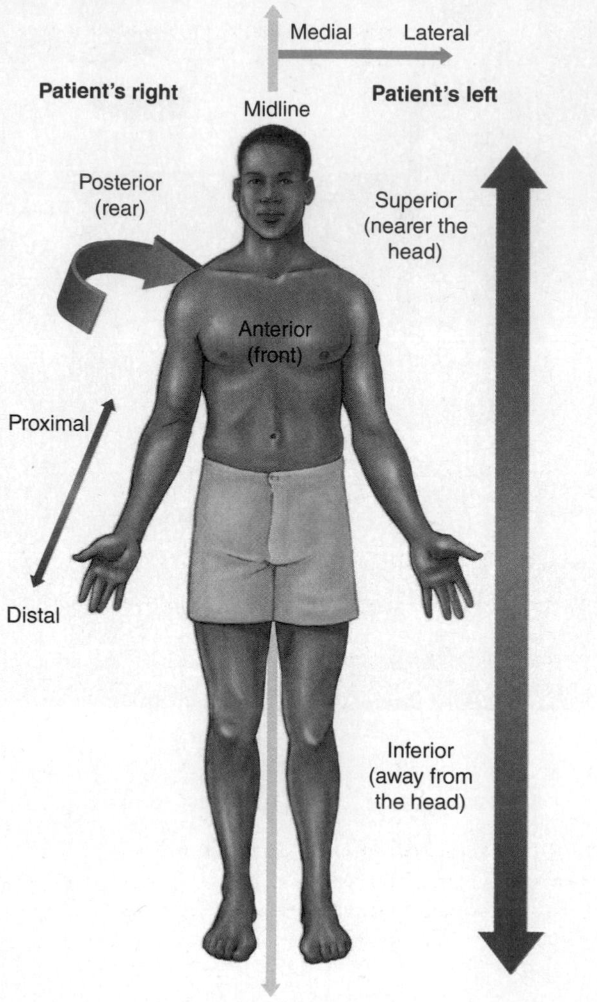

FIGURE 3-1 Directional terms indicate distance and direction from the middle of the body.

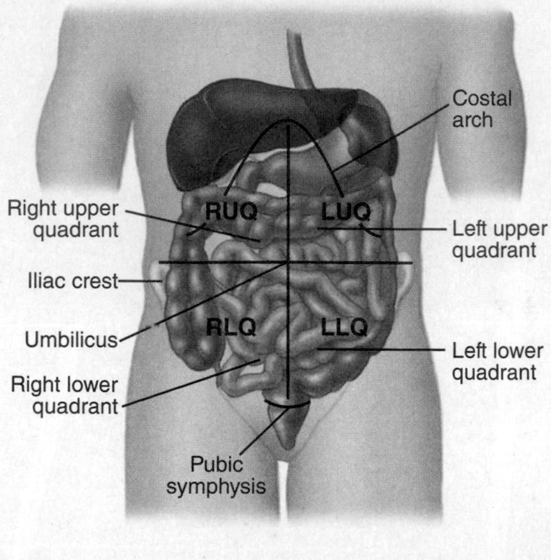

FIGURE 3-2 The abdomen is divided into four quadrants.

the body or to the point where the arm or leg is attached to the body. **Distal** (distant) refers to areas that are distant from the center of the body or from the point of attachment.

Superficial means closer to or on the skin. **Deep** means farther inside the body and away from the skin.

The term **quadrant** indicates a section of the abdominal cavity. Imagine a horizontal line and a vertical line intersecting at the umbilicus (navel), dividing the **abdomen** into four equal areas. These areas are referred to as the right upper quadrant (RUQ), left upper quadrant (LUQ), right lower quadrant (RLQ), and left lower quadrant (LLQ) **FIGURE 3-2**.

The Body Systems

In injuries and illnesses, most life-threatening conditions affect the respiratory, cardiovascular, and nervous systems. These three body systems include the most important and sensitive organs: the lungs, the heart, the brain, and the spinal cord. The other body systems are also important, and thorough assessment of the person can locate injury and/or sudden illnesses affecting them as well. The major body systems described in this chapter are the respiratory, cardiovascular, nervous, skeletal, and muscular systems. The skin is also described. The other body systems—including the endocrine, gastrointestinal, and genitourinary systems—are summarized in **TABLE 3-1**.

The Respiratory System

The body can store food to last several weeks and water to last several days, but it can store enough oxygen for only a few minutes. Ordinarily, this limited oxygen reserve is not a concern because we only have to inhale air to get the oxygen we need. However, if the body's oxygen supply is cut off, as in drowning, choking, or smothering, death will result in about 4 to 6 minutes unless the oxygen intake is restored. Oxygen from air is made available to the blood through the **respiratory system** **FIGURE 3-3** and then to the body cells by the cardiovascular system.

Nose

Air normally enters the body during inhalation through the nostrils. It is warmed, moistened, and filtered as it flows over the damp, mucous membrane (sticky lining) of the nose. When a person breathes through the mouth instead of the nose, there is less filtration and warming. After passing through the nasal passages, air enters the nasal portion of the **pharynx** (throat).

Pharynx and Trachea

From the back of the nose or the mouth, air enters the pharynx. The pharynx is a common passageway for food and air. At its lower end, the pharynx divides into two passageways: one for food and the other for air. Muscular control in the back of the throat routes food to the **esophagus** (food tube), which leads to the stomach; air is routed from the pharynx

TABLE 3-1 The Human Body Systems

System	Function	Major Components	Interactions With Other Systems
Digestive	■ Takes in food (ingestion) ■ Digests food into smaller molecules and absorbs nutrients ■ Removes indigestible food from body (feces)	■ Mouth ■ Esophagus ■ Stomach ■ Small intestine ■ Large intestine ■ Rectum ■ Anus ■ Salivary glands ■ Pancreas ■ Liver ■ Gallbladder	■ Cardiovascular system: Absorbs and delivers the digested nutrients to the cells ■ Muscular system: Controls the contractions of many of the digestive organs to pass food along ■ Nervous system: Hypothalamus maintains homeostasis by triggering appetite (stomach growling)
Cardiovascular	Transports materials (oxygen, nutrients, hormones, cellular waste products) to and from cells	■ Heart ■ Veins ■ Arteries ■ Capillaries ■ Blood	■ Respiratory system: Delivers O_2 from lungs to cells and transports CO_2 from cells to lungs ■ Digestive system: Absorbs and delivers digested nutrients to cells ■ Excretory system: Kidneys filter cellular waste out of blood for removal ■ Lymphatic system: Transports tissue fluid back to the cardiovascular system ■ Immune system: Transports WBCs throughout the body to fight disease ■ Nervous system: Brain controls heartbeat ■ Endocrine system: Transports hormones
Nervous	■ Gathers and interprets information ■ Responds to information ■ Helps maintain homeostasis	■ Brain ■ Spinal cord ■ Nerves ■ Neurons	■ Controls all other systems ■ Maintains homeostasis by working with all systems
Excretory	■ Removes waste products from cellular metabolism ■ Filters blood	■ Kidneys ■ Ureters ■ Bladder ■ Urethra ■ Lungs ■ Skin ■ Liver	■ Cardiovascular system: Filters waste out of blood ■ Lungs: Removes excretory waste ■ Integumentary system: Removes excretory waste
Respiratory	Takes in O_2 and removes CO_2 and water	■ Nose ■ Trachea ■ Bronchi ■ Bronchioles ■ Alveoli ■ Lungs	■ Cardiovascular system: Takes in O_2 for delivery to cells and removes CO_2 brought from cells ■ Excretory system: Removes excretory waste ■ Nervous system: Controls breathing ■ Muscular system: Diaphragm assists breathing
Skeletal	■ Protects organs ■ Provides shape and support ■ Stores materials (fats, minerals) ■ Produces blood cells ■ Allows movement	■ Bones ■ Cartilage ■ Ligaments	■ Muscular system: Allows movement ■ Cardiovascular system: Produces blood cells ■ Immune system: Produces WBCs ■ Cardiovascular and respiratory systems: Protects its organs
Muscular	Allows for movement by contracting	■ Skeletal muscle ■ Tendons	■ Skeletal system: Allows movement ■ Digestive system: Allows organs to contract to push food through ■ Respiratory system: Diaphragm assists breathing ■ Cardiovascular system: Controls pumping of blood ■ Nervous system: Controls all muscle contractions
Endocrine	Regulates body activities using hormones (slow response, long lasting)	■ Glands • Hypothalamus • Pituitary • Thyroid • Thymus • Adrenal • Pancreas • Ovaries • Testes	■ Cardiovascular system: Transports hormones to target organs ■ Nervous system: Maintains homeostasis, hormone release ■ Reproductive system: Controlled by hormones ■ Skeletal system: Controls growth of bones

Continues

TABLE 3-1 The Human Body Systems (*Continued*)

System	Function	Major Components	Interactions With Other Systems
Immune	Fights off foreign invaders in the body	■ WBCs ■ T cells ■ B cells ■ Macrophages ■ Skin	■ Cardiovascular system: Transports WBCs to fight invaders ■ Lymphatic system: Has lots of WBCs to fight invaders; spleen filters bacteria/viruses out of blood ■ Skeletal system: WBCs made in bone marrow ■ Integumentary system: Prevents invaders from getting in
Integumentary	■ Acts as barrier against infection ■ Helps regulate body temperature ■ Removes excretory waste ■ Protects against sun's ultraviolet rays ■ Produces vitamin D	■ Skin ■ Epidermis ■ Dermis	■ Excretory system: Removes cellular waste ■ Nervous system: Controls body temperature ■ Immune system: Prevents pathogens from entering
Lymphatic	■ Stores and carries WBCs that fight disease ■ Collects excess fluid and returns it to blood (acts as a second cardiovascular system; reaches places the cardiovascular system cannot)	■ Lymph (liquid part of blood) ■ Lymph vessels ■ Lymph nodes ■ WBCs	■ Immune system: Holds lots of WBCs to fight pathogens ■ Cardiovascular system: Transports materials from cells
Reproductive	Allows organisms to reproduce, which prevents their species from becoming extinct	■ Ovaries ■ Testes	■ Endocrine system: Controls production of sex cells ■ Muscular system: Uterus contracts to give birth; controlled by hormones

Abbreviations: CO_2, carbon dioxide; O_2, oxygen; WBCs, white blood cells

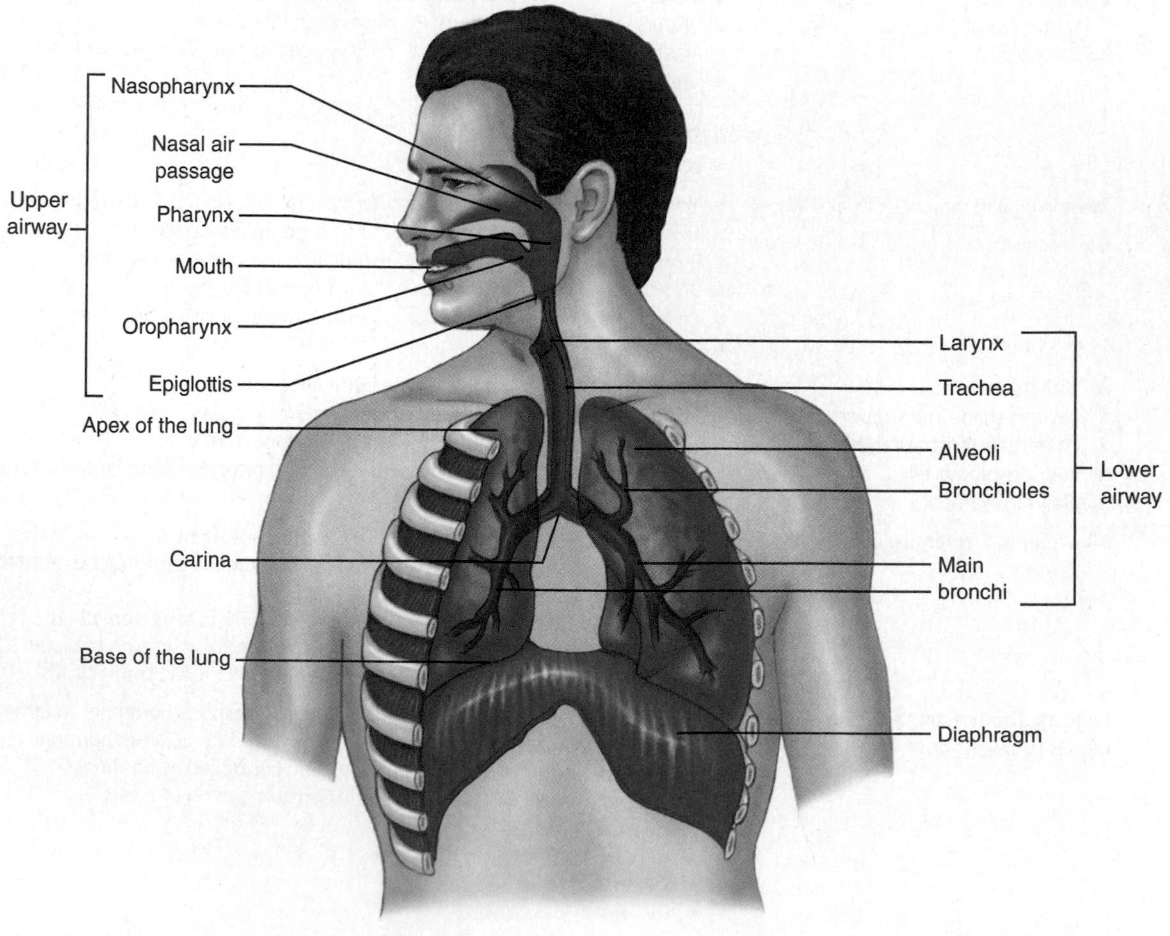

FIGURE 3-3 Respiratory system.

to the **trachea** (windpipe), which leads to the lungs. The trachea and the esophagus are separated by a small flap of tissue, the **epiglottis**, which diverts food away from the trachea. Usually this diversion works automatically to keep food out of the trachea and to prevent air from entering the esophagus. If the muscles of the pharynx and larynx are not coordinated, food or other liquid can enter the trachea instead of the esophagus.

Normal swallowing controls (gag reflex) do not operate if a person is unresponsive. That is why a first aid provider should never pour liquid into the mouth of an unresponsive person in an attempt to revive them. The liquid could flow into the trachea and suffocate the person. Foreign objects, such as false teeth or a piece of food, might also lodge in the throat or trachea and cut off the passage of air. In the upper 2 inches (5 cm) of the trachea, just below the epiglottis, is the **larynx** (voice box), which contains the vocal cords. The larynx can be felt in the front of the throat.

Lungs

The trachea branches into two tubes (**bronchial tubes** or bronchi), one for each lung. Each bronchus divides and subdivides somewhat like the branches of a tree. The smallest bronchioles end in thousands of tiny pouches (**alveoli**, or air sacs), just as the twigs of a tree end in leaves. Each air sac is enclosed in a network of capillaries. The walls that separate the air sacs and the capillaries are very thin. Through those walls, oxygen combines with the hemoglobin in red blood cells to form oxyhemoglobin, which is carried to all parts of the body. Carbon dioxide and certain other waste gases in the blood move across the capillary walls into the air sacs and are exhaled from the body. The lungs occupy most of the chest cavity.

Mechanics of Breathing

The passage of air into and out of the lungs is called respiration. Breathing in is called inhalation; breathing out is called exhalation. Ventilation is a mechanical process brought about by alternately increasing and decreasing the size of the chest cavity. When the **diaphragm** (the dome-shaped muscle dividing the chest from the abdomen) contracts, the chest expands, drawing air into the lungs (inhalation). An exchange of oxygen and carbon dioxide takes place in the lungs. When the diaphragm relaxes, it exerts pressure on the lungs, causing air to flow out (exhalation).

Infants and children differ from adults. Their respiratory structures are smaller and more easily obstructed than those of adults. Infants' and children's tongues take up proportionally more space in the mouth than do the tongues of adults. The trachea is more flexible in infants and children. The primary cause of cardiac arrest in infants and children is an uncorrected respiratory condition.

The average rate of breathing in an adult at rest is 12 to 20 complete respirations per minute **TABLE 3-2**. Normal rates for children are 18 to 40 respirations per minute; infant rates are 30 to 60 respirations per minute. Normally the rate slows when a person is lying down and speeds up during vigorous exercise. The rate of breathing is controlled by a nerve center in the brain. Signs of inadequate breathing include a rate of breathing outside the normal range, cool or clammy skin that is pale or cyanotic (blue-purple), and nasal flaring, especially in children.

TABLE 3-2 Typical Vital Signs Values Based on Age

Age	Pulse Rate (Heart Rate) (beats/min)	Respirations (breaths/min)
Infants (newborn to age 1 year)	90–180	25–60
Children (ages 1 to 12 years)	70–150	15–30
Adults	60–100	12–20

When a person performs hard muscular work, the lungs cannot get rid of carbon dioxide or take in oxygen fast enough at the normal rate of breathing. As carbon dioxide increases in the blood and tissues, the brain sends impulses along its nerves to cause deeper and more rapid respirations. At the same time, the heart rate increases. This faster heart rate increases the supply of oxygen available to the body as the heart pumps more blood through the lungs.

The Cardiovascular System

The **cardiovascular system** is made up of the blood, the heart, and the blood vessels **FIGURE 3-4**. Blood is the delivery system for cells throughout the body. It carries nutrients and other products from the digestive tract in its plasma, and it carries oxygen from the lungs in its hemoglobin. It also transports wastes produced by the cells to the lungs, kidneys, and other excretory organs for removal from the body.

Heart

The human cardiovascular system is a completely closed circuit of tubelike vessels through which blood flows. The **heart**, by contracting and relaxing, pumps blood through the vessels **FIGURE 3-5**. It is a powerful, hollow, muscular organ about as big as a man's clenched fist, shaped like a pear, and located in the left center of the chest, behind the sternum (breast bone). The heart is divided by a wall in the middle. Right and left compartments are divided into two chambers, the atrium above and the ventricle below. Valves are located between each atrium and its corresponding ventricle and at the exit of the major arteries leading out of each ventricle. The opening and shutting of these valves at just the right time in the heartbeat keeps the blood from backing up.

At each beat, or contraction, the heart pumps blood rich in carbon dioxide and low in oxygen from the right ventricle to the lungs and returns oxygen-rich blood to the left atrium of the heart from the lungs. The left ventricle pushes freshly obtained, oxygen-rich blood to the rest of the body and returns oxygen-poor blood to the right atrium. At each relaxation of the heart, blood flows into the left atrium from the lungs and into the right atrium from the rest of the body.

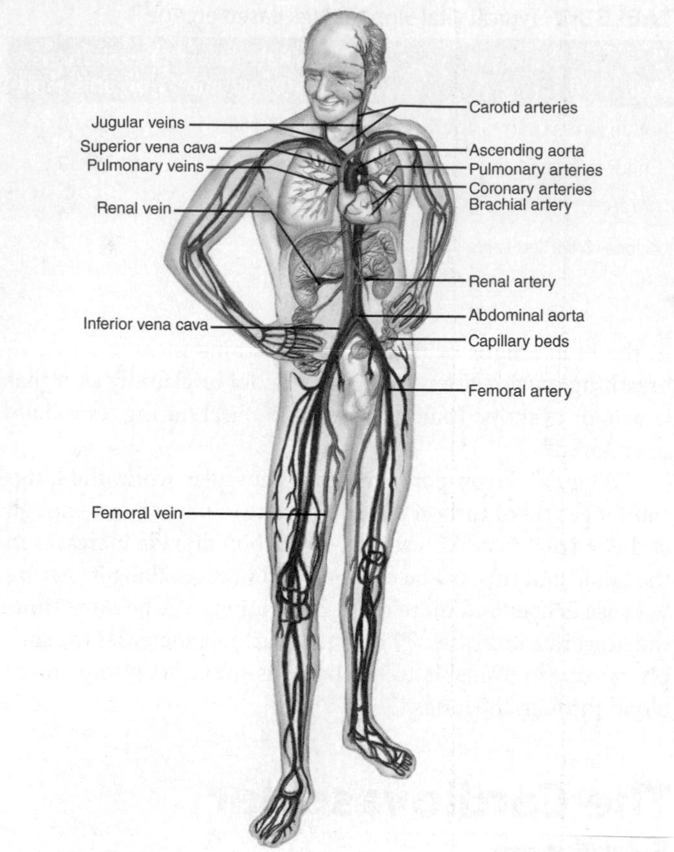

FIGURE 3-4 Cardiovascular system.

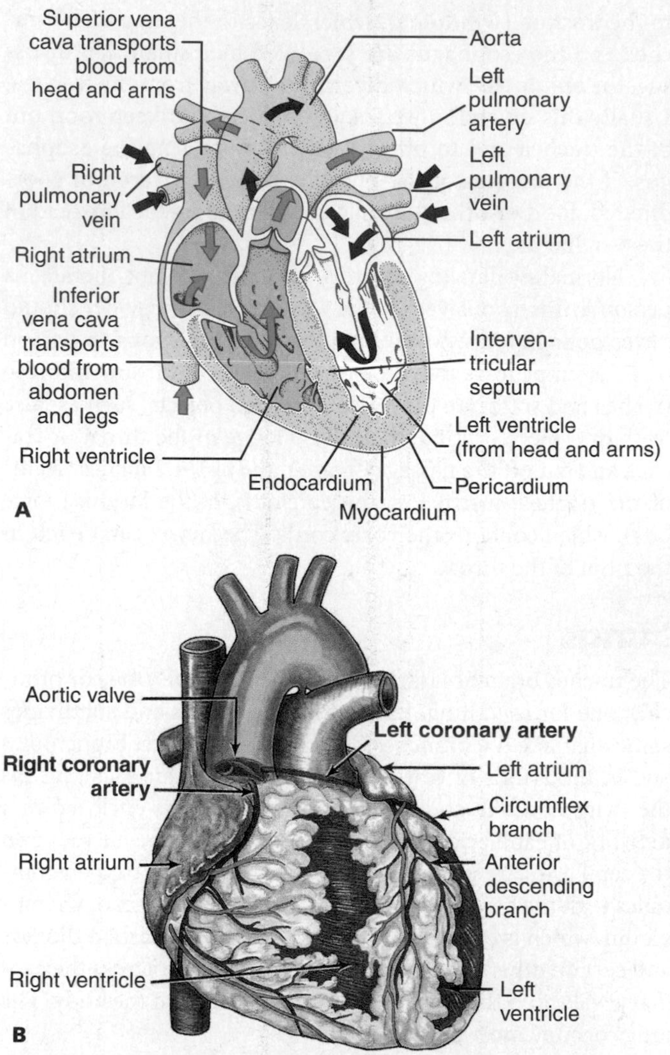

FIGURE 3-5 The heart. **A**. Circulation (internal view). **B**. The two main coronary arteries supply the heart with blood.

FYI

Did You Know?

The carotid arteries along the neck convey blood to the head, and if pressure is applied to them, the individual becomes unresponsive, seeming to drop off into a stupor or slumber. Hence, the Greeks called these arteries the karotides from the Greek word *karoun*, meaning "to stupefy."

Data from Skinner HA. *The Origin of Medical Terms*. 2nd ed. Baltimore, MD: Williams & Wilkins; 1961.

Blood Vessels

The **arteries** are elastic, muscular tubes that carry blood away from the heart **FIGURE 3-6**. They begin at the heart as two large tubes: the pulmonary artery, which carries blood to the lungs for the carbon dioxide and oxygen exchange, and the **aorta**, which carries blood to all the other parts of the body. The aorta divides and subdivides until it ends in networks of extremely fine vessels (**capillaries**) smaller than hairs. Through the thin walls of the capillaries, oxygen and nourishment pass out of the bloodstream into the stationary cells of the body, while the body cells discharge their waste products into the bloodstream. In the capillaries of the lungs, carbon dioxide is released and oxygen is absorbed. Capillaries, having reached their limit of subdivision, begin to join together again into veins. The **veins** become larger and larger and finally form major trunks that empty blood returning from the body into the right atrium and blood from the lungs into the left atrium.

FYI

Word Origins

Arteries received their name from the Greek term for windpipe because the Greek physician Praxagoras thought they carried air. In corpses, they are usually empty and that was probably where his observations were made.

Data from Skinner HA. *The Origin of Medical Terms*. 2nd ed. Baltimore, MD: Williams & Wilkins; 1961.

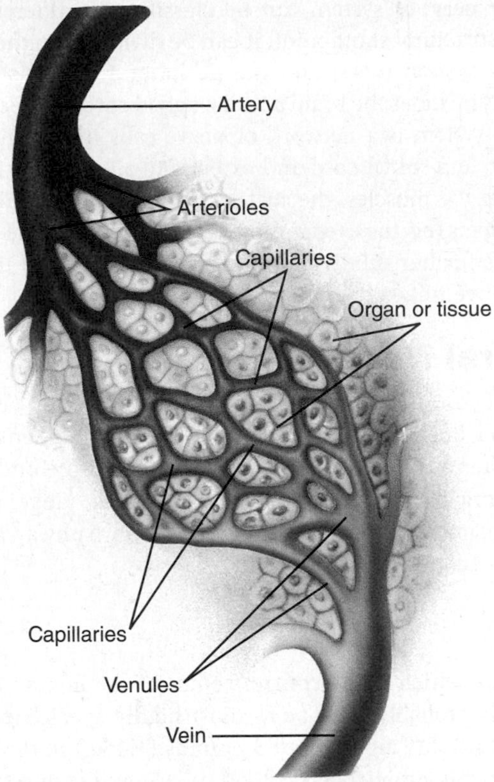

FIGURE 3-6 Blood enters an organ or tissue through the arteries and leaves through the veins. This process provides adequate blood flow to the tissue to meet the cells' needs.

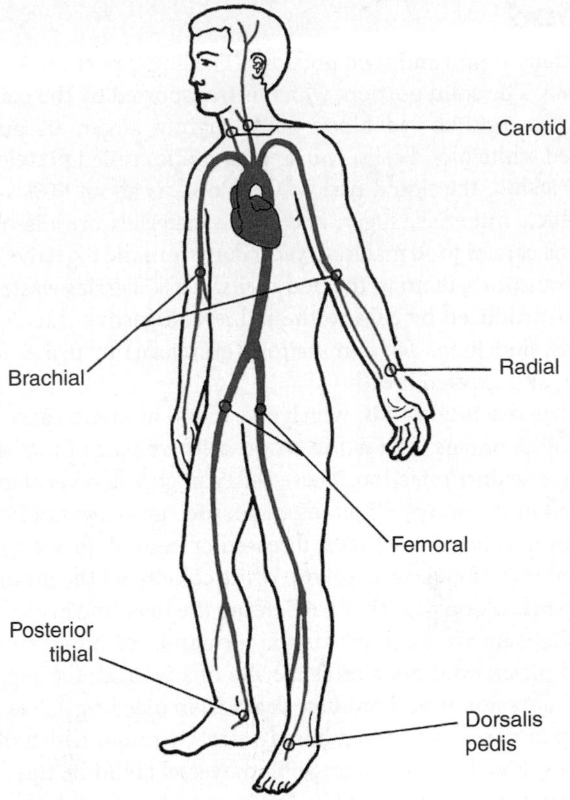

FIGURE 3-7 Locations for feeling pulses.

It is impossible to prick normal skin anywhere without puncturing capillaries. Because the flow of blood through the capillaries is relatively slow and under little pressure, blood merely oozes from a punctured capillary and usually has time to clot, promptly plugging the leak.

Each time the heart contracts, the surge of blood can be felt as a **pulse** at any point where an artery lies close to the surface of the body, near the skin surface and over a bone. When an artery is cut, blood spurts out. There is no pulse in a vein because the pressure wave is lost by the time the blood has passed through the capillaries. Hence, blood from a cut vein flows out in a steady stream. It has much less pressure behind it than blood from a cut artery. Blood makes its way back to the heart through a series of one-way valves in the veins.

Major locations for feeling pulses include the following **FIGURE 3-7**:

- **Carotid artery**: The major artery in the neck, which supplies the head with blood. Pulsations can be palpated (felt) on either side of the neck (do not try to feel both at the same time). Health care providers use the carotid artery to check an unresponsive person's pulse.
- **Femoral artery**: The major artery of the thigh, which supplies the thigh and leg with blood. There are two femoral arteries, one for each leg. Pulsations can be palpated in the groin area (the crease between the abdomen and the thigh).
- **Radial artery**: One of two main arteries of the lower arm (along with the ulnar artery). Pulsations can be palpated at the palm side of the wrist on the thumb side. Use the radial location to check an alert person's pulse.
- **Brachial artery**: An artery of the upper arm. Pulsations can be palpated on the inside of the arm between the elbow and the armpit. Health care providers use the brachial location to determine a pulse in an infant.
- **Posterior tibial artery**: Located behind the inside ankle knob (medial malleolus). Pulsations can be palpated behind the posterior surface of the medial malleolus.
- **Dorsalis pedis artery**: Pulsations can be palpated on the top surface of the foot (many people have no pulsations here).

Blood Pressure

Blood pressure is a measure of the pressure exerted by the blood on the walls of the arteries. Blood pressure might be high or low according to the resistance offered by the walls to the passage of blood. This difference in resistance could have several causes. For example, if blood does not fill the system, as occurs following a hemorrhage, the pressure will be low (hypotension). High blood pressure (hypertension) is when the blood is pushing too hard against the walls of the artery. It might be present when the arterial walls have become hard and cannot expand readily. A diet high in salt, fat, and/or cholesterol can lead to hardening of the arteries or atherosclerosis and cause high blood pressure.

Blood

Blood has liquid and solid portions. The liquid portion is called plasma. The solid portion, which is transported by the plasma, includes disklike red blood cells; slightly larger, irregularly shaped white blood cells; and smaller bodies called **platelets**.

Plasma, the liquid part of the blood, is about 90% water, in which minerals, sugar, and other materials are dissolved. Plasma carries food materials picked up from the digestive tract and transports them to the body cells. It also carries waste materials produced by cells to the kidneys, digestive tract, sweat glands, and lungs for elimination (excretion) in urine, feces, sweat, and expired breath.

The **red blood cells**, which give blood its color, carry oxygen to the organs. The **white blood cells** are part of the body's defense against infection. These cells can go wherever they are needed in the body to fight infection, such as to a wound in the skin or to other tissue that is diseased or injured. Pus, a sign of wound infection, gets its yellow-white color from the innumerable white blood cells that are fighting the invading bacteria.

Platelets are essential for the formation of blood clots. If blood plasma did not clot at the site of a wound, the slightest cut or abrasion would produce death from bleeding. Clots plug the openings of punctured blood vessels through which blood escapes. Bleeding from a large blood vessel could be too rapid to permit the formation of a clot. Hemorrhage is the term for profuse bleeding.

Perfusion refers to the circulation of blood through cells, organs, and organ systems. Hypoperfusion is the inadequate circulation of blood through an organ or a structure. An average-size person of approximately 150 to 180 pounds has about 4.5 to 6 quarts (12 pints [roughly 6 L]) of blood.

Inadequate circulation is known as shock (hypoperfusion). Shock is a state of profound depression of the vital processes of the body and may be characterized by the following signs and symptoms: pale or cyanotic (blue) skin; cool, clammy skin; rapid pulse; rapid breathing; restlessness, anxiety, or mental dullness; nausea and/or vomiting; reduction in total blood volume; low or decreasing blood pressure; and low body temperature.

The Nervous System

The **nervous system** is a complex collection of nerve cells (neurons) that coordinate the work of all parts of the human body and keep the individual in touch with the outside world. Neurons receive stimuli from the environment and transmit impulses to nerve centers in the brain and spinal cord. Then, through a complicated process that includes signals from the conscious thoughts of the person, in addition to reflex and automatic reactions, they produce nerve impulses that regulate and coordinate all bodily movements and functions and govern behavior and consciousness.

Once neurons have been destroyed, the body cannot regenerate them. Some limited nerve repair is possible, however, as long as the vital cell body is intact. If a nerve fiber is cut or injured, the section attached to the cell body remains alive, but the part beyond the injury will have no feeling or sensation and will not be able to function.

The nervous system can be classified in different ways. From a structural standpoint, it can be divided into the **central nervous system (CNS)** and the **peripheral nervous system**. The CNS includes the brain and the spinal cord. The peripheral nervous system is a network of nerve cells that originates in the brain and spinal cord and extends to all parts of the body, including the muscles, the surface of the skin, and the special sense organs (eg, the eyes and the ears). The peripheral nervous system is further subdivided into the voluntary and the autonomic (involuntary) nervous systems.

Central Nervous System

The CNS consists of the brain, which is enclosed within the skull, and the spinal cord, which is housed in a semiflexible bony column of vertebrae. The CNS serves as the body's controlling organ. The brain enables us to think, judge, and act. The spinal cord is a major communication pathway between the brain and the rest of the body.

Brain

The **brain**, which is the control center of the human nervous system, is probably the body's most highly specialized organ **FIGURE 3-8**. It weighs about 3 pounds (1.4 kg) in the average adult, is richly supplied with blood vessels, and requires considerable oxygen to perform effectively.

The brain has three main subdivisions: the **cerebrum** (large brain), which occupies nearly all (75%) of the cranial cavity; the **cerebellum** (small brain); and the **brainstem**. The cerebrum is divided into two hemispheres by a deep cleft. The outer surface of the cerebrum, the cerebral cortex, is about one-eighth of an inch (3.2 mm) thick, composed mainly of cell bodies of nerve cells, and often referred to as gray matter.

Certain sections of the cerebrum are localized to control specific body functions, such as sensation, thought, and associative memory, which allows us to store, recall, and make use of past experiences. The sight center of the brain is located at the back of the cerebrum, which is called the occipital lobe. The temporal lobes, at the sides of the skull, direct smell and hearing. The cerebellum is located at the back of the **cranium** and below the cerebrum. Its main function is to coordinate muscular activity and balance.

The third major area of the brain is the brainstem, which extends from the base of the cerebrum to the **foramen magnum** (a large opening at the base of the skull). The brainstem controls automatic functions such as breathing and heart rate.

Small cavities in the brain contain the **cerebrospinal fluid (CSF)**, a clear, watery solution similar to blood plasma. Circulating around the brain and the spinal cord, CSF serves as a protective cushion and exchanges food and waste materials. The total quantity of CSF in the brain–spinal cord system is 100 to 150 mL, although up to several liters can be produced daily. It is constantly being produced and reabsorbed.

Knowledge of nerve structure and function enables physicians to locate diseased brain sections. Because nerves from one side of the body eventually connect with the opposite side of the brain, a person whose left arm is paralyzed after a stroke will have suffered damage to the right side of the brain.

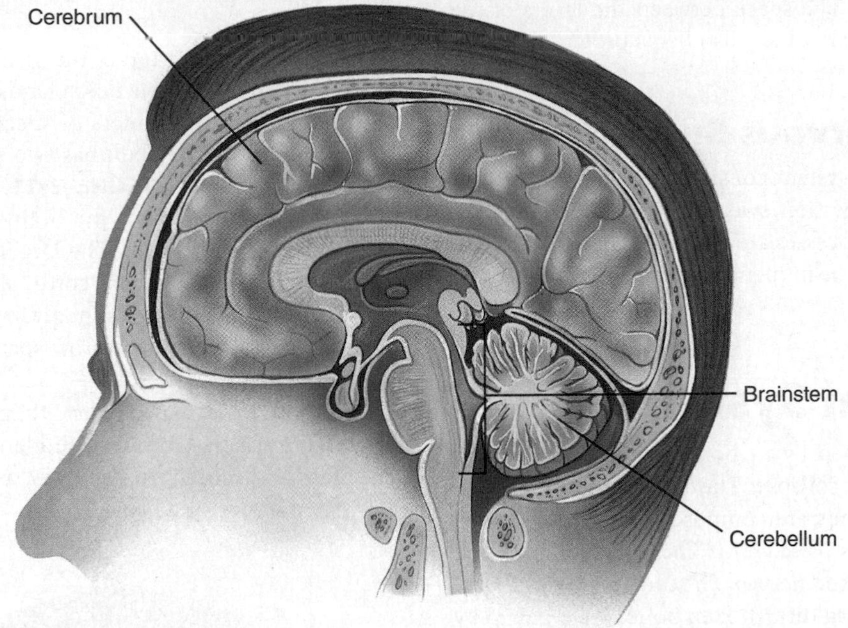

FIGURE 3-8 The brain lies well protected within the skull. Its principal subdivisions are the cerebrum, the cerebellum, and the brainstem.

Spinal Cord

The **spinal cord** is a soft column of nerve tissue continuous with the lower part of the brain that is enclosed in the bony vertebral column **FIGURE 3-9**. The spinal cord exits the brain through the foramen magnum, which is a hole in the base of the skull. Thirty-one pairs of spinal nerves branch from the spinal cord. These nerves are large trunks that are similar to telephone cables because they house many nerve fibers. Some fibers carry impulses into the spinal cord; others carry impulses away from it. Spinal nerves at different levels of the cord regulate activities of various parts of the body.

Because the spinal cord lies within the bony walls of the vertebrae, especially in the cervical (neck) and thoracic (chest) regions, it is particularly vulnerable to injury. Damage to the cord is almost always irreversible. An injury to the lumbar (lower back) spine causes paralysis and loss of sensation in the legs; an injury to the cervical cord causes paralysis and loss of sensation in the arms and the legs.

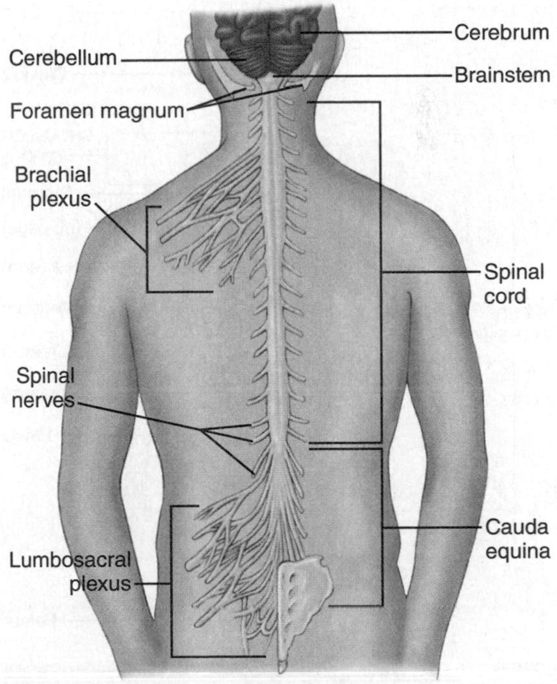

FIGURE 3-9 The spinal cord is a continuation of the brainstem.

Peripheral Nervous System

At each vertebral level and on each side of the spinal cord, a spinal nerve exits the spinal cord through an opening in the bony canal. These nerves make up the peripheral nervous system. The peripheral nervous system consists of the sensory and motor nerves. The sensory nerves carry sensations such as smell, touch, heat, and sound from the body to the brain and the spinal cord. The motor nerves carry information from the brain and the spinal cord to the muscles of the body.

If a nerve is cut or seriously damaged, disrupting the connection between the brain and the body, the body part will not be able to function. For example, if the motor nerve going to the right leg is cut, the leg will be unable to move. This loss of function may be permanent. Injuries to the nerves in the spinal cord can be very serious.

Fortunately, the CNS is well protected against injury. The brain is enclosed in the skull's cranial cavity. The spinal cord is contained in the hollow space of the vertebrae. The brain and the spinal cord are also protected by three layers of tissue known as the meninges. The space between the layers of the meninges is filled with CSF, which also helps protect the brain and spinal cord from injury.

Autonomic Nervous System

The autonomic nervous system consists of a group of nerves that control heart rate, digestion, sweating, and other automatic body processes. These processes are not controlled by the conscious mind, but they can be influenced by the CNS to a limited extent.

The Skeletal System

The human body is shaped by its bony framework. Without its bones, the body would collapse. The adult **skeleton** has 206 bones **FIGURE 3-10**. **Bones** are composed of living cells surrounded by hard deposits of calcium. The bone cells are well supplied by blood vessels and nerves. The calcium deposits give bones their strength and rigidity. Broken bones are repaired by bone-building cells within the bone and its covering sheath, the periosteum. New bone is formed at the site of the break, much as two pieces of steel are welded together.

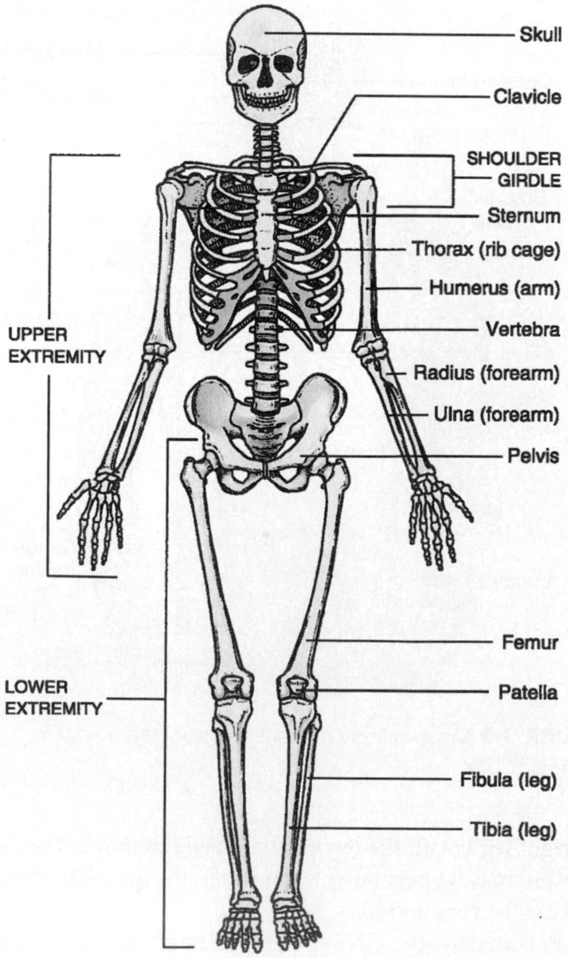

FIGURE 3-10 The bones of the skeleton give us our form, protect our vital organs, and allow us to move.

Skull

The skull rests at the top of the spinal column. It contains the brain, certain special-purpose glands (such as the pituitary and the pineal), and the centers of special senses—sight, hearing, taste, and smell. The skull has two parts, the brain case (cranium) and the face **FIGURE 3-11**. Blood vessels and nerve trunks pass to and from the brain through openings in the skull, mostly at the base. The largest opening is the foramen magnum, where the spinal cord exits the skull and joins the brain. The brain, which fits snugly in the cranium, is covered by the meninges. The very narrow spaces between the meninges are filled with CSF.

Although the skull is very tough, a blow can fracture it. Even if there is no fracture, a sudden impact can tear or bruise the brain and cause it to swell, just as any soft tissue swells following an injury or a bruise. Because the skull does not "give,"

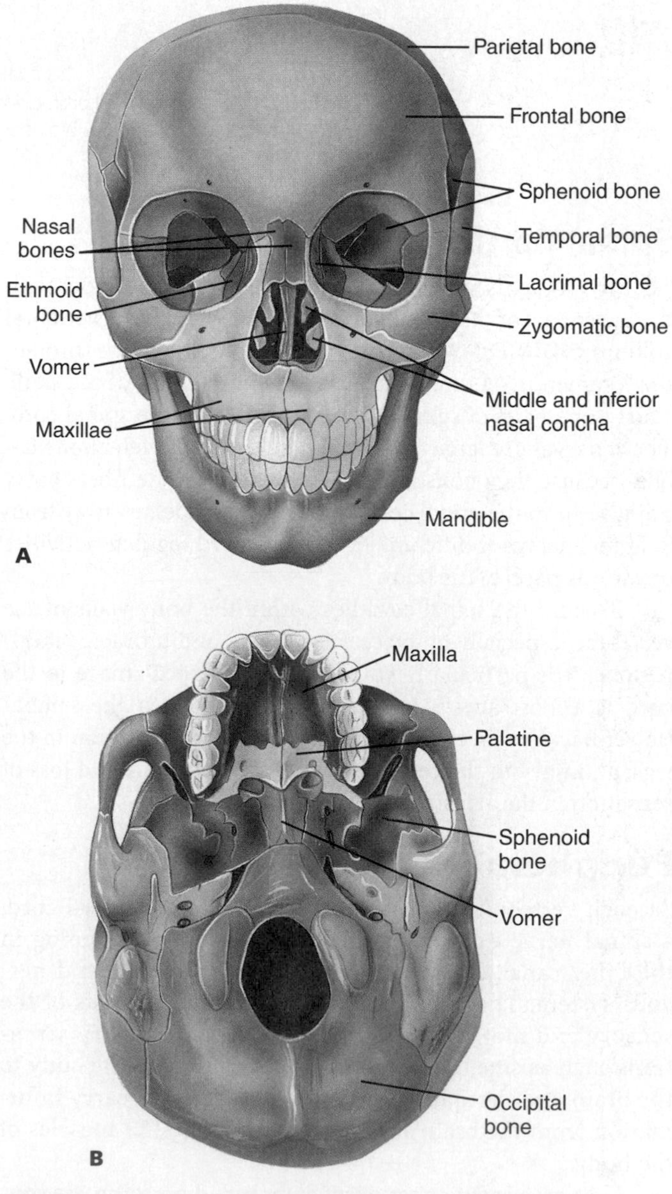

FIGURE 3-11 The skull. **A**. Anterior (front) view. **B**. Inferior (from bottom) view.

injury to the brain is magnified by the contained pressure within the skull. Unresponsiveness or even death could result from swelling (edema), a tearing wound (laceration), bleeding, or other damage to the brain. The face extends from the eyebrows to the chin and contains the eyes, nose, cheeks, mouth, and lower jaw (mandible).

Spinal Column

The spinal column is made up of irregularly shaped bones called **vertebrae** (singular is vertebra) **FIGURE 3-12**. Lying one on top of the other to form a strong, flexible column, the vertebrae are bound firmly together by strong **ligaments**. Between every two vertebrae is an intervertebral disk, a pad of tough elastic cartilage that acts as a shock absorber.

The spinal column can be damaged by disease or by injury. A crushed or displaced vertebra can squeeze, stretch, tear, or sever the spinal cord. Careless handling of an injured person by well-meaning but uninformed people or movement of the disabled part by the injured person can result in additional injury to the cord and possibly permanent paralysis. For that reason, a person with a back or neck injury must be handled with extreme care.

Thorax

The **thorax** (rib cage) is made up of ribs and the sternum (breast bone). The **sternum** is a flat, narrow bone in the middle of the front wall of the chest. The lowest portion of the sternum is the **xiphoid process**. Collarbones and certain ribs are attached to the sternum. The 24 ribs are semiflexible arches of bone. There are 12 on each side of the chest. The back ends of the 12 pairs of ribs are attached to the 12 thoracic vertebrae. Strong ligaments bind the back ends of the ribs to the spinal column but allow slight gliding or tilting movements. The front ends of the top 10 pairs of ribs are attached to the sternum by cartilage. The front ends of the last two pairs (pairs 11 and 12) hang free, giving them the name **floating ribs**.

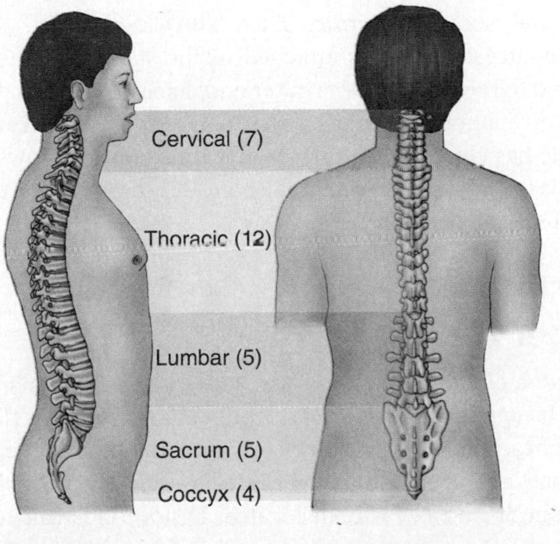

FIGURE 3-12 The spinal column (spine) is composed of 33 bones.

Fractures of the sternum or the ribs usually result from crushing or squeezing the chest. A fall, blow, or penetration of the chest wall by an object can have the same effect. The chief danger from such injuries is that the lungs might be punctured by the sharp ends of the broken bones.

Pelvis

The two hipbones and the sacrum form the pelvic girdle (pelvis). Muscles help connect the pelvic bones, the torso, the thighs, and the legs. The pelvis forms the floor of the abdominal cavity. The lower part of this cavity, sometimes called the pelvic cavity, holds the bladder, rectum, and internal parts of the reproductive organs. The floor of the pelvic cavity helps to support the intestines.

Leg Bones

Upper Leg (Thigh)

At the outer side of each hipbone is a deep socket into which the round head of the thigh bone (**femur**) fits, forming a ball-and-socket joint. The lower end of the femur is flat and has two knobs. These knobs articulate with the shin bone (tibia) at the knee joint. Although the femur is the longest and strongest bone in the skeleton, it is a common fracture site. A broken femur is always serious because it is difficult to align the broken or splintered ends. Because of the force required to break the femur, laceration of the surrounding tissues, pain, and blood loss could be extensive.

Knee

The knee joint is the largest joint in the body and is a strong hinge joint **FIGURE 3-13**. The joint is protected and stabilized in the front by the kneecap (patella). The **patella** is a small, triangular-shaped bone located in front of and between the femur and the tibia and within the tendon of the large muscle (the quadriceps) of the front of the thigh. Because the patella usually receives the force of falls or blows to the knee, it is frequently bruised or dislocated, and sometimes fractured.

Lower Leg

The lower leg refers to the portion of the lower extremity between the knee and the ankle. Its two bones are the tibia and the fibula **FIGURE 3-14**. The **tibia** (shin bone) is at the front and inner side of the leg. It is palpable throughout its length. Its broad upper surface receives the end of the femur to form the knee joint. The lower end, much smaller than the upper end, forms the inner rounded knob of the ankle (medial malleolus). The **fibula**, which is not a part of the true knee joint, is attached at the top to the tibia. Its lower end forms the outside ankle knob (lateral malleolus). The fibula is more often fractured alone than is the tibia.

Ankles, Feet, and Toes

The ends of the tibia and fibula form the socket of the ankle joint. Both ankle knobs are easily palpated. The seven ankle

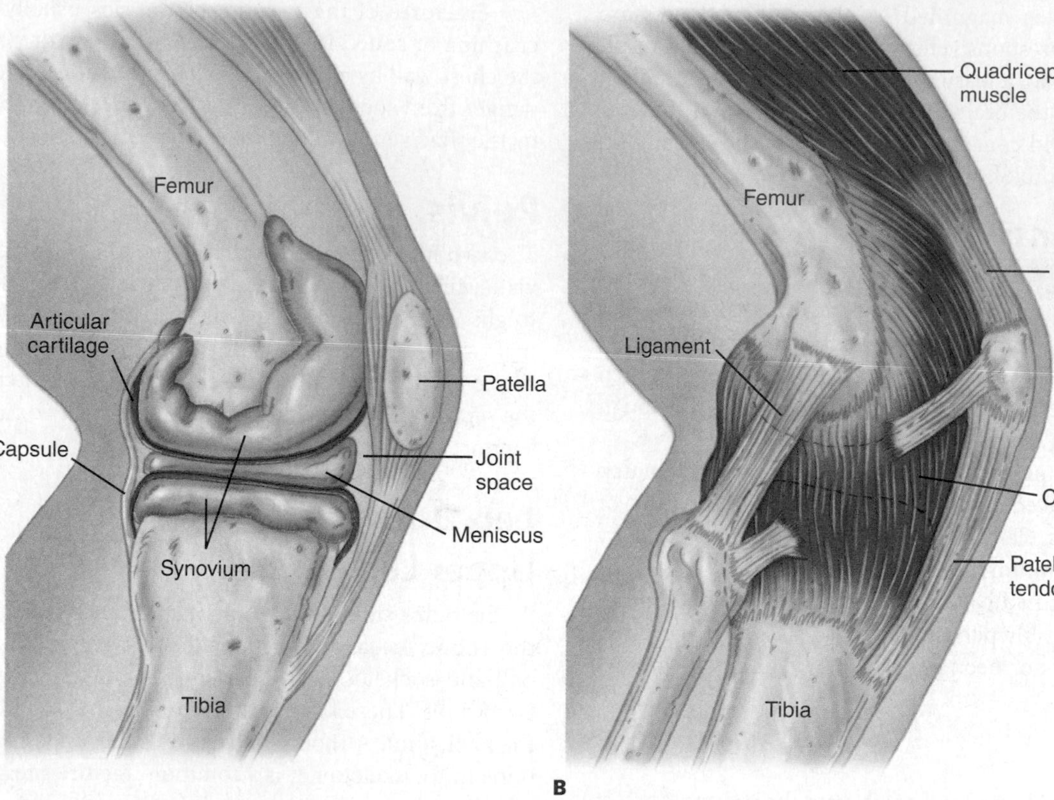

FIGURE 3-13 The knee joint. A joint consists of bone ends (**A**), the fibrous joint capsule, and ligaments (**B**).

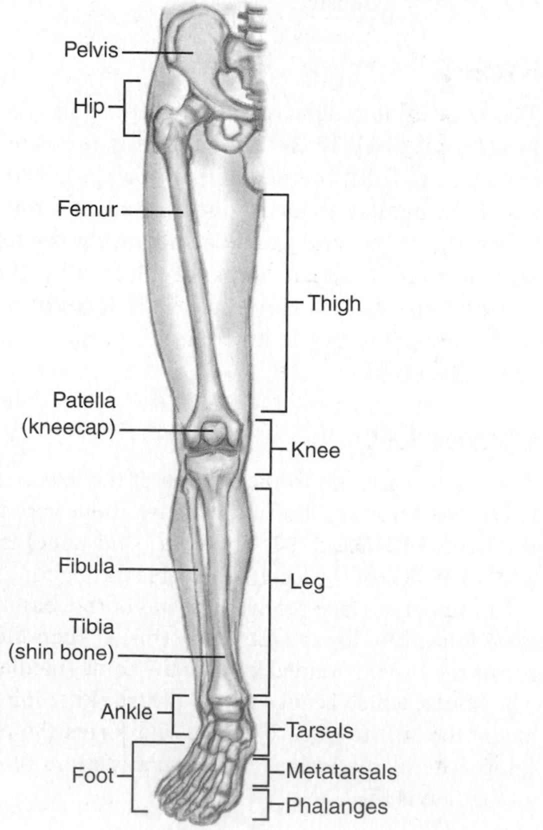

FIGURE 3-14 The principal parts of the lower extremity include the thigh, leg, and foot. The principal parts of the lower leg include the tibia and fibula.

bones (tarsals) are bound firmly together by tough ligaments. The heel bone (calcaneus) transmits the weight of the body to the ground and forms a base for the muscles of the calf of the leg when walking **FIGURE 3-15**. The sole and the instep of the foot are formed by the five long metatarsals. These bones articulate with the tarsals and with the front row of toe bones (phalanges).

Shoulder

The collarbone (clavicle) and the shoulder blade (scapula) form the shoulder girdle. Each **clavicle**—a long, slightly double-curved bone—is attached to the sternum at its inner end and to the scapula at its outer end. Each clavicle can be palpated throughout its length. Fractures are common because the clavicle lies close to the surface and must absorb blows. Each scapula—a large, flat, triangular bone—is located over the upper ribs at the back of the thorax.

Arm Bones

Upper Arm

The bone of the upper arm, the **humerus**, is the arm's largest bone. Its upper end (the head) is round; its lower end is flat. The round head fits into a shallow cup in the shoulder blade, forming a ball-and-socket joint. This is the most freely movable joint in the body and is easily dislocated. Dislocations can tear the capsule of the joint (synovial membrane) and cause damage. Improper manipulation during attempts to reduce or set the

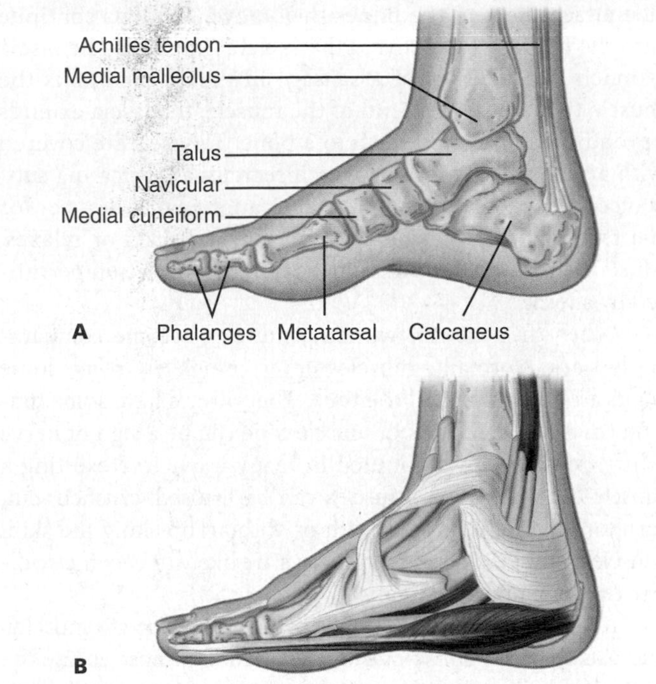

FIGURE 3-15 A. The surface landmarks of the foot and ankle include the medial malleolus, the calcaneus, and the phalanges. **B**. Soft tissue of the ankle.

dislocation could add to the damage. Therefore, it is important to treat dislocations of the shoulder with gentle care.

Forearm

The two bones of the forearm (radius and ulna) lie side by side. The larger of the two, the **ulna**, is on the little finger side, and part of it forms the elbow. The flat, curved lower end of the humerus fits into a big notch at the upper end of the ulna to form the elbow joint. This hinge joint permits movement in one direction only. The **radius**, shorter and smaller than the ulna, is on the thumb side of the forearm **FIGURE 3-16**.

Wrist, Hand, and Fingers

The wrist is composed of eight small, irregularly shaped bones (carpals) united by ligaments. Tendons extending from the muscles of the forearm to the bones of the hand and fingers pass down the front and the back of the wrist close to the surface. Wrist lacerations could sever these tendons, resulting in total or partial immobility of the fingers.

The palm of the hand has five long bones (metacarpals). The 14 bones of the fingers (phalanges) give the hand its great flexibility. The thumb is the most important digit. A functioning thumb and one or two fingers make a far more useful hand than four fingers minus the thumb **FIGURE 3-17**.

Joints

A **joint** is where two or more bones meet or join. Some joints, such as those in the cranium, allow little, if any, movement of the bones. Other joints, such as the hip and the shoulder, allow a wide range of motion. In a typical joint, a layer of cartilage,

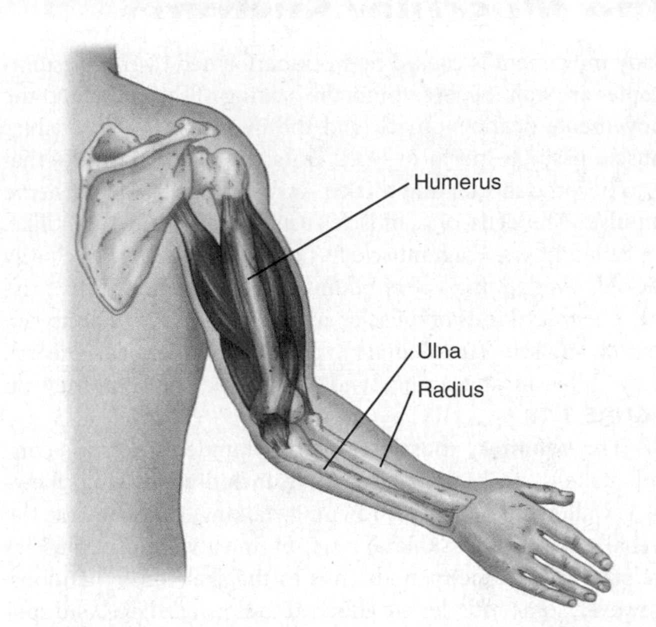

FIGURE 3-16 The principal bones in the arm and forearm include the humerus, the radius, and the ulna.

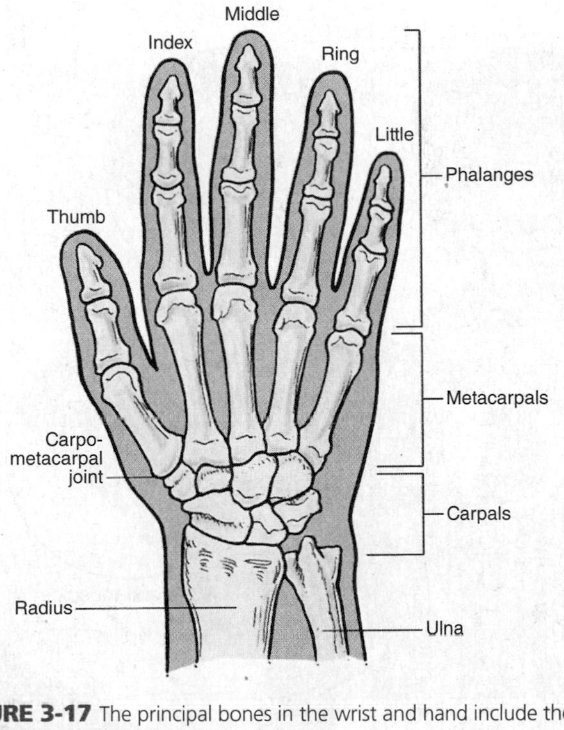

FIGURE 3-17 The principal bones in the wrist and hand include the carpals, the metacarpals, and the phalanges.

which is softer than bone, acts as a pad or buffer. The bones of such a joint are held in place by firmly attached ligaments, which are bands of dense, tough, but flexible connective tissue. Joints are enclosed in a capsule, a layer of thin, tough material, strengthened by the ligaments. The inner side of the capsule (synovial membrane) secretes a thick fluid (synovial fluid) that lubricates and protects the joint.

The Muscular System

Body movement is caused by work performed by muscles. Examples are walking, breathing, the beating of the heart, and the movements of the stomach and the intestines. What enables muscle tissue to perform work is its ability to contract—that is, to become shorter and thicker—when stimulated by a nerve impulse. The cells of a muscle, usually long and threadlike, are called fibers. Each muscle has countless bundles of closely packed, overlapping fibers bound together by connective tissue. The three kinds of muscles are skeletal muscle (voluntary), smooth muscle (involuntary), and cardiac muscle (heart). They differ in appearance and in the specific jobs they do **FIGURE 3-18**.

The **voluntary muscles**, which are under a person's control, make all deliberate acts possible, including walking, chewing, swallowing, smiling, frowning, talking, and moving the eyeballs. Also called **skeletal muscles**, most voluntary muscles are attached by one or both ends to the skeleton by tendons. However, some muscles are attached to skin, cartilage, and special organs (such as the eyeball) or to other muscles, such as the tongue.

Muscles help to shape the body and to form its walls. Most skeletal muscles end in tough, whitish cords (**tendons**) that attach them to the bones they move. Tendons continue into the fascia, which covers the skeletal muscles. The fascia is much like the skin of a sausage in that it surrounds the muscle tissue. At either end of the muscle, the fascia extends beyond the muscle to attach to a bone. Tendons are covered with a synovial membrane, which secretes a lubricating substance, the synovial fluid. This lubrication makes it easier for the tendon to move when the muscle contracts or relaxes. Muscular contraction pulls the bone in the direction permitted by a joint.

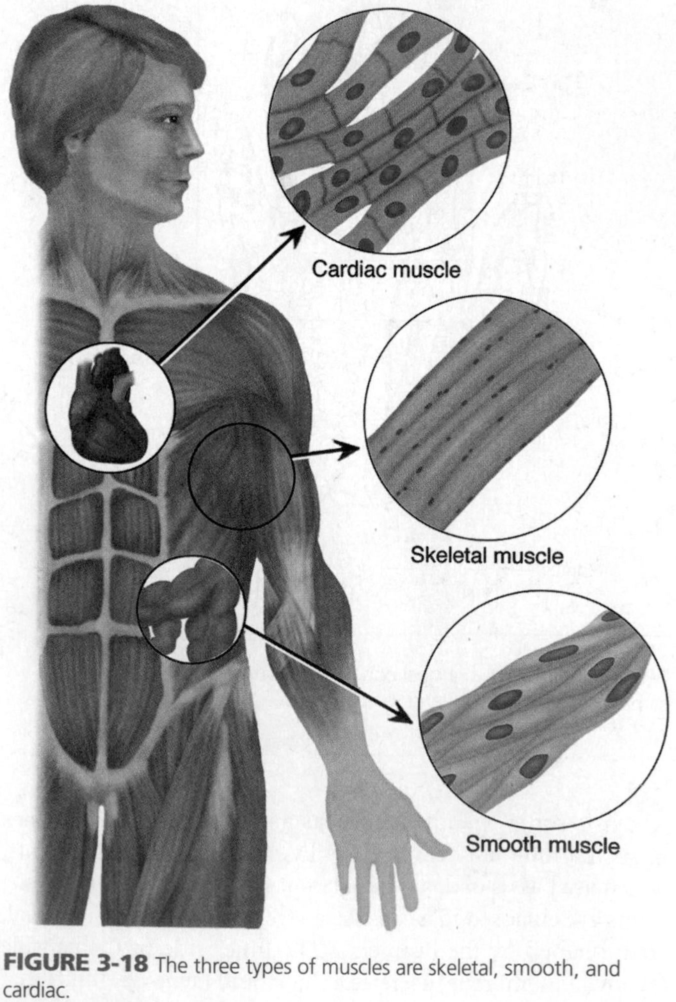

FIGURE 3-18 The three types of muscles are skeletal, smooth, and cardiac.

When they are not working, muscles become comparatively slack. Normally, muscles never completely relax; some fibers are contracting all the time. They always have some tension (muscle tone). Loss of muscle tone can be a sign of nerve injury. Muscles can be injured in many ways. Overexerting a muscle can tear fibers. Muscles can be bruised, crushed, cut, torn, or otherwise injured, with or without breaking the skin. Muscles injured in any of those ways are likely to become swollen, tender, painful, or weak.

A person has little or no control over the **smooth muscles** and usually is not conscious of them. Smooth muscles line the walls of tubelike structures such as the gastrointestinal tract, the urinary system, the blood vessels, and the bronchi of the lungs. **Cardiac muscle** is a specialized form of muscle found only in the heart. A continuous supply of oxygen and glucose is needed for cardiac muscle to work properly, otherwise it becomes irritable and may produce dangerous, potentially lethal beats.

The Skin

The skin covers the entire body, protecting the deep tissues from being injured, drying out, or being invaded by bacteria and other foreign bodies. The skin helps to regulate body temperature by aiding in the elimination of water and various salts. The skin senses heat, cold, touch, pressure, and pain and transmits that information to the brain and the spinal cord.

The skin consists of two layers: the outer layer (**epidermis**) and the inner layer (**dermis**) **FIGURE 3-19**. The epidermis varies in thickness in different parts of the body (the palms and the soles of the feet are thickest), and its dead cells are constantly worn off. The dermis has a rich supply of blood vessels and nerve endings. Hair grows from the dermis through openings called hair follicles. Sweat glands and oil glands in the dermis empty onto the surface of the epidermis through pores in the skin. Beneath the dermis is the subcutaneous (meaning "under the skin") layer, which is well supplied with fat cells and blood vessels.

Sweat glands, which create perspiration, occur in nearly all parts of the skin. Sweat contains essentially the same minerals as blood plasma and urine, but it is more dilute. Normally, only traces of the waste products excreted in urine are in sweat. But when sweating is profuse or when the kidneys are diseased, the amounts of such wastes excreted in the sweat could be considerable. Several mineral salts are removed from the body in sweat. Chief among those in quantity is sodium chloride (the same mineral as common table salt).

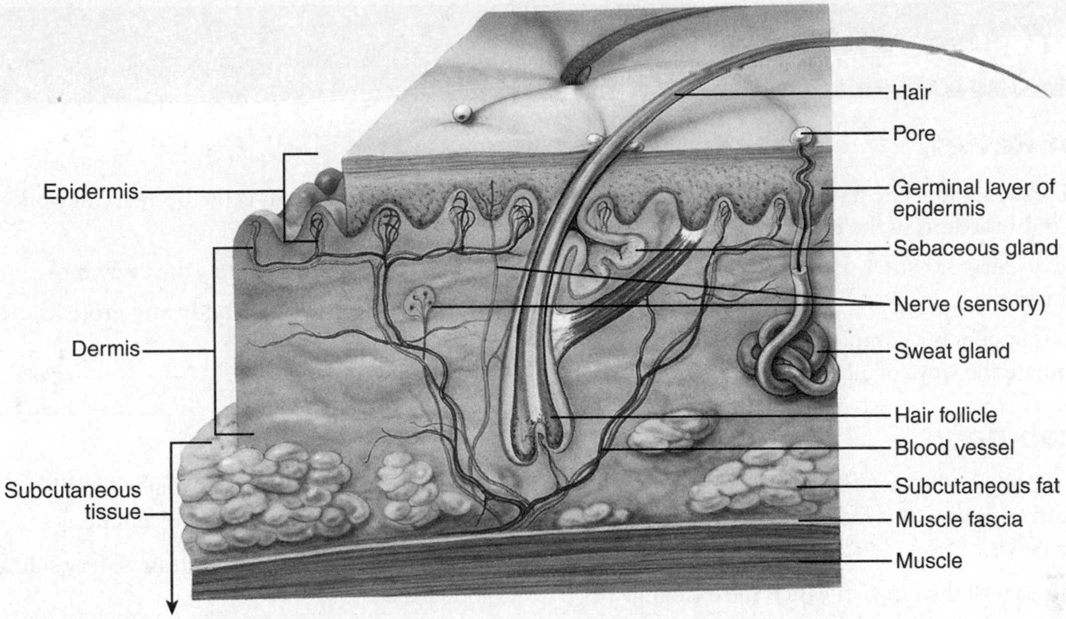

FIGURE 3-19 The skin has two main layers: the epidermis and the dermis. Below the skin is a layer of subcutaneous tissue.

PREP KIT

Ready for Review

- A first aid provider must be familiar with the basic structure and functions of the human body.
- The cardiovascular system is made up of the blood, heart, and blood vessels.
- The nervous system is a complex collection of nerve cells that coordinate the work of all parts of the human body.
- The skeletal system is the bony framework that shapes the body.
- The muscular system lets the body move.
- Skin covers the entire body and protects the deep tissues.

Vital Vocabulary

abdomen The body cavity that contains the major organs of digestion and excretion. It is located below the diaphragm and above the pelvis.

alveoli The air sacs of the lungs in which the exchange of oxygen and carbon dioxide takes place.

anterior The front surface of the body.

aorta The principal artery leaving the left side of the heart and carrying freshly oxygenated blood to the body.

artery A blood vessel, consisting of three layers of tissue and smooth muscle, that carries blood away from the heart.

blood The fluid that circulates through the heart, arteries, capillaries, and veins, carrying nutrients and oxygen to the body cells and removing waste products such as carbon dioxide and various metabolic products for excretion.

bones The hard form of connective tissue that constitutes most of the skeleton in humans.

brachial artery The artery of the arm that branches at the elbow into the radial and ulnar arteries; used to determine an infant's pulse.

brain The soft, large mass of nerve tissue that is contained in the cranium.

brainstem The area of the brain between the spinal cord and cerebrum, surrounded by the cerebellum; controls automatic functions that are necessary for life, such as respirations.

bronchial tubes The passageways from the trachea to the lungs.

capillaries The small blood vessels through whose walls various substances pass into and out of the tissues and on to the cells.

cardiac muscle The heart muscle.

cardiovascular system The arrangement of connected tubes, including the arteries, arterioles, capillaries, venules, and veins, that moves blood, oxygen, nutrients, carbon dioxide, and cellular waste throughout the body.

carotid artery The major arteries that supply blood to the head and brain.

central nervous system (CNS) The brain and spinal cord.

cerebellum One of the three major subdivisions of the brain; coordinates voluntary body movements.

cerebrospinal fluid (CSF) A clear, watery solution similar to blood plasma.

cerebrum The largest part of the three subdivisions of the brain, made up of several lobes that control movement, hearing, balance, speech, visual perception, emotions, and personality.

clavicle The collarbone.

cranium The area of the head above the ears and eyes; the part of the skull that contains the brain.

deep Located farther inside the body and away from the skin.

dermis The inner layer of the skin, containing hair follicles, sweat glands, nerve endings, and blood vessels.

diaphragm A muscular dome that forms the undersurface of the thorax, separating the chest from the abdominal cavity. Contraction of the diaphragm brings air into the lungs. Relaxation allows air to be expelled from the lungs.

distal Located away from the center of the body or from the point of attachment, such as the point where the arm or leg attaches to the body.

dorsalis pedis artery The artery on the anterior (top) surface of the foot between the first and second metatarsals.

epidermis The outer layer of the skin, which is made up of cells that are sealed together to form a watertight protective covering for the body.

epiglottis A small flap of tissue that allows air to pass into the trachea but prevents food and liquid from entering.

esophagus A collapsible tube that extends from the pharynx to the stomach. Contractions of the muscle in the wall of the esophagus propel food and liquids through it to the stomach.

femoral artery The principal artery of the thigh. It supplies blood to the lower abdominal wall, external genitalia, and leg. There are two, one in each leg. It can be palpated in the groin area.

femur The thigh bone; the longest and one of the strongest bones in the body.

PREP KIT continued

fibula The outer and smaller bone of the two bones of the lower leg.

floating ribs The 11th and 12th ribs, which do not attach to the sternum.

foramen magnum A large opening at the base of the skull through which the brain connects to the spinal cord.

heart A hollow, muscular organ that receives blood from the veins and propels it into the arteries.

humerus The bone of the upper arm.

inferior Located closer to the feet.

joint The place where two bones come into contact.

larynx The voice box.

lateral Located farther from the middle of the body.

ligament A band of the fibrous tissue that connects bones to bones. It supports and strengthens a joint.

medial Located closer to the middle of the body.

nervous system The system that controls virtually all activities of the body, both voluntary and involuntary.

patella The kneecap; a specialized bone that lies within the tendon of the quadriceps muscle.

perfusion The circulation of oxygenated blood within an organ or tissue in adequate amounts to meet the cells' current needs.

peripheral nervous system A network of nerve cells that originates in the brain and spinal cord and extends to all parts of the body, including the muscles, the surface of the skin, and the special sense organs, such as the eyes and the ears.

pharynx The throat.

plasma A sticky, yellow fluid that carries the blood cells and nutrients and transports cellular waste material to the organs of excretion.

platelets Tiny, disk-shaped elements that are much smaller than cells. They are essential in the initial formation of a blood clot, the mechanism that stops bleeding.

posterior The back surface of the body.

posterior tibial artery The artery just posterior to the medial malleolus; supplies blood to the foot.

proximal Located closer to the center of the body or to the point of attachment, such as the point where the arm or leg attaches to the body.

pulse The wave of pressure created as the heart contracts and forces blood out of the left ventricle and into the major arteries.

quadrant A section of the abdominal cavity. Imagine a horizontal and a vertical line intersecting at the umbilicus, dividing the abdomen into four equal areas.

radial artery A main artery in the forearm. It is palpable at the wrist on the thumb side.

radius The bone on the thumb side of the forearm.

red blood cells Cells that carry oxygen to the body tissues; also called erythrocytes.

respiratory system All the structures of the body that contribute to the process of breathing, consisting of the upper and lower airways and their component parts.

skeletal muscle Muscle that is attached to bones and usually crosses at least one joint. It is striated, or voluntary, muscle.

skeleton The framework that gives us our recognizable form; also designed to allow motion of the body and protection of vital organs.

smooth muscle Muscle that constitutes the bulk of the gastrointestinal tract and is present in nearly every organ to regulate automatic activity. It is nonstriated, or involuntary, muscle.

spinal cord An extension of the brain, composed of virtually all the nerves carrying messages between the brain and the rest of the body. It lies inside of and is protected by the spinal canal.

sternum The breast bone.

superficial Located closer to or on the skin.

superior Located closer to the head.

tendons The fibrous connective tissue that attaches muscle to bone.

thorax The chest cavity that contains the heart, lungs, esophagus, and great vessels.

tibia The shin bone; the larger of the two bones of the lower leg.

trachea The windpipe; the main trunk for air passing to and from the lungs.

ulna The inner bone of the forearm, on the side opposite the thumb.

vein Any blood vessel that carries blood from the tissues to the heart.

vertebrae The 33 bones that make up the spinal column.

voluntary muscle Muscle that is under direct voluntary control of the brain and can be contracted or relaxed at will; skeletal or striated muscle.

white blood cells Blood cells involved in the body's immune defense mechanisms against infection.

xiphoid process The lowest part of the sternum.

PREP KIT continued

Assessment in Action

You are helping a friend with her human anatomy and physiology homework during your lunch break. Having taken the same class, you feel confident that you can help explain how the human body works. Your friend seems impressed when you explain different types of muscles. After taking a bite of her lunch, your friend clutches her throat and appears to be choking. You ask her if she is choking and she nods her head "yes." You ask her to say something but she cannot and continues clutching her throat. You notice that she had been eating a hot dog.

Directions: Circle Yes if you agree with the statement; circle No if you disagree.

1. You should not panic. Your friend is young and with a little more time the hot dog will pass into her esophagus.

   YES NO

2. Because your friend is alert and responsive, she can survive without breathing for over 10 minutes.

   YES NO

3. Her face begins to turn blue and she collapses to the floor. Her chest is not moving, which is a sign that she is not breathing.

   YES NO

4. If your friend is not breathing, her tissues and organs are not getting enough carbon dioxide.

   YES NO

Check Your Knowledge

Directions: Circle Yes if you agree with the statement; circle No if you disagree.

1. A first aid provider does not have to understand how the human body works in order to effectively provide care.

   YES NO

2. The human body can store oxygen for hours.

   YES NO

3. Blood is the delivery system for cells throughout the body.

   YES NO

4. The heart is a pear-shaped, muscular organ.

   YES NO

5. Once neurons have been destroyed, the body can replace them.

   YES NO

6. The autonomic nervous system consists of a group of nerves that control heart rate, digestion, sweating, and other automatic body processes.

   YES NO

7. The adult skeleton has 228 bones.

   YES NO

8. A joint is where two or more bones meet or join.

   YES NO

9. There are three kinds of muscle: skeletal, smooth, and cardiac.

   YES NO

10. Skin transmits information to the brain and helps regulate body temperature.

    YES NO

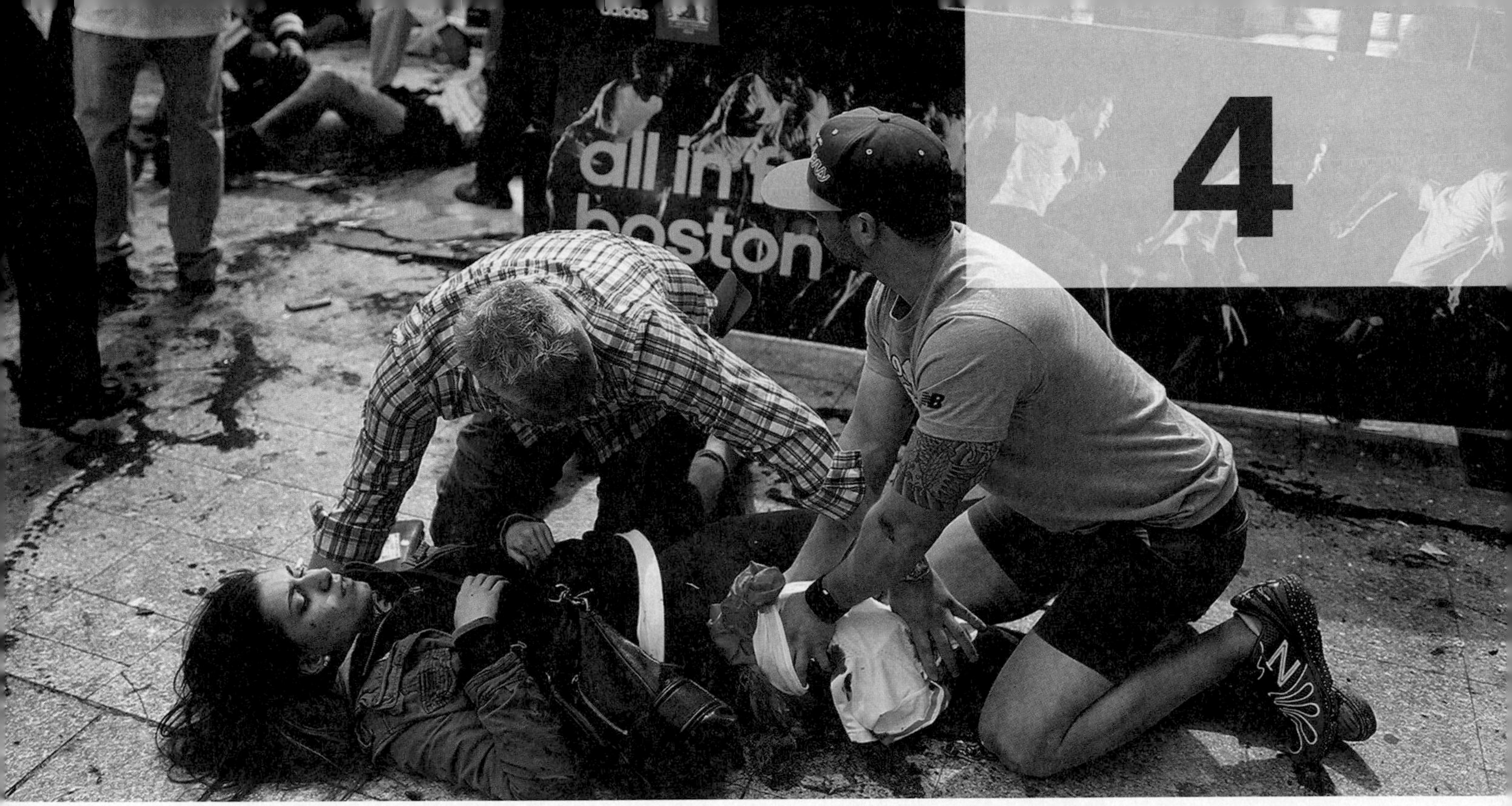

4

Finding Out What Is Wrong

CHAPTER AT A GLANCE

- Assessment Overview
- Scene Size-up
- Primary Assessment
- History Taking (SAMPLE)
- Secondary Assessment (Physical Exam)
- Reassessment
- Special Considerations
- Optional Assessments

Assessment Overview

During emergency situations when panic exists, knowing what to do and what not to do is crucial. An assessment is a sequence of actions that helps determine what is wrong, and thus helps provide safe and appropriate first aid. Becoming familiar with the process of assessment will enable you to act quickly and decisively in hectic emergency situations. Assessment is an important first aid skill. It requires an understanding of each assessment step as well as decision-making skills.

Finding out what is wrong with a person will be influenced by whether the person is suffering from an illness or an injury, whether the person has an altered mental status and whether life-threatening conditions exist.

Different conditions require different approaches for determining what is wrong. Not all parts of an assessment apply to every person, and the sequencing can vary depending on the person's medical condition. Most people do not require a complete assessment. For example, a person who cut a finger while whittling a stick will not require a complete assessment; however, a person who cut a finger while sliding down a mountainside will require a full assessment because this person might have sustained other injuries.

An assessment can provide important information about a condition and help you determine how to treat it and whether professional medical care is needed **FLOWCHART 4-1**. If the person

Flowchart 4-1 Finding What Is Wrong

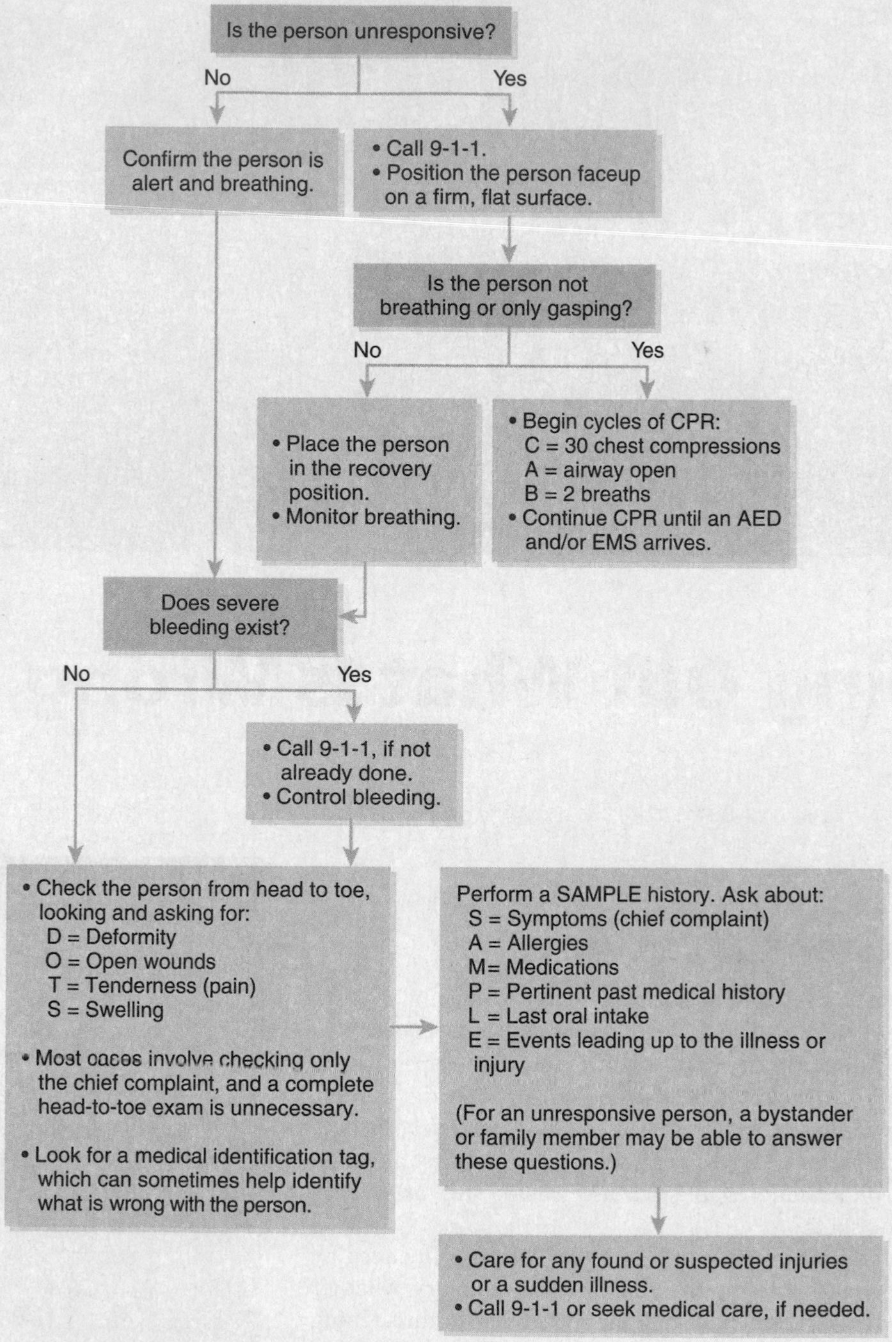

requires professional medical care, pass what you found during the assessment to the emergency medical services (EMS) personnel or health care providers. Call 9-1-1 for any person with a significant **cause of injury** (sometimes called mechanism of injury [MOI]) or **nature of illness (NOI)**, and for any unresponsive person.

Assessment Format

You should assess the person systematically. You can do this by performing these steps:

1. Perform a scene size-up.
2. Perform a primary assessment.

3. Obtain the person's SAMPLE history.
4. Perform a secondary assessment.
5. Perform a reassessment.

A **scene size-up** is a crucial first step that must be taken to make sure the scene is safe. Quickly, but carefully, examine the area for any potential hazards, which can include dangerous people as well as dangerous situations.

The **primary assessment** consists of identifying and treating life-threatening conditions involving airway, breathing impairments, and circulation (ie, severe bleeding, pulse). People with immediate, life-threatening conditions can die within minutes unless the cause is quickly recognized and treated.

A **SAMPLE history** allows an injury to be found and cared for sooner when it comes before the physical exam. The SAMPLE history allows you to gain detailed information about the person's injury (eg, a painful ankle or bleeding nose) or **chief complaint** (eg, chest pain or itchy skin).When caring for a stranger, having a conversation as you gather the person's SAMPLE history may alleviate their anxiety about having you conduct a physical exam. Also, in cases of illness, performing the SAMPLE history before the physical exam can indicate which part of the physical exam should be performed first.

A secondary assessment, which consists of a physical exam, generally follows the primary assessment and SAMPLE history. (For a critically injured person, you might not go beyond the primary assessment.) These procedures can reveal information that will help you identify the injury or illness, judge its severity, and determine what first aid is needed.

Perform a reassessment after the most critical illness or injuries have been cared for.

Scene Size-up

Every time you encounter a person with an injury or illness, first check out the scene. The **scene size-up** determines the safety of the scene, the cause of injury or nature of illness, and the number of people involved. (Refer to Chapter 2, *Action at an Emergency*, for additional information.)

Without a scene size-up, a potentially hazardous situation could result in further injury to the person or injury to you and bystanders. Hazards come in many different forms (eg, chemicals, electricity, water, fires, explosions, carbon monoxide). They exist at most motor vehicle crash scenes. Some scenes have the potential for violence—violent people, distraught family members, angry bystanders, gangs, and unruly crowds. Be observant for weapons. If the scene appears hazardous, do not enter the area. You cannot help a person if you become injured or ill yourself.

Reduce exposure to potentially dangerous body substances that can carry disease. Disease transmission is very rare; however, you should wear medical exam gloves and assume that all people are infected.

Determining whether an injury or an illness exists is also an important step. Making this distinction gives you a starting point. If the scene size-up suggests serious illness or injury, call 9-1-1.

Primary Assessment

The purpose of the primary assessment is to identify life-threatening conditions so you can immediately take action to treat the conditions. The primary assessment includes checking the person's responsiveness, checking for breathing, and checking for circulation and severe external bleeding.

Form a General Impression

While approaching the person, form an immediate first impression, or **general impression**. The general impression is sometimes referred to as the look test or gut reaction. Using the scene size-up and your general impression of the person, determine the following:

1. Is there a chance of exposure to the person's blood or other body fluids?
2. Is there any danger to you, the person, or bystanders at the scene?
3. Does the person appear to have an injury or an illness? If you are unable to determine whether the person is ill or injured, proceed as though they are injured.
4. Does the person appear to be responsive or unresponsive?
5. Is the person obviously breathing adequately or normally? If the person is able to talk, there is a good chance they are breathing adequately.
6. Are signs of obvious bleeding present—blood spurting, blood-soaked clothing, blood pooled on the ground or floor?

Assess Responsiveness

Shortly after reaching the person, determine the person's mental status or responsiveness. A person's level of responsiveness can range from fully responsive (conscious) to unresponsive (unconscious). Not all responsive people are fully alert, and they may respond to different levels of stimulation.

Assessing a Responsive Person

For an alert person, begin by introducing yourself. Tell the person that you are trained in first aid and ask permission to help. For an alert, responsive person, you can evaluate the person's ability to remember by asking about the following:

- Person—What is your name?
- Place—Do you know where you are?
- Time—What is the month and year?
- Event—What happened?

If the person is motionless, gently tap their shoulder and ask loudly, "Are you okay?" Beyond this point, how and in what order you conduct the assessments will largely depend on the answer to this question. If the person answers, moans, or moves, the person is responsive.

All people who have been injured need a primary assessment. Even a responsive person could be developing an airway obstruction, may have severe bleeding, may be having a heart attack, or may be in the early stages of shock or some other serious condition. Each of these conditions is considered a medical emergency, and immediate care must be provided if you suspect any of them.

Assessing an Unresponsive, Motionless Person

For an unresponsive person, the steps resemble the steps used when beginning to perform CPR—which are remembered with the mnemonic RAB-CAB—although most unresponsive people do not need CPR (see Chapter 5, *CPR*):

R = *Responsive?* For any motionless person, check responsiveness by gently tapping the person's shoulder and shouting, "Are you okay?" Speak loudly enough to wake the person if they are sleeping.

A = *Activate EMS.* If there is no response, activate EMS by calling 9-1-1.

B = *Breathing?* After activating EMS, position the person on their back on a flat, firm surface. Check for no breathing or only gasping. If the person is breathing, place them in the recovery position and check for severe bleeding. If the person is not breathing, give CPR.

An unresponsive, breathing person can receive other first aid, especially to control severe bleeding. Providing care would be covered by implied consent. (Refer to Chapter 1, *Introduction*.)

Q&A

When should I interrupt a primary assessment?

When a life-threatening condition is identified during the primary assessment, immediately begin first aid. For example, if a person has an obstructed airway, treat the obstruction before going through the other assessment steps. Once the life-threatening condition (eg, choking) has been cared for and/or corrected, continue the primary check of the person until completed.

Assessing Breathing

Check for adequate breathing by looking for chest (neck to waist) rise and fall and listening for normal or abnormal breath sounds. Distinguish between effective and ineffective breathing efforts. Cyanosis (blue discoloration around lips and mouth) and ashen (gray) skin are signs of inadequate oxygenation. See **TABLE 4-1** for breathing sounds that may indicate inadequate breathing.

TABLE 4-1 Abnormal Breathing Sounds

Breathing Sound	Possible Cause
Snoring	Airway partially blocked (usually by tongue)
Gurgling (breaths passing through liquid)	Fluids in throat
Crowing (noisy creak or squeak)	Spasm of the larynx, foreign body
Wheezing	Spasm or partial obstruction in bronchi (asthma, emphysema)

Check for Severe Bleeding

When assessing severe bleeding, is there any life-threatening external bleeding to control? Check for severe bleeding by quickly looking over the person's entire body for blood (eg, blood-soaked clothing or blood pooling on the floor or the ground). This is not a head-to-toe exam, but rather a search for large amounts of blood around the person or in the person's clothing. In most cases, placing a sterile dressing over the wound and applying direct pressure with a hand or a pressure bandage controls the bleeding. Life-threatening external bleeding is rare, but when found, it must be controlled immediately or the person can bleed to death. Avoid contact with the

Q&A

How should an injured person be positioned?

Most people should not be moved, especially if a spinal injury is suspected. However, you may need to safely reposition the person if the position in which you find the person is impeding the primary assessment or if repositioning can otherwise improve the person's recovery. Such circumstances include the following:

- When the person and first aid provider or providers are in an unsafe location, you may move the person only as needed to reach a safe location.
- When an unresponsive person is facedown (prone position) and needs CPR, turn the person faceup (supine position) on a firm, flat surface to be in a position to receive CPR.
- In some cases, when the person has difficulty breathing because of vomiting or secretions, or if you are alone and must leave to get help, it is best to place the person in the recovery position **FIGURE 4-1**. (See Chapter 5, *CPR*, for additional information on the recovery position.) While rolling the person into the side position, keep the person's nose and navel pointing in the same direction to avoid twisting the spine. When signs of shock develop, place the person on their back (supine position). **DO NOT** move the person if suspected leg fractures or head or spinal injuries exist.

Most people with no suspected spinal injuries may be placed in the position in which they are most comfortable. People with chest pain, nausea, or difficulty breathing fare better in a half-sitting (semi-sitting) position at about a 45° angle. During an asthma attack, a person may prefer the tripod position, which is sitting up and leaning forward with the hands on the knees and elbows out.

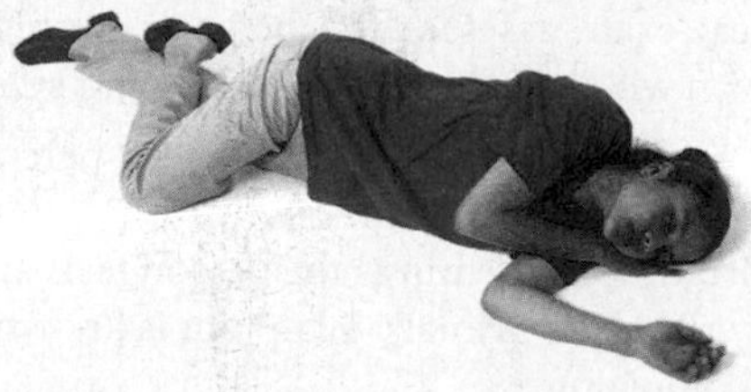

FIGURE 4-1 Recovery position.

person's blood whenever possible by using medical exam gloves or plastic bags if gloves are not available. Extra layers of dressings or cloth can be used but note that they will not protect against bloodborne pathogens if blood contact occurs.

History Taking (SAMPLE)

Gather information using the mnemonic SAMPLE. The information in a SAMPLE history may help you identify what is wrong with the person and what first aid is needed **TABLE 4-2**.

In the best of circumstances, the person will be able to answer all questions about their chief complaint and medical history. In other cases, you may obtain this information from family, friends, bystanders, medical identification tag, or other medical information sources.

TABLE 4-2 SAMPLE History

Description	Questions
S = Symptoms	What is wrong? Where do you hurt?
A = Allergies	Are you allergic to anything?
M = Medications	Are you taking any prescription, nonprescription, herbal, or recreational medications? What are they for? When were they last taken?
P = Pertinent past medical history	Have you had this problem before? Have you had recent medical conditions? Are you under a doctor's care?
L = Last food or drink	When did you last eat or drink anything? What was it? How much?
E = Events leading up to the illness or injury	Injury: How did you get hurt? Illness: What led to this condition?

Checking for Medical Identification Tags

Look for a medical identification tag or for a medical information card in the person's wallet or purse. (Note that this search might be illegal in some states.) Such information can be beneficial in identifying allergies, medications, or medical history **FIGURE 4-2**. A medical identification tag, worn as a necklace or as a bracelet, contains the wearer's medical condition or conditions and a 24-hour telephone number that offers, in case of an emergency, access to the person's medical history plus names of physicians and close relatives. These sources of information can be especially useful when the wearer is unresponsive or not old enough to answer questions. Necklaces and bracelets are durable, instantly recognizable, and less likely than cards to be separated from the person in an emergency. If looking through a person's wallet or purse, always do so in the presence of another person at the scene to protect yourself against later accusations, should money or credit cards be missing.

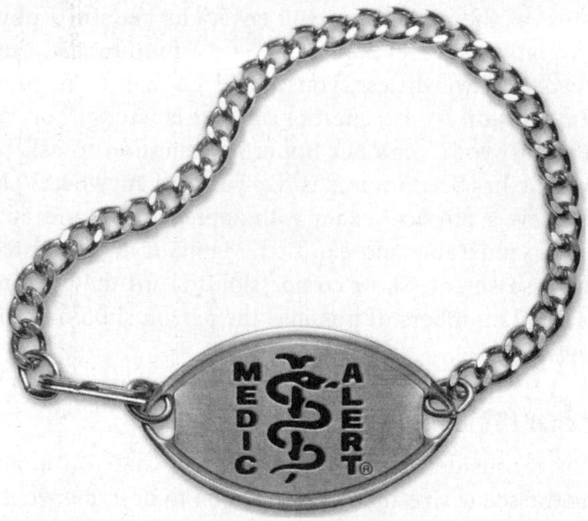

FIGURE 4-2 Medical identification tag. Front of tag.

FYI

Check for Clues

In addition to a medical identification tag, you may find other clues in determining the cause of the person's injury or illness. A medicine bottle label gives the name of the medication, but you may not know why the medication was prescribed. Suspect a diabetic emergency if you find glucose tablets or gel or insulin with a person. An inhaler indicates that a person has asthma. An auto-injector could point to a person's susceptibility to severe, life-threatening allergic reactions.

The mechanism of injury (such as a sharp object, broken glass, or bent steering wheel) can provide crucial details about an injury. Additionally, objects at the scene that are not the cause of an injury can offer a clue as to what may be wrong with a person. Examples include a fallen ladder or an open medicine bottle.

Secondary Assessment (Physical Exam)

Complete a **physical exam** after the SAMPLE history. This secondary assessment is where you will focus on the chief complaint and immediately treat any life-threatening conditions. The goal of doing a physical exam is to identify any potentially life-threatening sudden illness or injury requiring first aid. A good physical exam is essential in discovering what is wrong. The adage of "Find it, fix it" stresses the fact that you cannot provide first aid unless you know what is wrong. And, you will not know what is wrong until you do an assessment.

Most of the people you will encounter require a physical exam of only the chief complaint, and a full physical exam is not needed. Nevertheless, you should know how to perform one. In addition to the question, "What is wrong?" or "What happened to you?" another important question to ask of the person who has been injured is "Do you hurt anywhere?" Many people view a physical exam with apprehension and anxiety. They feel vulnerable and exposed. Maintain dignity throughout the assessment. Show compassion toward the person and their family members. If possible, the person should be sitting or lying down.

Perform a Physical Exam

Start by reconsidering the cause of injury that you identified during the scene size-up. Ask the person to describe what happened in detail, so that you can use the cause of the injury to predict possible injured areas—especially head, neck, spine, and internal injuries (see Chapter 2, *Action at an Emergency*). Establishing the cause of injury helps to determine which first aid procedures to use.

Determine whether the cause of injury was significant **TABLE 4-3**. In addition to the significant causes of injury, assume that a person with a head injury also has a spinal injury until proven otherwise.

For a responsive person, check for a spinal injury. Ask the person the questions in Chapter 12, *Head and Spinal Injuries*.

Stabilize the person against any movement, and tell them not to move.

For an unresponsive person whom you suspect has a spinal injury, do not move the person's head or neck.

Q&A

Do I have to perform a complete assessment for every person with an injury or sudden illness?

No. Perform a primary assessment for every person and acquire as much of each person's SAMPLE history as you can. Performing a complete head-to-toe physical exam is crucial for the person with an altered mental status or significant MOI. However, for the alert person with an illness or nonsignificant injury, the physical exam focuses primarily on the body system of the person's chief complaint.

TABLE 4-3 Significant Causes of Injury

- Falls of more than 15 ft (4.6 m) for adults, more than 10 ft (3 m) for children, or more than three times the person's height
- Falls headfirst from the person's height or greater distance
- Vehicle collisions involving ejection, a rollover, high speed, a pedestrian, a motorcycle, or a bicycle
- Head trauma with altered mental status
- Penetrations of the head, chest, or abdomen (eg, stab or gunshot wounds)
- Major burn injury
- Vehicle collisions involving death of an occupant in the same vehicle
- Pedestrian hit by a vehicle

A physical exam assesses the person's entire body from head to toe; you will note the person's signs and symptoms:

- **Signs** refer to your observations of the person's conditions—what you can see.
- **Symptoms** refer to things the person feels and is able to describe. The primary symptom is known as the chief complaint.

To check a part of the body, look for and ask about the following signs and symptoms of injury: deformities, open wounds, tenderness, and swelling. The mnemonic **DOTS** is helpful for remembering the signs and symptoms of an injury **FIGURE 4-3**:

D = *Deformity.* The shape of the body part is abnormal. Compare the body part to the opposite uninjured part, if applicable. Deformities occur when bones are broken or joints are dislocated.

O = *Open wounds.* The skin is broken and bleeding is present.

T = *Tenderness.* The person reports sensitivity, discomfort, or pain. Be sure to press or have the person press on an area to check for tenderness.

S = *Swelling.* The area looks larger than usual. Swelling is caused by excess fluid in the tissue.

Q&A

When might an assessment be unreliable?

Use caution when assessing any person who has an altered mental status or a painful injury that could distract from other injuries or illness (eg, femur fracture), or who has ingested alcohol or drugs.

Person With a Significant Cause of Injury

For a person with a significant cause or mechanism of injury, perform a head-to-toe physical exam. The person may be responsive or unresponsive. Assume that an unresponsive person, with an MOI, has a spinal injury and protect the head and neck against movement. When a man examines a woman, it is wise, if possible, to have another woman present.

Person With No Significant Cause of Injury

When a person has no significant cause of injury, a head-to-toe physical exam may not be needed. Instead, focus the assessment on the chief complaint (the cut right finger as opposed to the rest of the body). For most first aid providers, this will be the more frequently performed type of assessment.

Checking a Person

Before helping, take the appropriate actions described on pages 12–13. Persons needing first aid may fit into one of two types: an injury or a sudden illness. If while following the plan, you find a life-threatening condition, stop and treat it before continuing on with the assessment.

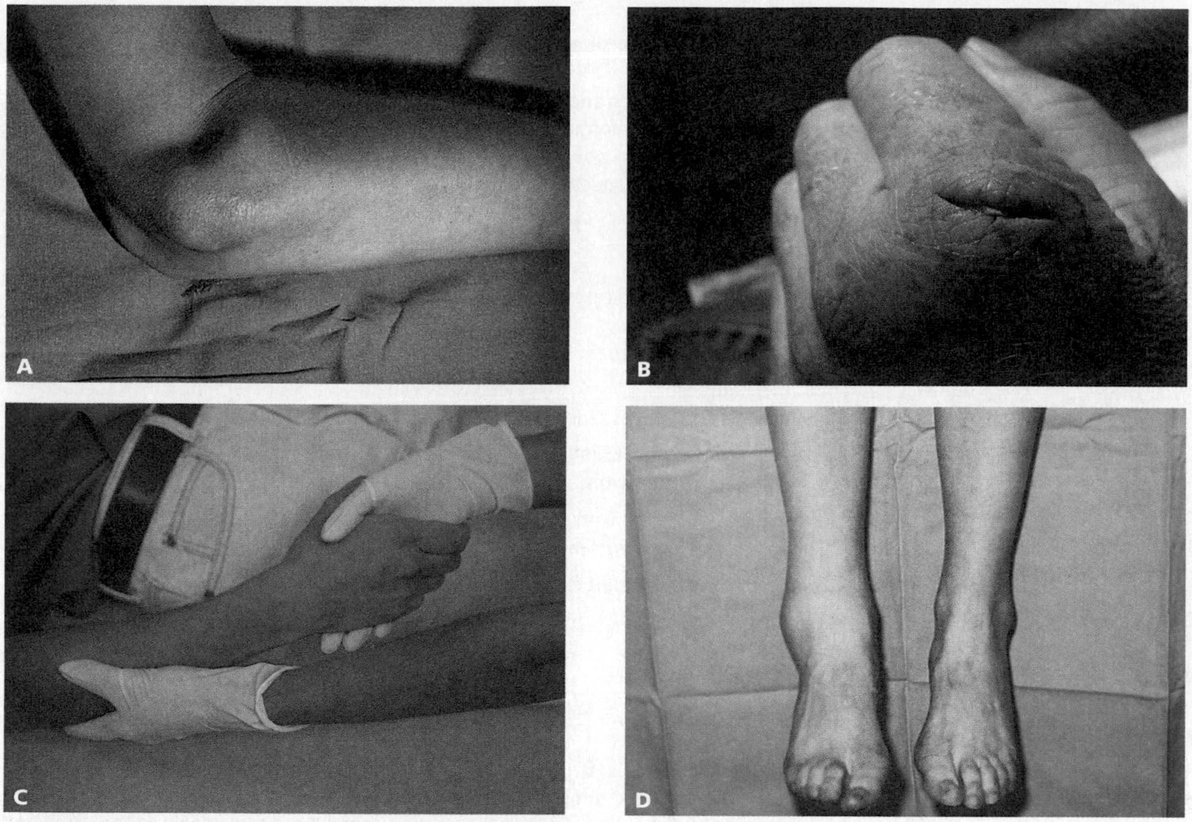

FIGURE 4-3 Examine an area by looking for and asking about DOTS: D = deformity (**A**), O = open wounds (**B**), T = tenderness (**C**), and S = swelling (**D**).

If the person is . . .	Then . . .
Motionless	**1.** Tap the person on the shoulder and shout, "Are you OK?" **2.** If the person does not respond, shout for help. ▪ If someone arrives to help, have them call 9-1-1 and retrieve a first aid kit and AED. ▪ If no one arrives to help and you have a mobile phone, put the phone on speaker and call 9-1-1. Follow the dispatcher's instructions. Retrieve the first aid kit and AED yourself. ▪ If no one arrives to help and you do not have a mobile phone, find a phone and call 9-1-1. **3.** For an unresponsive person, check for breathing ▪ If the person is breathing normally, place the person onto their side into the recovery position (see page 49), call 9-1-1, and stay with the person until EMS arrives. ▪ If the person is not breathing normally or is only gasping, call or have someone call 9-1-1. Begin CPR and use an AED see Chapter 5, *CPR*, and Chapter 6, *Automated External Defibrillation*. **4.** Scan the body looking for external bleeding. If found, control it immediately. Look for a medical identification tag.
Alert and awake First aid providers are more likely to see this type of injured or suddenly ill person.	**1.** Introduce yourself. Ask for the person's name and use it when speaking to them. Tell them that you are first aid trained. Obtain their consent to give care by asking if you can help them. Ask the person, where they are now and for the day or date. Their answers can reflect their mental status. **2.** Make a quick check for any breathing difficulty. **3.** Scan the body looking for external bleeding. If found, control it immediately (see page 48). **4.** If any life-threatening conditions are found or suspected, treat them. ▪ If someone arrives to help, have them call 9-1-1 and retrieve a first aid kit. ▪ If no one arrives for help and you have a mobile phone, after treating life-threatening conditions, call 9-1-1 and put the phone on speaker. Follow the dispatcher's instructions. ▪ If no one arrives to help and you do not have a mobile phone, find a phone and call 9-1-1. **5.** Look for or ask about a medical identification tag. Such tags show if the person has a serious medical condition.

Continues

Continued

If the person is . . .	Then . . .
Interview the alert person	**1.** Gather history information and the chief complaint using the mnemonic SAMPLE, which helps you remember what to ask. Information from a SAMPLE history may help identify what is wrong. The person can usually answer your SAMPLE questions, but if unable, the information may be obtained from family, friends, bystanders, or a medical identification tag. **S** = **S**ymptoms? **A** = **A**llergies? **M** = **M**edications? **P** = **P**ertinent past medical problems? **L** = **L**ast food or drink? **E** = **E**vents leading up to the condition the injury or illness? **2.** For a chief complaint involving an illness, you probably cannot determine the exact cause of the condition. Instead, decide if it is serious enough to require professional medical care. **3.** Be sure to give the SAMPLE information to the EMS personnel when they arrive. What you find may help determine what is wrong and what professional medical care the person needs.
Perform physical exam: Check the person from head to toe	**1.** Most people require only a physical exam of a specific body system (related to the chief complaint); a full body physical exam is usually not needed. **2.** Any life-threating conditions found should be immediately treated before continuing. **3.** Check a body area by *looking for* and *asking about* DOTS: **D** = **D**eformity **O** = **O**pen wounds **T** = **T**enderness **S** = **S**welling **4.** Before starting the check, tell the person what you are going to do and obtain their consent. Start at the head and examine each body area by *looking for* and *asking about* DOTS. Check the body areas in the following sequence—starting at the head and checking the arms and hands last: ▪ Head and neck ▪ Shoulders ▪ Chest and abdomen ▪ Hips ▪ Legs and feet ▪ Arms and hands

FYI

Verbal First Aid: What to Say to a Person With an Injury or Illness

Use these guidelines for gaining rapport and calming an alert and responsive person with an injury or illness:

- Avoid negative statements that could add to a person's distress and anxiety.
- Your first words to a person are very important because they set the tone of your interaction.
- Do not ask unnecessary questions unless it aids treatment or satisfies the person's need to talk.
- Tears and/or laughter can be normal. Let the person know this if such responses seem to make them feel embarrassed.
- Stress the positive. For example, instead of saying, "You will not have any pain," say, "You are doing great."
- Do not deny the obvious. For example, instead of saying, "There is nothing wrong," say, "You have had quite a fall and probably do not feel too well, but we are going to look at you."
- Use the person's name while providing first aid.

Reassessment

The primary assessment, SAMPLE history, and secondary assessment or physical exam are done quickly so that injuries and illnesses can be identified and given first aid. After the most serious conditions have been cared for, regularly recheck the person who has a serious injury or illness such as breathing difficulties or major blood loss, or who has experienced a significant cause of injury. When in doubt, keep checking the person as frequently as possible. Simply remaining calm and reassuring the person that help is on the way may be the best treatment you can provide for the person.

Q&A

Can I make a diagnosis as to what is wrong?

No. Diagnosing a medical condition is best left to a physician. A layperson diagnosing a medical condition could be accused of practicing medicine without a license, which has legal consequences. However, a first aid provider can suspect what may be wrong based on the signs and symptoms found. Additionally, EMS providers can obtain a differential diagnosis—a short list of potential problems the patient may be experiencing. But an official diagnosis should wait until after the person has been assessed in a hospital.

Reassessment may not be necessary since EMS may arrive quickly. The first aid provider should be prepared to report to EMS personnel what was found and what was done.

Special Considerations

Exposing the Injury

You might have to remove items of clothing from the person to check for an injury and to give proper first aid. If you need to remove clothing, explain what you intend to do (and why) to the person and any family members or bystanders. Ask for the person's consent before removing any clothing. Once it is received, remove only as much clothing as necessary. Be sure to try to maintain privacy and prevent exposure to cold. Cover the person back up with a warm blanket if possible. Damage clothing only if necessary, and do so by cutting along the seams **FIGURE 4-4**.

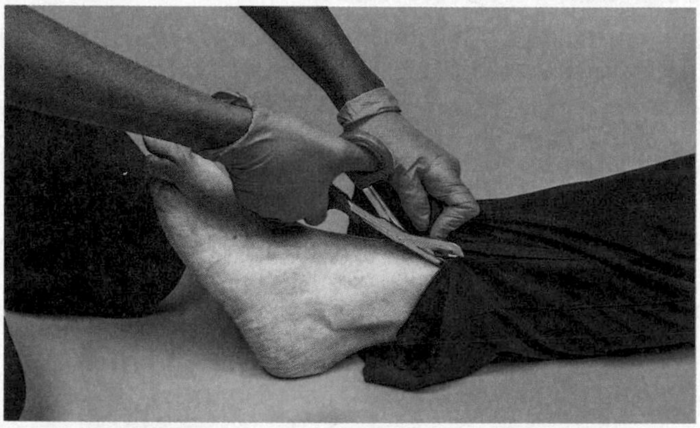

FIGURE 4-4 Expose the injury. Remove as much clothing from the person as necessary, while trying to maintain privacy.

Avoiding Contact During a Physical Exam

First aid providers will find it difficult to avoid close contact with an injured or sick person. However, during a physical exam, first aid providers should avoid, whenever possible, touching or feeling a person they are helping. Not touching or feeling another person during a physical exam represents a major change and is the result of two situations:

- The COVID-19 pandemic highlights the importance of maintaining a physical distance of 6 feet (about two arm lengths). New and reemerging diseases with the potential to be life threatening should be expected. Refer to page 22 for the COVID-19 infection risk to first aid providers from persons in cardiac arrest.
- Actual or potential physical or sexual abuse or molestation accusations during a physical exam increase when touching and feeling is taught and practiced.

To avoid touching or feeling a person, the physical exam uses these instructions: *Look for and ask about DOTS.* Three of these four conditions can be accomplished by looking, while the other, tenderness, involves asking about and/or having the person you're helping press or feel a body area for pain or tenderness if they are able to. During a physical exam's head-to-toe check, the first aid provider checks one part of the body at a time by looking for and asking about DOTS.

Of course, exceptions for not touching or feeling exist. While this may not be a complete list, the following offers examples of potential exceptions, with several involving minimal touching or feeling:

- Checking for responsiveness by tapping the shoulder of a motionless person
- Placing a person onto their side in the recovery position
- Applying direct pressure to stop bleeding
- Placing a person in a faceup position for CPR
- Using the head tilt–chin lift maneuver to open the airway when giving rescue breaths
- Appling chest compressions during CPR
- Attaching AED pads on a unresponsive, nonbreathing person
- Checking for a spinal injury
- Rescuing and/or moving a person
- Giving back blows and abdominal thrusts

Optional Assessments

First aid providers are not expected to take vital signs (eg, heart rate, breathing rate, blood pressure, etc). Some first aid classes may teach otherwise but are usually reserved for emergency medical responders, emergency medical technicians, and health care professionals. The following sections describe optional assessments that may be considered.

Heart Rate

The heart rate (also known as the pulse rate) is the number of heartbeats per minute. The normal rate for an adult at rest is between 60 and 100 beats per minute. An exception is an athlete in good health, with a normal resting heart rate between 40 and 50 beats per minute. Be concerned about the adult whose heart rate stays above 100 or below 60 beats per minute. If the heart rate is taken several times and it continues above 120 beats or below 50 beats per minute, something may be seriously wrong that requires professional medical care. Measure the heart rate by placing the flat part of the ends of your index and middle fingers 2 inches above the base of the thumb on the inside of the wrist (known as the radial pulse site). **DO NOT** use your thumb, because you might feel your own pulse. Count the beats for 30 seconds, then multiply by two to get the heart rate in beats per minute. A heartbeat felt at the wrist (radial pulse) indicates that enough blood pressure exists to saturate all the body tissues with oxygenated blood.

Breathing Rate

One breath consists of one inhalation and one exhalation. The breathing rate (also known as the respiration rate) is the number of breaths taken in 1 minute. The normal breathing rate of an adult at rest is 12 to 20 breaths per minute. A rate less than 8 or greater than 24 is abnormal and may indicate a problem requiring supplemental oxygen.

Count the breathing rate by watching the person's chest rise and fall for 30 seconds, counting each time the person inhales and then multiplying this number by two. Some persons may deliberately change their breathing rate if they know you are counting them. Try to count the breathing without the person's knowledge by pretending to be taking the heart rate. Abnormal sounds can indicate a medical problem.

Skin Condition

A quick check of the person's skin can also provide information about the person's condition. When assessing the head, check skin temperature, color, and moisture. Skin color, especially in light-skinned people, reflects the circulation under the skin as well as oxygen status. For those with dark complexions, changes might not be readily apparent but can be assessed by the appearance of the nail beds, the inside of the mouth, and the inner eyelids.

Check the Eyes

Compare the pupils, the black center of the eye. Pupils should be the same size and react to light **FIGURE 4-5**. Use a flashlight to determine whether the pupils are reactive. If a flashlight is not present, cover one of the person's eyes with your hand and observe the pupil's reaction when the eye is uncovered. Normally, the pupil constricts (gets smaller) within 1 second. No pupil reaction to light could mean death, coma, cataracts (in older people), or an artificial eye. Pupil dilation happens within 30 to 60 seconds of cardiac arrest. Look for unequal pupils. A difference in the size of the two pupils is almost always a sign of a medical emergency, such as a stroke or a brain injury. However, the unequal condition occurs normally in 2% to 4% of the population. Also, an artificial eye may give the appearance of unequal pupils.

You can get a rough idea of skin temperature by putting the back of your hand or wrist on the person's forehead to determine whether the temperature is elevated or decreased. Dry skin is normal. Skin that is wet, moist, or excessively dry and hot suggests a medical condition.

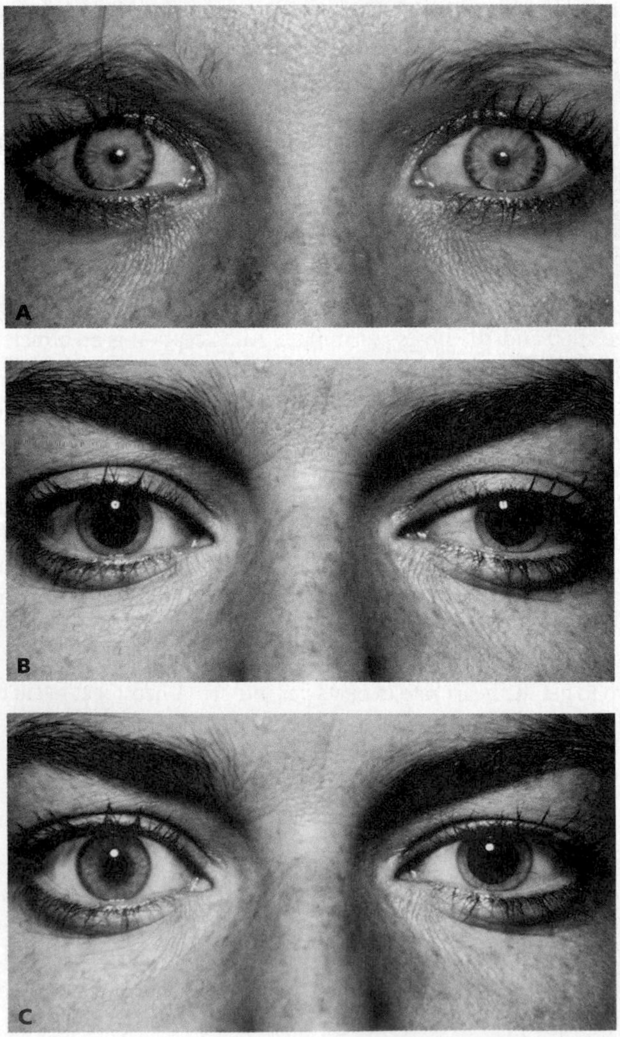

FIGURE 4-5 A. Constricted pupils. **B**. Dilated pupils. **C**. Unequal pupils.

A, B, C: © American Academy of Orthopaedic Surgeons.

Capillary Refill Test

Some first aid providers use the capillary refill technique to check adequacy of blood circulation in an extremity. To perform the technique, gently press a fingernail or toenail for a few seconds and then release the pressure **FIGURE 4-6**. When released, the blanched skin should return to its normal color within 2 seconds. A refill time of greater than 2 seconds indicates poor circulation, which requires professional medical care.

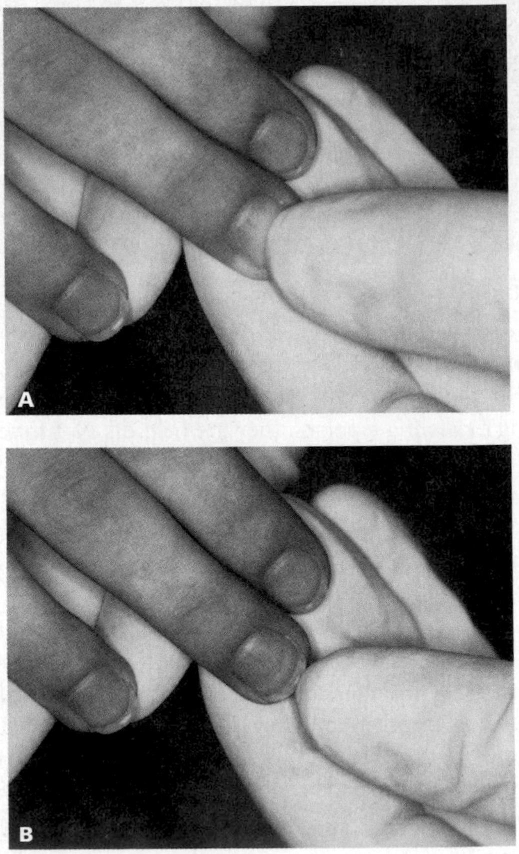

FIGURE 4-6 A. To test capillary refill, gently compress the fingertip until it blanches. **B**. Release the fingertip and count until it returns to its normal pink color.

A, B: © American Academy of Orthopaedic Surgeons.

PREP KIT

Ready for Review

- Assessment is a sequence of actions that helps determine what is wrong, and thus ensures safe and appropriate first aid.
- Every time you encounter a person, first perform a scene size-up.
- Assessment will be influenced by whether the person is suffering from an illness or an injury, whether the person is responsive or unresponsive, and whether life-threatening conditions are present.
- The primary assessment determines whether there are life-threatening conditions requiring quick care.
- The information in a SAMPLE history can help you identify what is wrong with the person and can indicate the needed first aid.
- Look for medical identification tags on the person.
- The goal of a secondary assessment is to identify any potentially life-threatening illness or injury, as well as get a history and perform the appropriate physical exam and obtain vital signs.
- A reassessment is performed to regularly check a person who has experienced a severe injury or illness for further problems.

Vital Vocabulary

cause of injury The force that causes an injury; sometimes called mechanism of injury or MOI.

chief complaint The primary symptom a person complains about; also, the person's response to questions such as "What is wrong?" or "What happened?"; the reason EMS or professional medical care was called for in the patient's own words when possible.

DOTS A mnemonic for assessment in which each area of the body is evaluated for deformities, open wounds, tenderness, and swelling.

general impression The part of the assessment that helps identify any immediately or potentially life-threatening conditions.

nature of illness (NOI) The general type of illness a person is experiencing.

physical exam A part of the secondary assessment process in which a detailed exam is performed, based on the body system of the chief complaint, on people whose conditions cannot be readily identified or when more specific information is needed about a condition.

primary assessment When a first aid provider checks for life-threatening injuries and gives care for any that are found.

SAMPLE history A brief history of a person's condition to determine signs and symptoms, allergies, medications, pertinent past medical history, last oral intake, and events leading to the illness/injury.

scene size-up A quick assessment of the scene and the surroundings for safety issues, the mechanism of injury or nature of illness, and the number of people; completed before starting first aid.

sign Evidence of an injury or disease that can be seen, heard, or felt; objective findings.

symptom What a person tells a first aid provider about what they feel; subjective findings.

Assessment in Action

You are in a crowded mall doing some last-minute holiday shopping. You hear someone yell for help at a nearby store. You are the first to arrive on the scene. Bystanders begin to approach and ask what is going on. The person who called for help witnessed a man collapse.

Directions: Circle Yes if you agree with the statement; circle No if you disagree.

1. The first thing you should do is conduct a physical exam.

   YES NO

2. Your primary assessment of the man includes identifying and treating immediate life-threatening conditions such as issues with his breathing and severe bleeding.

   YES NO

3. The man is responsive and alert. Ask permission from him before beginning first aid.

   YES NO

4. The man asks you to stay until medical help arrives. You should continue to do regular checks of him until medical help arrives.

   YES NO

PREP KIT continued

Check Your Knowledge

Directions: Circle Yes if you agree with the statement; circle No if you disagree.

1. The purpose of a primary assessment is to find life-threatening conditions.

   YES **NO**

2. Most injured people require a complete physical exam.

   YES **NO**

3. For a physical exam, you usually begin at the head and work down the body.

   YES **NO**

4. The mnemonic DOTS helps in remembering what information to obtain about the person's history that could be useful.

   YES **NO**

5. For all injured and suddenly ill people, look for a medical identification tag during a physical exam.

   YES **NO**

6. The mnemonic SAMPLE can remind you how to examine an area for signs of an injury.

   YES **NO**

7. A gurgling sound heard while checking for breathing indicates possible fluid in the throat.

   YES **NO**

8. The letter M in the mnemonic SAMPLE represents a person's movement.

   YES **NO**

9. The letter S in the mnemonic DOTS represents splinting.

   YES **NO**

10. Medical identification tags are available only as necklaces.

    YES **NO**

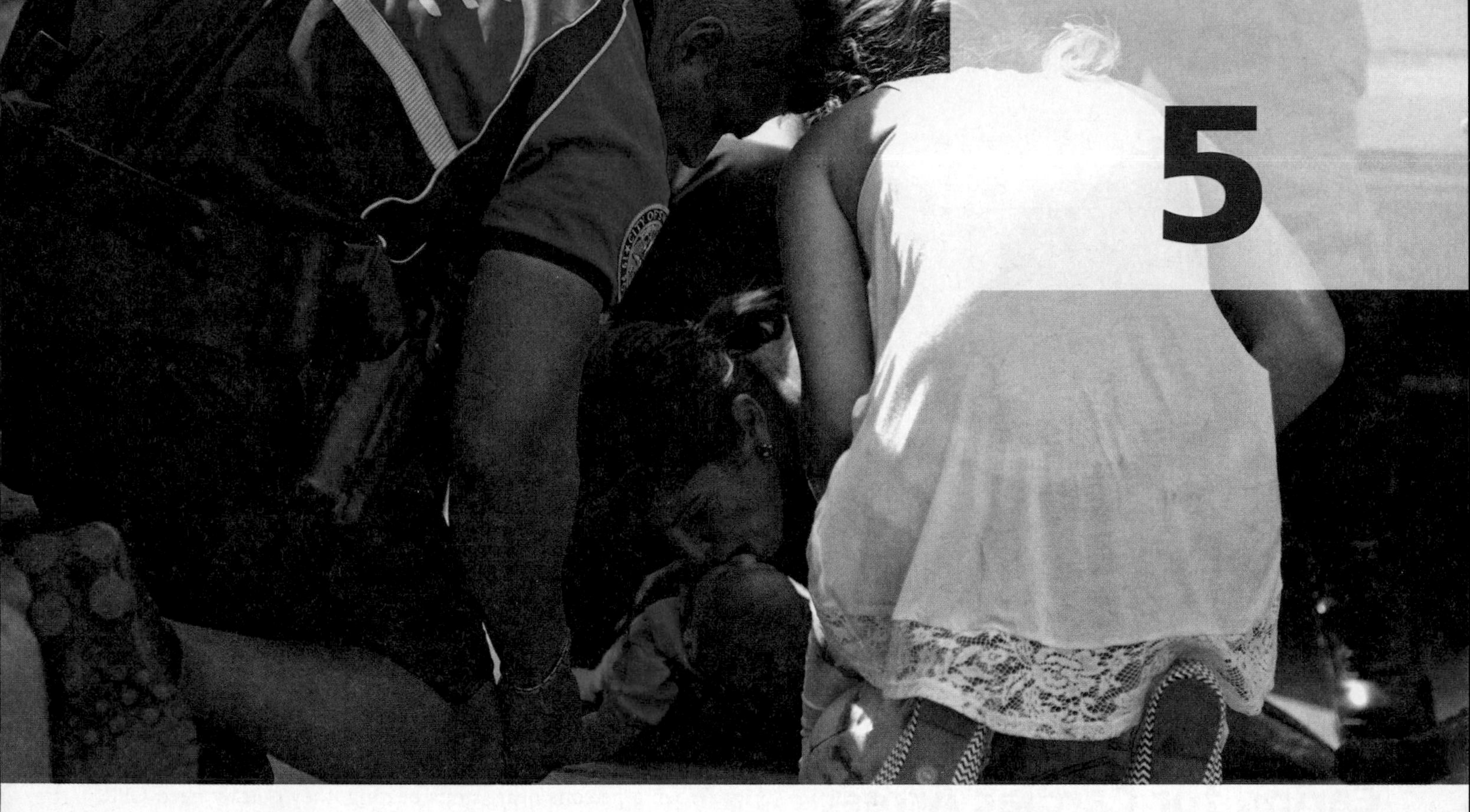

5

CPR

CHAPTER AT A GLANCE

What Is a Cardiac Arrest?

The meaning of these two terms—*heart attack* and *cardiac arrest*—confuses many people.

A **heart attack** occurs when the blood supply to the heart muscle is suddenly reduced or blocked. If the blocked artery is not reopened quickly, the affected part of the heart muscle begins to die. The longer a person goes without treatment, the greater the damage, and this can result in a **cardiac arrest**, where the heart stops beating due to severe damage. The first aid for a heart attack is found in Chapter 17, *Sudden Illness*.

In the absence of adequate oxygen to the heart muscle tissue, the muscle becomes irritable and can produce life-threatening irregular "beats," which can lead to ventricular fibrillation (VF) or ventricular tachycardia (VT), both producing a sudden cardiac arrest (SCA). The focus of the care of these patients involves strengthening the links in the out-of-hospital chain of survival (discussed later). This chapter focuses on the skills of cardiopulmonary resuscitation (CPR).

CPR is the set of skills necessary to help a person in cardiac arrest until EMS arrives to take over. Some people worry about hurting the person (eg, breaking ribs), which is very unlikely. Any harm done is less of a problem than having a nonfunctioning heart.

CPR for a child is almost identical to that given for an adult, with a few differences. See page 62, *Differences Between Adult and Child CPR*.

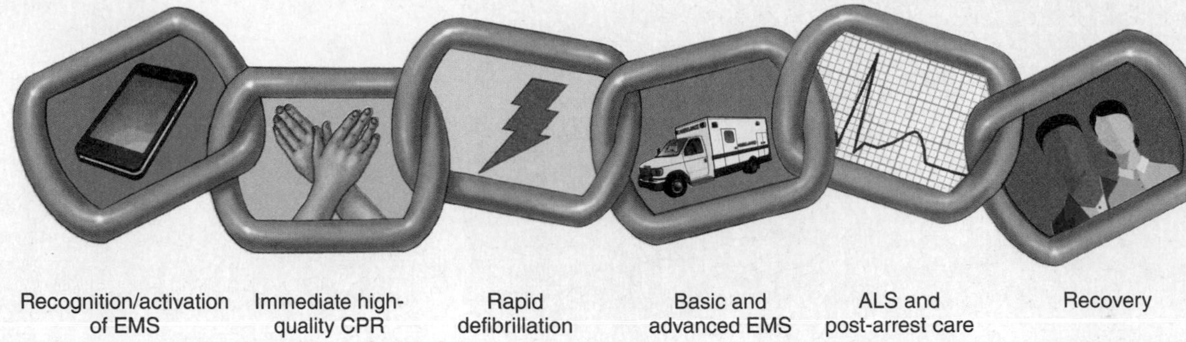

FIGURE 5-1 Out-of-hospital chain of survival.

For a life-threatening condition such as cardiac arrest, doing something is better than doing nothing! Another reason for performing CPR may be for your, the first aid provider's, benefit. Even if unsuccessful, you will know that you tried saving a person's life.

Caring for Cardiac Arrest

Few people experiencing SCA outside of a hospital survive unless a rapid sequence of events takes place. One way of describing the ideal sequence of care that should take place when a cardiac arrest occurs is to compare it to the links in a chain. Each link is dependent on the others for strength and success. In this way, the links form a **chain of survival**.

The six events (links) that must occur rapidly and in an integrated manner during cardiac arrest outside of a hospital are as follows **FIGURE 5-1**:

1. *Recognition and action.* First aid providers must recognize the early warning signs of cardiac arrest and immediately call 9-1-1 to activate emergency medical services (EMS).
2. *CPR.* The chest compressions delivered during **cardiopulmonary resuscitation (CPR)** circulate blood to the heart and brain. Effective chest compressions are critical to buying time until a defibrillator and EMS personnel are available.
3. *Defibrillation.* Administering a shock to the heart can restore the heartbeat in some people. Time is a critical factor. The earlier the shock, the better the chance of success. Automated external defibrillators (AEDs) are found in many government buildings, health clubs, airports, and sports complexes.
4. *Advanced care.* Paramedics provide advanced cardiac life support to people experiencing SCA. This support includes providing intravenous fluids, medications, advanced airway devices, and rapid transport to the hospital.
5. *Post-arrest care.* A specialty cardiac hospital can provide life-saving medications, surgical procedures, and advanced professional medical care to enable the person who experienced SCA to survive and recover.
6. *Recovery.* Identifies the system of care to support recovery and plan treatment and rehabilitation for cardiac arrest survivors as they transition from the hospital to home and return to their daily activities.

Adult and Child CPR

When a person's heart stops beating, they quickly need CPR, defibrillation, and the help of EMS professionals. CPR consists of moving blood to the heart and brain by giving **chest compressions** and providing periodic breaths (ventilations) to place oxygen into the person's lungs. CPR techniques are similar for infants (birth to 1 year), children (1 year to puberty), and adults (puberty and older), with just slight variations.

Use the RAB-CAB mnemonic to remember the sequence of performing CPR. RAB-CAB stands for:

R = Responsive?
A = Activate EMS and get an AED
B = Breathing?
C = Chest Compressions
A = Airway open
B = Breaths

Q&A

For CPR purposes, what defines a person as an adult, child, or infant?

- Infants are less than 1 year of age.
- A child's age ranges from 1 year to puberty. (Puberty can be recognized by hair in the armpits of boys and breast development in girls.)
- Adults include those at puberty and older.

R = Responsive?

In a motionless person, check for responsiveness by tapping the person's shoulder and asking if they are okay. If the person does not respond (ie, does not answer, move, or moan), they are said to be unresponsive.

Tap the person's shoulder and shout, "Are you okay?" to decide if the person is responsive or unresponsive.

If...	Then...
The person is responsive (eg, speaks, moves).	▪ Ask if you can help them. ▪ If they agree, use the SAMPLE mnemonic (symptoms, allergies, medications, pertinent past medical history, last oral intake, events leading up to the injury or illness) to obtain relevant medical information. See page 49. ▪ If they appear to have been injured, look for and ask about DOTS (deformities, open wounds, tenderness, swelling). See page 50. ▪ Provide care for what is found and, if necessary, call 9-1-1.
The person is unresponsive (eg, does not answer, move, or moan).	▪ Continue to the next step, A = Activate.

A = Activate EMS and Obtain an AED

After you check for responsiveness, shout for nearby help. Activate the EMS system by calling or asking a bystander to call 9-1-1. Using a mobile phone, you can call EMS without leaving the person's side. If a mobile phone is used, it should be kept by the person's side, if possible. Use the mobile phone's speaker mode so the dispatcher can monitor your performance. If a mobile phone is not available, leave the person to call 9-1-1 and get an AED. If you are alone with a child or infant, give CPR for five sets of 30 compressions and 2 breaths (2 minutes); then call 9-1-1. Shout for help.

If...	Then...
Someone is coming to help or is nearby.	▪ Have them activate EMS by calling 9-1-1 and obtain an AED while you continue to provide care. ▪ If a mobile phone is used, put it on speaker mode and place it at the person's side to hear the dispatcher's directions.
You are alone and the person is an adult.	▪ Call 9-1-1 and obtain an AED. ▪ After making the call, continue providing care. ▪ If a phone is not available, leave the person to call 9-1-1 and get an AED. After making the call, return and continue providing care.
The person is a child (between age 1 and puberty).	▪ If you are alone, give five sets (about 2 minutes) of 30 chest compressions and 2 breaths before calling 9-1-1.

B = Breathing?

Check breathing for 5 to 10 seconds by looking for the rise and fall of the person's chest from neck to waist. No breathing and occasional gasps (may sound like a groan or snore) indicate that a person needs CPR.

Observe the person from neck to waist for movement (rise an fall); take 5 to 10 seconds.

If...	Then...
The person is breathing normally.	▪ Place the person on their side in the recovery position to keep the airway open. If you suspect a neck or back injury, **DO NOT** move the person. ▪ Stay with the person and monitor their breathing until EMS arrives.
The person is not breathing or is only gasping (may sound like a quick inhalation or like a groan or snore).	▪ Place the person faceup on a flat, firm surface. ▪ Continue to the next step, C = Chest Compressions.

C = Chest Compressions

Place the person faceup on a firm, flat surface. Expose the chest by removing clothing. This will enable you to locate the correct hand position for chest compressions and apply an AED when it arrives on the scene. Give chest compressions as follows:

1. Move enough clothing to locate the correct hand position for compressions and apply an AED when it arrives on the scene.
2. For an adult, place the heel of one hand on the center of the person's chest and on the lower half of their breastbone (sternum).
3. Place your other hand on top of the first one with your fingers interlocked. Hold your fingers off the person's chest and point them directly away from you. **DO NOT** cross your hands **FIGURE 5-2**. For a child, use one hand; however, depending upon the child's size and your size, using two hands may be necessary.
4. Keep your arms straight and elbows locked, with your shoulders positioned directly over your hands.
5. Push hard: straight down on the sternum, at least 2 inches (5 cm) to 2.4 inches (6 cm) for an adult, or about 2 inches (5 cm) or one-third depth of the chest

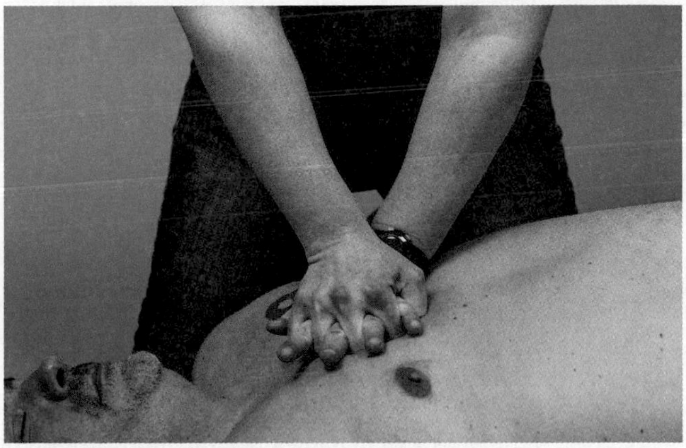

FIGURE 5-2 The hand position for chest compressions is in the center of the chest.

for a child. Use your upper body's weight to compress the chest. **DO NOT** rock back and forth.

6. Push fast: Give 30 compressions at a rate of 100 to 120 compressions per minute. Follow the beats of the Bee Gees' song "Stayin' Alive," the beats from a smartphone app that was previously installed and is quickly accessible, or a dispatcher's directions heard over a mobile phone speaker.
7. Push smoothly: **DO NOT** bounce or jab, and **DO NOT** stop at the top or bottom of a compression.
8. Allow the chest to fully recoil after each compression. **DO NOT** lean on the chest.

A = Airway Open

Before giving breaths during CPR, open the airway using the head tilt–chin lift maneuver. **DO NOT** use this maneuver if you suspect a neck or back injury.

To perform the **head tilt–chin lift maneuver**, follow these steps:

1. Place one hand on the person's forehead and the fingertips of the other hand on the bony part of the chin nearest you.
2. While applying firm backward pressure with your hand, lift the chin upward with the other hand to help tilt the person's head back.

FYI

Oxygen Use in First Aid

Supplemental oxygen is useful for various medical conditions; however, its use is not considered a first aid skill and requires special training. If using supplemental oxygen, be sure to keep any possible source of fire (eg, glowing cigarette, spark) away from the area.

B = Breaths

Breathing for a person who is not breathing is known as rescue breathing. Keep the person's airway open using the head tilt–chin lift maneuver **FIGURE 5-3**.

To perform rescue breaths, follow these steps:

1. Pinch the person's nose shut and make a tight seal with your mouth on the mouth-to-barrier device or the person's mouth. When possible, use a mouth-to-barrier device to prevent potential disease transmission. If unwilling or unable to give breaths (ie, seriously injured mouth, ineffective seal, mouth cannot be opened), give compression-only CPR (see pages 66–67).
2. Give 2 breaths, each lasting 1 second (take a normal breath for yourself after each breath). **DO NOT** blow too forcefully or for too long.
3. Watch for chest rise to determine if your breaths go in.
4. Allow for chest deflation after each breath.
5. Follow the actions in the table that follows.

If . . .	Then . . .
The first breath does not cause the chest to rise.	Retilt the person's head and give a second breath.
After retilting the head, the second breath does not make the chest rise.	▪ An object may be blocking the person's airway. ▪ Give CPR with one change: after each set of compressions and before giving breaths, open the mouth, look for an object, and if seen, remove it. **DO NOT** use blind finger sweeps in those with a foreign body airway obstruction.
You see the chest rise after the 2 breaths.	Give sets of 30 chests compressions followed by 2 breaths.
You cannot use the person's mouth (eg, seriously injured mouth, ineffective seal, mouth cannot be opened, person is in water).	▪ Use the head tilt–chin lift maneuver. ▪ Seal your mouth around the person's nose and breathe. Use a barrier device when possible. ▪ Alternately, use compression-only CPR.
The person vomits or there is fluid in the mouth.	Roll the person onto their side and clear the mouth using a gloved finger or piece of gauze. Then, roll the person onto their back and continue care.

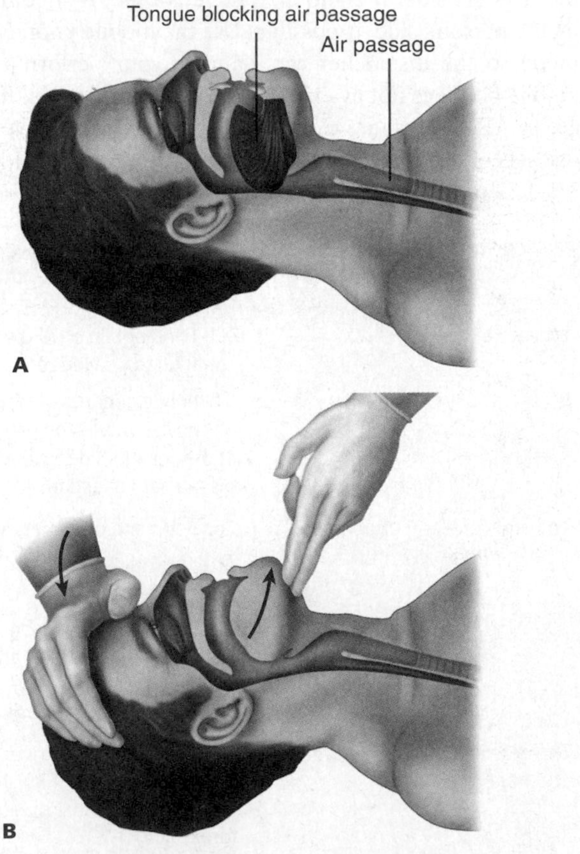

FIGURE 5-3 **A**. Relaxation of the tongue back into the throat causes airway obstruction. **B**. To perform the head tilt–chin lift maneuver, place one hand on the person's forehead and apply firm backward pressure with your palm to tilt the head back. Next, place the tips of the index and middle fingers of your other hand under the lower jaw near the bony part of the chin. Lift the chin upward, bringing the entire lower jaw with it, helping to tilt the head back.

6. Continue sets of 30 chest compressions and 2 breaths until:
   - An AED arrives and the voice prompts you to stop so it can analyze and shock if necessary.
   - The person begins breathing.
   - Someone of equal or higher training takes over.
   - The scene becomes unsafe. The person should be moved to a nearby safer location before continuing CPR.
   - You are alone and become physically exhausted and unable to continue.
7. If another person is present, they could help by giving chest compressions while you give breaths, or vice versa. If the other person is not trained in CPR, you can coach them on how to perform chest compressions and how to give breaths. Switching places after every five sets (about every 2 minutes) helps avoid fatigue.

The concern about contracting a disease from giving breaths can be remedied by: (1) giving compression-only CPR or (2) having both rescuers using their own mouth-to-barrier device while giving breaths.

Refer to **SKILL SHEET 5-1** and **FLOWCHART 5-1** for the appropriate steps and techniques for adult or child CPR.

Barrier Devices

A barrier device (eg, face mask or shield) is a protective device used during rescue breathing; it features a plastic barrier placed on a person's face to prevent contact with secretions, vomitus, and gases. This device is a safety precaution to prevent possible disease transmission. Provide mouth-to-mouth breathing without a barrier device only when a barrier device is unavailable.

Mouth-to-Mouth Breathing

To perform mouth-to-mouth breathing, follow these steps:

1. Position yourself beside the person's head.
2. Pinch the person's nostrils together with a thumb and index finger.
3. Open the airway with the head tilt–chin lift maneuver. Press on the forehead to maintain a backward tilt of the head.
4. Place your mouth over the person's mouth and gently breathe into the person's mouth for 1 second. The person's chest should rise.
5. Remove your mouth and take a breath for yourself before giving the next breath.

SKILL SHEET 5-1 Adult and Child CPR

Note: Whenever possible, use a mouth-to-barrier device to prevent disease transmission. Use RAB-CAB to remember what to do.

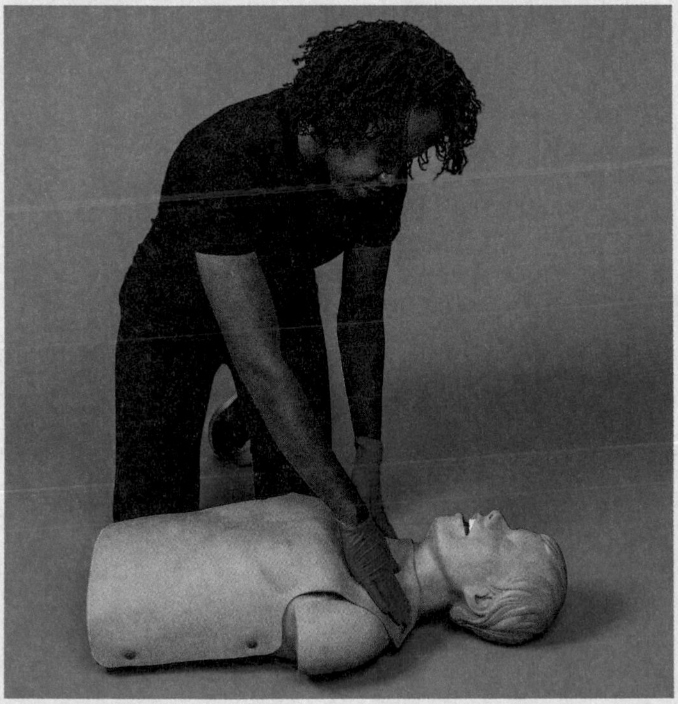

1 R = Responsive?

Tap the person on the shoulder and shout, "Are you okay?"

a. If the person responds, ask SAMPLE history questions and look for and ask about DOTS.

b. If the person does not respond, continue to the next step, *Activate.*

Continues

SKILL SHEET 5-1 Adult and Child CPR (*Continued*)

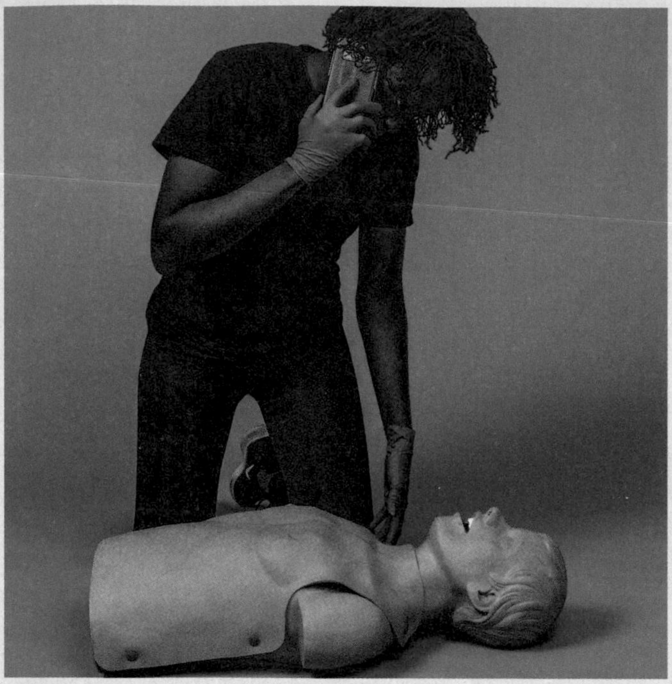

© Aleksandra Gigowska/Shutterstock.

2 A = Activate EMS and get an AED.

a. Shout for nearby help.

b. If someone responds, have them call 9-1-1 and get an AED while you provide care.

c. If no one comes and you are alone with an adult, call 9-1-1. If a phone is not available, leave the person to locate a phone and get an AED.

d. If no one comes and you are alone with a child, give five sets of 30 chest compressions and 2 breaths before calling 9-1-1.

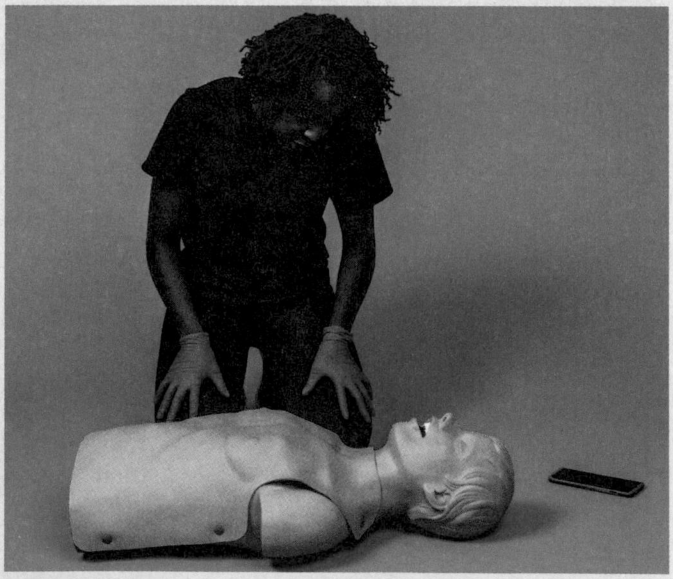

© Jones & Bartlett Learning.

3 B = Breathing?

a. Place the person faceup on a flat, firm surface.

b. Take 5 to 10 seconds to observe the person from the neck to waist for movement (rise and fall).

c. If the person is not breathing or is only gasping, continue to the next step, *Compressions*.

SKILL SHEET 5-1 Adult and Child CPR (*Continued*)

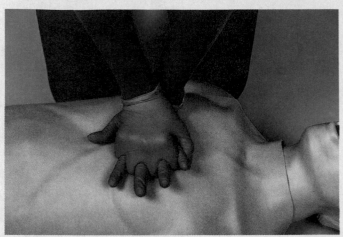

© Jones & Bartlett Learning.

4 **C = Chest compressions.**

Provide chest compressions.

a. Move enough clothing to locate the correct hand position for compressions and where to apply an AED when it arrives on the scene.

b. For an adult:

- Place the heel of one hand on the center of the person's chest and on the lower half of their breastbone (sternum).
- Place your other hand on top of the first one with your fingers interlocked. Hold your fingers off the person's chest and point them directly away from you; **DO NOT** cross your hands.

c. For a child:

- Use one hand; however, depending upon the child's size and your size, using two hands may be necessary.

d. Keep your arms straight and elbows locked, with your shoulders positioned directly over your hands.

e. Push hard and straight down on the breastbone (sternum), at least 2 inches (5 cm) for an adult and about 2 inches (5 cm) or about one-third the depth of the chest for a child. Use your upper body's weight to compress the chest. **DO NOT** rock back and forth.

f. Push fast: 100 to 120 compressions per minute. It may be easier to push to the beat of the Bee Gees' song "Stayin' Alive" or the beat from a CPR smartphone app that was previously installed and is quickly accessible.

g. Push smoothly: **DO NOT** bounce or jab, and **DO NOT** stop at the top or bottom of a compression.

h. Allow the chest to fully recoil after each compression. **DO NOT** lean on the chest.

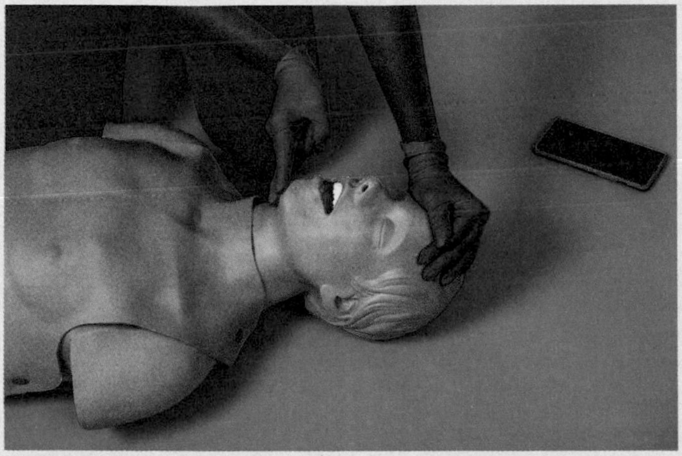

© Jones & Bartlett Learning.

5 **A = Airway open.**

Open the person's airway:

a. Take your hand nearest the person's head and place it on their forehead; apply pressure to tilt the head back.

b. Place two fingers of your other hand under the bony part of the person's jaw (near the chin) and lift. Avoid pressing on soft tissues under the jaw.

c. Tilt the head backward.

Continues

SKILL SHEET 5-1 Adult and Child CPR (*Continued*)

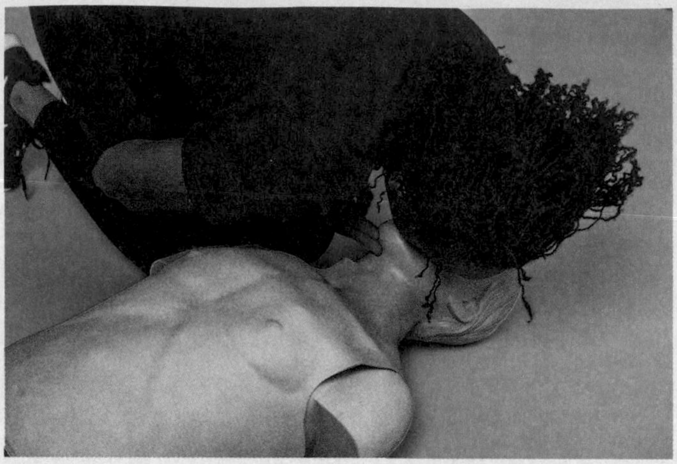

© Jones & Bartlett Learning.

6 **B = Breaths.**

Give two breaths.

a. Pinch the person's nose shut and make a tight seal with your mouth on the mouth-to-barrier device or the person's mouth. If unwilling or unable to give breaths, give compression-only CPR instead.

b. Give 2 breaths, each lasting 1 second. **DO NOT** blow too forcefully or for too long. (Take a normal breath for yourself after each breath.)

c. Watch for chest rise to determine if your breaths go in.

d. Allow for chest deflation after each breath.

e. If you see chest rise after the 2 breaths, give 30 chest compressions.

f. If the first breath does not make the chest rise, retilt the person's head and give a second breath. If the second breath does not make the chest rise, begin CPR (30 compressions and 2 breaths). Each time before giving the first of the two breaths, open the mouth and look for an object; if seen, remove it.

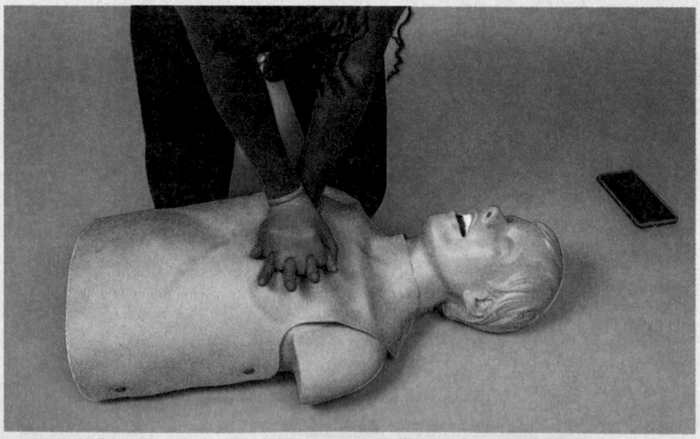

© Jones & Bartlett Learning.

7 Continue sets of 30 chest compressions and 2 breaths until an AED arrives and voice prompts you to stop so it can analyze and shock if necessary. (If a bystander is present, they could help by giving chest compressions while you perform rescue breathing, or vice versa.)

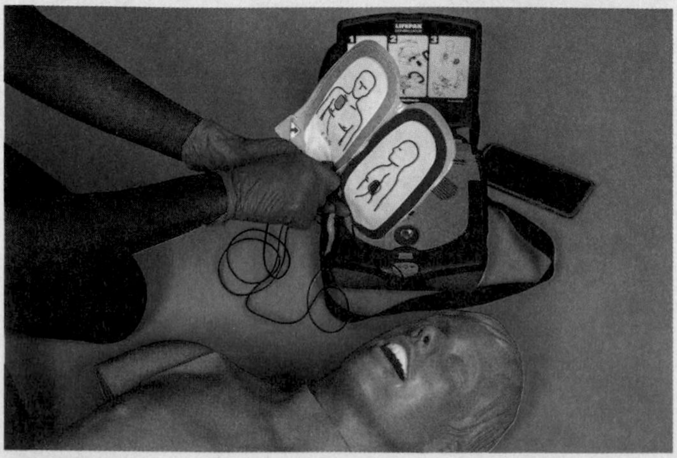

© Jones & Bartlett Learning.

8 When an AED becomes available, use it as soon as possible. (See Chapter 6, *Automated External Defibrillation.*)

Flowchart 5-1 Adult and Child CPR

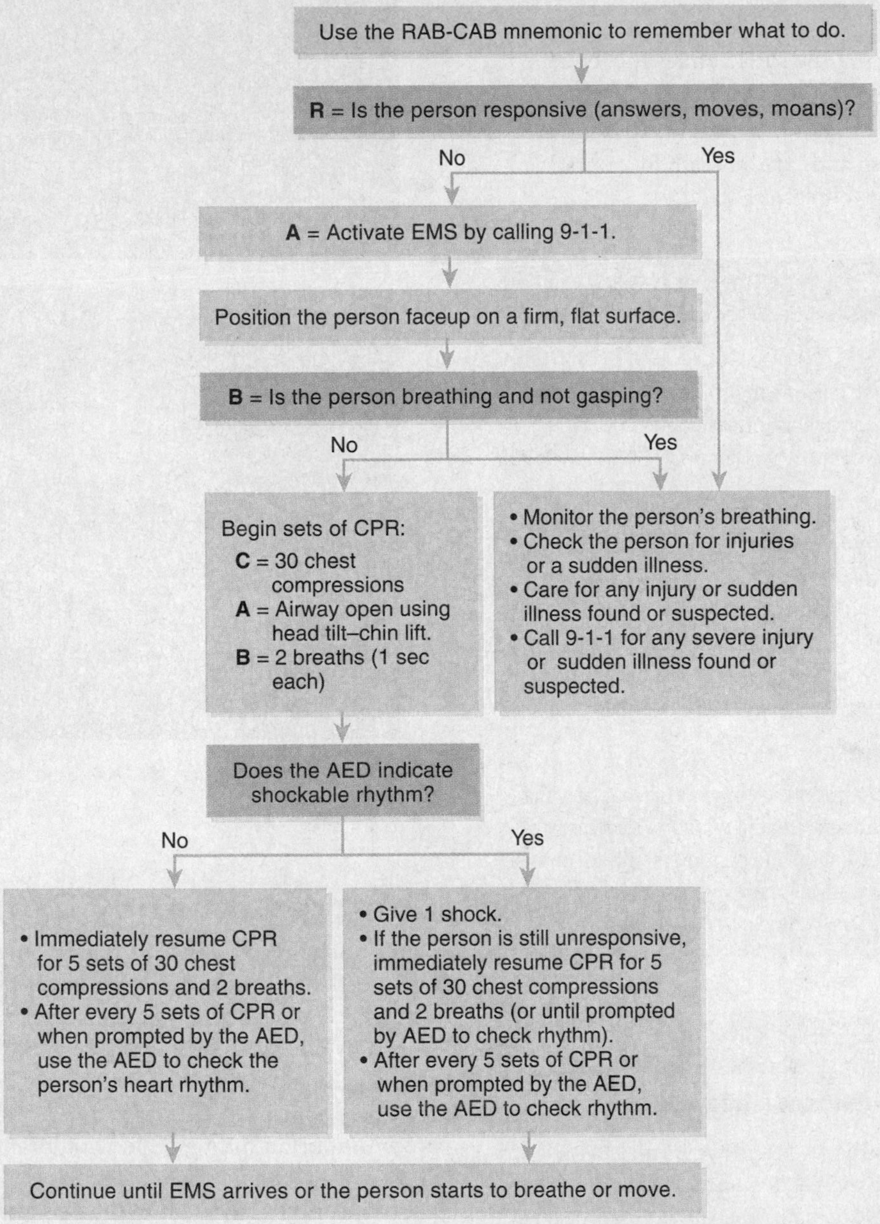
Use the RAB-CAB mnemonic to remember what to do.
R = Is the person responsive (answers, moves, moans)?
No
Yes
A = Activate EMS by calling 9-1-1.
Position the person faceup on a firm, flat surface.
B = Is the person breathing and not gasping?
No
Yes
Begin sets of CPR:
C = 30 chest compressions
A = Airway open using head tilt–chin lift.
B = 2 breaths (1 sec each)
• Monitor the person's breathing.
• Check the person for injuries or a sudden illness.
• Care for any injury or sudden illness found or suspected.
• Call 9-1-1 for any severe injury or sudden illness found or suspected.
Does the AED indicate shockable rhythm?
No
Yes
• Immediately resume CPR for 5 sets of 30 chest compressions and 2 breaths.
• After every 5 sets of CPR or when prompted by the AED, use the AED to check the person's heart rhythm.
• Give 1 shock.
• If the person is still unresponsive, immediately resume CPR for 5 sets of 30 chest compressions and 2 breaths (or until prompted by AED to check rhythm).
• After every 5 sets of CPR or when prompted by the AED, use the AED to check rhythm.
Continue until EMS arrives or the person starts to breathe or move.

Mouth-to-Mask Breathing

To perform mouth-to-mask breathing, follow these steps:

1. Position yourself beside the person's head.
2. Place the mask over the person's mouth and nose. The mask's nose notch should be on the nose and not on the chin.
3. Open the airway with the head tilt–chin lift maneuver. Press on the forehead to maintain a backward tilt of the head.
4. Place your mouth on the mouthpiece and gently breathe into the mouthpiece for 1 second. The person's chest should rise.
5. Remove your mouth and take a breath for yourself before giving the next breath.

Mouth-to-Face Shield Breathing

To perform mouth-to-face shield breathing, follow these steps:

1. Position yourself beside the person's head.
2. Place the shield over the person's mouth.

3. Pinch the person's nostrils together with a thumb and index finger.
4. Open the airway with the head tilt–chin lift maneuver. Press on the forehead to maintain a backward tilt of the head.
5. Place your mouth over the shield and gently breathe into the person's mouth for 1 second. The person's chest should rise.
6. Remove your mouth and take a breath for yourself before giving the next breath.

FYI

Mouth-to-Barrier Device

A barrier device is placed in the person's mouth or over the person's mouth and nose as a precaution against disease transmission. There are several different types of barrier devices **FIGURE 5-4**.

Mouth-to-Nose Method

If you cannot open the person's mouth, the person's mouth is severely injured, or you cannot make a good seal with the person's mouth (eg, because there are no teeth), use the mouth-to-nose method. With the head tilted back, push up on the person's chin to close the mouth. Make a seal with your mouth over the person's nose and provide rescue breaths. Use a barrier device when possible.

Mouth-to-Stoma Method

Some diseases of the vocal cords may result in surgical removal of the larynx. People who have this surgery breathe through a small permanent opening in the neck called a stoma. To perform mouth-to-stoma breathing, close the person's mouth and nose and breathe through the opening in the neck. Use a small round mask when possible.

FYI

Differences Between Adult and Child CPR

- A *child* is defined as those between age 1 year and puberty. Puberty signs: males with chest and/or underarm hair and females with any breast development. When unsure, provide care the same as for an adult.
- If you are alone and do not have a phone, give five sets of 30 compressions and 2 breaths. After five sets of CPR, leave the child to find a phone, call 9-1-1, and get an AED. When you return, use the AED on the child as soon as possible.
- Compress the chest to a depth of *about 2 inches* (about one-third the depth of the child's chest) instead of compressing to *at least 2 inches*. Pushing too hard or too deep is better than not hard enough.
- Compress a small child's chest with one hand. For a large child, or if unable to press deep enough, use two hands to compress the chest.

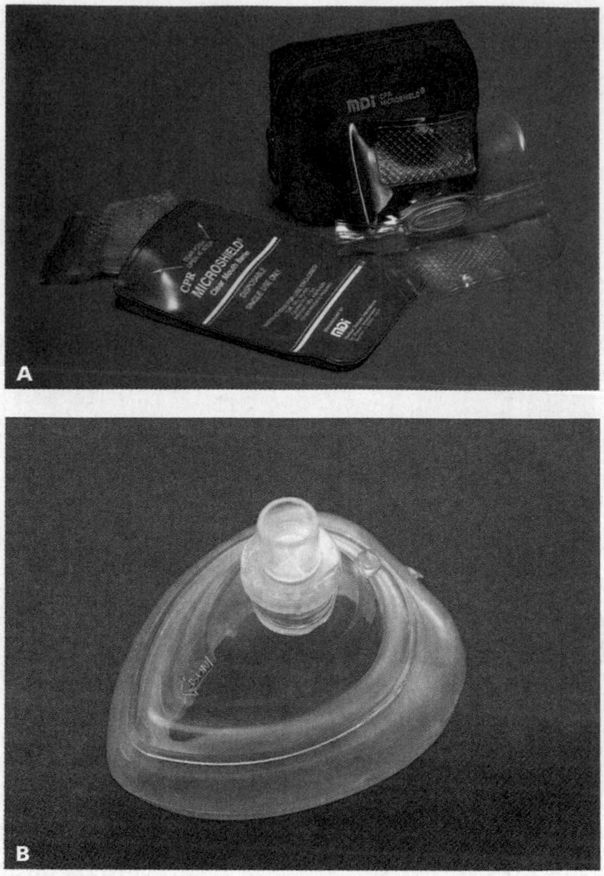

FIGURE 5-4 Barrier devices. **A**. Face shield. **B**. Pocket face mask.

Compression-Only CPR

Compression-only CPR, or hands-only CPR, is CPR without breaths. It is intended to increase bystander involvement when CPR is needed for a person in cardiac arrest. Compression-only CPR is easy to teach, remember, and perform compared with conventional CPR. It may be used with adults or children, but not infants. It is important to note that breaths are an important part of CPR with infants. Compression-only CPR in infants is *not* as effective as CPR with breaths. Compression-only CPR can even be detrimental for infants. Therefore, compression-only CPR should only be used with adults and children.

A bystander who sees a person who has suddenly collapsed and is not breathing but who is unable or unwilling to make mouth-to-mouth contact or unable to perform CPR can:

1. Ask another person to call 9-1-1 or an emergency response number.
2. Place the person faceup on a flat, firm surface.
3. Push the center of the chest hard and fast (faster than 1 per second or use the beat of the Bee Gees' song "Stayin' Alive", the beats from a smartphone app that was previously installed and is quickly accessible, or a dispatcher's directions heard over a mobile phone speaker).

If...	Then...
The first aid provider is willing and able to provide compression-only CPR or can follow a dispatcher's instructions over a mobile phone's speaker.	1. If available, use a barrier device. 2. If barrier device is not available, cover your own and the person's nose and mouth with a mask or cloth. 3. Give continuous chest compressions only (also known as hands-only CPR). Push hard, push fast! See page 63. 4. Continue chest compressions until: ▪ An AED arrives and the voice prompts you to stop so it can analyze and shock if necessary. The AED will advise if CPR should be continued. ▪ The person begins breathing normally. ▪ Someone of equal or higher training replaces you and takes over CPR. ▪ The scene becomes unsafe. The person should be moved to a nearby safer location before continuing CPR. ▪ You are alone and become physically exhausted and unable to continue. 5. If another person is present, they could help by giving chest compressions. If the other person is not trained in CPR, you can coach them on how to perform chest compressions. Switching places after about every 2 minutes helps avoid fatigue.

4. Continue chest compressions without stopping until help arrives or as long as possible. If another person is available, trade off about every 2 minutes.

COVID-19 and CPR

COVID-19 is an illness caused by a virus that can spread from person to person. A person can become infected from inhaling respiratory droplets when an infected person coughs, sneezes, or speaks. It may also be spread by touching a surface or object that has the virus on it and then touching your mouth, nose, eyes, or face. Everyone is at risk of getting COVID-19. In addition to the COVID-19 pandemic, other respiratory-related epidemics and pandemics have occurred in the past and will continue to occur in the future.

This presents a dilemma for a first aid provider who is concerned about compromising their own health and perhaps life, yet wants to give CPR as an attempt to save the life of a COVID-19 victim in cardiac arrest. If a person known to be infected with the COVID-19 virus is in cardiac arrest, perform compression-only CPR as described previously, with the addition of covering the person's nose and mouth with a cloth or face mask and the first aid provider wearing a mask to cover their own nose and mouth. If there is only one face mask or covering available, place it on the victim.

Infant CPR

To perform CPR on an infant, follow the steps in **SKILL SHEET 5-2** and **FLOWCHART 5-2**.

SKILL SHEET 5-2 Infant CPR

Note: Use the RAB-CAB mnemonic.

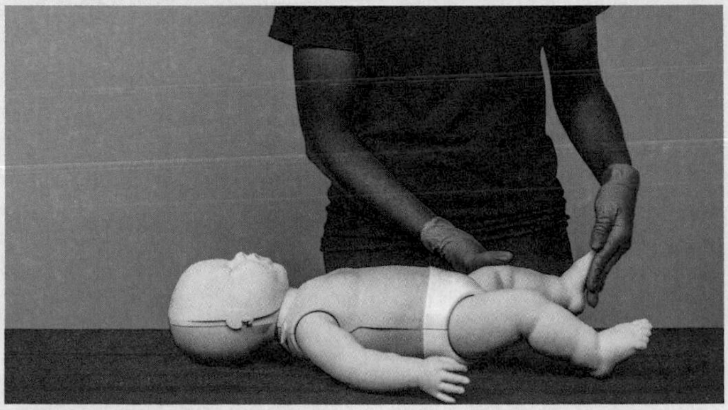

1 R = Responsive?

Tap the bottom of the infant's foot and shout their name. Take 5 to 10 seconds to check for no breathing or only gasping.

Continues

SKILL SHEET 5-2 Infant CPR (*Continued*)

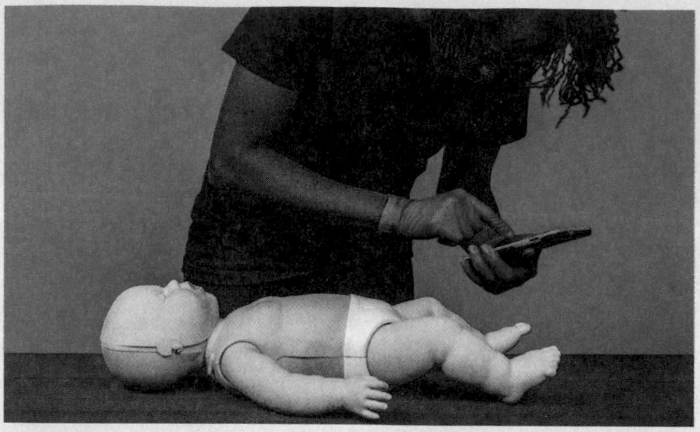

© Aleksandra Gigowska/Shutterstock.

2 A = Activate EMS and get an AED.

a. Shout for nearby help.

b. If someone responds, have them call 9-1-1 and get an AED while you start CPR.

c. If you are alone, perform CPR (30 chest compressions and 2 breaths for five cycles), call 9-1-1, and then get an AED. **DO NOT** call 9-1-1 until after giving five sets of CPR. If a phone is not available, perform CPR and get an AED.

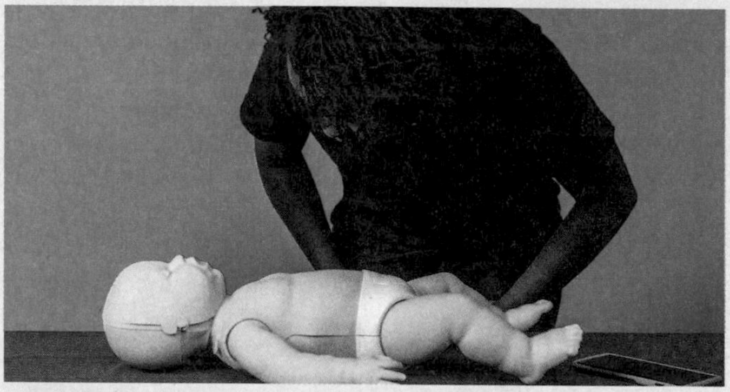

© Jones & Bartlett Learning.

3 B = Breathing?

Take 5 to 10 seconds to check for breathing or only gasping by observing the infant's face and chest movement. If the infant is not breathing or only gasping, continue to the next step, *Compressions*.

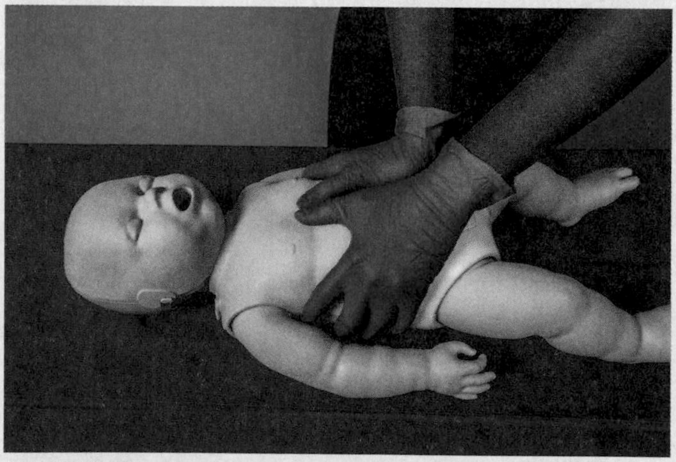

© Jones & Bartlett Learning.

4 C = Chest compressions.

Place the infant faceup on a flat, firm surface. If possible, use an elevated surface (eg, table, cabinet top). Single rescuers can use either the two-finger technique or the encircling thumbs (two-thumbs) technique.

4a. Encircling thumbs (two-thumbs) technique:

a. Place both thumbs on the lower third of the breastbone (sternum), both touching the imaginary nipple line and the fingers encircling around the infant's back and chest.

b. Give 30 chest compressions:

- Push hard: about 1.5 inches (4 cm) or about one-third the depth of the chest diameter straight down.
- Push fast: to the beat of the Bee Gees' song "Stayin' Alive", the beats from a smartphone app that was previously installed and is quickly accessible, or a dispatcher's directions heard over a mobile phone speaker.
- At the end of each compression, let the infant's chest come back up to its normal position.

or

SKILL SHEET 5-2 Infant CPR (*Continued*)

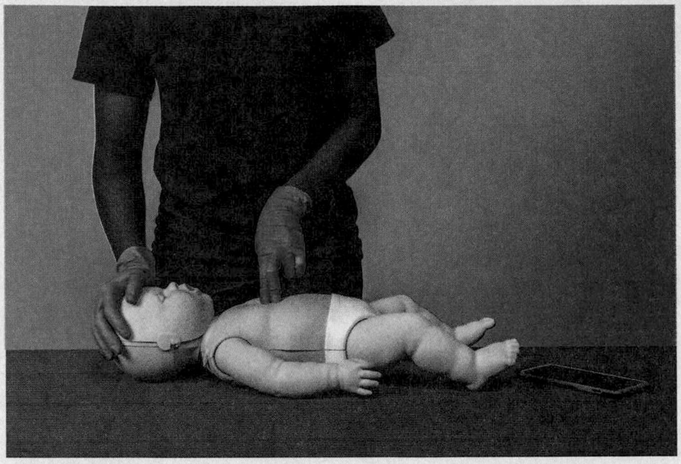

© Jones & Bartlett Learning.

4b. *Two-finger technique:*

a. Place the pads of two fingers on the infant's breastbone (sternum), with one touching and both below the imaginary nipple line.

b. Give 30 chest compressions:

- Push hard: about 1.5 inches (4 cm) or about one-third the depth of the chest diameter straight down. If unable to the achieve the appropriate depth, use the heel of one hand instead of two fingers.
- Push fast: to the beat of the Bee Gees' song "Stayin' Alive", the beats from a smartphone app that was previously installed and is quickly accessible, or a dispatcher's directions heard over a mobile phone speaker.
- At the end of each compression, let the infant's chest come back up to its normal position.

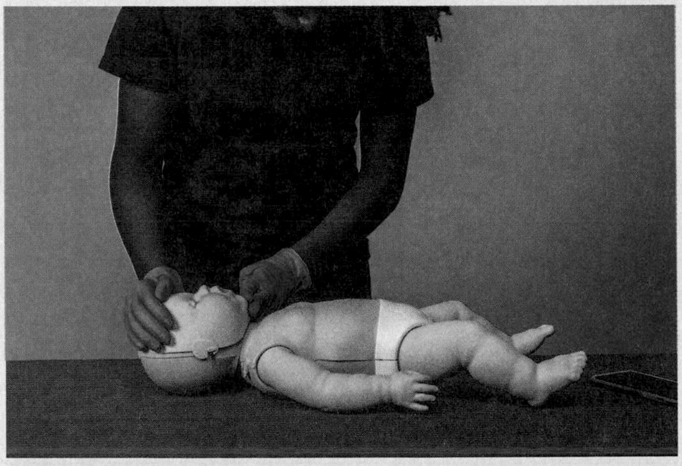

© Jones & Bartlett Learning.

5 **A = Airway open.**

Open the infant's airway using the head tilt–chin lift maneuver. **DO NOT** tilt the head back too far (less than for an adult or child).

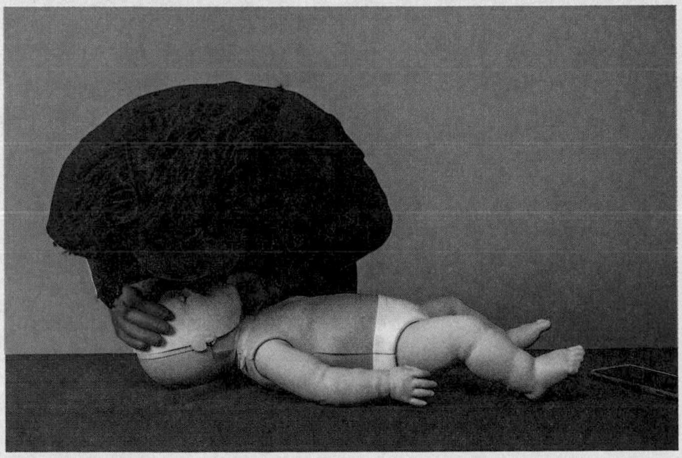

© Jones & Bartlett Learning.

6 **B = Breaths.**

a. Cover the infant's mouth and nose with your mouth and make an airtight seal. If this does not work, try either mouth-to-mouth or mouth-to-nose breaths.

b. Give two breaths, each lasting 1 second, to make the infant's chest rise.

c. Take a breath between giving the two breaths.

d. Continue CPR until one of the following occurs:

- The infant begins breathing.
- Someone of equal or higher training replaces you and takes over CPR.
- You become physically exhausted and unable to continue.

e. If another person is available, trade off about every five sets of CPR (2 minutes).

Flowchart 5-2 Infant CPR

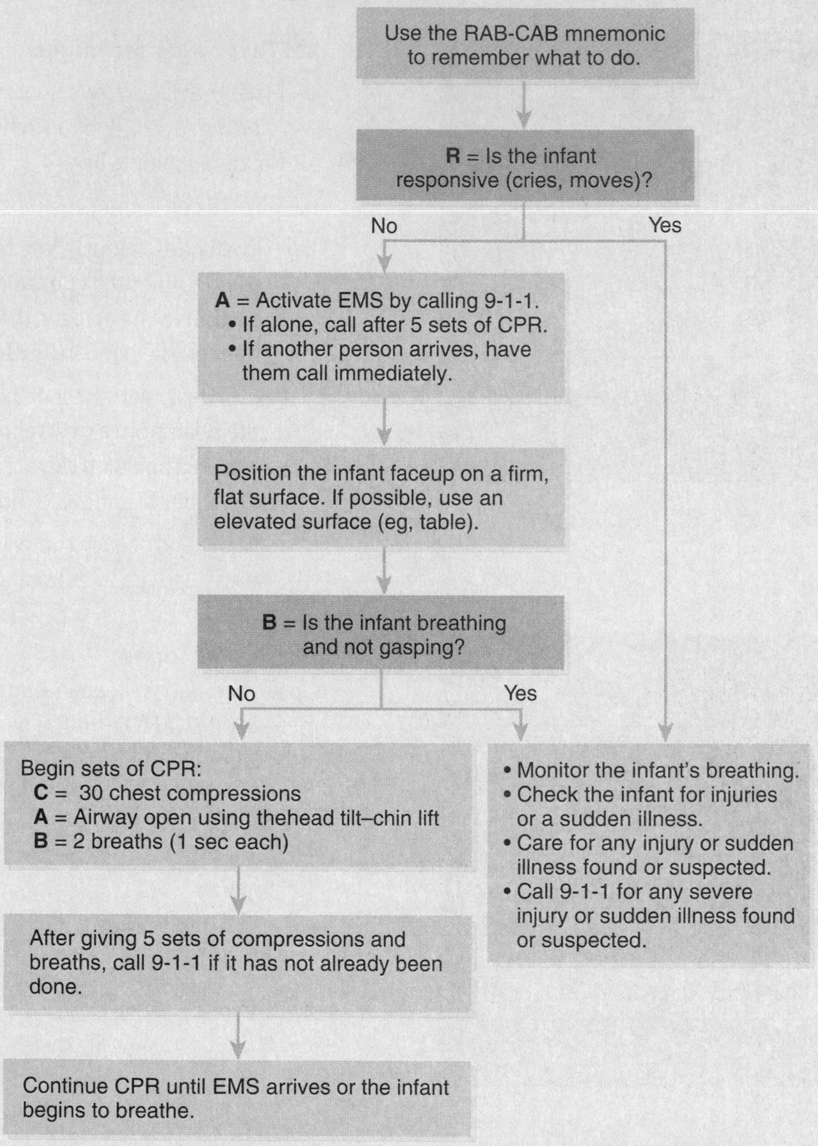
Use the RAB-CAB mnemonic to remember what to do.
R = Is the infant responsive (cries, moves)?
No
Yes
A = Activate EMS by calling 9-1-1.
• If alone, call after 5 sets of CPR.
• If another person arrives, have them call immediately.
Position the infant faceup on a firm, flat surface. If possible, use an elevated surface (eg, table).
B = Is the infant breathing and not gasping?
No
Yes
Begin sets of CPR:
C = 30 chest compressions
A = Airway open using thehead tilt–chin lift
B = 2 breaths (1 sec each)
After giving 5 sets of compressions and breaths, call 9-1-1 if it has not already been done.
Continue CPR until EMS arrives or the infant begins to breathe.
• Monitor the infant's breathing.
• Check the infant for injuries or a sudden illness.
• Care for any injury or sudden illness found or suspected.
• Call 9-1-1 for any severe injury or sudden illness found or suspected.

Recovery Position

If a person is unresponsive and breathing, place them in the side-lying recovery position **FIGURE 5-5**. This position provides the following advantages:

- Helps keep the airway open.
- Allows fluids (eg, blood, vomit, mucus) to drain out of the nose and mouth and not into the throat.
- Allows the first aid provider, when alone, to leave to call for help.

Place the person (usually by rolling) on their side, using the following points:

- Bottom arm: Extend outward.
- Top arm: Rest arm on bicep of bottom arm.
- Top hand: Keep under the person's cheek to cushion it, keep the airway open, and allow fluids to drain.
- Top leg: Adjust so both the knee and hip are bent at right angles to serve as a prop.
- Head: Attempt to extend the chin while pointing the mouth downward.

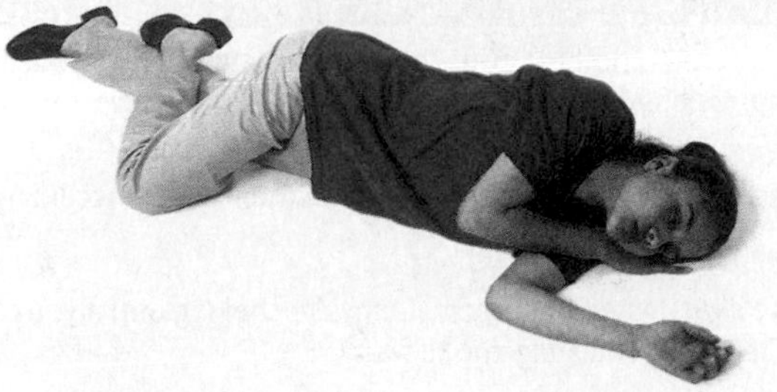

FIGURE 5-5 Recovery position.

If a neck, back, hip, or pelvic injury is suspected:

- **DO NOT** move the person. Leave the person in the position in which they were found.
- If the airway is blocked or the area is unsafe, move the person only as needed to open the airway or to reach a safe location. If moving them is necessary, support the head and neck while keeping the person's nose and navel pointing in the same direction.

Airway Obstruction

People can choke on all kinds of objects. Foods such as candy, peanuts, and grapes are major offenders because of their shapes and consistencies. Nonfood choking deaths are often caused by balloons, balls and marbles, toys, and coins inhaled by children and infants.

Recognizing Airway Obstruction

An object lodged in the airway can cause a mild or severe **airway obstruction**. In a mild airway obstruction, good air exchange is present and the person is able to make forceful coughing efforts in an attempt to relieve the obstruction. The person should be encouraged to cough.

A person with a severe airway obstruction will have poor air exchange. The signs of a severe airway obstruction include the following:

- Increased breathing difficulty
- Weak and ineffective cough
- Inability to speak or breathe
- Blue-gray skin, fingernail beds, and inside of the mouth (indicating **cyanosis**)

People who are choking may clutch their throats to communicate that they are choking **FIGURE 5-6**. This motion is known as the universal distress signal for choking. The person may also be pointing at their mouth indicating that they are choking. The person may become panicked and desperate.

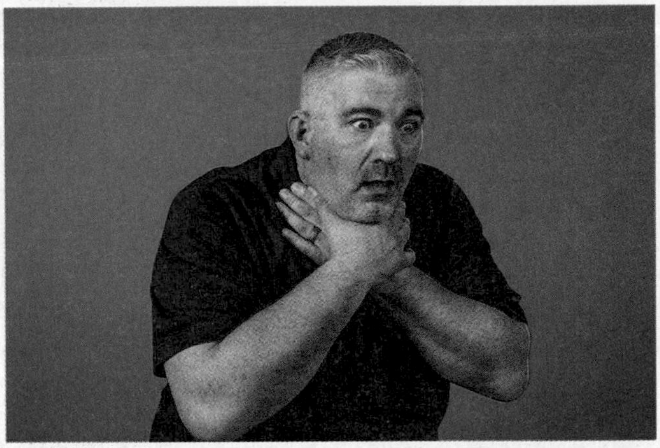

FIGURE 5-6 The universal sign of choking: holding the neck with one or both hands.

Caring for Airway Obstruction

Adult and Child Airway Obstruction

The American Heart Association (AHA) recommends providing abdominal thrusts for dislodging an airway obstruction (choking) in a responsive adult or child older than 1 year. The International Liaison Committee on Resuscitation (ILCOR) recommends a combination of back blows and abdominal thrusts (5 back blows followed by 5 abdominal thrusts, known as the 5 and 5 approach) for airway obstruction.

Past editions of this book have not included back blows for dislodging an airway obstruction because the AHA does not take a stance on them. However, back blows are recommended by ILCOR, which conducts rigorous and continuous reviews of scientific literature focused on resuscitation, cardiac arrest, and conditions requiring first aid. This organization's 2020 guidelines provide the justification for delivering back blows or a combination of back blows and abdominal thrusts for choking.

Some training organizations do not teach the back blow technique, only the abdominal thrust procedure. However, both approaches can be effective. An airway obstruction is a life-threatening event, so it is a good idea to know several procedures that can be taken if others have failed.

If...	Then...
The person is responsive and shows signs of mild airway obstruction (choking): ▪ Good air exchange is present ▪ Able to make forceful coughing efforts in an attempt to relieve the obstruction	▪ Encourage continued coughing, but do nothing else. Aggressive treatment (eg, back blows, abdominal thrusts, chest compressions) may cause complications and could worsen the airway obstruction. ▪ Monitor the person until they improve, since a severe airway obstruction can occur anytime.
The person is responsive and shows signs of complete airway obstruction: ▪ Difficulty breathing ▪ Unable to cough forcefully ▪ Unable to talk ▪ Skin, fingernail beds, or lips turn blue or gray ▪ Appears panicky and desperate ▪ Pointing to their mouth or grasps at their throat *Note:* It is important to distinguish choking from fainting, heart attack, seizure, anaphylaxis, and other conditions that may cause sudden respiratory distress or loss of responsiveness.	**1.** **DO NOT** ask them if they are okay. Instead, ask them if they are choking and if you can help them. If they nod "yes," tell them you are going to help. **2.** Have someone call 9-1-1. **3.** Stand to the side and slightly behind the choking person. **4.** Support the person by placing one hand on the upper chest or over the navel and have the person bend over at the waist to a 90° angle (their upper body should be parallel to the ground or floor). **DO NOT** keep them in an upright or vertical position. If they are not bending over when the jolt of the back blow dislodges the object, the object may become stuck deeper in the airway. **5.** Give 5 hard back blows with the heel of the hand that is not supporting the person. Aim for the area in between their shoulder blades **SKILL SHEET 5-3**. **DO NOT** just pat them on the back; use hard blows (eg, like driving or hitting a nail into a thick board with a hammer). Each back blow should be a separate and distinct effort to dislodge the object. **6.** Check to see if each back blow has dislodged the obstruction. The aim is to relieve the object with a blow, not to necessarily give all 5 back blows.
The 5 back blows fail to dislodge the airway obstruction	**1.** Stand behind the person or kneel behind a child. If the person is a lot taller than you, have them kneel or sit. **2.** Put one foot in front of the other foot; this provides stability during the thrusts and if the person becomes unresponsive and collapses, they can slide down your leg to the ground or floor. **3.** Wrap your arms around the person's waist. Locate the person's navel (belly button) using two fingers (right-handed people will usually use their left hand). If your arms cannot encircle the person's waist (eg, pregnant woman, or a very large person and you are smaller than them), use chest thrusts. See below for chest thrust directions. **4.** Make a fist and with the other hand (right-handed people will usually use their right hand to make a fist). Place the thumb side of the fist just above the person's navel and below the tip of the breastbone (sternum). Grab the fist with the other hand. **5.** Give up to 5 abdominal thrusts by quick inward and upward pulling of the fist into the person's abdomen **SKILL SHEET 5-4**. Each thrust should be a separate and distinct effort to dislodge the object, not to necessarily give all 5 abdominal thrusts.
The obstruction does not get dislodged and is still in place	Repeat alternating between back blows and abdominal thrusts until: ▪ The person can cough forcefully, breathe, or speak, or ▪ The person becomes unresponsive, or ▪ EMS or someone with more advanced training takes over.
The person becomes unresponsive or is found unresponsive	▪ Support the person while carefully lowering them to the ground. ▪ If EMS have not arrived or have not been called, call them immediately. ▪ Begin CPR, starting with chest compressions.
Solid material or an object can be seen in the airway	Remove the solid material or object only if seen. **DO NOT** use a blind finger sweep.
The person is pregnant, very large, or if you are small	Provide chest thrusts **FIGURE 5-7**: **1.** Position yourself behind the person. **2.** Put your arms under the person's armpits and your hands on the lower half of the breastbone (sternum). **3.** Pull your hands straight back into the chest.
The object has been dislodged and the person has a persistent cough or feels something is stuck in their throat	Seek professional medical care because injuries may have occurred.

Infant Airway Obstruction

For a responsive infant with an airway obstruction, give back blows and chest thrusts instead of abdominal thrusts to relieve the obstruction **SKILL SHEET 5-5**.

SKILL SHEET 5-3 Adult and Child Choking: Back Blows

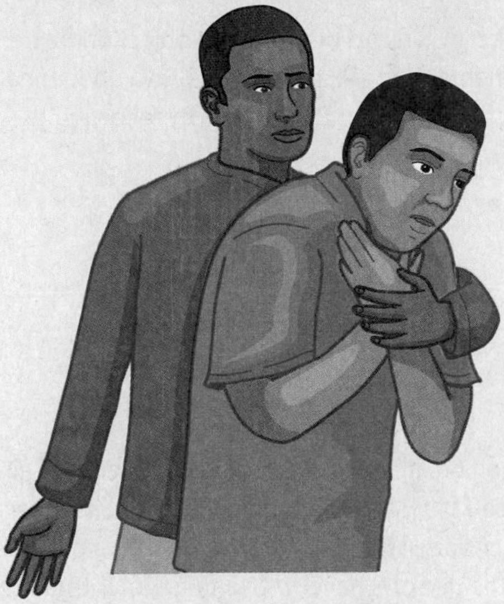

© Jones & Bartlett Learning.

1 Stand behind the person and slightly to one side. Reach across the person's chest by wrapping one arm either over the person's arm or under their armpit. Place the palm of that hand on the person's upper chest or shoulder. Another option is to place your hand over the person's navel. Leave your other hand free.

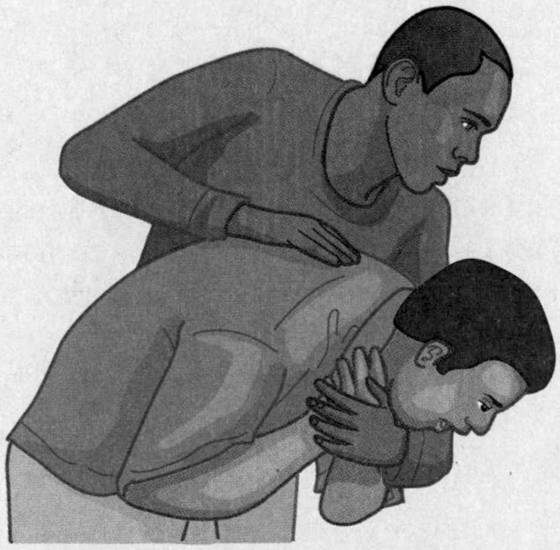

© Jones & Bartlett Learning.

2 Have the person bend over at the waist to a 90° angle (their upper body should be parallel to the ground or floor). **DO NOT** keep them in an upright or a vertical position. If they are not bending over when the jolt of the back blow dislodges the object, the dislodged object may become stuck deeper in the airway.

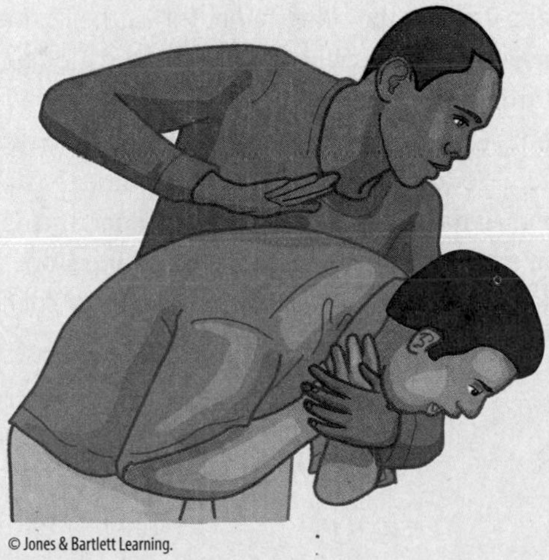

© Jones & Bartlett Learning.

3 With your fingertips up, use the heel of your hand to firmly strike the person between their shoulder blades.

4 If 5 back blows do not dislodge the object, give up to 5 abdominal thrusts (see Skill Sheet 5-4).

SKILL SHEET 5-4 Adult and Child Choking: Abdominal Thrusts

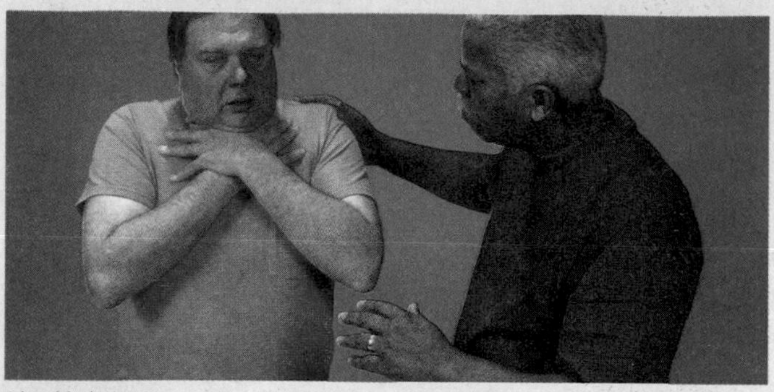

1 If 5 back blows fail to dislodge the object or the person is still unable to speak, then give up to 5 abdominal thrusts. Do the abdominal thrusts by following the remaining steps.

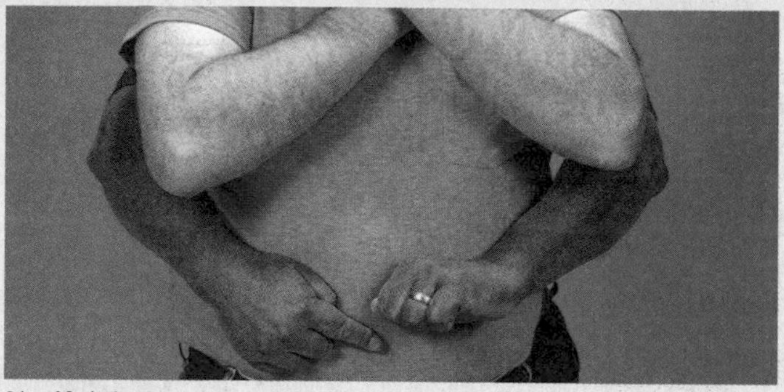

2 Stand behind an adult; stand or kneel behind a child. (If the person is a lot taller than you, have them kneel or sit in front of you). Wrap your arms around the person's waist. Locate the person's navel with a finger (right-handed people will usually use their left hand).

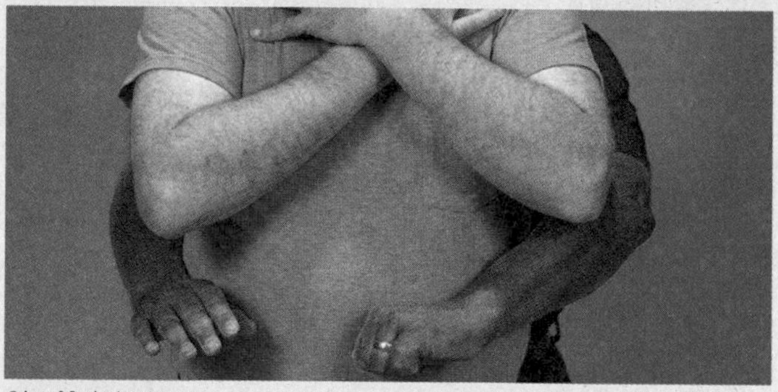

3 Make a fist with the other hand (right-handed people will usually use their right hand) and place the thumb side of the hand just above the person's navel and below the tip of the breastbone (sternum).

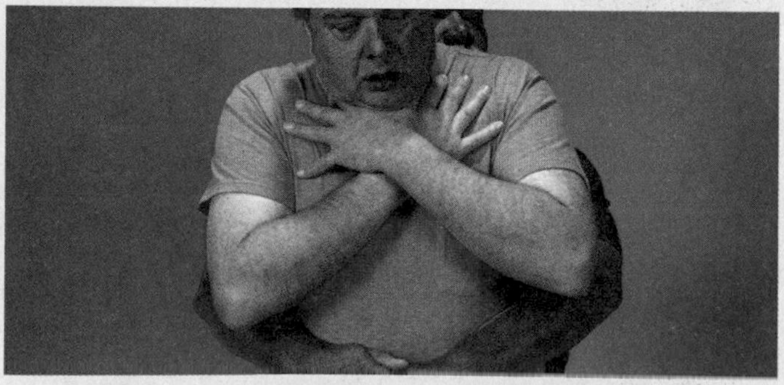

4 Grasp the fist with the other hand. Thrust the fist into the person's abdomen with a quick upward motion. (Use chest thrusts on a person who is choking and very large or pregnant.) Each thrust should be a separate and distinct effort to dislodge the object. After each thrust, quickly determine if the abdominal thrust dislodged the object. The aim is to dislodge the object with a thrust, not to necessarily give all 5 abdominal thrusts before checking.

SKILL SHEET 5-4 Adult and Child Choking: Abdominal Thrusts (*Continued*)

5 If the 5 abdominal thrusts did not dislodge the object, give up to 5 back blows again. Repeat a combination of 5 back blows and 5 abdominal thrusts until:

- The object is dislodged and the person starts breathing.
- EMS arrives and takes over.
- Another person is available you take turns giving back blows and abdominal thrusts.
- The person becomes unresponsive and collapses to the ground or floor.

6 If the person becomes unresponsive or a person is found unresponsive, provide CPR with the addition of a step:

a. Give 30 chest compressions.

b. Open the mouth, look for an object, and if seen, remove it.

c. Give 2 breaths. If the first breath does not cause the chest to rise, retilt the head and attempt a second breath.

d. Continue sets of 30 chest compressions and 2 breaths. Each time before giving the first of the 2 breaths, look into the mouth for an object; if seen, remove it.

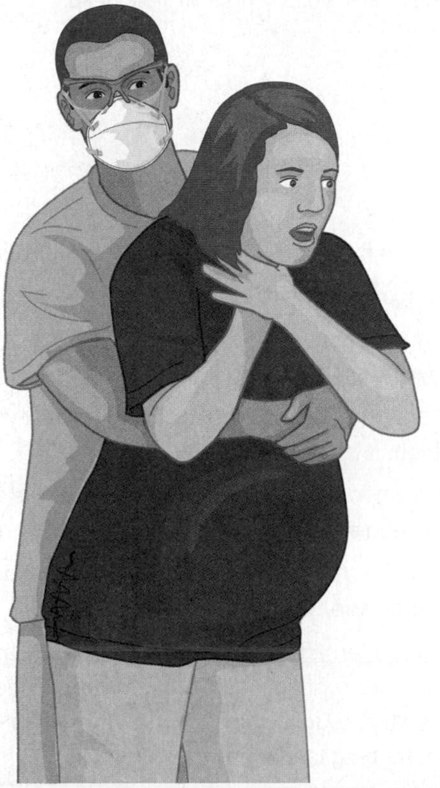

FIGURE 5-7 Chest thrusts are similar to CPR chest compressions, but are sharper and delivered at a slower rate. Hands are placed on the lower half of the breastbone (sternum).

Q&A

What are the types of upper airway obstruction?

- *Tongue.* Unconsciousness produces relaxation of soft tissues, and the tongue can fall into the airway. Swallowing one's tongue is impossible, but the widespread belief that it can happen is explained by slippage of the relaxed tongue into the airway. The tongue is the most common cause of airway obstruction in an unresponsive person.
- *Foreign body.* People, especially children, inhale all kinds of objects. Foods such as hot dogs, candy, peanuts, and grapes are major offenders because of their shapes and consistencies. According to the *Journal of Forensic Science*, meat is the main cause of choking in adults. Coins and toys are the top causes of nonfood choking deaths in children, as reported by the American Academy of Pediatrics. Unresponsive people's airways can also be obstructed by a foreign material such as vomit and teeth.
- *Swelling.* Severe allergic reactions (anaphylaxis) and irritants (eg, smoke, chemicals) can cause swelling. Even a nonallergic person who is stung inside the throat by a bee, yellow jacket, or other flying insect can experience swelling in the airway.
- *Spasm.* Water that is suddenly inhaled can cause a spasm in the throat.
- *Vomit.* Many people vomit when they are near death. Whenever performing CPR, expect vomit before or during CPR.

FYI

The Tongue and Airway Obstruction

Airway obstruction in an unresponsive person lying on their back is usually the result of the tongue relaxing in the back of the mouth, restricting air movement. Opening the airway with the head tilt–chin lift method may be all that is needed to correct this condition.

Q&A

Why isn't the pulse checked?

Studies show that first aid providers as well as health care providers take too long to check for a pulse and have difficulty determining whether a pulse is present. Taking too long delays giving chest compressions.

Data from Berg RA, Hemphill R, Abella BS, et al. Part 5: adult basic life support. *Circulation*. 2010;122:S689.

SKILL SHEET 5-5 Infant Choking

Note: An infant is not breathing if they are unable to cry or make a sound.

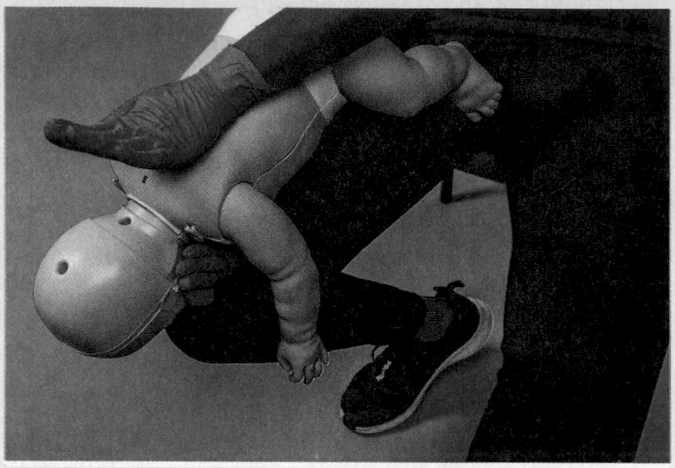

1 Give up to five separate and distinct back blows.

- **a.** Support the infant's head with your hand.
- **b.** Lay the infant facedown over your forearm, with the head lower than their chest.
- **c.** Brace your forearm and the infant against your thigh.
- **d.** Give the back blows between the infant's shoulder blades with the heel of your other hand.
- **e.** If the object does not come out, turn the infant onto their back while supporting the head.

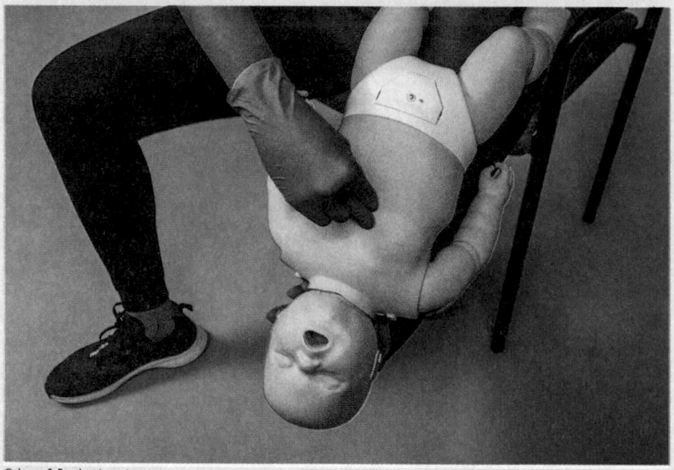

2 Give up to five separate and distinct chest thrusts.

- **a.** Support the infant's head with your hand.
- **b.** Lay the infant faceup over your forearm, with the head lower than their chest.
- **c.** Brace your forearm and the infant against your other thigh.
- **d.** Place two fingers of your other hand in the same location as for giving CPR compressions.
- **e.** Give the thrusts 1 second apart; this is not as fast as CPR compressions.

3 Continue alternating the 5 back blows and 5 chest thrusts without interruption until the infant stops responding or can breathe, cough, or cry, or until someone of equal or higher training takes over.

4 If the infant is found or becomes unresponsive:

- **a.** Give 30 chest compressions.
- **b.** Look into the infant's mouth for an object; if seen, remove it.
- **c.** Give 2 breaths.

PREP KIT

Ready for Review

- A heart attack occurs when heart muscle tissue dies because the blood supply is severely reduced or stopped.
- The six links in the chain of survival are recognition and activation of EMS, CPR, defibrillation, advanced care, post-arrest care, and recovery.
- CPR consists of moving blood to the heart and brain by giving chest compressions and breathing oxygen into a person's lungs.
- The signs of a severe airway obstruction include difficulty breathing, weak and ineffective cough, inability to speak or breathe, and signs of cyanosis.

Vital Vocabulary

airway obstruction A blockage, often the result of a foreign body, in which airflow to the lungs is reduced or completely blocked.

cardiac arrest Stoppage of the heartbeat.

cardiopulmonary resuscitation (CPR) The act of providing chest compressions and rescue breaths for a person in cardiac arrest.

chain of survival A concept involving six critical links (recognition and activation of EMS, CPR, defibrillation, advanced care, post-arrest care, recovery) to help improve survival from cardiac arrest.

chest compression The act of depressing the chest and allowing it to return to its normal position as part of CPR.

cyanosis A blue-gray skin color that is caused by a reduced level of oxygen in the blood.

head tilt–chin lift maneuver A combination of two movements to open the airway by tilting the forehead back and lifting the chin.

heart attack Death of a part of the heart muscle.

Assessment in Action

You are having dinner in a very crowded restaurant with your family on New Year's Eve. An older man is pushing a piano into the restaurant as part of the entertainment that evening. As he passes your table, he clutches his chest and falls to the floor. He is not moving.

Directions: Circle Yes if you agree with the statement; circle No if you disagree.

1. If he is not breathing or is breathing abnormally, you should call 9-1-1.

   YES NO

2. The man must be choking because he is in a restaurant.

   YES NO

3. If the man is choking, you should perform abdominal thrusts.

   YES NO

4. If the man is choking, you should perform sets of 30 chest compressions and 2 breaths.

   YES NO

5. Check for breathing before giving any breaths to the person.

   YES NO

6. Continue CPR until the AED's voice prompt tells you to stop so it can analyze and shock if necessary or EMS personnel arrive.

   YES NO

Check Your Knowledge

Directions: Circle Yes if you agree with the statement; circle No if you disagree.

1. Gasping in an unresponsive person can indicate that the person is not breathing.

   YES NO

2. After you determine that an adult is unresponsive, the next step is for someone to call 9-1-1.

   YES NO

3. Tilting the head back and lifting the chin helps move the tongue and open the airway.

   YES NO

4. If you determine that a person is not breathing, begin chest compressions.

   YES NO

PREP KIT continued

5. Do not start chest compressions until you have checked for a pulse.
   YES **NO**
6. For all people (adult, child, infant) needing CPR, give 30 compressions followed by 2 breaths.
   YES **NO**
7. Use two fingers when performing CPR on an infant.
   YES **NO**
8. A sign of choking is that the person is unable to speak or cough.
   YES **NO**
9. To give abdominal thrusts to a responsive choking person, place your fist below the person's navel.
   YES **NO**
10. When giving abdominal thrusts to a responsive choking person, repeat the thrusts until the object is removed or the person becomes unresponsive.
    YES **NO**

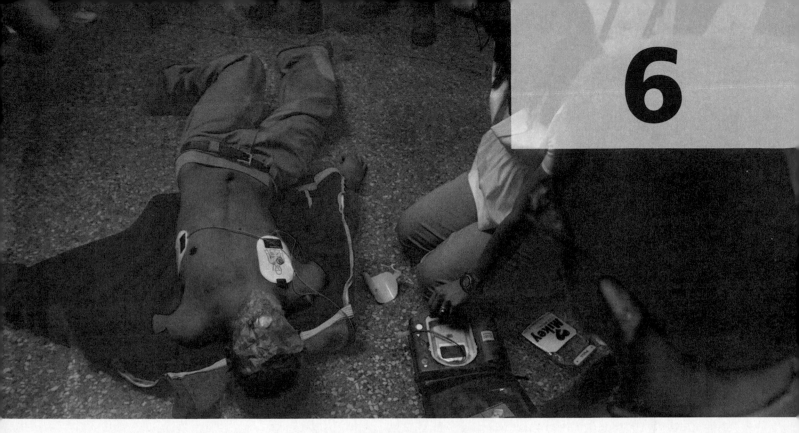

6

Automated External Defibrillation

Public Access Defibrillation

A person's chance of survival after cardiac arrest dramatically improves through early cardiopulmonary resuscitation (CPR) and early **defibrillation** with the use of an **automated external defibrillator (AED)**. To be effective, defibrillation must be used in the first few minutes following cardiac arrest. The implementation of state public access defibrillation laws and the Food and Drug Administration's approval of home-use AEDs have made this important care step available to many first aid providers in many places, including the following **FIGURE 6-1**:

- Airports and airplanes
- Stadiums
- Health clubs
- Golf courses
- Schools
- Government buildings
- Offices
- Homes
- Shopping centers/malls

CHAPTER AT A GLANCE

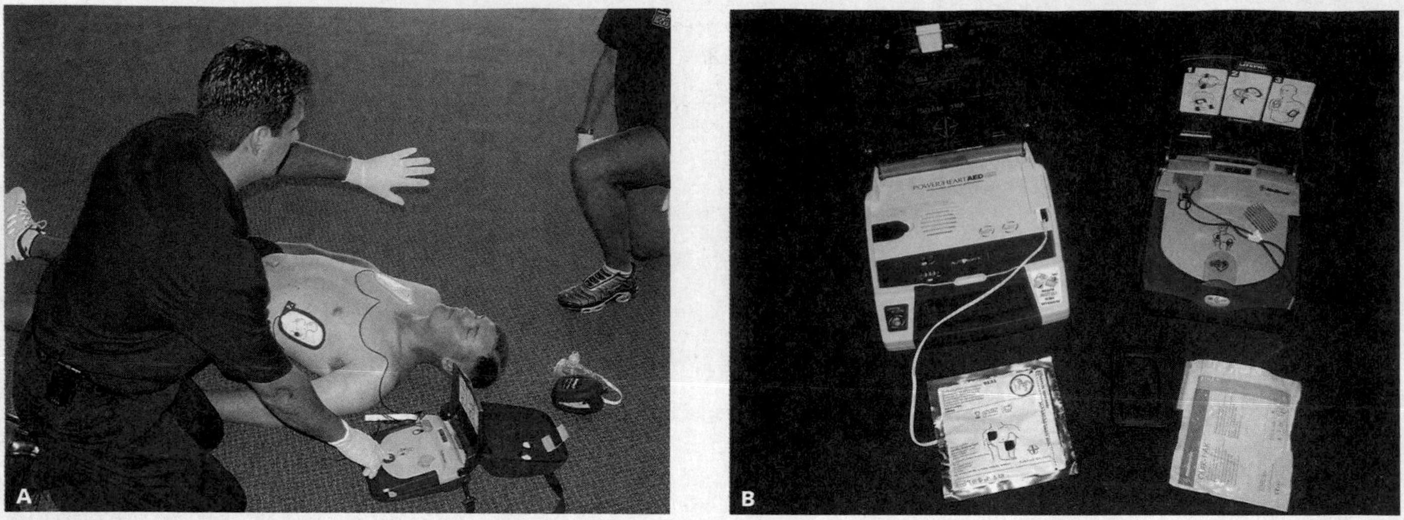

FIGURE 6-1 A. Automated external defibrillators (AEDs) are available in many places for use by trained first aid providers. **B**. Various AED devices.

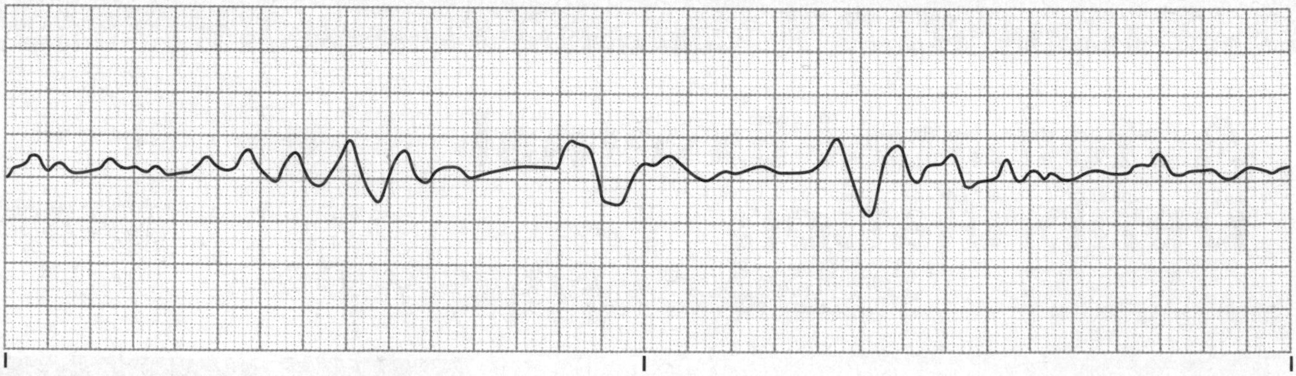

FIGURE 6-2 Ventricular fibrillation (VF) is disorganized electrical activity.

How the Heart Works

The heart is an organ with four hollow chambers. The two chambers on the right side receive blood from the body and send it to the lungs for oxygen. The two chambers on the left side receive freshly oxygenated blood from the lungs and send it back out to the body.

The heart has a unique electrical system that controls the rate at which the heart beats and the amount of work the heart performs. In the right upper chamber of the heart, there is a collection of special pacemaker cells. These cells emit electrical impulses about 60 to 100 times a minute that cause the other heart muscle cells to contract in a coordinated manner.

Because the heart contracts approximately every second, it needs an abundant supply of oxygen, which it gets through the coronary arteries. These arteries run along the outside of the heart muscle and branch into smaller vessels. These arteries sometimes become diseased (atherosclerosis), resulting in a lack of oxygen to the pacemaker cells, which can cause abnormal electrical activity in the heart.

When Normal Electrical Activity Is Interrupted

Ventricular fibrillation (VF) is the most common abnormal heart rhythm in cases of sudden cardiac arrest in adults **FIGURE 6-2**.

The organized wave of electrical impulses that cause the heart muscle to contract and relax in a regular fashion is lost when the heart is in VF. As a result, the lower chambers of the heart quiver and cannot pump blood, so circulation is lost (no pulse).

A second, potentially life-threatening, electrical condition is **ventricular tachycardia (VT)**, in which the heart beats too fast to pump blood effectively **FIGURE 6-3**. Both of these conditions could lead to a complete stoppage of the heart, which is known as cardiac arrest.

Care for Cardiac Arrest

When the heart stops beating, the blood stops circulating, cutting off all oxygen and nourishment to the entire body. Vital organs will start to die when they lose their supply of oxygen-rich

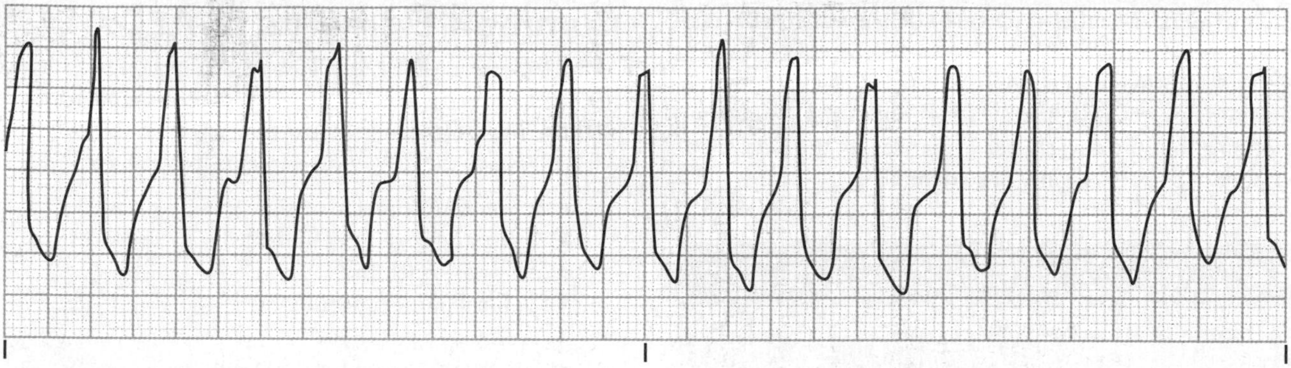

FIGURE 6-3 Ventricular tachycardia (VT) is very rapid electrical activity.

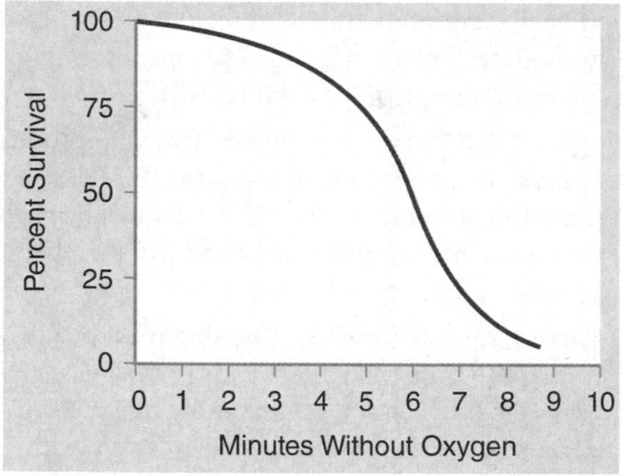

FIGURE 6-4 A person's chance of survival decreases with every minute that passes without proper care.

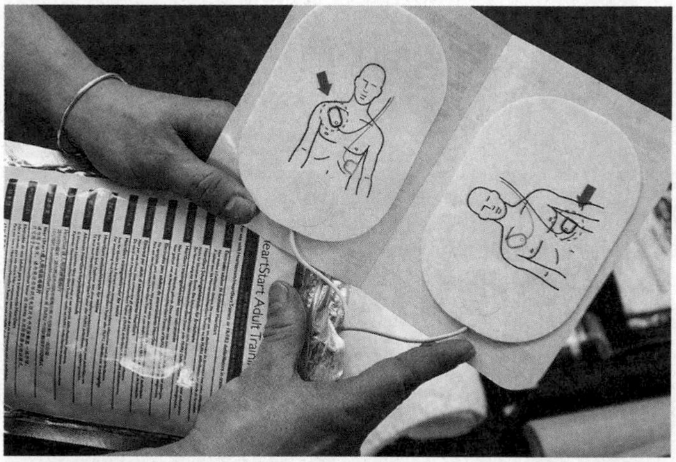

FIGURE 6-5 Two adhesive pads are placed on the person's chest and connected by a cable to the automated external defibrillators.

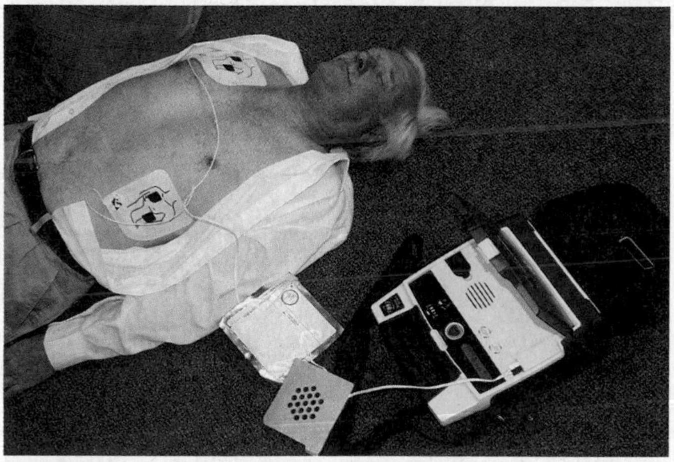

FIGURE 6-6 The pad-and-cable system sends the electrical signal from the heart into the device for analysis and delivers the electric shock to the person as directed by the operator.

blood. The brain, for example, will start to die within minutes. In this situation, time is a crucial factor. For every minute that defibrillation is delayed, the person's chance of survival decreases by 7% to 10% **FIGURE 6-4**.

CPR is the initial care for cardiac arrest. Perform cycles of chest compressions and breaths until an AED becomes available and is attached to the person. The AED's voice prompts will tell you to stop so that the AED can analyze and shock if necessary.

Automated External Defibrillation

Many out-of-hospital cardiac arrests involve an irregular heart electrical rhythm or beat called VF. An AED is an electronic device that analyzes the heart rhythm and, if necessary, recommends the operator deliver an electric shock, known as defibrillation, to the heart of a person in cardiac arrest. The purpose of this shock is to correct an abnormal electrical disturbance and reestablish a heart rhythm that will result in normal electrical and pumping function. Using an AED as soon as possible increases the person's chance of survival.

All AEDs are attached to the person by a cable connected to two adhesive pads (electrodes) placed on the person's chest **FIGURE 6-5**. The pad-and-cable system sends the electrical signal from the heart into the device for analysis and delivers the electric shock to the person when needed **FIGURE 6-6**.

AEDs have built-in rhythm analysis systems that determine whether the person needs a shock. This system enables first aid providers and other rescuers to deliver early defibrillation with only minimal training.

AEDs also provide a record of the person's heart rhythm (known as an electrocardiogram [ECG]), shock data, and other information about the device's performance (eg, the date, time, and number of shocks supplied) **FIGURE 6-7**.

Q&A

How does an AED work?

A microprocessor inside the defibrillator interprets (analyzes) the person's heart rhythm through adhesive electrodes. The computer analyzes the heart rhythm and advises the rescuer whether a shock is needed. The AED advises a shock only if it detects VF or VT. The AED delivers electrical energy from one pad to the other, then back to the first pad. This electrically stuns the heart and allows the heart to resume normal function.

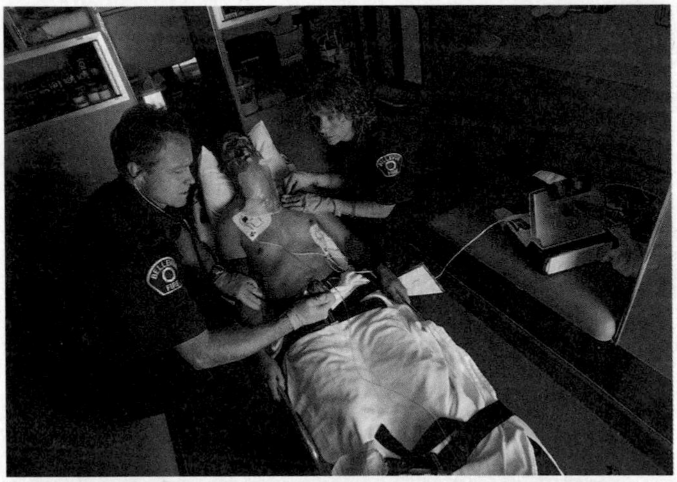

FIGURE 6-7 Automated external defibrillators store information, including heart rhythms and shock data.

Common Elements of AEDs

Many different AED models exist. The principles for use are the same for each, but the displays, controls, and options vary slightly. You will need to know how to use your specific AED. All AEDs have the following elements in common:

- Power on/off mechanism
- Cable and pads (electrodes)
- Analysis capability
- Defibrillation capability
- Prompts to guide you
- Battery operation for portability

Using an AED

Once you have determined the need for the AED (person unresponsive and not breathing), the basic operation of all AED models follows the sequence in **SKILL SHEET 6-1**.

1. Some AEDs power on by pressing an on/off button. Others power on when opening the AED case lid. Once the power is on, the AED will quickly go through some internal checks and will then begin to provide voice and screen prompts.
2. Expose the person's chest. The skin must be fairly dry so that the pads will adhere and conduct electricity properly. If necessary, dry the skin with a towel. Because excessive chest hair may interfere with adhesion and electrical conduction, you may need to quickly shave the area where the pads are to be placed.
3. Remove the backing from the two AED pads and apply them firmly to the person's bare chest according to the diagram on the pads or the manufacturer's directions. Place one pad on the upper right side of the sternum (breastbone) and just beneath the clavicle (collarbone). Place the second pad on the left size, above the lowest rib and to the left of the left nipple. If another person is giving chest compressions, do not

SKILL SHEET 6-1 Using an AED

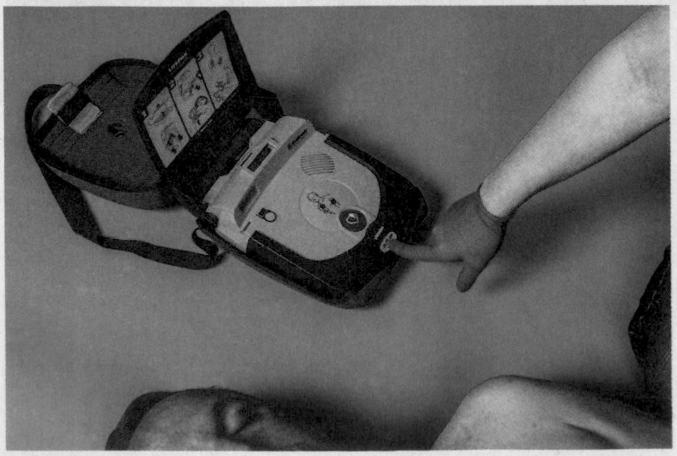

1 Turn on the AED. This is done by lifting the lid or pressing an "On" button. Follow the AED's prompts.

SKILL SHEET 6-1 Using an AED (*Continued*)

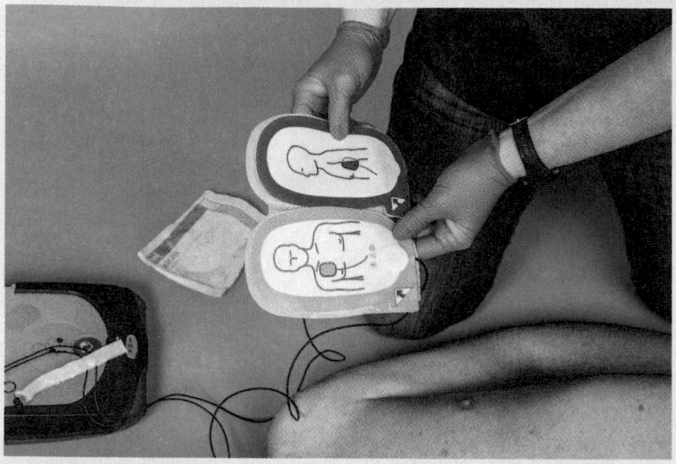

2 Attach the pads to the person's bare, dry chest (as shown on the pads). If needed, plug the cables into the AED.

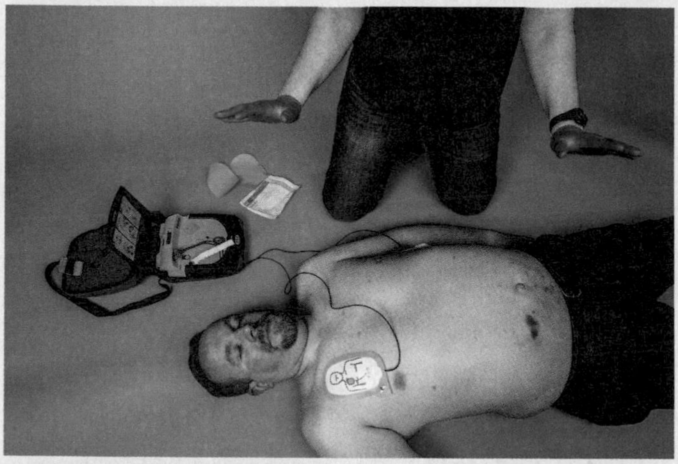

3 Stay clear of the person. Make sure no one, including you, is touching the person. Say, "Clear!"

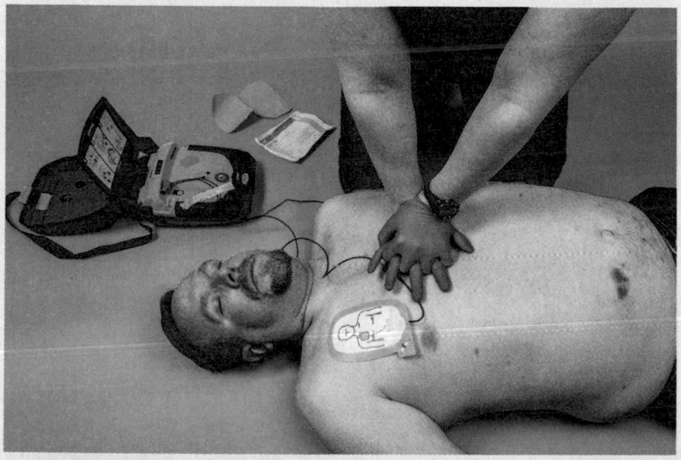

4 Allow the AED to analyze the heart rhythm. The AED will prompt one of two actions:

a. Stay clear and press the "Shock" button to deliver a shock.

b. Do not shock, but give CPR starting with chest compressions, leaving the pads in place.

5 After either one of the two actions, give CPR starting with chest compressions immediately for five cycles (about 2 minutes) unless the person moves, begins to breathe, or wakes up. Even if the person wakes up, leave the AED pads on until EMS arrives.

6 Repeat Steps **3**, **4**, and **5** until the person moves or begins to breathe, or until someone of equal or higher training replaces you and takes over.

interrupt the compressions when applying the AED pads.

4. Stop compressions and make sure no one, including you, is touching the person. Allow the AED to analyze the heart rhythm by pushing the "Analyze" button on the AED.
5. If the AED advises a shock, continue CPR while the AED is charging. If no shock is advised, resume CPR for five cycles (about 2 minutes) until prompted by the AED to allow for a rhythm check, and then reanalyze the cardiac rhythm.
6. Say "Clear" and make sure that no one, including you, is touching the person. Deliver the shock by pushing the "Shock" button.
7. After a shock is given, immediately resume CPR, starting with chest compressions.
8. After five cycles (about 2 minutes), stop compressions and allow the AED to reanalyze the rhythm.
9. Repeat steps 4 through 7 until advanced life support personnel arrive or the person starts to move.

Q&A

Will I get zapped if a person is shocked in the rain or near water?

It is remotely possible to get shocked or to shock bystanders if standing water is present around and under the person. Try to move the person to a dry area and cut off wet clothing. Also be sure that the skin has been dried off so that the electrode pads will stick to the skin. No one should be touching any part of the person while the device emits an electrical current.

If the first aid provider sees a person . . .	Then . . .
With wet skin, lying in shallow water or on snow	▪ Move the person out of the water or off the snow. ▪ Wipe the chest dry before attaching the pads.
Who has chest hair	Remove hair that may prevent the pads from sticking to the skin. Do this by either: ▪ Shaving the area where pads will be placed, or ▪ Applying adhesive tape (eg, duct, masking, bandage) firmly onto the hair and ripping the hair off. It may be necessary to repeat this action several times.
With medication patches (eg, nitroglycerin, nicotine, pain medication)	▪ **DO NOT** place an AED pad over a medicine patch. ▪ Remove the patch while wearing medical exam gloves or using a paper towel or cloth.
Implanted devices seen or felt when chest is exposed (devices include pacemakers or defibrillators)	▪ **DO NOT** place an AED pad directly over the implanted device. Apply at least 2 inches (5 cm) from the device/battery. ▪ Allow the implanted device to stop twitching before using an AED.
Who is a child or infant	The procedure is the same as for an adult. Some AEDs may have pediatric AED pads. If the pads may touch each other, place one pad in the middle of the chest and the other pad on the back, between the shoulder blades. If pediatric equipment is not available, use the adult equipment.

Special Considerations

There are several special situations that you should be aware of when using an AED. These include the following:

Water

Because water conducts electricity, it may provide an energy pathway between the AED and you or bystanders. First remove the person from free-standing water. Quickly dry the chest before applying the pads. The risk to you and bystanders is very low if the chest is dry and the pads are secured to the chest.

Children

Cardiac arrest in children is usually caused by an airway or breathing condition, rather than a primary heart condition as in adults. AEDs can deliver energy levels appropriate for children and infants. If your AED has special pediatric pads and cable, use these for the child **FIGURE 6-8**. If pediatric equipment is not available, use the adult equipment.

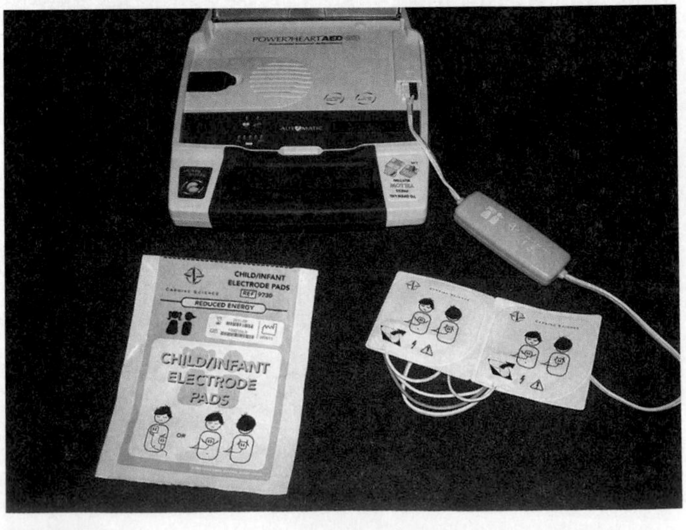

FIGURE 6-8 If your automated external defibrillator has pediatric pads, use them according to the manufacturer's instructions.

Medication Patches

Some people wear an adhesive patch containing medication (eg, nitroglycerin, nicotine, pain medication) that is absorbed through the skin. Because these patches may block the delivery of energy from the pads to the heart, they need to be removed and the skin wiped dry before attaching the AED pads **FIGURE 6-9**.

Chest Hair

Chest hair may prevent the pads from sticking to the skin. If necessary, remove the hair by doing either of the following:

- Shaving the area where pads will be placed
- Applying adhesive tape (eg, duct tape, masking tape, bandage) firmly onto the hair and ripping the tape off. It may be necessary to repeat this action several times.

Implanted Devices

Implanted pacemakers and defibrillators are small devices placed underneath the skin of people with certain types of heart disease **FIGURE 6-10**. These devices or their battery can often be seen or felt when the chest is exposed. Avoid placing the pads directly over these devices whenever possible. If an implanted defibrillator is discharging, you may see the person twitching periodically. You may also feel small jolts of electricity while performing compressions if the defibrillator discharges. Allow the implanted unit to stop before using your AED.

AED Maintenance

Periodic inspection of an AED ensures that the device has the necessary supplies and is in proper working condition **FIGURE 6-11**. AEDs conduct automatic internal checks and provide visual indications that the unit is ready and functioning properly. You do not need to turn the device on daily to check it. Doing so will only wear down the battery.

AED supplies should include items such as the following:

- Two sets of electrode pads with expiration dates that are not expired
- An extra battery

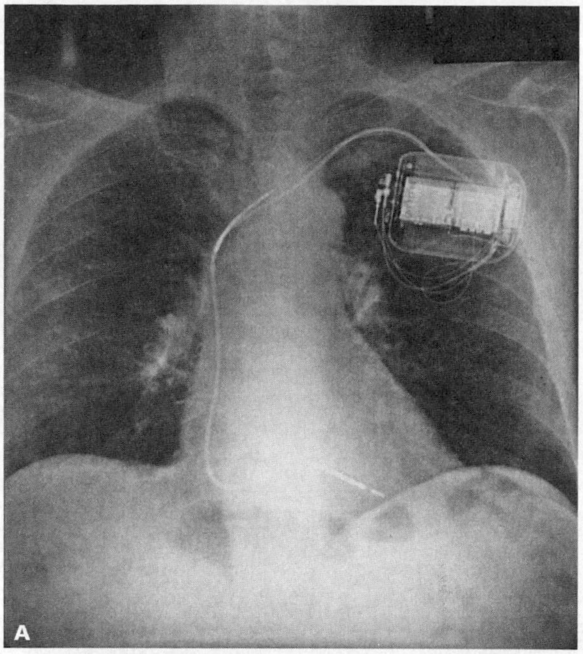

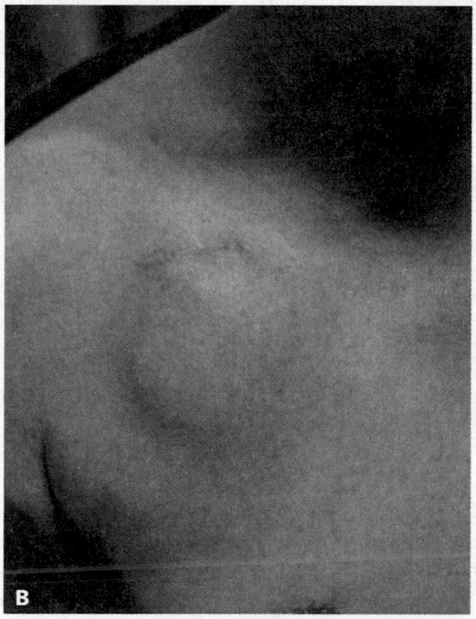

FIGURE 6-10 Implanted defibrillator. **A**. Radiograph. **B**. External view.
Photo A: © American Academy of Orthopaedic Surgeons. Photo B: © Chaikom/Shutterstock.

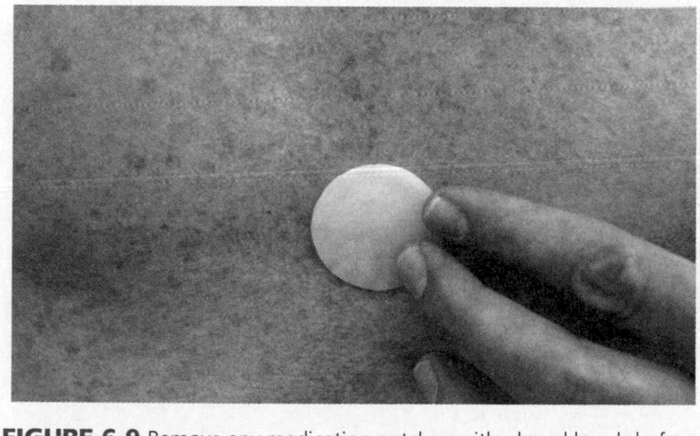

FIGURE 6-9 Remove any medication patches with gloved hands before applying automated external defibrillator pads.
© Van D. Bucher/Science Source.

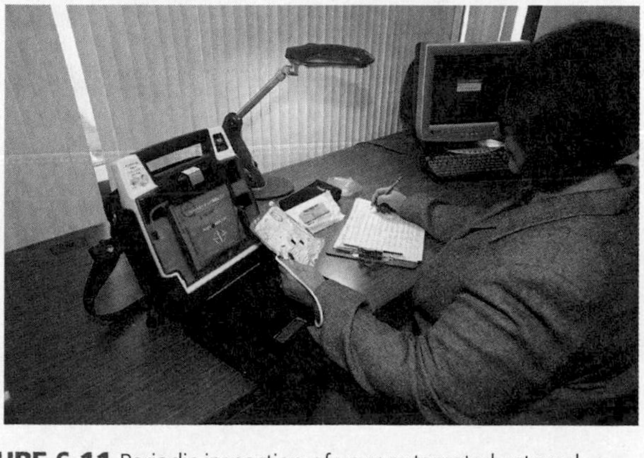

FIGURE 6-11 Periodic inspection of your automated external defibrillator supplies ensures that all items are in working condition.
© American Academy of Orthopaedic Surgeons.

- A razor
- A hand towel
- Mouth-to-barrier device
- Medical exam gloves

CPR and AED Review

TABLE 6-1 provides a review of CPR and AED procedures using the **RAB-CAB** sequence.

TABLE 6-1 Quick Review of CPR and AED Procedures Using the RAB-CAB Procedure

Steps/Action	Adults (at or past puberty)	Child (1 year to puberty)	Infant (younger than 1 year)
R = Responsive?			
Technique	■ Tap a shoulder and shout, "Are you OK?" ■ A person who is responsive will answer, move, or moan.		Tap the bottom of a foot and shout their name.
A = Activate EMS and get an AED.			
When?	■ If you are alone, call 9-1-1 and get an AED. When you return, use the AED. ■ If another person is with you, send them to call and get an AED while you begin CPR.	■ If you are alone, and before calling 9-1-1, give five sets of 30 chest compressions and 2 breaths (CPR). ■ After five sets of CPR, leave the child or infant to call 9-1-1 and get an AED. ■ When you return, use the AED.	
B = Breathing? Check for no breathing or any gasping.			
■ Place person faceup on a flat, firm surface. ■ Take 5 to 10 seconds to observe face and chest (from neck to waist) movement for breathing.	If the person is not breathing or is only occasionally gasping, CPR is needed. If the person is breathing but not responding, CPR is not needed; place the person in the recovery position to keep their airway clear, and monitor breathing.		
C = Chest compressions			
Where to place person?	Firm, flat surface		Can be placed on table or cabinet top
Where to place hands?	Center of chest and lower half of breastbone (sternum)		Pads of two fingers in the center of chest on the breastbone with one touching and both below the imaginary nipple line *or* Place both thumbs on the lower third of the breastbone with both thumbs touching the imaginary nipple line and the fingers encircling around the infant's back and chest.
	Two hands: ■ Heel of one hand on breastbone; other hand on top ■ Fingers of both hands interlocked ■ Arms straight with shoulders directly over the hands	One hand for very small child: Heel of one hand only Two hands: ■ Same as for an adult ■ Arms straight with shoulders directly over the hands	
Depth	At least 2 in. (5 cm) but no more than 2.4 in. (6 cm)	About 2 in. (5 cm) or at least one-third depth of chest	About 1.5 in. (4 cm) or at least one-third depth of chest
	After each compression, allow full recoil of the chest. **DO NOT** lean on the chest of an adult or child.		
Rate	100 to 120 per minute (Follow the beat of the Bee Gees song "Stayin' Alive," the beats from a smartphone application that was previously installed and is quickly accessible, or a dispatcher's directions heard over a mobile phone's speaker.)		
Ratio of chest compressions to breaths	30:2		
A = Airway open			
Technique	Head tilt–chin lift		

<table>
<tr><th>Steps/Action</th><th>Adults (at or past puberty)</th><th>Child (1 year to puberty)</th><th>Infant (younger than 1 year)</th></tr>
<tr><td colspan="4">B = Breaths. Use a CPR mask or face shield for adult, child, or infant when possible.</td></tr>
<tr><td>Technique</td><td colspan="2">■ Pinch the nose shut, and, with your mouth, make an airtight mouth-to-mouth seal.
■ Perform the head tilt–chin lift maneuver.
■ Give two breaths:
• Each breath should last 1 s.
• Blow enough to make the chest rise.

If first breath does not cause chest to rise, retilt head and give second breath. If second breath does not make chest rise, begin CPR (30 compressions and 2 breaths). Each time before giving a breath, open the mouth and look for an object; if seen, remove it.</td><td>Perform the head tilt–chin lift maneuver (DO NOT tilt the head back too far).
■ Cover the infant's mouth and nose with your mouth, making an airtight seal. If this does not work, try either mouth-to-mouth or mouth-to-nose breaths.
■ Give two breaths:
• Each breath should last 1 s.
• Blow enough to make the chest rise.</td></tr>
<tr><td colspan="4">Continue CPR until:
1. The person begins breathing.
2. Replaced by a person of equal or higher training.
3. An AED arrives and is used.
4. You become physically exhausted and unable to continue.
If a bystander is available, they could help by giving chest compressions while you perform rescue breathing, or vice versa.</td></tr>
<tr><td colspan="4">Defibrillation</td></tr>
<tr><td colspan="4">If available, use an AED as soon as possible.
1. Turn on the AED.
2. Attach the pads to the person's bare, dry chest (shown on the pads' diagrams). If needed, plug the cables into the AED. Child-sized pads may be available.
3. Stay clear of the person. Make sure no one, including you, is touching the person. Say, "Clear!"
4. Allow the AED to analyze the heart rhythm (push the Analyze button, if necessary). The AED will prompt one of two actions:
■ Stay clear and press the Shock button.
■ DO NOT shock but give CPR, starting with chest compressions with the pads staying in place.
After any one of the actions, give five sets of CPR unless the person moves, begins to breathe, or wakes up.
Repeat defibrillation steps 3 and 4 until the person moves, begins to breathe, or wakes up, or a person of equal or higher training takes over.</td></tr>
</table>

PREP KIT

Ready for Review

- A person's chances for survival after cardiac arrest improve dramatically with early CPR and early defibrillation.
- Because the heart contracts approximately every second, it needs an abundant supply of oxygen.
- CPR is the initial care for cardiac arrest until a defibrillator is available.
- An AED is an electronic device that analyzes the heart rhythm and prompts the operator to deliver an electrical shock to the heart of a person in cardiac arrest.
- There are several special situations to be aware of when using an AED, including water, children, medication patches, and implanted devices.
- Periodic inspection of the AED can ensure that the device has the necessary supplies and is in proper working condition.

Vital Vocabulary

automated external defibrillator (AED) A device capable of analyzing the heart rhythm and providing a shock.

defibrillation The electrical shock administered by an AED to reestablish a normal heart rhythm.

ventricular fibrillation (VF) A potentially life-threatening electrical condition, in which the heart muscle contracts and relaxes in a disorganized fashion; the lower chambers of the heart quiver and cannot pump blood.

ventricular tachycardia (VT) A potentially life-threatening electrical condition, in which the heart beats too fast to pump blood effectively.

Assessment in Action

Your workplace has recently implemented an AED program. You and several other employees have been trained to locate and use an AED. While at work, a coworker collapses. She is around 50 years old and you know she has a history of heart conditions. You tell a coworker to call 9-1-1 and to bring the AED.

Directions: Circle Yes if you agree with the statement; circle No if you disagree.

1. You should establish unresponsiveness before starting anything else.
   YES NO
2. You should begin chest compressions as soon as possible and stop only to apply the AED pads to the chest or to give two breaths.
   YES NO
3. AED pads can be applied over the top of the person's blouse.
   YES NO
4. The AED will alert you about improper pad placement.
   YES NO
5. You should deliver a shock even if the AED has not alerted you to do so.
   YES NO

Check Your Knowledge

Directions: Circle Yes if you agree with the statement; circle No if you disagree.

1. The earlier defibrillation occurs, the better the person's chance of survival.
   YES NO
2. An AED is to be applied only to a person who is unresponsive and not breathing.
   YES NO
3. CPR is not needed if you are sure an AED will be available in 3 to 4 minutes.
   YES NO
4. AEDs require the operator to know how to interpret heart rhythms.
   YES NO

PREP KIT continued

5. Because all AEDs are different, the basic steps of operation are also different.

   YES NO

6. The AED pads (electrodes) need to be attached to a dry chest.

   YES NO

7. Two electrode pads are placed on the left side of the person's chest.

   YES NO

8. Batteries and pads have expiration dates of which you should be aware.

   YES NO

9. You can still use an AED if an implanted pacemaker is present.

   YES NO

10. You need to turn the AED on daily as part of a routine inspection.

    YES NO

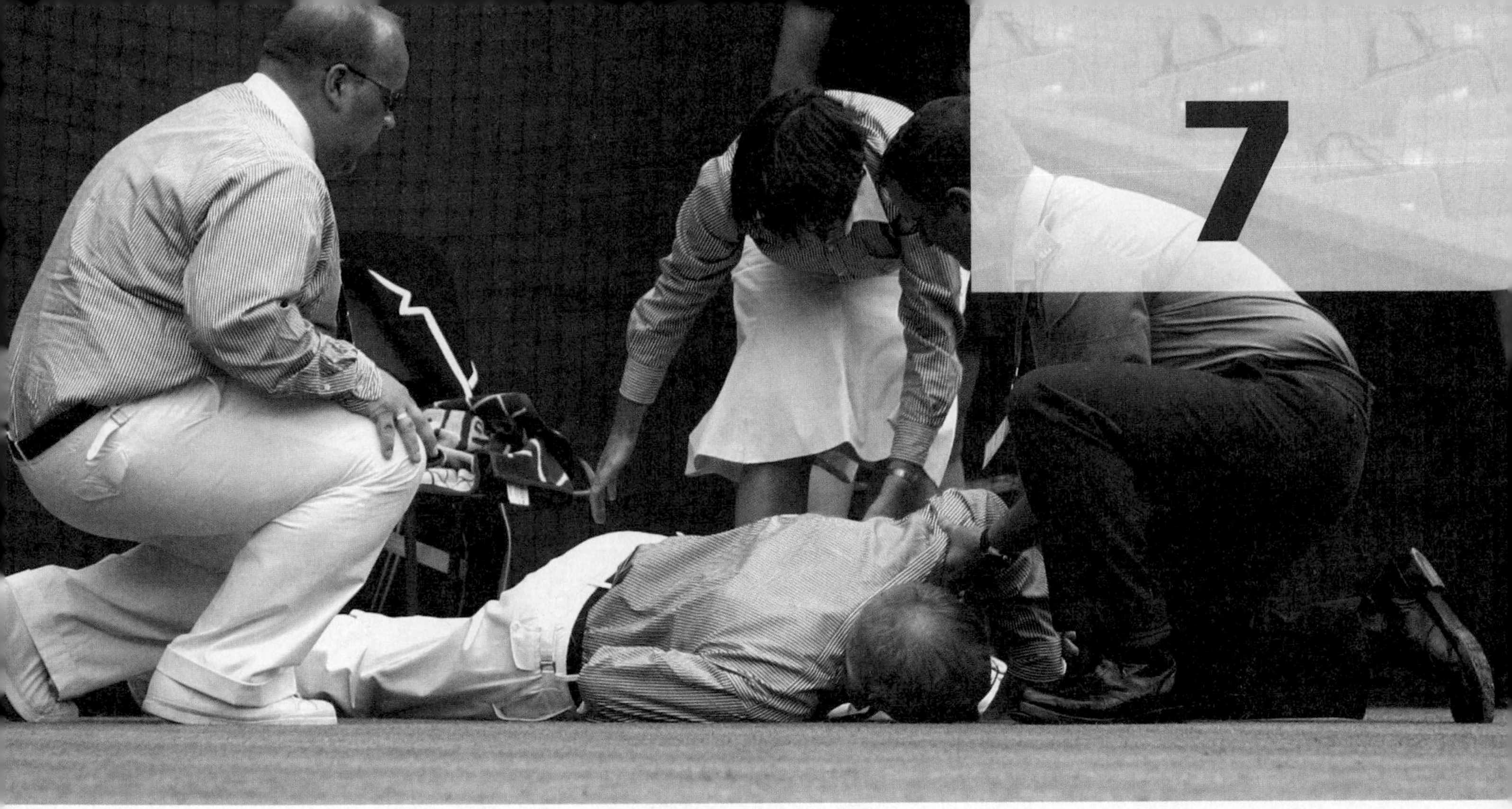

7

Shock

CHAPTER AT A GLANCE

- Shock
- Causes of Shock
- The Progression of Shock
- General Care for Shock
- Care for Anaphylaxis
- Care for Fainting (Psychogenic Shock)

Shock

Shock occurs when the body cells do not receive enough oxygen-rich blood. Do not confuse this type of shock with electric shock or being shocked, as in being scared or surprised. Perfusion is the delivery of blood and oxygen to all of the cells in the body's tissues and organs. **Shock** (hypoperfusion) describes a state of collapse and failure of the cardiovascular system in which blood circulation decreases and eventually ceases. Shock can be associated with a wide variety of conditions—from a heart attack, to major blood loss, to a severe allergic reaction.

Causes of Shock

Understanding the basic physiologic causes of shock will better prepare you to treat it. The damage caused by shock depends on which tissues or organ is deprived of oxygen and for how long. For example, without oxygen, the brain will be irreparably damaged in 4 to 6 minutes, the abdominal organs in 45 to 90 minutes, and the skin and muscle cells in 3 to 6 hours.

To understand shock, think of the cardiovascular system as having three components: a working pump (the heart), a network of pipes (the blood vessels), and an adequate amount of fluid (the blood) pumped through the pipes. Damage to any of these components can

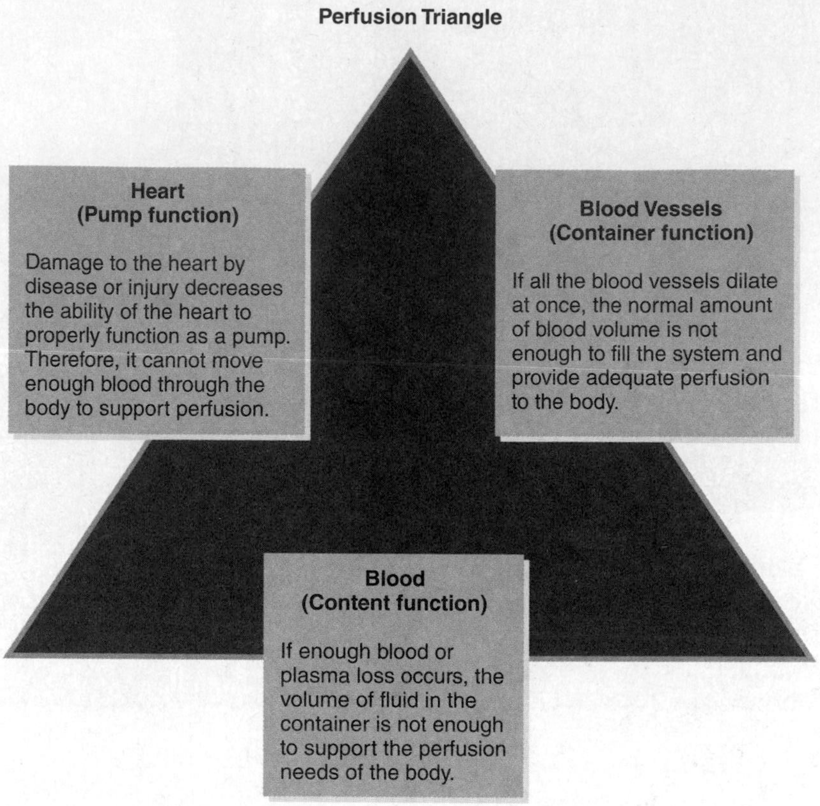
Perfusion Triangle
Heart
(Pump function)
Damage to the heart by disease or injury decreases the ability of the heart to properly function as a pump. Therefore, it cannot move enough blood through the body to support perfusion.
Blood Vessels
(Container function)
If all the blood vessels dilate at once, the normal amount of blood volume is not enough to fill the system and provide adequate perfusion to the body.
Blood
(Content function)
If enough blood or plasma loss occurs, the volume of fluid in the container is not enough to support the perfusion needs of the body.

FIGURE 7-1 The perfusion triangle.

deprive cells of blood and produce shock. These three parts can be referred to as the perfusion triangle **FIGURE 7-1**. When a person is in shock, one or more of the three sides of the triangle is not working properly.

Causes of shock can be both cardiovascular and noncardiovascular. The noncardiovascular causes of shock are respiratory insufficiency, neurogenic shock, **psychogenic shock**, and **anaphylaxis**, an extreme allergic reaction to a foreign substance. There are three major cardiovascular causes of shock, as outlined in **FIGURE 7-2**.

Cardiovascular Causes of Shock

- *Pump failure.* Cardiogenic shock is caused by inadequate function of the heart, or pump failure. Circulation requires the constant pumping action of a normal heart muscle. Many diseases can cause destruction or inflammation of this muscle. The heart can adapt somewhat to these conditions, but if too much muscle damage occurs, as sometimes happens in a heart attack, the heart no longer functions well. The major effect is the backup of blood into the lungs. The resulting buildup of fluid in the lungs is called pulmonary edema.
- *Loss of fluid or blood.* In injuries, shock is most often the result of fluid or blood loss. This type of shock is called hypovolemic (low-volume) shock or hemorrhagic shock. The loss can be due to internal or external bleeding. Hypovolemic shock also occurs with severe thermal burns. Plasma, the fluid portion

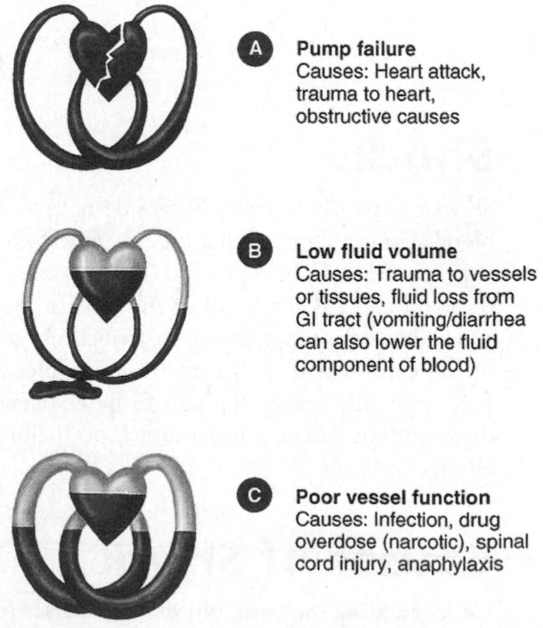
A
Pump failure
Causes: Heart attack, trauma to heart, obstructive causes
B
Low fluid volume
Causes: Trauma to vessels or tissues, fluid loss from GI tract (vomiting/diarrhea can also lower the fluid component of blood)
C
Poor vessel function
Causes: Infection, drug overdose (narcotic), spinal cord injury, anaphylaxis

FIGURE 7-2 There are three basic cardiovascular causes of shock and the resulting impaired tissue perfusion. **A.** Pump failure occurs when the heart is damaged by disease, injury, or obstructive causes. The heart may not generate enough force to move the blood through the system. **B.** Low fluid volume, often a result of bleeding or in other cases severe sweating, leads to inadequate perfusion. A common cause of low fluid volume is fluid loss in the gastrointestinal (GI) tract. **C.** The blood vessels can dilate excessively so that the blood within them, even though it is of normal volume, is inadequate to fill the system and provide efficient perfusion.

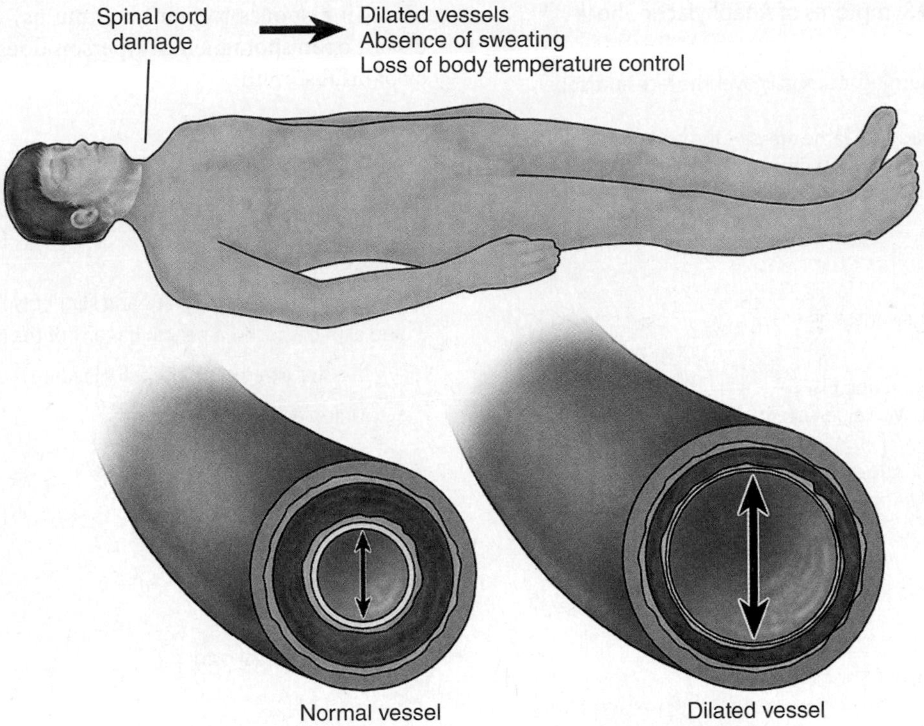

FIGURE 7-3 Neurogenic shock.

of the blood, leaks from the cardiovascular system into burned tissues. Dehydration aggravates shock. In all these circumstances, the common factor is an insufficient volume of blood within the vascular system to provide adequate perfusion to the tissues.

- *Poor vessel function.* Spinal cord damage can injure the part of the nervous system that controls blood vessel size and muscle tone. This can cause cardiovascular failure and widespread blood vessel dilation, known as **neurogenic shock**. Cut off from their impulses to contract, muscles in the blood vessels dilate (relax) widely, increasing the size and capacity of the vascular system. The blood in the body can no longer fill the enlarged vessels **FIGURE 7-3**.
- *Combined vessel and content failure.* Septic shock is seen in people who have severe bacterial infections that produce toxins (poisons). The toxins damage the vessel walls, causing them to become leaky and unable to contract. Widespread vessel dilation, combined with the loss of plasma through injured vessel walls, results in shock. Infections that result in septic shock can be associated with serious illness, injury, or surgery.

Noncardiovascular Causes of Shock

- *Respiratory insufficiency.* A severe chest injury or an airway obstruction can make a person unable to breathe adequately. Insufficient oxygen in the blood can produce shock as rapidly as vascular causes, even when cardiovascular function is normal. Circulation of nonoxygenated blood will not benefit the person.
- *Anaphylactic shock.* Anaphylaxis, or anaphylactic shock, occurs when the immune system reacts violently to a substance to which it has already been sensitized. Severe allergic reactions commonly follow exposure to one of the following:
  - Medications (penicillin and related drugs, aspirin, sulfa drugs)
  - Food (shellfish, nuts—especially peanuts, eggs)
  - Insect stings (honeybee, wasp, yellow jacket, hornet, fire ant)

  Anaphylactic reactions can develop in minutes or even seconds after contact with the substance to which a person is sensitized. The signs of such allergic reactions are distinct from those of other forms of shock. **TABLE 7-1** shows the signs and symptoms of anaphylactic shock.

  In anaphylactic shock, although there is no loss of blood, no vascular damage, and only a slight possibility of cardiac muscular injury, the widespread vascular dilation causes poor oxygenation and poor perfusion of tissues, which can easily cause death.
- *Psychogenic shock.* Psychogenic shock is a sudden nervous system reaction that produces a temporary vascular dilation, resulting in fainting, or syncope. Blood pools in the dilated vessels, reducing the blood supply to the brain, and the person becomes unresponsive. Causes of fainting (psychogenic shock) include fear, bad news, or unpleasant sights, such as the sight of blood.

TABLE 7-1 Signs and Symptoms of Anaphylactic Shock

Skin
■ Flushing, itching, or burning, especially over the face and upper chest
■ Hives, which can spread over large areas of the body
■ Swelling, especially of the face, tongue, and lips
■ Blue discoloration around lips and mouth (cyanosis)
Cardiovascular System
■ Rapid pulse
■ Dizziness
■ Fainting and unresponsiveness
Respiratory System
■ Sneezing or itching in the nostrils
■ Tightness in the chest, with a persistent, dry cough
■ Breathing difficulty
■ Secretions of fluid and mucus into the throat and lungs
■ Wheezing
■ Breathing stoppage

TABLE 7-2 Progression of Shock

Compensated Shock
■ Agitation
■ Anxiety
■ Restlessness
■ Feeling of impending doom
■ Altered mental status (verbal on AVPU scale)
■ Clammy (pale, cool, moist) skin
■ Paleness, with cyanosis about the lips
■ Shallow, rapid breathing
■ Shortness of breath
■ Nausea or vomiting
■ Capillary refill longer than 2 seconds in infants and children
■ Thirst
Decompensated Shock
■ Difficulty breathing
■ Ashen, mottled, or cyanotic skin
■ Dull eyes, dilated pupils
■ Altered mental state (P on AVPU scale)
■ Unresponsive (U on AVPU scale

The Progression of Shock

Although shock itself cannot be seen, you can see its signs and symptoms progress **TABLE 7-2**. The early stage of shock, when the body can still compensate for blood loss, is called compensated shock. The late stage, when blood pressure is falling, is decompensated shock. The final stage, when shock is terminal, is called irreversible shock. Even transfusion may not save the person's life at this point. The AVPU scale can be used to measure responsiveness in a person experiencing shock. In this system you check if a person is alert (aware and can respond to their surrounding environment), verbally responsive (eyes do not open spontaneously, but open in response to verbal stimulus), painfully responsive (eyes do not open spontaneously, person responds by moving, moaning, or making noise in response to painful stimulus), or unresponsive (eyes do not open spontaneously, person does not respond to verbal or painful stimuli).

FYI

Red Flags for Shock

Shock is seen in both injured and suddenly ill people. Anticipate and expect shock if a person has any of the following conditions:

- Massive external or internal bleeding
- Multiple severe fractures
- An abdominal or chest injury
- A severe infection
- Any signs of a heart attack
- Anaphylaxis
- Severe burns
- Severed spinal cord

General Care for Shock

Automatically treat any injured person for shock, because every injury affects the cardiovascular system to some degree. Shock is one of the most common causes of death in an injured person. Provide care for shock even if an injured person does not have signs or symptoms of shock. You can prevent shock from getting worse, but you cannot reverse it.

Refer to **FLOWCHART 7-1** for additional information regarding the care of a person in shock.

What to Look For	What to Do
Injuries	Treat the injuries.
Responsive and breathing normally	▪ Keep the person flat (horizontal) on their back. ▪ If there is no sign of a leg injury and it does not cause pain feet can be raised 6 to 12 inches (15 to 30 cm) **FIGURE 7-4**. ▪ **DO NOT** give anything to eat or drink unless medical help is delayed over 1 hour, in which case, sips of water can be given if fluids do not cause nausea and/or vomiting.
Unresponsive and breathing	▪ Roll the person onto their side (recovery position; see pages 48–49). **DO NOT** roll the person if there is a neck, back, hip, or pelvic injury; leave in the position found unless it is unsafe. ▪ Call 9-1-1. ▪ Prevent heat loss by putting blankets or coats under and over the person.

Flowchart 7-1 Shock

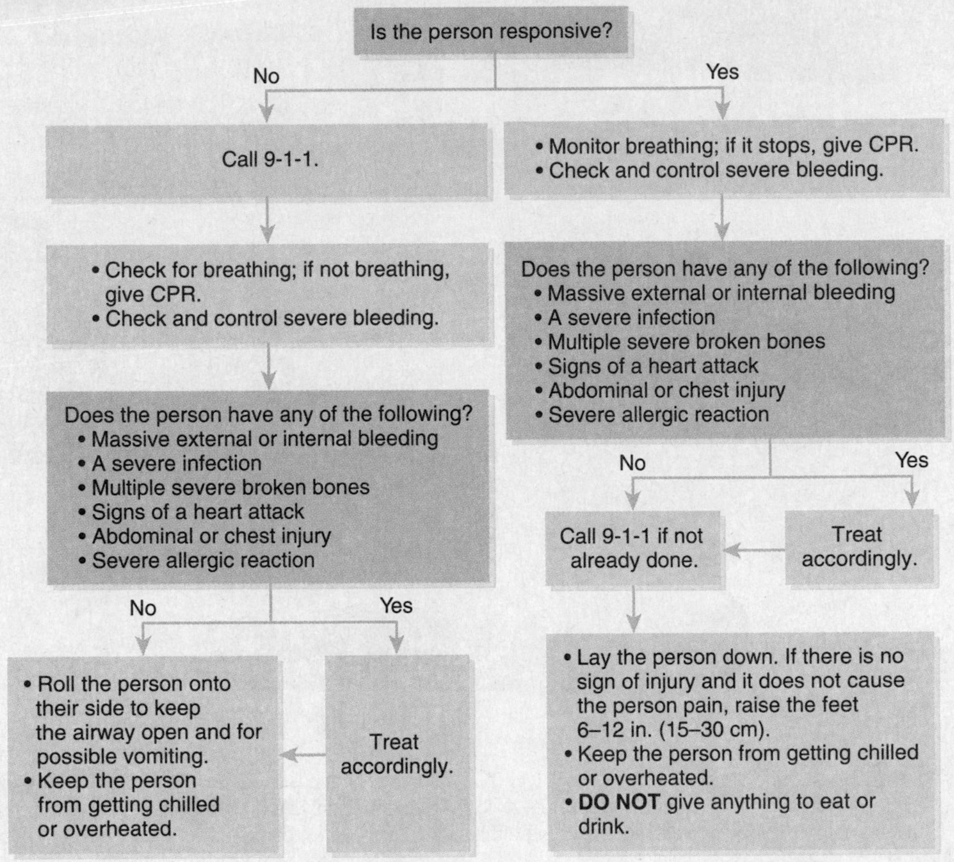
Is the person responsive?
No
Yes
Call 9-1-1.
• Monitor breathing; if it stops, give CPR.
• Check and control severe bleeding.
• Check for breathing; if not breathing, give CPR.
• Check and control severe bleeding.
Does the person have any of the following?
• Massive external or internal bleeding
• A severe infection
• Multiple severe broken bones
• Signs of a heart attack
• Abdominal or chest injury
• Severe allergic reaction
Does the person have any of the following?
• Massive external or internal bleeding
• A severe infection
• Multiple severe broken bones
• Signs of a heart attack
• Abdominal or chest injury
• Severe allergic reaction
No
Yes
Call 9-1-1 if not already done.
Treat accordingly.
No
Yes
• Roll the person onto their side to keep the airway open and for possible vomiting.
• Keep the person from getting chilled or overheated.
Treat accordingly.
• Lay the person down. If there is no sign of injury and it does not cause the person pain, raise the feet 6–12 in. (15–30 cm).
• Keep the person from getting chilled or overheated.
• DO NOT give anything to eat or drink.

Q&A

What is the optimal position for a person in shock? Does elevating the legs improve outcome?

Most people who have experienced an injury or sudden illness should not be moved. However, first aid providers are often taught to raise the feet of people whom they suspect to be in shock. The theory is that doing so will return blood volume to the person's central circulation, thus raising cardiac output and blood pressure. While raising the feet 6 to 12 inches (15 to 30 cm) can be beneficial in some cases (eg, fainting, dehydration, heat exhaustion), the evidence is mixed on the effects of leg elevation, and no studies demonstrate improved outcome in the medical literature. Elevating the legs of a person with a pelvic or lower extremity injury may worsen the person's outcome. Therefore, the legs should not be raised if a leg is injured or if moving an injured leg causes pain.

CAUTION

DO NOT place people with breathing difficulties, chest injuries, penetrating eye injuries, or heart attacks on their backs. Place them in a half-sitting position or position of comfort.

DO NOT give the person anything to eat or drink. It could cause nausea and vomiting. It could also cause complications if surgery is needed.

DO NOT lift the foot of a bed or stretcher. Lifting the end of the bed or stretcher (Trendelenburg position) moves internal organs against the diaphragm and can affect breathing.

DO NOT raise the legs of a person with head injuries, stroke, chest injuries, or breathing difficulty, or those of a person in whom a heart attack is suspected.

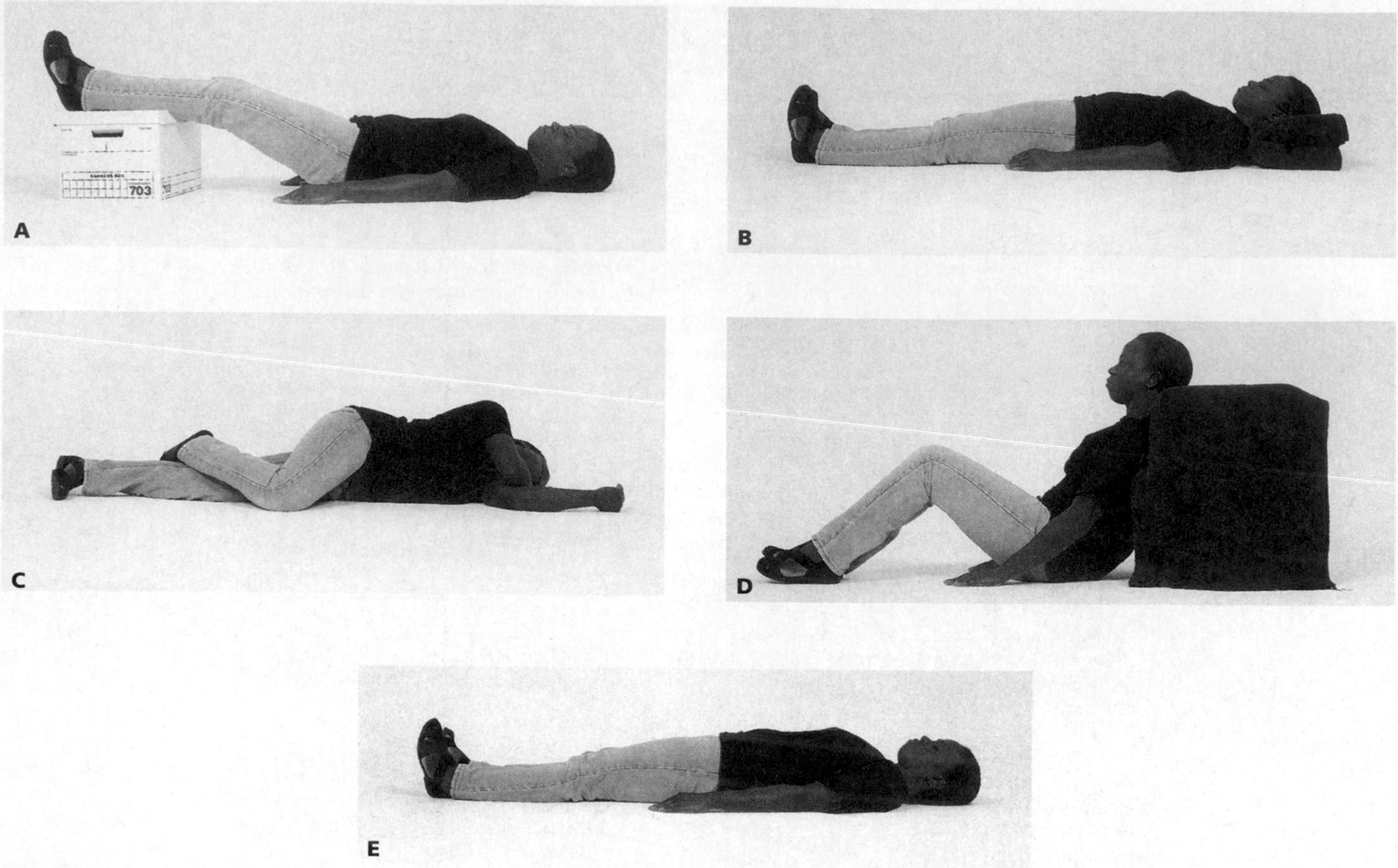

FIGURE 7-4 Shock positions. **A**. Feet can be raised 6 to 12 inches (15 to 30 cm) if it does not cause pain or if the legs or pelvis are not injured. **B**. For a person with head injury, elevate the head (if spinal injury is not suspected). **C**. Position a person who is unresponsive or has experienced a stroke in the recovery position. **D**. Use a half-sitting position for people with breathing difficulties, chest injuries, or a heart attack. **E**. Keep the person flat if a spinal injury or leg fracture is suspected.

Q&A

When can a person be moved?

DO NOT move a person unless necessary. This is especially true for a person whose spine might be injured. People can be moved in the following circumstances:

- When hazards exist (eg, burning building, potential explosion, hazardous materials, vehicular traffic, landslide, avalanche), you can move the person to a safer area.
- When a person is facing downward (prone position) and is unresponsive, you can roll the person to face upward (supine position).
- When a person is having breathing difficulty due to vomit or other body fluids (eg, blood) or when you are alone and must leave an unresponsive person to get help, you can place the person in the recovery position. Roll the body, as a single unit, until the person is on their side. Support the head by resting it on the extended arm.
- When shock becomes apparent, keep the person in a supine position. The feet can be raised about 6 to 12 inches (15 to 30 cm) if there are no injuries. If pain occurs while moving or positioning the person, do not raise the feet.

Data from Markenson D, et al. Part 13: First aid: 2010 consensus on first aid science. *Circulation* 2010;122(suppl):S532–S605.

Care for Anaphylaxis

Many people have allergies and react to certain triggers (eg, certain foods, certain medicines, insect stings, latex). When they come into contact with these triggers, they can develop such symptoms such as sneezing, a stuffy or runny nose, and itchy eyes, nose, or skin.

When the body overreacts to allergy triggers and releases chemicals to protect itself, a severe allergic reaction occurs called anaphylaxis. Anaphylaxis happens quickly and can be life threatening.

Epinephrine is a medication that can stop anaphylaxis. This medication is available with a physician's prescription and can be self-administered via an **epinephrine auto-injector**

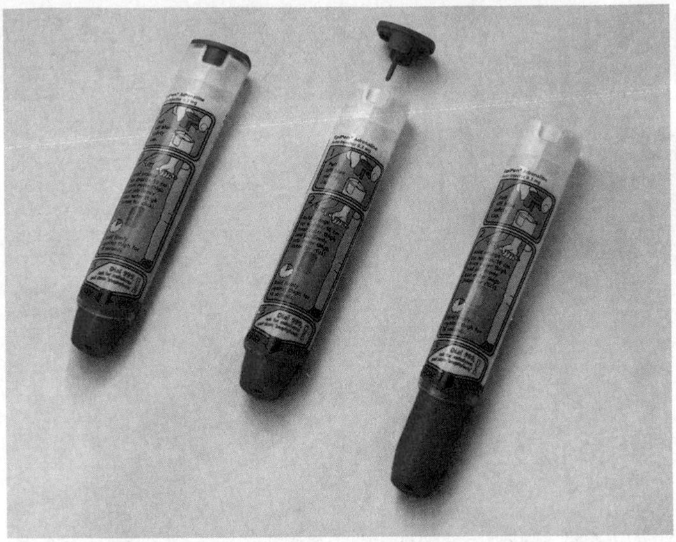

FIGURE 7-5 Epinephrine auto-injector. Left, EpiPen intact before use; Center, blue safety cap removed; Right, after injection, the orange cover automatically extends to ensure the needle is never exposed.

FIGURE 7-5. It is highly recommended that two such auto-injectors be available to those with a past or potential anaphylactic emergency (such as a past reaction to Novocain in a dentist's office). Replacements should be obtained once the device's expiration date occurs or the device is empty.

Most allergic reactions do not require epinephrine, but a small portion of reactions can progress to life-threatening anaphylaxis.

Antihistamines such as Benadryl are not lifesaving because they take too long to work, but they are helpful for mild allergic reactions (eg, seasonal allergies).

Always suspect anaphylaxis if a person shows signs of a severe allergic reaction within minutes or even seconds of eating, taking medicine, or being stung by an insect. However, anaphylaxis can also occur up to an hour or more after exposure to an allergen.

Refer to **FLOWCHART 7-2** for additional information regarding the care of a person with anaphylaxis.

Care for Fainting (Psychogenic Shock)

In most cases of fainting, once the person collapses and is lying down, blood circulation to the brain is restored and responsiveness usually returns. Refer to Fainting on pages 256–258 for what to look for and what to do.

What to Look For	What to Do
Severe allergic reaction (anaphylaxis): ▪ Mouth: swelling of the lips, tongue, mouth, nose ▪ Throat: swelling, itching, difficulty swallowing and speaking ▪ Skin: swelling around the eyes, flushing, severe itching, hives ▪ Breathing: trouble breathing, coughing, or wheezing (whistling sound during breathing) ▪ Abdomen: cramps, nausea, vomiting ▪ Unresponsive ▪ Medical identification tag	**1.** Call 9-1-1 immediately. It is important seek professional medical care or go to the emergency department even after successfully using an auto-injector because the effects of epinephrine will wear off. **2.** Ask about any previous severe allergic reactions. **3.** Look or ask about a medical identification tag. **4.** If the person has their own medically prescribed epinephrine auto-injector, they will usually know when and how to use it. If the person asks for help and your state law allows giving an injection, use their prescribed auto-injector **SKILL SHEET 7-1**. ▪ If there is not an epinephrine auto-injector available, use an asthma inhaler or nasal decongestant spray. If the person can swallow, give an antihistamine (eg, Benadryl). These are not lifesaving because they take too long to work, but they can help prevent further reactions. Monitor until professional medical care arrives. ▪ After administering an epinephrine auto-injector stay with the person and continue to reassure and monitor them until EMS arrives. **5. DO NOT** inject another dose right after the first one. Wait 5 to 10 minutes. **6.** If the person does not get better 5 to 10 minutes after the first dose *or* the EMS arrival will exceed 5 to 10 minutes, consider giving a second dose if you have a second injector. About 20% of people receiving a first dose will require a second dose. When in doubt, administer a second dose. **7.** If there are no signs of breathing, call 9-1-1 if not already done and begin CPR. See Chapter 5, *CPR*.
Mild allergic reaction: ▪ Red, itchy eyes ▪ Itchy, sneezing, stuffy, or runny nose ▪ Rash on skin, itching, usually on one part of body	Help the person: ▪ Self-administer their asthma rescue inhaler, and/or ▪ Take an antihistamine.

Flowchart 7-2 Anaphylaxis

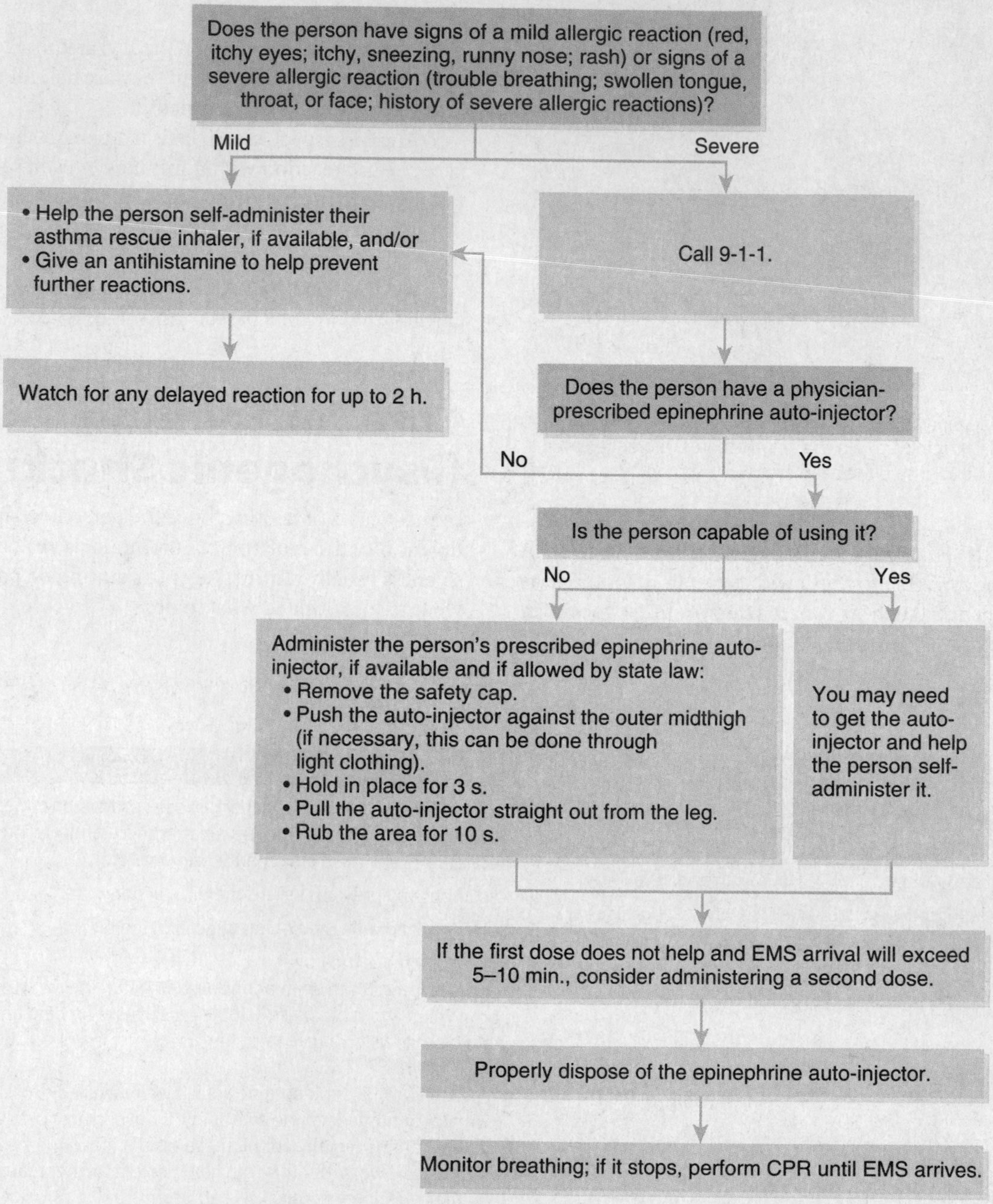
Does the person have signs of a mild allergic reaction (red, itchy eyes; itchy, sneezing, runny nose; rash) or signs of a severe allergic reaction (trouble breathing; swollen tongue, throat, or face; history of severe allergic reactions)?
Mild
Severe
• Help the person self-administer their asthma rescue inhaler, if available, and/or
• Give an antihistamine to help prevent further reactions.
Watch for any delayed reaction for up to 2 h.
Call 9-1-1.
Does the person have a physician-prescribed epinephrine auto-injector?
No
Yes
Is the person capable of using it?
No
Yes
Administer the person's prescribed epinephrine auto-injector, if available and if allowed by state law:
• Remove the safety cap.
• Push the auto-injector against the outer midthigh (if necessary, this can be done through light clothing).
• Hold in place for 3 s.
• Pull the auto-injector straight out from the leg.
• Rub the area for 10 s.
You may need to get the auto-injector and help the person self-administer it.
If the first dose does not help and EMS arrival will exceed 5–10 min., consider administering a second dose.
Properly dispose of the epinephrine auto-injector.
Monitor breathing; if it stops, perform CPR until EMS arrives.

SKILL SHEET 7-1 Using an Epinephrine Auto-injector

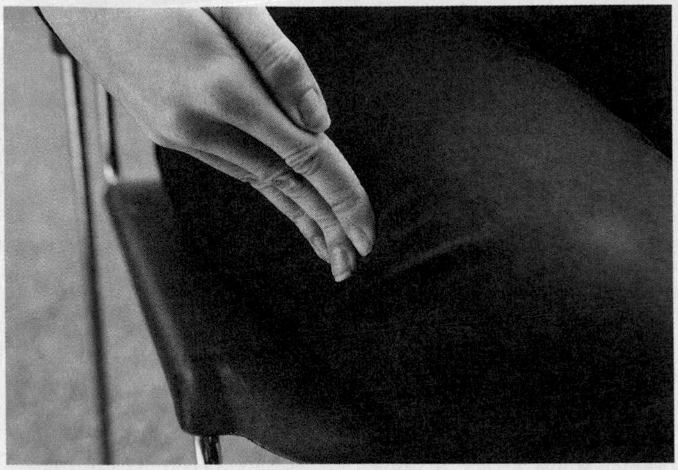

© Jones & Bartlett Learning.

1 Find the injection site on the outer side of the person's midthigh, halfway between the knee and the hip. Removing clothing is not necessary because the needle can go through thin clothing. Check for coins, keys, and pant seams, which could obstruct the needle.

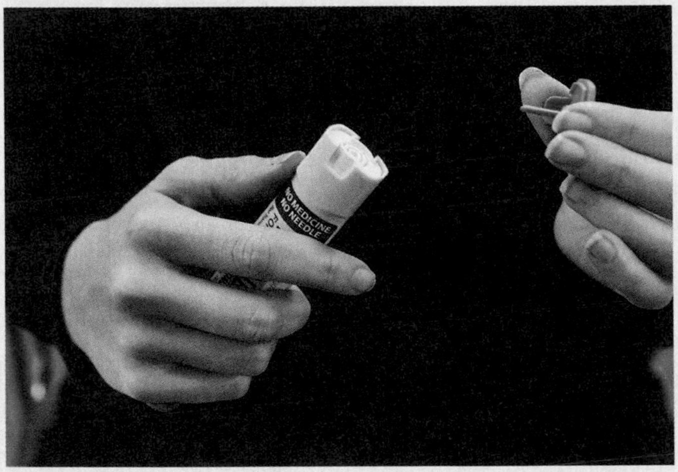

© Jones & Bartlett Learning.

2 Take the auto-injector out of its package and remove the safety cap by pulling it straight out. Hold the auto-injector in your fist without touching either end of the pen, with the tip pointing downward. Depending on the type of auto-injector, the tip may be orange (EpiPen), black (Auvi-Q), red (Adrenaclick), or another color.

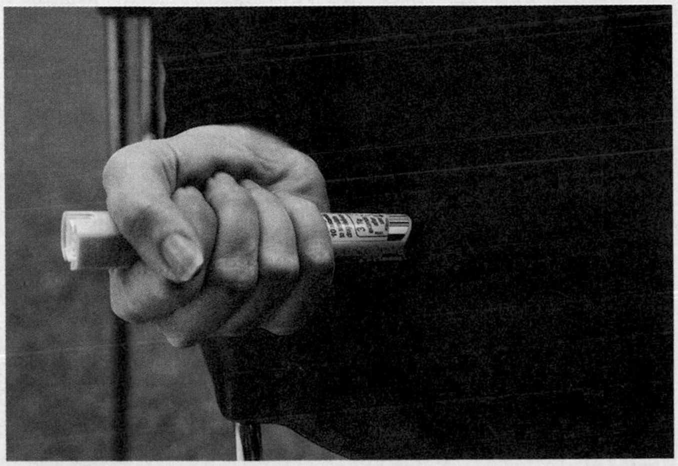

© Jones & Bartlett Learning.

3 While holding the leg firmly in place, push the auto-injector firmly against the thigh until you hear a click. Hold in place for about 3 seconds.

4 Pull the auto-injector straight out from the leg. Rub the injection site for about 10 seconds.

5 Put the auto-injector back into its safety case, and give it to EMS when they arrive.

PREP KIT

Ready for Review

- Shock is a state of collapse and failure of the cardiovascular system in which blood circulation decreases and eventually ceases.
- The damage caused by shock depends on which organ is deprived of oxygen and for how long.
- Causes of shock can be both cardiovascular and noncardiovascular.
- Anaphylaxis occurs when the immune system reacts violently to a substance to which it has already been sensitized.
- Although shock itself cannot be seen, you can see the progression of its signs and symptoms.
- First aid providers should automatically treat people for shock.

Vital Vocabulary

anaphylaxis A life-threatening allergic reaction.

epinephrine auto-injector A prescribed device used to administer an emergency dose of epinephrine to a person experiencing anaphylaxis.

neurogenic shock Cardiovascular failure caused by paralysis of the nerves that control the size of the blood vessels, leading to widespread dilation; seen in people with spinal cord injuries.

psychogenic shock A sudden nervous system reaction that produces a temporary vascular dilation, resulting in fainting, or syncope.

shock Inadequate tissue perfusion resulting from serious injury or illness.

Assessment in Action

You are walking up a popular canyon trail on a cool fall afternoon. You hear someone call for help farther up the trail, near a cliff. You jog up the trail and find a hiker bent over another person at the base of a cliff. The hiker says the person lying motionless fell about 20 feet (6 m) while climbing the cliff with no ropes or harness. There are no obvious signs of injury. The person appears to be breathing, and no serious bleeding is seen.

Directions: Circle Yes if you agree with the statement; circle No if you disagree.

1. You should suspect spinal injury.

YES **NO**

2. Do not allow the person to move or attempt to move if a spinal injury is suspected.

YES **NO**

3. You should offer the person something to eat and drink.

YES **NO**

4. There is no need to seek professional medical care for this situation.

YES **NO**

Check Your Knowledge

Directions: Circle Yes if you agree with the statement; circle No if you disagree.

1. Place all people with severe injuries in the recovery position.

YES **NO**

2. Prevent the loss of body heat by putting blankets under and over the person.

YES **NO**

3. A person in shock with possible spinal injuries should be placed in a seated position.

YES **NO**

4. A person in shock with breathing difficulty or chest injury should be placed on their back.

YES **NO**

5. Anxiety and restlessness can be signs of shock.

YES **NO**

6. An epinephrine auto-injector can be used for people experiencing anaphylaxis.

YES **NO**

PREP KIT continued

7. All people with severe injuries or illnesses should be treated for shock.

YES **NO**

8. Treat people with severe injuries for shock even if there are no signs of it.

YES **NO**

9. Anaphylaxis is a life-threatening condition.

YES **NO**

10. People in shock have hot skin.

YES **NO**

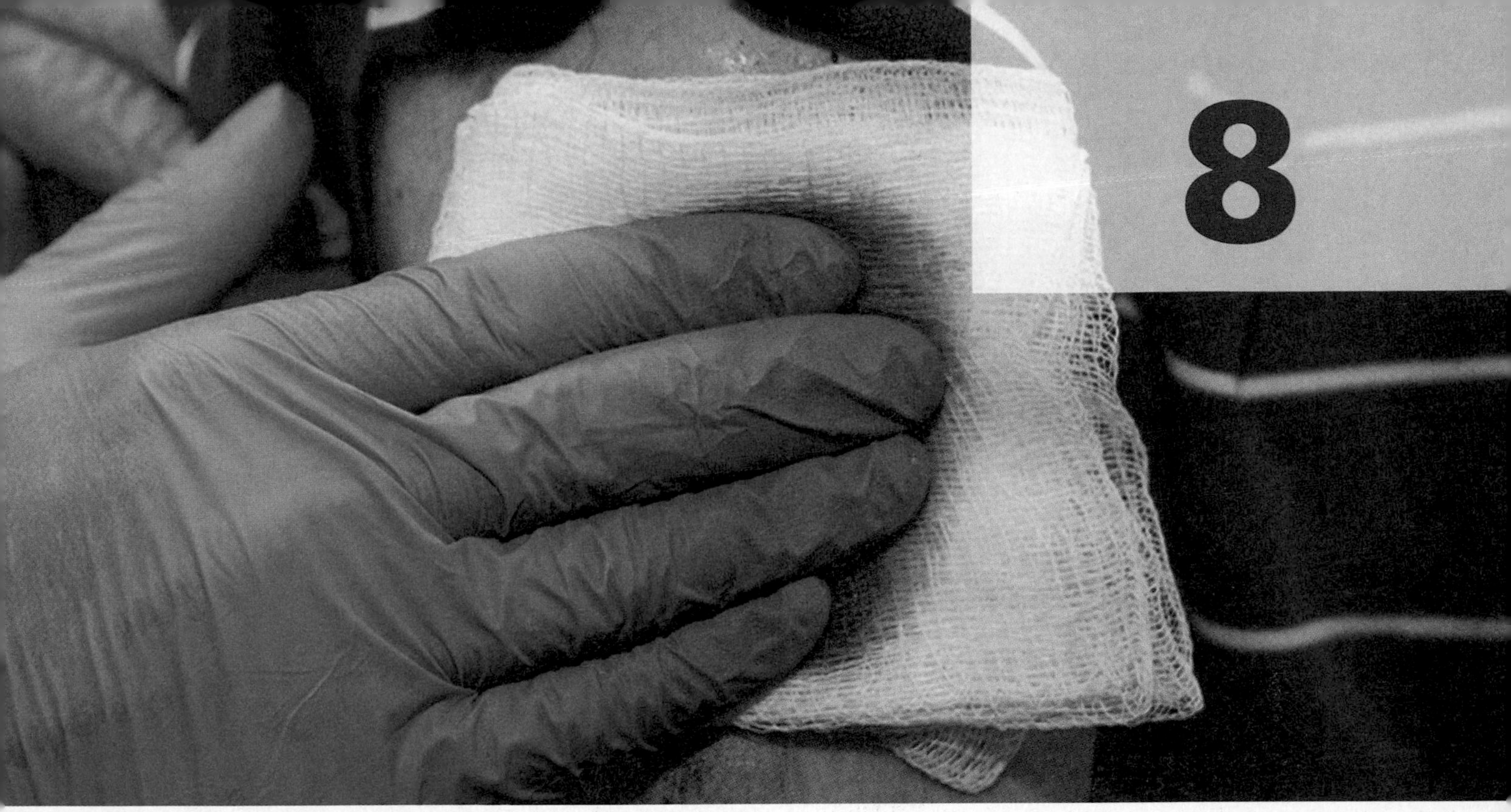

8

Bleeding

CHAPTER AT A GLANCE

Bleeding

An average-size adult has 5 to 6 quarts (about 5 to 6 L) of blood and can safely donate one-half quart (0.5 L). However, rapid blood loss of 1 quart (about 1 L) or more can lead to shock and death. A child who has lost one-half quart (0.5 L) of blood is in extreme danger.

External Bleeding

External bleeding refers to blood coming from an open wound. The term **hemorrhage** refers to a large amount of bleeding in a short time and can be life-threatening. External bleeding can be classified into three types, according to the type of blood vessel that is damaged: an artery, a vein, or a capillary **FIGURE 8-1**.

In **arterial bleeding**, initially blood spurts (up to several feet) from the wound. Arterial bleeding is the most serious type of bleeding because a large amount of blood loss can occur in a very short time. This type of bleeding does not clot well because the high flow of the blood reduces the ability of a clot to adhere to the damaged vessel.

In **venous bleeding**, blood from a vein flows steadily or gushes. Venous bleeding is easier to control than arterial bleeding. Even though small cuts bleed a lot at first, by the time you treat a bleeding person,

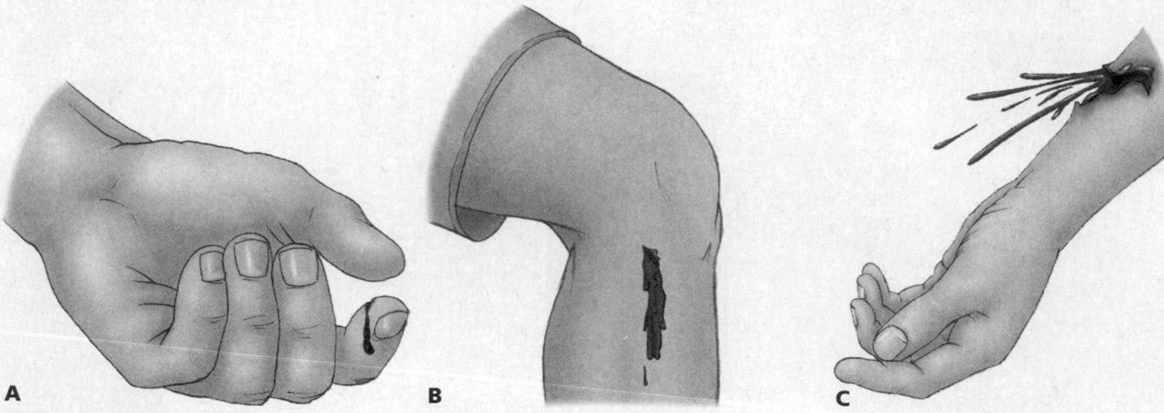

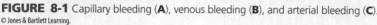

FIGURE 8-1 Capillary bleeding (**A**), venous bleeding (**B**), and arterial bleeding (**C**).

most bleeding will have already slowed or stopped. Most veins collapse when cut. Bleeding from deep veins, however, can be as massive and as hard to control as arterial bleeding.

In **capillary bleeding**, the most common type of bleeding, blood oozes from capillaries. It usually is not serious and can be controlled easily. Quite often, this type of bleeding will clot and stop by itself.

Each type of blood vessel—artery, vein, or capillary—contains blood of a different shade of red. An inexperienced person may have difficulty detecting the color difference but would still be able to identify the type of bleeding by its flow. The body naturally responds to bleeding in the following ways:

- *Blood vessel spasm.* Arteries contain small amounts of muscle tissue in their walls. If a blood vessel is completely severed, it draws back into the tissue, constricts its diameter, and slows the bleeding dramatically. If an artery is only partially cut across its diameter, however, constriction is incomplete. The vessel may not contract, and the loss of blood may not slow as dramatically.
- *Clotting.* Special elements in blood, called platelets, form a clot. Clotting serves as a protective covering for a wound until the tissues underneath can repair themselves. In a healthy person, initial clot formation normally takes about 10 minutes. Clotting time is longer in people who have a great deal of blood loss over a prolonged time, are taking aspirin or anticoagulants, are anemic, or have hemophilia or severe liver disease.

An alert and responsive person can often tell and show where they are bleeding. Ask the person, "Are you bleeding?" Look for wet spots on clothing, which may be blood. Thick clothing may hide visible traces of blood, but severe bleeding can soak through clothing and appear on its surface. For an unresponsive, injured person, you may also need to feel for blood; be sure to wear medical exam gloves when doing so. Blood's stickiness will differentiate it from other fluids.

Q&A

What are the largest artery and the largest vein in the human body?

The aorta is the largest artery in the human body. In adults, it is about the size of a garden hose. Its internal diameter is 1 inch (2.5 cm) and its wall is 0.0790 inch (0.2 cm) thick.

The largest vein in the human body is the inferior vena cava, the vein that returns blood from the lower half of the body back to the heart.

CAUTION

DO NOT come in contact with blood with your bare hands. Protect yourself with medical exam gloves, extra gauze pads, or clean cloths, or have the injured person apply direct pressure. After the bleeding has stopped and the wound has been cared for, vigorously wash your hands with soap and water.

DO NOT use direct pressure on an eye injury, a wound with an embedded object, or a skull fracture.

Dressings and Tourniquets

A dressing directly touches and covers an open wound **FIGURE 8-2**. A **hemostatic gauze dressing** is a special type of dressing that is stuffed or packed into a wound to help clot the blood **FIGURE 8-3** (more on how to use these later). Whenever possible, a dressing should be sterile, larger than the wound, thick, soft and compressible, and lint-free. A bandage holds the dressing in place over an open wound. A bandage is used to apply pressure to control bleeding. It also prevents or reduces swelling and provides stability for an extremity or joint. Direct pressure stops most bleeding.

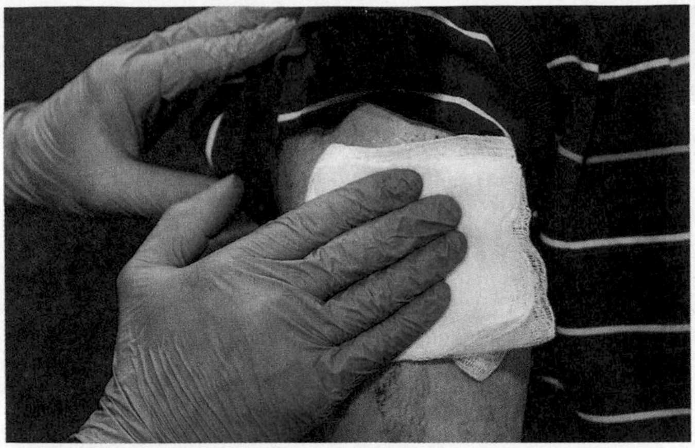

FIGURE 8-2 Dressing.

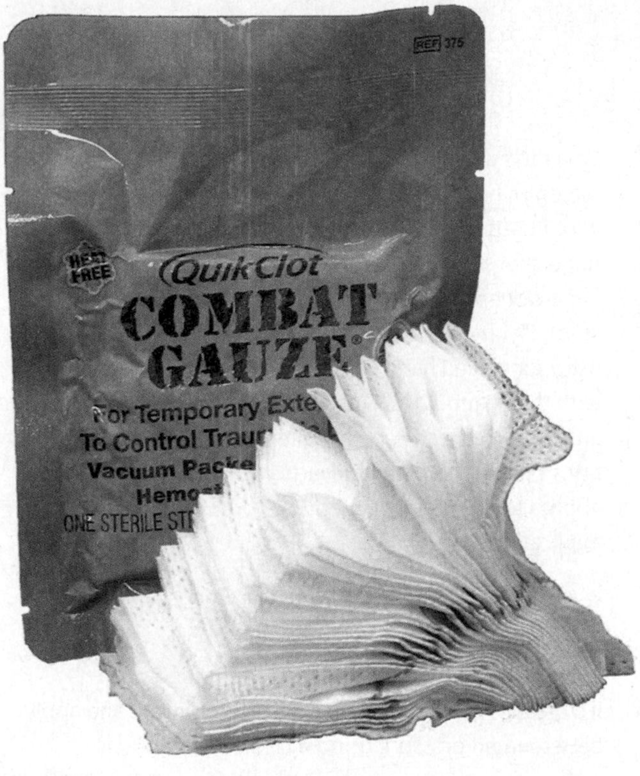

FIGURE 8-3 Hemostatic gauze dressings.

If bleeding does not stop with direct pressure, a tourniquet may be needed. A **tourniquet** is a device that is wrapped tightly around an extremity to stop blood flow **FIGURE 8-4**. It may be manufactured or improvised.

External Bleeding Control

Many different types of injuries may involve blood, so it is important to know how to control bleeding. In some cases, the first aid provider should consider massive bleeding control before airway management.

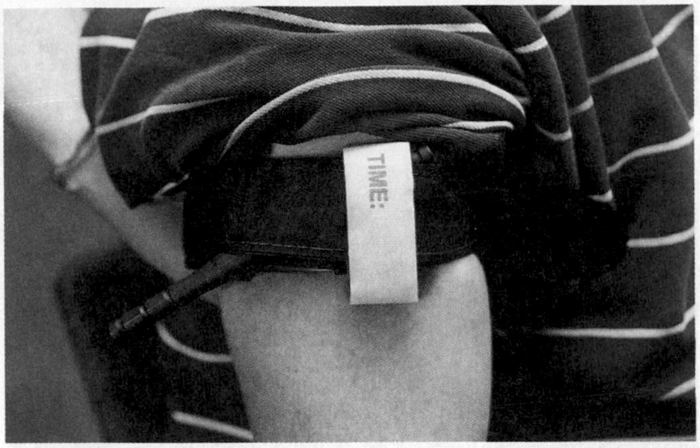

FIGURE 8-4 Tourniquet.

Examples of life-threatening bleeding include the following:

- Blood spurting out of a wound
- Blood-soaked clothing
- Blood pooling on the ground
- Arm or leg partially or completely amputated

To control bleeding, take the following steps and see **SKILL SHEET 8-1**:

1. Find the source of bleeding and, if necessary, remove or cut the clothing to see it.
2. Depending on the size of the wound and amount of bleeding, place a sterile gauze pad or a clean cloth (eg, handkerchief, washcloth, towel) over the entire wound. If the wound is large and deep, try to "stuff" the cloth down into the wound (further directions for controlling massive bleeding are discussed later).
3. For small wounds, apply well-aimed direct pressure with your fingers. For large wounds, apply pressure with the palm of one or both hands. Dressings that quickly become blood-soaked indicate that adequate pressure has not been applied to the bleeding site. Simply adding more dressings on top of the wound will not help control bleeding. If a dressing becomes blood-soaked, remove it and apply better aimed pressure with a clean dressing. No evidence exists that removing a blood-soaked dressing will dislodge any clot that has formed or cause the clotting to start over. Direct pressure stops most bleeding—even major arterial bleeding. **DO NOT** apply pressure on an eye injury, an embedded object, or a skull fracture.
4. For an arm or leg, a pressure bandage may be applied when the first aid provider cannot keep pressure on the wound (eg, going to help other injured people at the scene). A pressure bandage consists of wrapping a roller bandage (eg, elastic or self-adhering gauze) firmly over the dressings and the extremity. To apply a pressure bandage, make a series of turns or wraps progressing up the arm or leg with each turn

SKILL SHEET 8-1 Bleeding Control

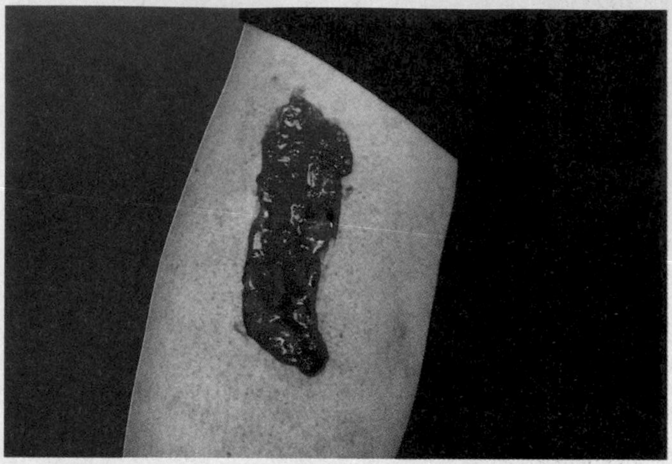

© Jones & Bartlett Learning.

1 Put on medical exam gloves and expose the wound. If gloves are not available, improvise a barrier (eg, plastic bag, plastic wrap, extra dressings, cloths). If those are not available, have the person apply pressure with their hand. **DO NOT** remove or apply any pressure on an impaled object.

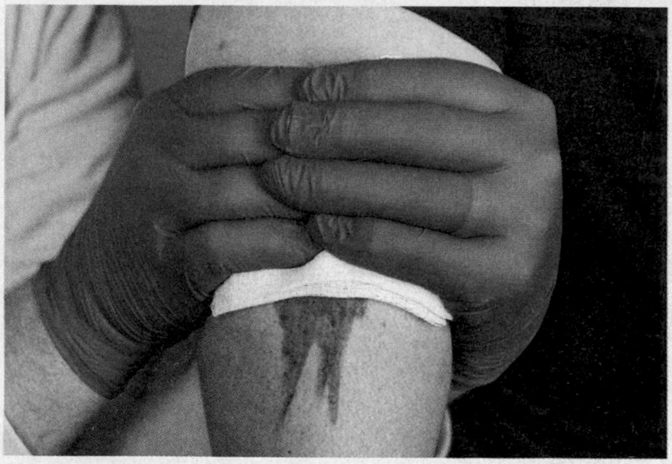

© Jones & Bartlett Learning.

2 Cover the wound with a sterile dressing or any clean cloth (eg, shirt, handkerchief, washcloth, towel). Apply firm, continuous direct pressure using the flat part of your fingers for small wounds or with the palm of your hand for large wounds. Keep applying pressure until the bleeding stops. If you do *not* have a sterile dressing or clean cloth, use your gloved hand or have the person apply pressure with their hand. **DO NOT** remove or apply any pressure on an impaled object. For extremities, if direct pressure does not stop a massive hemorrhage within the first minute, apply a tourniquet (see Step **5** for proper tourniquet application).

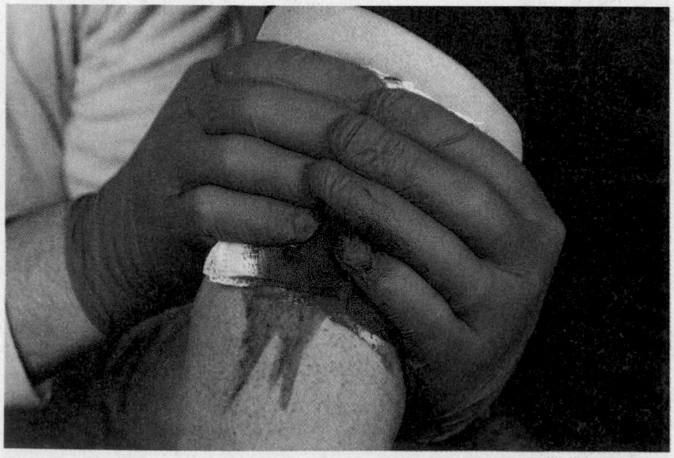

© Jones & Bartlett Learning.

3 If a dressing becomes blood-soaked, remove it and apply better-aimed pressure using a clean dressing.

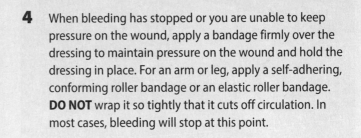

SKILL SHEET 8-1 Bleeding Control (*Continued*)

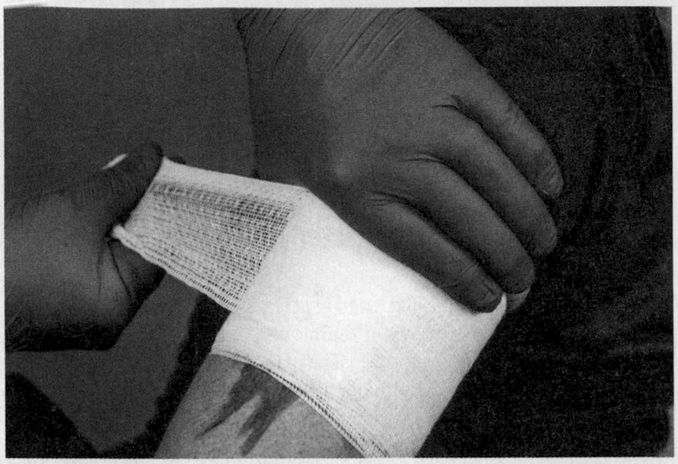
© Jones & Bartlett Learning.

4 When bleeding has stopped or you are unable to keep pressure on the wound, apply a bandage firmly over the dressing to maintain pressure on the wound and hold the dressing in place. For an arm or leg, apply a self-adhering, conforming roller bandage or an elastic roller bandage. **DO NOT** wrap it so tightly that it cuts off circulation. In most cases, bleeding will stop at this point.

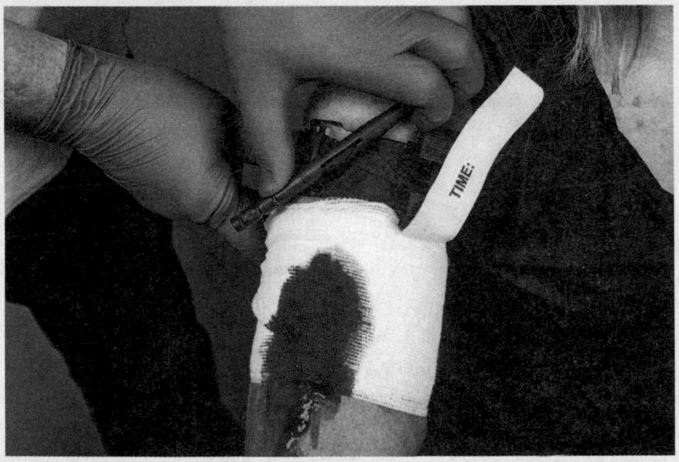

© Jones & Bartlett Learning.

5 If direct pressure fails to immediately stop bleeding from an arm or leg, apply a manufactured tourniquet (see Skill Sheet 8-2). For other body areas where a tourniquet placement is impossible (eg, neck, shoulders, groin) or when a tourniquet is ineffective or not available, stuff a hemostatic gauze dressing (special dressing that helps clot the blood) directly into the wound (ie, not merely applying it as a cover) and apply hard, direct pressure over it for 5 minutes or until bleeding stops.

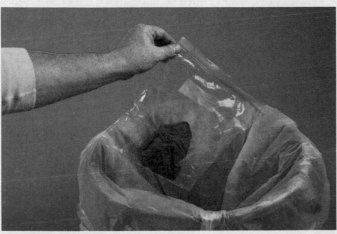
© Jones & Bartlett Learning.

6 After the bleeding stops:

a. Care for the wound (refer to Chapter 9 for details).

b. Properly dispose of the medical exam gloves and any blood-contaminated clothing.

c. Wash your hands.

d. If needed, seek professional medical care for cleaning, sutures, or a tetanus immunization. For massive, life-threatening bleeding, call EMS.

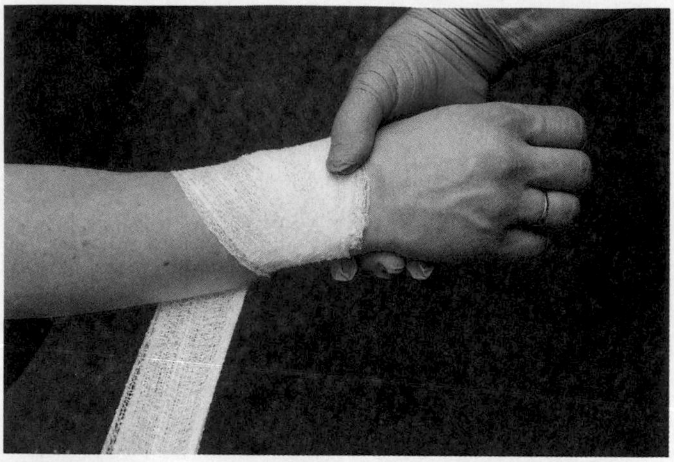

FIGURE 8-5 To apply a roller bandage, wrap upward toward the wider part of the arm or leg to make the bandage more secure.

overlapping the previous wrap **FIGURE 8-5**. Wrap the arm or leg with crisscross (figure-eight) turns in overlapping turns ending tightly over the dressing and above and below the wound. **DO NOT** wrap a pressure bandage so tightly that it cuts off blood flow.

5. When direct pressure will not stop the bleeding (eg, blood-soaked dressings) or life-threatening bleeding was seen before direct pressure was applied, take the following steps:

If . . .	Then . . .
Bleeding is from an arm or leg and a manufactured tourniquet *is* available.	Apply the manufactured tourniquet (see Skill Sheet 8-2).
Bleeding is from an arm or leg and a manufactured tourniquet is *not* available but hemostatic dressing(s) are.	Apply a hemostatic dressing into the wound (see Skill Sheet 8-1).
Bleeding is from an arm or leg and a manufactured tourniquet or a hemostatic gauze dressing are *not* available.	▪ Stuff any clean cloth or gauze into the wound and apply pressure on the wound as hard as you can, and/or ▪ Apply an improvised tourniquet (see Skill Sheet 8-3).
Bleeding is from other body areas where a tourniquet should not be applied or is impossible to apply (eg, neck, shoulder, groin).	▪ Apply a hemostatic dressing into the wound, or ▪ Stuff any clean cloth or gauze into the wound, and apply pressure on the wound as hard as you can.

Some people panic when they see even the smallest amount of blood. The sight of more than a couple of tablespoons of blood, especially on white or light-colored clothing, generally is enough to frighten an injured person and bystanders. Take time to reassure the person that everything possible is being done, but do not belittle the person's concerns.

If . . .	Then . . .
Bleeding is controlled.	**1.** Care for the wound see Chapter 9, *Wounds*. **2.** If needed, seek professional medical care for cleaning, stitches, or a tetanus immunization.
Bleeding continues.	**1.** Apply a manufactured tourniquet about 2 to 3 inches (5 to 8 cm) above the wound **SKILL SHEET 8-2**. ▪ Tourniquets are used only on arms and legs **TABLE 8-1**. ▪ Tighten the tourniquet until the bleeding stops, then secure it in place. If bleeding continues, apply a second tourniquet 2 to 3 inches (5 to 8 cm) above or near the first one. **2.** Manufactured tourniquets are preferred over improvised tourniquets, which often fail to stop the bleeding. They are also designed to be applied with one hand, if necessary, for self-rescue. **3. DO NOT** cover, release, or remove a tourniquet. Write "TQ" or "TK" (for tourniquet) and the time it was applied on a piece of tape and stick it on the person's forehead. Manufactured tourniquets also have a tab for writing the time it was applied. *Note*: Unsafe conditions (eg, active shooter, military combat), inability to see the wound (eg, darkness), and a large-scale event involving more than one person needing care (eg, natural disasters, explosions, motor vehicle and air crashes) can warrant placing a tourniquet as quickly as possible. Placing a tourniquet in a "high and tight" location (near armpit for an arm and near the groin for the leg) allows for fast evacuation and caring for life-threatening injuries.
Bleeding still continues.	**1.** Apply a hemostatic gauze dressing if: ▪ Direct pressure is not effective in controlling bleeding. ▪ A manufactured tourniquet is not available, is ineffective, or cannot be applied (eg, wound is on neck, shoulder, groin). **2.** Stuff (pack) a hemostatic gauze dressing (special dressing that helps clot the blood) into the wound, then apply direct and firm continuous pressure. If a hemostatic gauze dressing is not available, stuff any gauze or clean cloth into the wound. Apply a hemostatic gauze dressing as follows: ▪ Wipe pooled blood from the wound. ▪ Stuff (pack) a hemostatic gauze dressing (or clean cloth or gauze) directly into the wound (ie, do not merely apply it as a cover) **FIGURE 8-6**. ▪ Apply hard, direct pressure over the wound and packing for 5 minutes or until bleeding stops. **3.** Call 9-1-1 if it has not already been done. **4.** Consider using an improvised tourniquet if a manufactured tourniquet is not available or if direct pressure and a hemostatic dressing fail to stop life-threatening bleeding **SKILL SHEET 8-3**.

FYI

Prevent Infection

Applying a dressing not only controls bleeding, it also prevents infection. Capillary bleeding is most prone to infection because the wound is usually quite large (eg, road rash, etc).

CAUTION

DO NOT apply a pressure bandage so tightly that it cuts off blood flow. Check the radial pulse if the bandage is on an arm; for a leg, check the posterior tibial pulse between the medial malleolus (the inner ankle knob) and the Achilles tendon. Pulses are hard to feel. Other signs that the dressing is too tight are increasing pain, numbness or tingling, loss of color in the skin, and loss of muscle function.

TABLE 8-1 Common Tourniquet Mistakes

Not using a tourniquet when you should
Using a tourniquet for minimal bleeding
Placing the tourniquet too far from the bleeding site
Not making the tourniquet tight enough to stop bleeding
Not using a second tourniquet if needed
Using anything narrow such as rope, wire, string, cords, or belt
Waiting too long to put the tourniquet on life-threatening bleeding
Periodically loosening the tourniquet to allow blood flow to the injured extremity
Not monitoring its effectiveness

FYI

Application of a Hemostatic Dressing

A hemostatic dressing is best used when a tourniquet cannot be applied to the body part (eg, neck, shoulder, groin), when a tourniquet is not available, or when a tourniquet is unable to stop the bleeding. When applying a hemostatic gauze dressing, the skin tissue may need to be spread open to place the dressing into a deeper portion of the wound. If blood soaks through the first dressing, remove and insert another dressing, but deeper. If the wound is deep, place a bulky dressing over the hemostatic gauze dressing. If a nonhemostatic dressing has already been applied and is not working, remove all of it. Hemostatic dressings are designed to be placed directly into the bleeding wound.

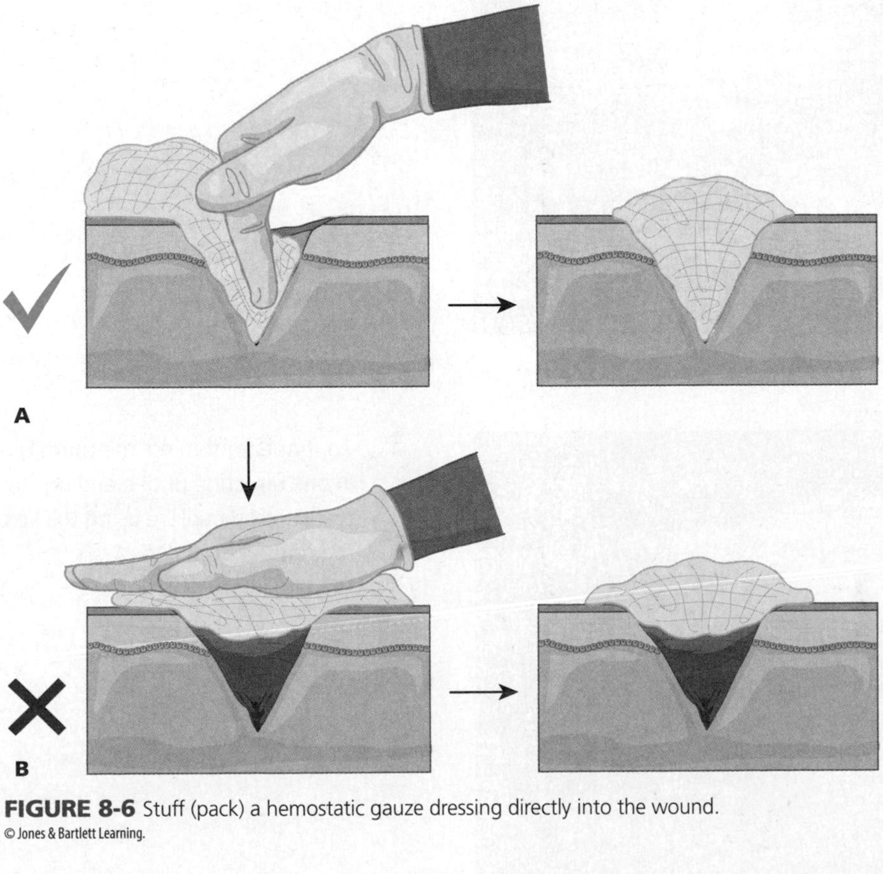

FIGURE 8-6 Stuff (pack) a hemostatic gauze dressing directly into the wound.

SKILL SHEET 8-2 Massive Bleeding Control: Applying a Manufactured Tourniquet

Apply a manufactured tourniquet to save a life when direct pressure cannot stop the bleeding (see Skill Sheet 8-1, *Bleeding Control*). Call 9-1-1 if it has not already been done.

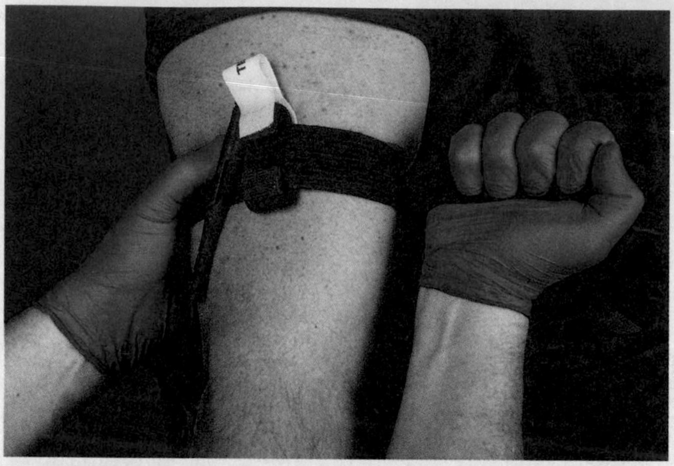

1 Place the tourniquet firmly in place about 2 to 3 inches (5 to 8 cm) above the wound. **DO NOT** apply it anywhere other than an arm or leg. **DO NOT** apply it on the (eg, elbow, wrist, knee)—apply it above the joint.

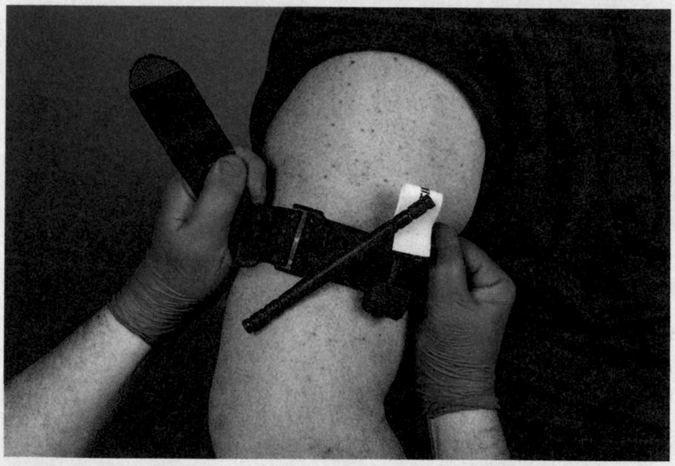

2 Pull the free end of the tourniquet to make it as tight as possible and secure the free end. Thread the Velcro strap through the buckle and pull firmly on the end strap to tighten the tourniquet.

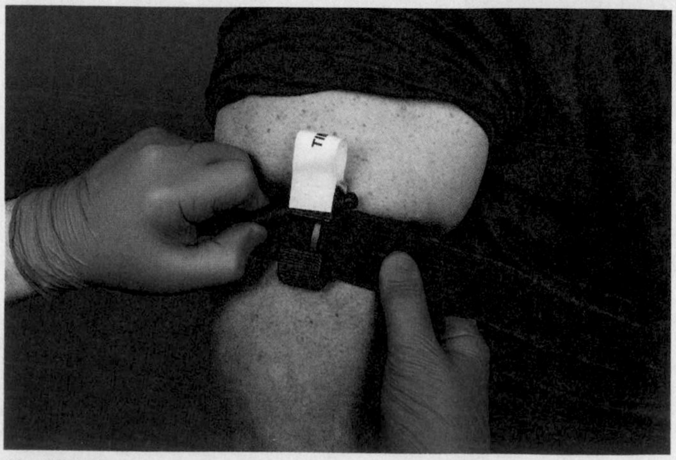

3 Continue tightening the tourniquet by twisting the rod in one direction until bleeding stops. Then, secure the twisting rod in place using the Velcro or holder so that the rod does not unwind.

SKILL SHEET 8-2 Massive Bleeding Control: Applying a Manufactured Tourniquet (*Continued*)

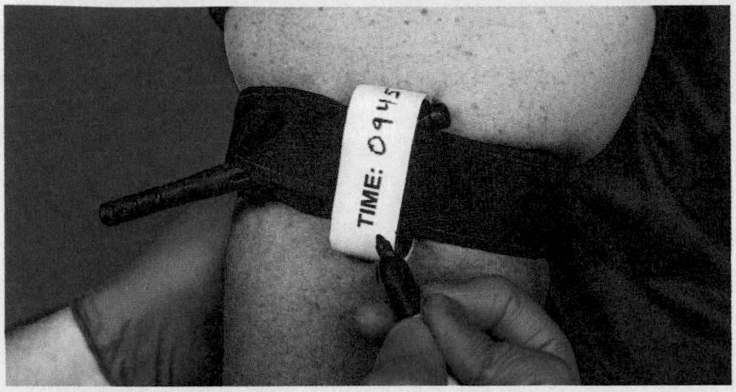

4 Write the time it was applied on the tourniquet's tag. If a tag is not available, write on a piece of tape "TQ" or "TK" for tourniquet and the time applied, and stick it on the person's forehead. **DO NOT** cover, release, or remove the tourniquet.

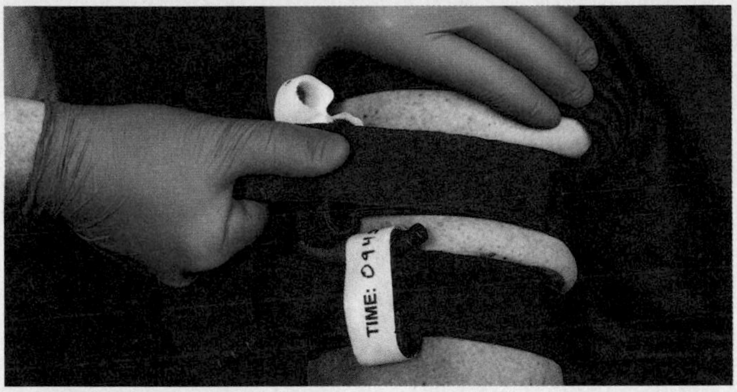

5 If massive bleeding continues, the tourniquet is not tight enough. Tighten the tourniquet. If it is still ineffective, apply a second tourniquet near the first, above it if possible. A second tourniquet is rarely needed.

SKILL SHEET 8-3 Massive Bleeding Control: Applying an Improvised Tourniquet

Improvise a tourniquet to save a life when direct pressure cannot stop the bleeding (see Skill Sheet 8-1) and a manufactured tourniquet and hemostatic dressing are not available (see SKILL SHEET 8-2). Call 9-1-1 if it has not already been done.

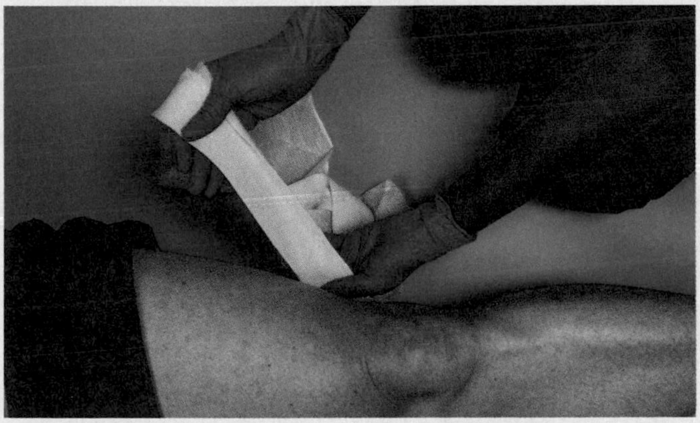

1 Expose the wound. Use a folded triangle bandage, wide roller bandage, or similar cloth folded into a long band about 2 inches (5 cm) wide and several layers thick. **DO NOT** use narrow materials (eg, wire, rope, cord).

Continues

SKILL SHEET 8-3 Massive Bleeding Control: Applying an Improvised Tourniquet (*Continued*)

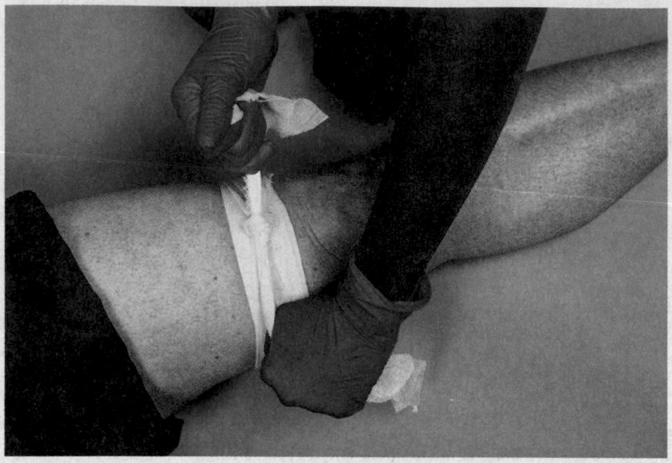

2 Wrap the folded band twice above the wound, about 2 to 3 inches (5 to 8 cm) and tie an overhand knot. **DO NOT** apply it anywhere other than the arm or leg. **DO NOT** apply it over a joint.

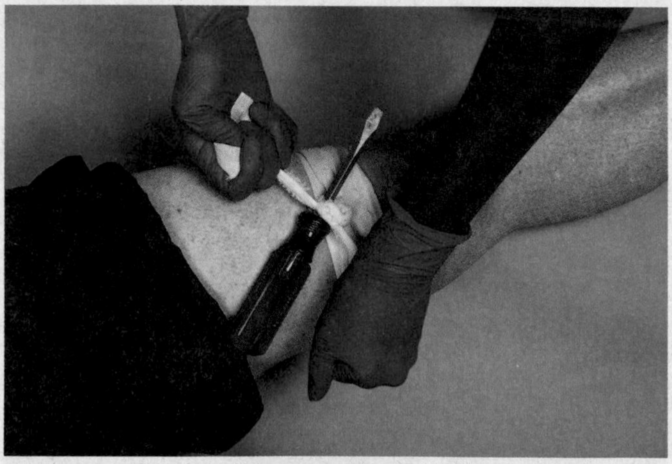

3 Place a short, rigid object (eg, screwdriver, stick) on top of the knot. Then tie a square knot over the rigid object with the ends of the cloth band.

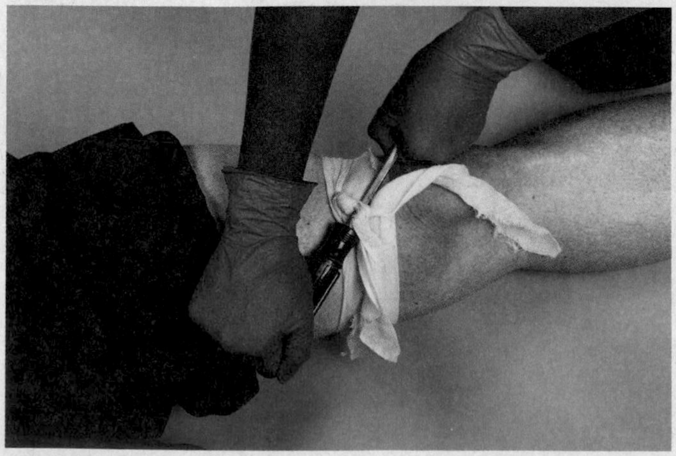

4 Twist the rigid object in one direction until the bleeding stops. Then, secure the rigid object in place with another cloth band or tape to prevent the tourniquet from untwisting.

SKILL SHEET 8-3 Massive Bleeding Control: Applying an Improvised Tourniquet (*Continued*)

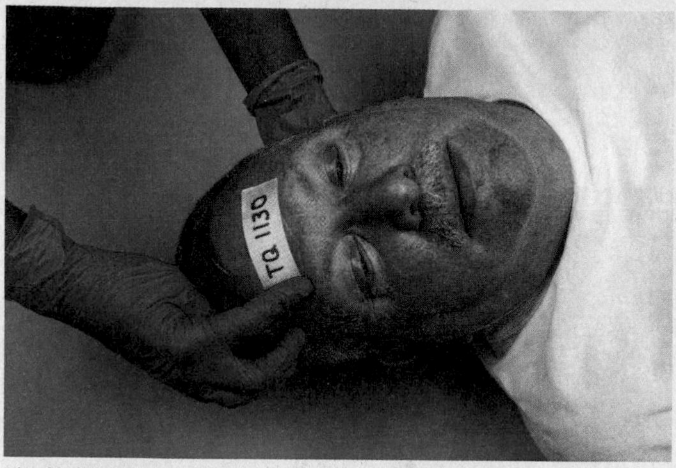

5 Write on a piece of tape "TQ" or "TK" for tourniquet and the time applied and stick it on the person's forehead. **DO NOT** cover, release, or remove the tourniquet.

6 If massive bleeding continues, the tourniquet is not tight enough. Tighten the tourniquet. If it is still ineffective, apply a second tourniquet near the first, above it if possible. A second tourniquet is rarely needed.

Internal Bleeding

Internal bleeding occurs when the skin is not broken and blood is not seen. It can be difficult to detect and can be life threatening. A person with bleeding stomach ulcers, a lacerated liver, or a ruptured spleen may have a considerable amount of blood loss into the abdomen with no outward sign of bleeding other than the presence of shock (see Chapter 7, *Shock*). Broken bones can also cause serious internal blood loss. A broken femur can easily result in a loss of 1 or more quarts (about 1 L or more) of blood.

Refer to **FLOWCHART 8-1** for additional information regarding care for bleeding.

CAUTION

DO NOT give the person anything to eat or drink. It could cause nausea and vomiting, which could result in aspiration. Food or liquids could also cause complications if surgery is needed.

What to Look For	What to Do
▪ Bright red blood from the mouth or rectum, or blood in the urine ▪ Nonmenstrual vaginal bleeding ▪ Vomited blood; may be bright red or dark red, or look like coffee grounds ▪ Black, foul-smelling, tarry stools ▪ Pain, tenderness, bruising, or swelling ▪ Broken ribs, bruises over the lower chest, or a rigid abdomen	**1.** Monitor breathing. **2.** Expect vomiting. If vomiting occurs, keep the person lying on their side to allow drainage and to prevent inhalation (aspiration) of vomitus. **3.** Treat for shock and cover the person with a coat or blanket for warmth. See Chapter 7, *Shock*, for when to use other body positions. **4.** Treat suspected internal bleeding in an extremity by applying a splint. See Chapter 16, *Splinting Extremities*. **5.** Seek immediate professional medical care.
Bruises (indicating non–life-threatening internal bleeding)	**1.** Apply an ice pack over the injury for 20 minutes. **2.** If an arm or a leg is involved, apply an elastic bandage for compression. Several layers of gauze pads or other cloth could be placed between the bandage and the injury to concentrate the compression to a specific location.

Flowchart 8-1 Bleeding Control

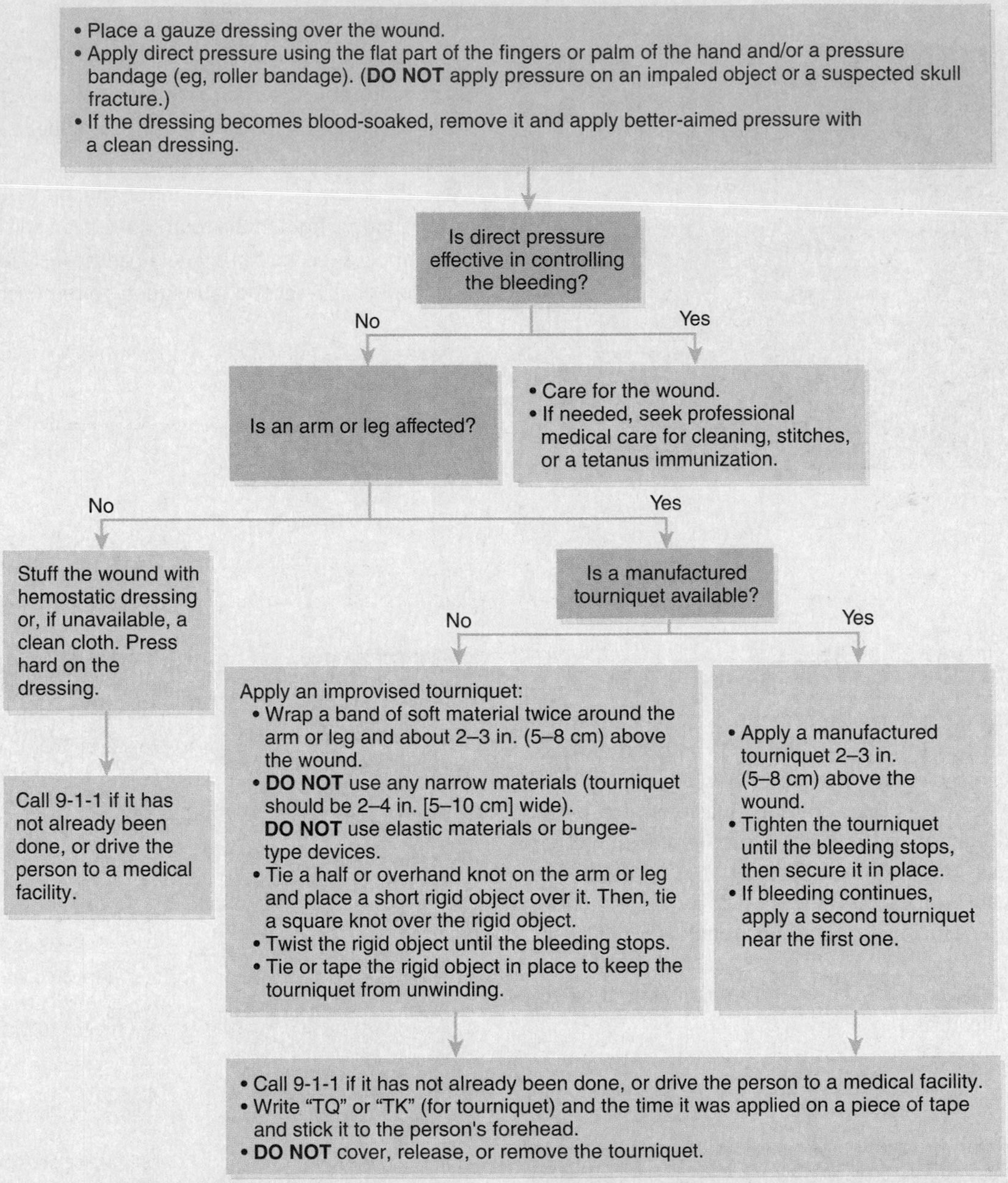
• Place a gauze dressing over the wound.
• Apply direct pressure using the flat part of the fingers or palm of the hand and/or a pressure bandage (eg, roller bandage). (DO NOT apply pressure on an impaled object or a suspected skull fracture.)
• If the dressing becomes blood-soaked, remove it and apply better-aimed pressure with a clean dressing.
Is direct pressure effective in controlling the bleeding?
No
Yes
Is an arm or leg affected?
• Care for the wound.
• If needed, seek professional medical care for cleaning, stitches, or a tetanus immunization.
No
Yes
Stuff the wound with hemostatic dressing or, if unavailable, a clean cloth. Press hard on the dressing.
Call 9-1-1 if it has not already been done, or drive the person to a medical facility.
Is a manufactured tourniquet available?
No
Yes
Apply an improvised tourniquet:
• Wrap a band of soft material twice around the arm or leg and about 2–3 in. (5–8 cm) above the wound.
• DO NOT use any narrow materials (tourniquet should be 2–4 in. [5–10 cm] wide). DO NOT use elastic materials or bungee-type devices.
• Tie a half or overhand knot on the arm or leg and place a short rigid object over it. Then, tie a square knot over the rigid object.
• Twist the rigid object until the bleeding stops.
• Tie or tape the rigid object in place to keep the tourniquet from unwinding.
• Apply a manufactured tourniquet 2–3 in. (5–8 cm) above the wound.
• Tighten the tourniquet until the bleeding stops, then secure it in place.
• If bleeding continues, apply a second tourniquet near the first one.
• Call 9-1-1 if it has not already been done, or drive the person to a medical facility.
• Write "TQ" or "TK" (for tourniquet) and the time it was applied on a piece of tape and stick it to the person's forehead.
• DO NOT cover, release, or remove the tourniquet.

PREP KIT

Ready for Review

- Rapid blood loss of 1 quart (about 1 L) or more can lead to shock and death.
- External bleeding can be classified into three types according to the type of blood vessel that is damaged: artery, vein, or capillary.
- Regardless of the type of bleeding or the type of wound, the first aid is the same. First and foremost, you must control the bleeding.

Vital Vocabulary

arterial bleeding Bleeding from an artery. This type of bleeding initially spurts up to several feet from the wound.

capillary bleeding Bleeding that oozes from a wound steadily but slowly.

hemorrhage A large amount of bleeding in a short time.

hemostatic gauze dressing A gauze-style dressing that is saturated with an agent that stops bleeding.

tourniquet A bleeding control device that is wrapped tightly around an extremity to stop blood flow from a wound.

venous bleeding Bleeding from a vein. This type of bleeding tends to flow steadily.

Assessment in Action

You are enjoying a bike ride on a paved trail with your friend. As she rounds the next bend, her bike tires slide out on the gravel and she falls to the ground. She gets up but has a large scrape on her knee and part of her lower leg. Blood is oozing from the wound.

Directions: Circle Yes if you agree with the statement; circle No if you disagree.

1. This person is experiencing capillary bleeding.
   YES **NO**
2. This type of bleeding is the most common type.
   YES **NO**
3. This type of bleeding is difficult to control and usually does not clot and stop by itself.
   YES **NO**
4. Direct pressure will control this type of bleeding.
   YES **NO**

Check Your Knowledge

Directions: Circle Yes if you agree with the statement; circle No if you disagree.

1. Most cases of bleeding require more than direct pressure to stop the bleeding.
   YES **NO**
2. Remove any blood-soaked dressings before applying additional ones.
   YES **NO**
3. Applying a pressure bandage over a wound can allow you to attend to another injury or another injured person.
   YES **NO**
4. If a bleeding arm wound is not controlled through direct pressure, apply pressure to the brachial artery.
   YES **NO**
5. Dressings are placed directly on a wound.
   YES **NO**
6. Internal bleeding is normal.
   YES **NO**
7. Dressings should be sterile or as clean as possible.
   YES **NO**
8. Clotting is the body's way of stopping bleeding.
   YES **NO**
9. If the person feels sick to the stomach and may vomit, roll them onto their left side.
   YES **NO**
10. When applying a tourniquet to control bleeding, place the tourniquet about 2 to 3 inches above the wound.
    YES **NO**

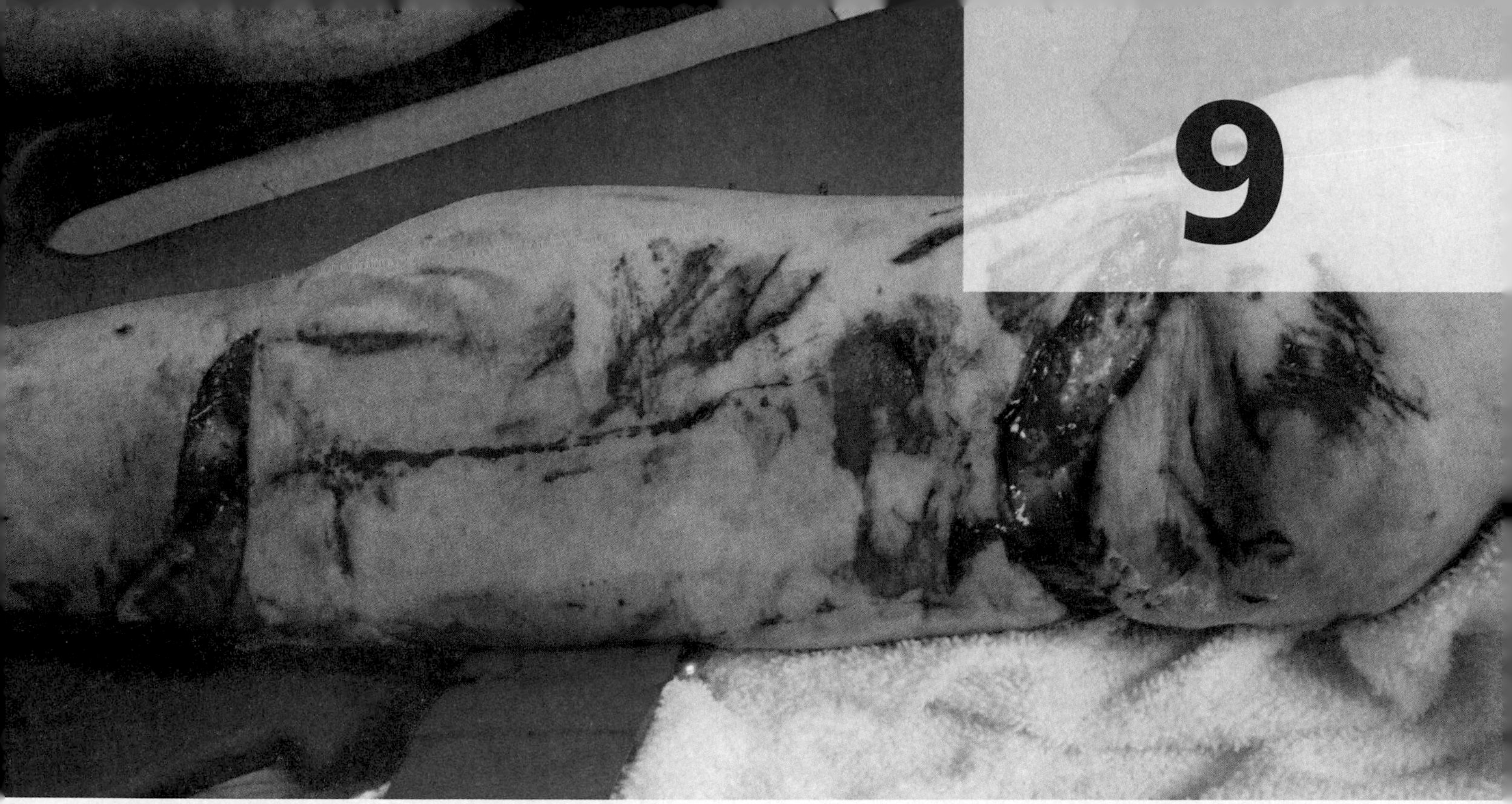

9

Wounds

CHAPTER AT A GLANCE

- Open Wounds
- Amputations and Avulsions
- Blisters
- Impaled (Embedded) Objects
- Closed Wounds
- Wounds Requiring Professional Medical Care
- Gunshot Wounds

Open Wounds

An open wound is a break in the skin's surface resulting in external bleeding. It may allow bacteria to enter the body, causing an infection. There are several types of open wounds. Recognizing the type of wound helps you give proper first aid. With an **abrasion**, the top layer of skin is removed, with little or no blood loss **FIGURE 9-1**. Abrasions tend to be painful because the nerve endings often are abraded along with the skin. Ground-in debris may be present. This type of wound can be serious if it covers a large area or becomes embedded with foreign matter. Other names for an abrasion are "scrape" and "road rash."

A **laceration** is cut skin with jagged, irregular edges **FIGURE 9-2**. This type of wound is usually caused by a forceful tearing away of skin tissue. **Incisions** have smooth edges and resemble a surgical or paper cut **FIGURE 9-3**. The amount of bleeding depends on the depth, the location, and the size of the wound. **Punctures** are usually deep, narrow wounds in the skin and underlying organs such as a stab wound from a nail or a knife **FIGURE 9-4**. The entrance is usually small, and the risk of infection is high. The object causing the injury may remain impaled in the wound.

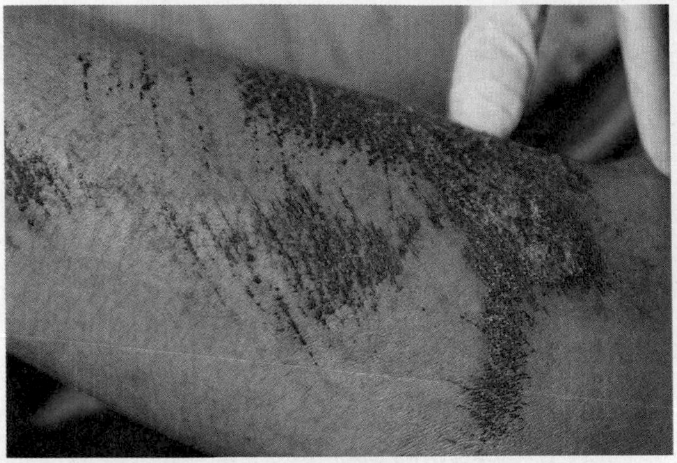

FIGURE 9-1 Abrasion.

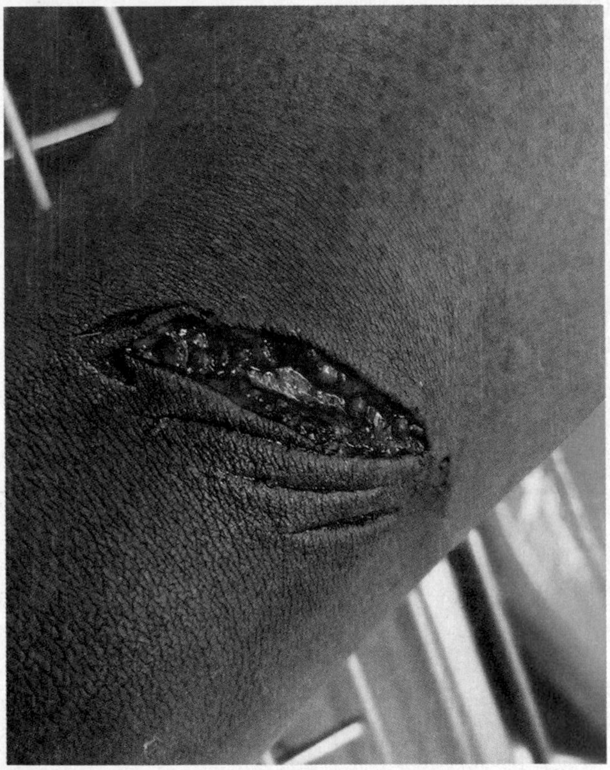

FIGURE 9-2 Laceration.

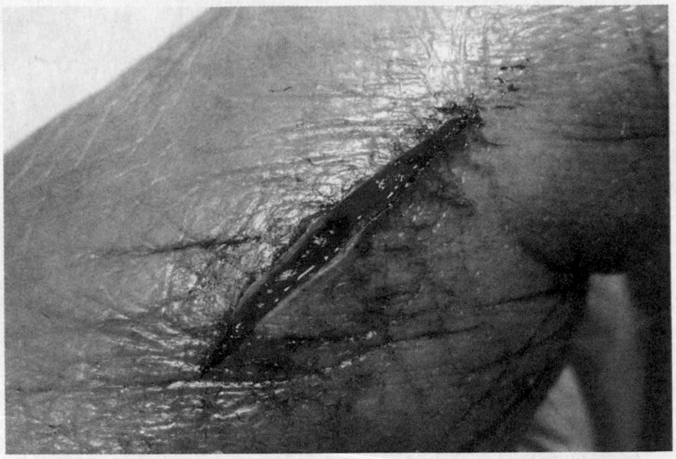

FIGURE 9-3 Incision.

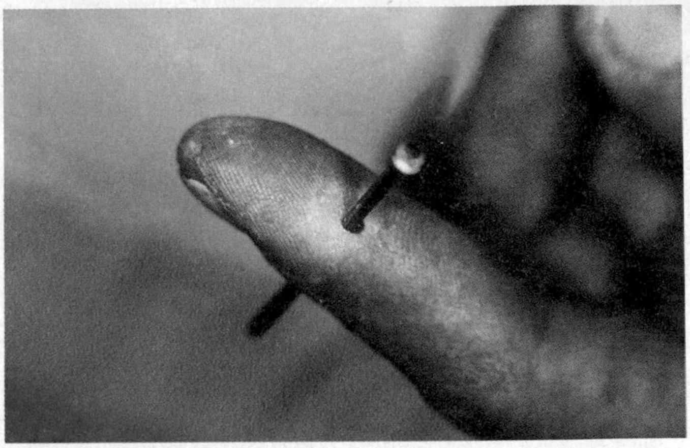

FIGURE 9-4 Puncture.

Care for Open Wounds

1. Protect yourself against disease by wearing medical exam gloves. If gloves are not available, use several layers of gauze pads, clean cloths, plastic wrap or bags, sanitary napkins, or waterproof material. If none of these items is available, have the person apply pressure to the wound with a clean cloth to their hand. **DO NOT** use your bare hand.
2. Expose the wound by removing or cutting away the clothing to find the source of the bleeding.
3. Control the bleeding by using direct pressure and, if needed, other methods. (See Chapter 8, *Bleeding*.)

CAUTION

DO NOT clean large, extremely dirty, or life-threatening wounds. Let the hospital emergency department personnel do the cleaning.

DO NOT scrub a wound. The benefit of scrubbing a wound is debatable, and it can bruise the tissue.

FYI

High-Risk Wounds

The following types of wounds have a high potential for infection:

- Bite wounds
- Very dirty or contaminated wounds
- Crushing, ragged wounds
- Deep wounds over an injured bone, joint, or tendon
- Puncture wounds

Cleaning a Wound

A person's wound should be cleaned to help prevent infection. Wound cleaning usually restarts the bleeding by disturbing the clot, but it should be done anyway for shallow wounds. For wounds with a high risk for infection, leave the pressure bandage in place because professional medical personnel will clean the wound.

1. Scrub your hands vigorously with soap and water if available. Put on medical exam gloves.
2. Expose the wound.
3. Clean the wound.

If...	Then...
The wound is shallow.	▪ Wash inside the wound with soap and water. ▪ Flush the wound with running water (use water clean enough to drink) **FIGURE 9-5**. Run water directly into the wound and allow the water to run over the wound and out, thus carrying the dirty particles away from the wound. Water from a faucet provides sufficient pressure and quantity. Irrigation with water is the most important factor in preventing infection.
The wound is deep or has a high risk of infection (such as animal bite or a very dirty or ragged wound or puncture).	▪ Seek professional medical care for wound cleaning. ▪ If you are in a remote location (more than 1 hour from professional medical care), clean the wound as best you can using the technique described for shallow wounds.

4. Anything not flushed out by irrigation should be removed manually (eg, sterile tweezers). A wound that is not properly cleaned has a high risk for infection.
5. If bleeding restarts, apply direct pressure over the wound.

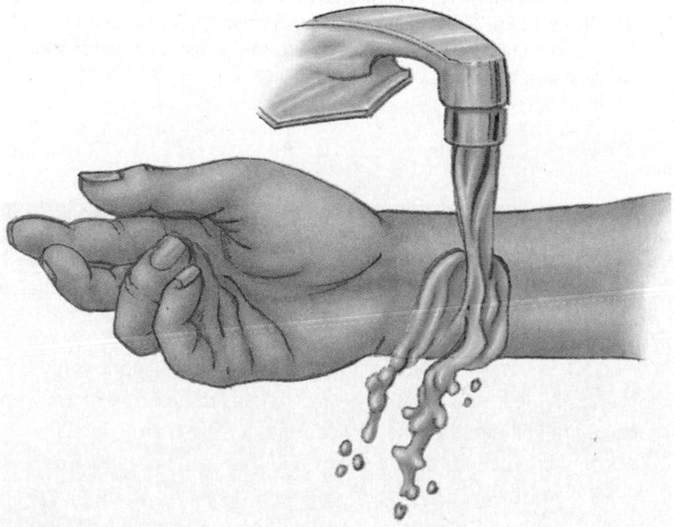

FIGURE 9-5 Irrigate a wound with copious amounts of water.

Q&A

Is a dirty wound the same as a contaminated wound?

No. For example, road rash (an abrasion resulting from road gravel) may be dirty, but it has a low bacterial count and would not be considered contaminated. In contrast, wounds that occur in a barnyard or that are exposed to soil contaminated with fecal material have a high bacterial count and are contaminated.

Covering a Wound

Dressings and bandages are two different kinds of first aid supplies. A **dressing** is applied over a wound to control bleeding and prevent contamination. A **bandage** holds the dressing in place. Dressings should be sterile or as clean as possible; bandages need not be.

If...	Then...
The wound is small and does not require sutures.	▪ Cover it with a thin layer of antibiotic ointment. These ointments can kill many bacteria and rarely cause allergic reactions. No prescription is needed. ▪ Cover the wound with a sterile dressing.
The wound is large.	▪ **DO NOT** close gaping or dirty wounds with tape or butterfly bandages. Bacteria may remain, leading to a greater chance of infection. Large, deep, or contaminated wounds should be managed by a medical professional. ▪ Cover the wound with a sterile dressing.
The wound bleeds after a dressing has been applied and the dressing becomes stuck to the wound.	▪ Leave the dressing on as long as the wound is healing. Pulling the scab loose to change the dressing retards healing and increases the chance of infection. ▪ If you must remove a dressing that is sticking, soak it in warm water to help soften the scab and make removal easier.
The dressing becomes wet or dirty.	Remove and apply new sterile dressing. Dirt and moisture are both breeding grounds for bacteria.

When to Seek Professional Medical Care

Wounds that have a high risk for an infection or other problem while healing should receive professional medical care. Examples of high-risk wounds include those with embedded foreign material (such as gravel), animal and human bites, puncture wounds, and ragged wounds. Large or deep wounds should receive professional medical care. Any wounds with edges that do not come together spontaneously should receive professional medical care. Any wounds that have visible bone, joint, muscle, fat, or tendons, and wounds that may have entered a joint or body cavity, should receive professional medical care. A particularly high-risk wound is the "fight bite," a wound over the knuckle caused by punching a person in the teeth. Anyone who has not had a tetanus vaccination within 10 years (5 years in the case of a dirty wound) should seek medical attention within 72 hours to update their tetanus inoculation status.

Refer to **FLOWCHART 9-1** for additional information regarding wound care.

FYI

Wound Irrigation

A study compared the effectiveness of tap water with saline solution for irrigating simple skin lacerations to remove bacteria. The results showed no significant difference between bacterial counts in wounds irrigated with normal saline and those irrigated with tap water. The removal of bacteria from a wound depends more on the mechanical effects (speed and pressure) than on the type of solution. Tap water has these advantages over saline: It is readily available; it is more continuous and, therefore, takes less time; it is less expensive; and it does not require other materials such as sterile syringes or splash guards. Other irrigation solutions with antibacterial properties and detergents have an anticellular effect that impairs wound healing and/or resistance to infection. Irrigation pressures above the 20- to 30-psi (138- to 207-kPa) range are discouraged because the higher pressure can damage tissue.

Data from Moscati R, Mayrose J, Fincher L, Jehle D. Comparison of normal saline with tap water for wound irrigation. *Am J Emerg Med*. 1998;164(4):379–381.

CAUTION

DO NOT irrigate a wound with full-strength iodine preparations such as povidone iodine (10%) or isopropyl alcohol (70%). They kill body cells as well as bacteria and are painful. Also, some people are allergic to iodine.

DO NOT use hydrogen peroxide. It does not kill bacteria well, it adversely affects capillary blood flow, and it extends wound healing.

DO NOT use antibiotic ointment on wounds that require sutures or on puncture wounds (the ointment may prevent drainage). Use an antibiotic ointment only on abrasions and shallow wounds.

DO NOT soak a wound to clean it. No evidence supports the effectiveness of soaking.

DO NOT close gaping wounds with tape such as butterfly tape. Infection is more likely when bacteria are trapped in the wound. If a wound requires closure, this should be done by medical personnel. Extremity wounds are best sutured within 6 hours of the injury.

DO NOT breathe or blow on a wound or the dressing.

FYI

Wound Care: What the Medical Literature Says

- Soaking wounds is not effective and can impair healing.
- The benefit of scrubbing wounds is debatable. Scrubbing can bruise the tissues and skin.
- All wound surfaces should be irrigated; this may require opening wound edges for exposure.
- Wound irrigation is the most important step for optimal wound healing, as long as there is sufficient pressure and volume.
- Irrigating wounds requires a minimum pressure of 5 to 8 psi (34 to 55 kPa) for tissue cleansing.
- Decontamination (brushing off any dry chemicals prior to copious irrigation) is essential.
- Not closing a wound (eg, with butterfly bandages, elastic skin closures), especially a dirty wound, reduces the risk of infection.
- Applying antiseptic solutions such as Merthiolate, Mercurochrome, iodine, isopropyl alcohol, and hydrogen peroxide can injure wounded tissues.
- Applying an antibiotic ointment such as Neosporin or Polysporin reduces the risk of infection in shallow wounds or abrasions.
- A moist wound healing environment (achieved with antibiotic ointment and a dressing) helps to promote healing, reduce pain, and improve cosmetic outcome.
- Centers for Disease Control and Prevention guidelines recommend a tetanus vaccine based on vaccination history and wound severity.
- Sunscreen should be used on a new wound for 3 to 6 months.
- You should consider each wound individually to create optimal conditions for wound healing.

Data from Howell JM, Chisholm CD. Outpatient wound preparation and care: a national survey. *Ann Emerg Med*. 1992;21(8):976–981; Nicks BA, Ayello EA, Woo K, Nitzki-George D, Sibbald RG. Acute wound management: revisiting the approach to assessment, irrigation, and closure considerations. *Int J Emerg Med*. 2010;3:399–407.

Q&A

When should wounds be closed by a physician or physician assistant?

Generally, a wound should be closed by one of several options (eg, sutures, staples, topical skin adhesives) when (1) the edges of the skin do not fall together and/or (2) the cut is more than 1 inch (3 cm) long and is deep. Closing the wound speeds the healing process, lessens the risk of infection, and lessens scarring. If sutures are needed, they should be made by a physician or physician assistant within 6 hours of the injury.

Flowchart 9-1 Wound Care

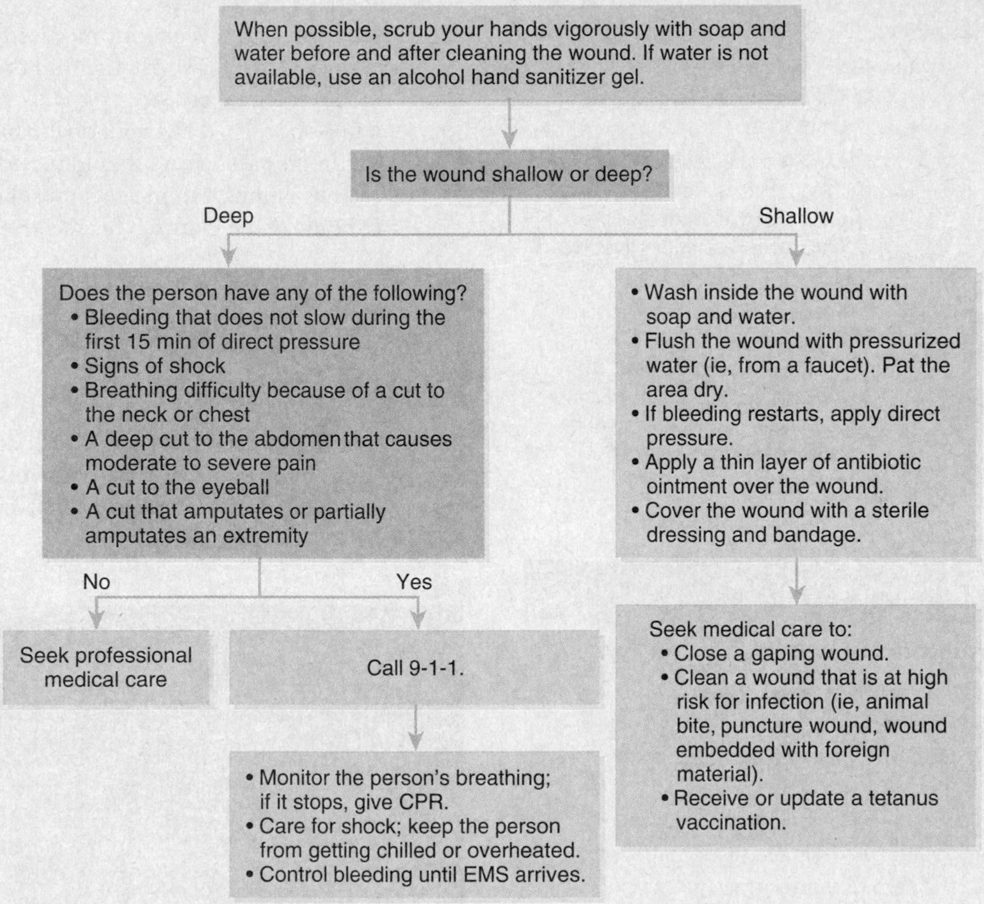
When possible, scrub your hands vigorously with soap and water before and after cleaning the wound. If water is not available, use an alcohol hand sanitizer gel.
Is the wound shallow or deep?
Deep
Shallow
Does the person have any of the following?
• Bleeding that does not slow during the first 15 min of direct pressure
• Signs of shock
• Breathing difficulty because of a cut to the neck or chest
• A deep cut to the abdomen that causes moderate to severe pain
• A cut to the eyeball
• A cut that amputates or partially amputates an extremity
No
Yes
Seek professional medical care
Call 9-1-1.
• Monitor the person's breathing; if it stops, give CPR.
• Care for shock; keep the person from getting chilled or overheated.
• Control bleeding until EMS arrives.
• Wash inside the wound with soap and water.
• Flush the wound with pressurized water (ie, from a faucet). Pat the area dry.
• If bleeding restarts, apply direct pressure.
• Apply a thin layer of antibiotic ointment over the wound.
• Cover the wound with a sterile dressing and bandage.
Seek medical care to:
• Close a gaping wound.
• Clean a wound that is at high risk for infection (ie, animal bite, puncture wound, wound embedded with foreign material).
• Receive or update a tetanus vaccination.

FYI

Myths About Wound Care

Myth: Wounds should be kept dry.
Fact: Although wet dressings should be changed, some moisture is good. Healing is faster and infection rates are lower when wounds are kept moist. Keep them moist by applying an antibiotic ointment and a dressing.
Myth: Redness is a sign of an infected wound.
Fact: Although redness can signal an infected wound, it does indicate an inflammatory reaction. When you see it, check for the other signs and symptoms of infection: fever and pus coming from the wound.
Myth: Saline solution should be used instead of tap water to irrigate a wound.
Fact: Saline solution is no more effective in preventing wound infections than is tap water.
Myth: A cut should not be covered—it needs to "breathe."
Fact: If a cut is not covered, it dries out and scabs over. Keep a cut moist and prevent a scab from forming. Apply an antibiotic ointment and cover with a dressing.

Infected Wound

Any wound, large or small, can become infected. Once an infection begins, damage can be extensive, so prevention is the best way to avoid infection. A wound should be cleaned using the procedures described earlier in this chapter.

It is important to know how to recognize and treat an infected wound **FIGURE 9-6**. Factors that increase the likelihood for wound infection include the following:

- Dirty and foreign material left in the wound
- Ragged or crushed tissue
- Injury to an underlying bone, joint, or tendon
- Bite wounds (human or animal)
- Hand and foot wounds
- Puncture wounds or other wounds that cannot drain

Tetanus

Tetanus is an illness caused by bacteria entering a wound and producing a poisonous toxin that causes muscles to tighten and contract, usually to the point of pain. Tetanus is not communicable from one person to another.

What to Look For	What to Do
▪ Swelling and redness around wound ▪ Feeling of increased temperature compared to surrounding area (eg, wound feels warmer) ▪ Throbbing pain ▪ Pus discharge ▪ Fever ▪ Swelling of lymph nodes ▪ One or more red streaks leading from the wound toward the heart (this is a serious sign that the infection is spreading and could cause death)	**1.** Soak the wound in warm water, or apply warm, wet packs over the infected wound. Separate the wound edges to allow pus to escape. **2.** Apply an antibiotic ointment. **3.** Change the dressings several times a day. **4.** Give over-the-counter pain medication such as acetaminophen or ibuprofen. Follow dosage instructions. Avoid aspirin because it can delay wound healing. **5.** Seek professional medical care if the infection becomes worse. If chills and fever develop, the infection has reached the cardiovascular system and immediate professional medical care is needed.

FYI

Using Topical Antibiotics to Improve Wound Healing

The use of topical triple-antibiotic ointment significantly decreases infection rates in minor wounds that are contaminated. Topical antibiotics are effective for minor wounds but not for major wounds.

Many studies support the use of topical antibiotics on wounds that are clean. Topical bacitracin zinc (Bacitracin); a triple ointment of neomycin sulfate, bacitracin zinc, and polymyxin B sulfate (Neosporin); and silver sulfadiazine (Silvadene) were compared with petrolatum as a control in patients with minor wounds. Wound infection rates were 17.6% for petrolatum, 5.5% for Bacitracin, 4.5% for Neosporin, and 12.1% for Silvadene.

Data from Diehr S, Hamp A, Jamieson B, Mendoza M. Clinical inquiries: do topical antibiotics improve wound healing? *J Fam Pract*. 2007;56(2):140–144.

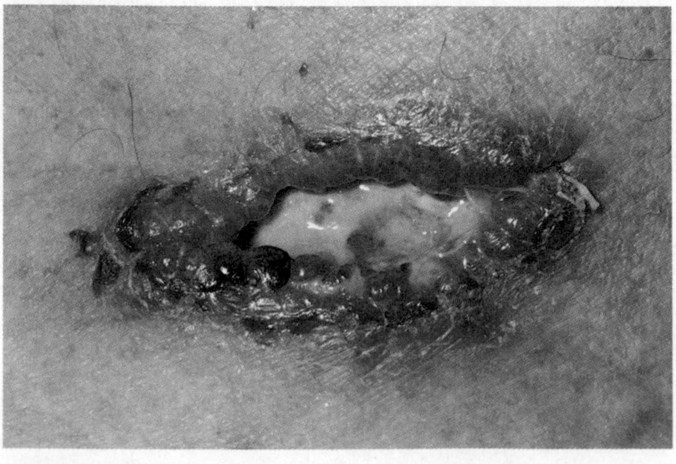

FIGURE 9-6 Infected wound.

Seek professional medical care to prevent tetanus for the following:

- Anyone with a wound who has never been immunized against tetanus should be given a tetanus vaccine and booster immediately.
- A person who was once immunized but has not received a tetanus booster within the last 10 years should receive a booster.
- A person with a dirty wound who has not had a booster within the past 5 years should receive a booster.
- Tetanus immunization shots must be given within 72 hours of the injury to be effective.

Amputations and Avulsions

An **amputation** is an injury in which part of the body is completely severed **FIGURE 9-7**. An **avulsion** is an injury in which the skin is torn completely loose or hanging as a flap **FIGURE 9-8**.

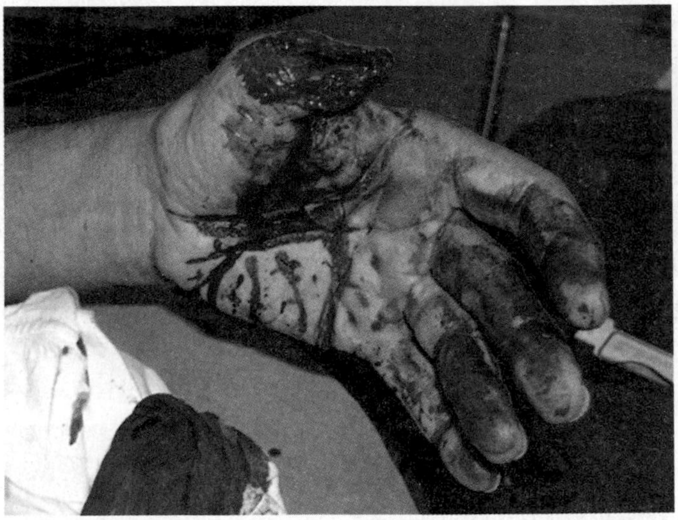

FIGURE 9-7 Clean amputation.

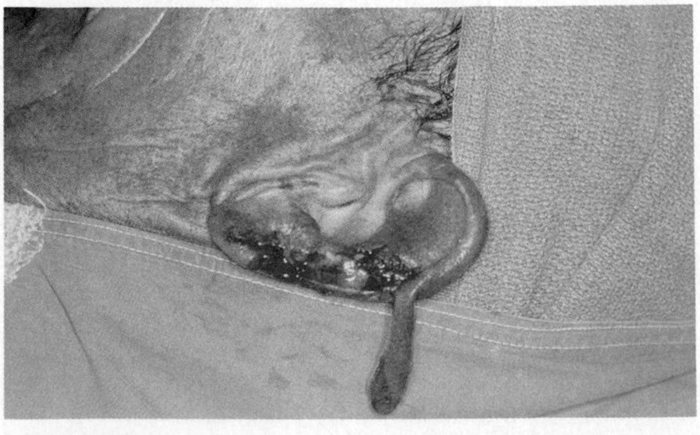

FIGURE 9-8 Avulsion.

In a **crushing amputation**, an extremity is separated by being crushed or mashed off, such as when a hand is caught in a roller machine. Crushing amputations are the most common type and the chance of reattachment is poor. In a **clean amputation**, the chance of reattachment is much better because it is clean cut and completely detached (see Figure 9-7). Many amputations can be reattached by an experienced surgeon, and time is a critical element in success. Function may be nearly normal in some cases. Do not give false hopes to a person with an amputation that the part will definitely be reattached at the hospital. Many amputated parts are not reattached after a surgeon's evaluation. It is better to tell the person that you are carefully handling the amputated part for the potential that it may be reattached.

An amputation may not involve heavy blood loss because blood vessels tend to go into spasms, recede into the injured

What to Look For	What to Do
Amputation	**1.** Call 9-1-1. **2.** If a body part is amputated, immediate action is needed for reattachment. Amputated body parts that are left uncooled for more than 6 hours have little chance of survival. **3.** Control bleeding by using direct pressure; if unsuccessful, apply a tourniquet or a hemostatic dressing, if available. **4.** Care for the amputated part: ▪ Wrap the severed part in a sterile gauze or a clean cloth that has been wet with water (make sure the excess water has been squeezed out). ▪ Put the wrapped part in a waterproof container (eg, plastic bag, plastic wrap) **FIGURE 9-9**. ▪ Keep the part cool by placing the wrapped part in a container of ice. **DO NOT** bury the part in the ice or allow the tissue to touch the ice. **DO NOT** submerge it in water. ▪ Send the part to the medical facility with the injured person. **5.** If the amputated part was not found, ask others to search for it and, if located, to take it to the medical facility where the person is going.
Avulsion (skin flap is torn loose but still attached and hanging from the body)	**1.** Gently move the skin flap back to its normal position. **2.** Cover with a sterile or clean dressing and apply pressure. **3.** If bleeding continues, apply a tourniquet or a hemostatic dressing, if available.

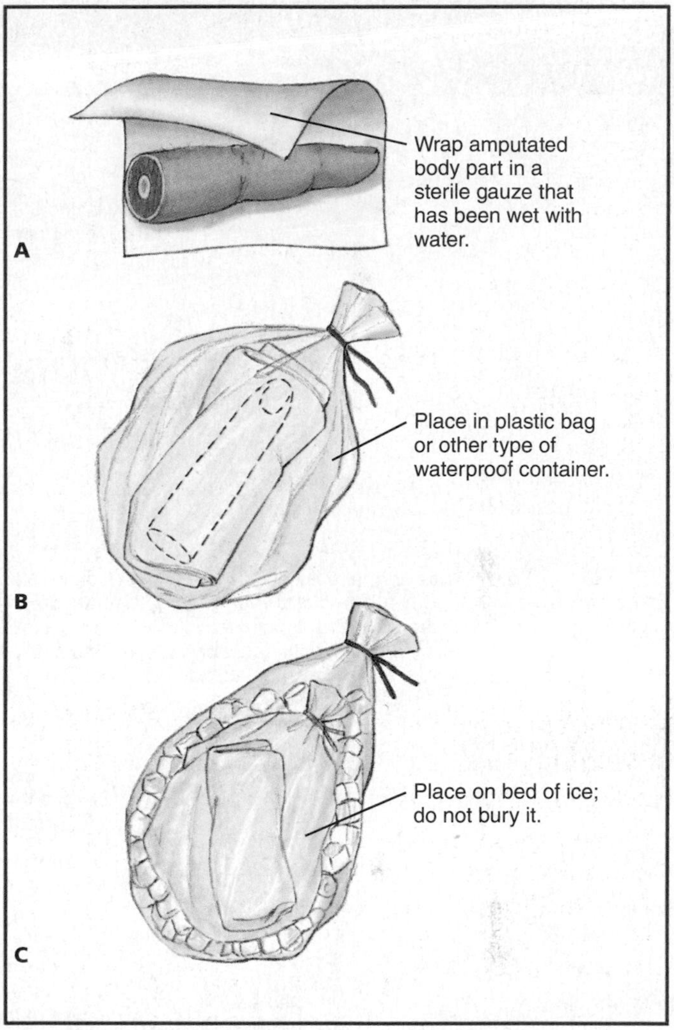

FIGURE 9-9 Care of an amputated part includes wrapping it in moist a sterile gauze or a clean cloth (**A**), placing it in a waterproof container (**B**), and placing it on a mixture of ice and water (**C**).

FYI

NEWS: Amputations

Ronald Malt, MD, performed the first successful reattachment in 1962 on a young boy's severed arm. Today, the reattachment success rate ranges from 80% to 90% due to improved microsurgical techniques and when appropriate actions are taken as follows:

- Minimize the time interval between amputation and replantation.
- Provide hypothermic preservation of the amputated part (39°F [4°C]).
- Avoid freezing or directly immersing the severed part in water.
- Preservation of the amputated part is key to successful replantation.

Data from Maricevich M, Carlsen B, Mardini S, Moran S. Upper extremity and digital replantation. *Hand*. 2011;6(4):356–363.

Flowchart 9-2 Amputations and Avulsions

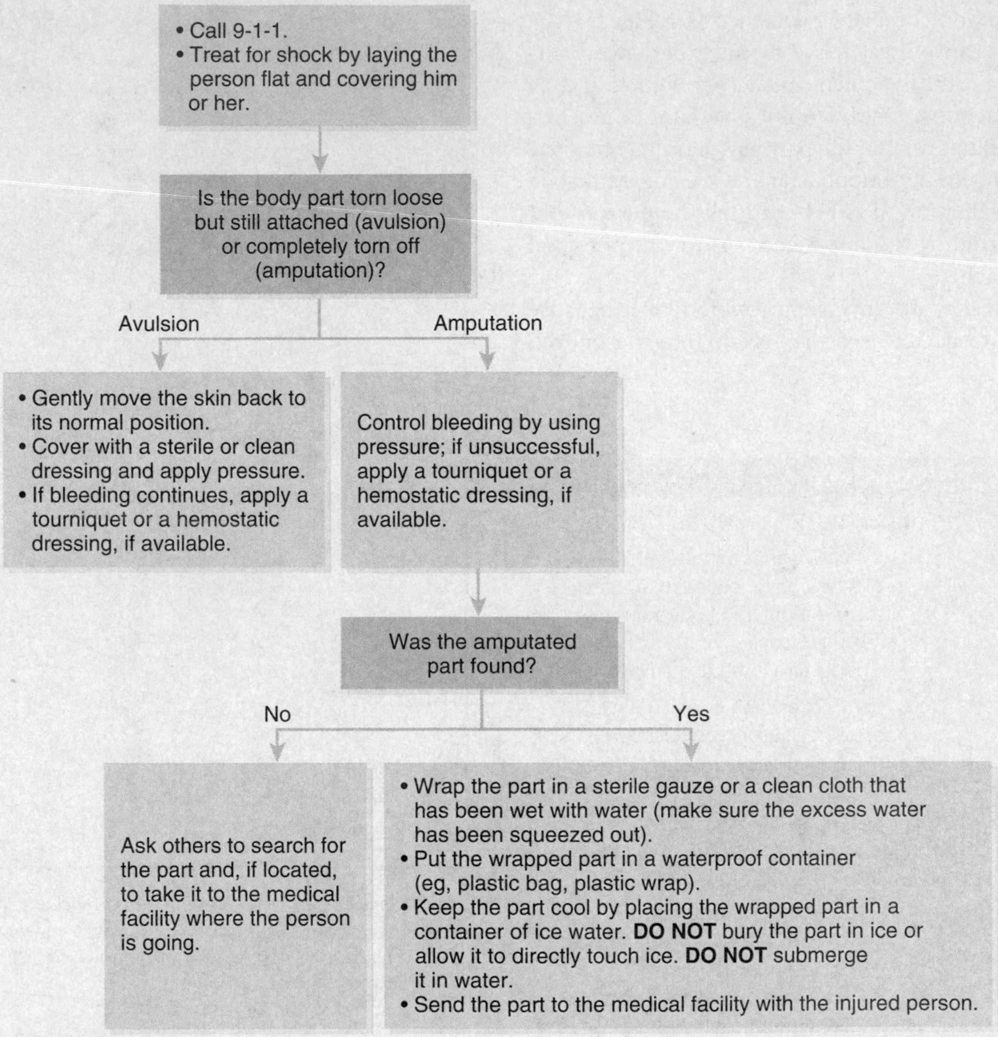
• Call 9-1-1.
• Treat for shock by laying the person flat and covering him or her.
Is the body part torn loose but still attached (avulsion) or completely torn off (amputation)?
Avulsion
Amputation
• Gently move the skin back to its normal position.
• Cover with a sterile or clean dressing and apply pressure.
• If bleeding continues, apply a tourniquet or a hemostatic dressing, if available.
Control bleeding by using pressure; if unsuccessful, apply a tourniquet or a hemostatic dressing, if available.
Was the amputated part found?
No
Yes
Ask others to search for the part and, if located, to take it to the medical facility where the person is going.
• Wrap the part in a sterile gauze or a clean cloth that has been wet with water (make sure the excess water has been squeezed out).
• Put the wrapped part in a waterproof container (eg, plastic bag, plastic wrap).
• Keep the part cool by placing the wrapped part in a container of ice water. DO NOT bury the part in ice or allow it to directly touch ice. DO NOT submerge it in water.
• Send the part to the medical facility with the injured person.

CAUTION

DO NOT try to decide whether a body part is salvageable or too small to save. Leave that decision to a physician.

DO NOT offer false hopes to the person with an amputation that the part can be reattached. Tell the person that you are handling the part for the potential that it may be reattached.

DO NOT wrap an amputated part in a soaking wet dressing or cloth. Using a soaking wet wrap on the part can cause waterlogging and tissue softening, which will make reattachment more difficult.

DO NOT bury an amputated part in ice; instead, place it on ice. Reattaching frostbitten parts is usually unsuccessful.

DO NOT use dry ice.

DO NOT cut a skin "bridge," a tendon, or other structure that is connecting a partially attached part to the rest of the body. Instead, reposition the part in the normal position, wrap the part in a dry, sterile dressing or clean cloth, and place an ice pack on it.

body parts, and shrink in diameter, resulting in a surprisingly small amount of blood loss.

Refer to **FLOWCHART 9-2** for additional information regarding the care of amputations and avulsions.

Blisters

A blister is a collection of fluid in a bubble under the outer layer of skin. (Note: This section applies only to friction blisters and does not apply to blisters from burns, frostbite, drug reactions, insect or snake bites, or contact with a poisonous plant.)

Repeated rubbing of a small area of the skin will produce a blister **FIGURE 9-10**. Blisters are so common that many people assume they are a fact of life. However, blisters are avoidable, and life for many people could be more comfortable if they knew how to treat and prevent blisters.

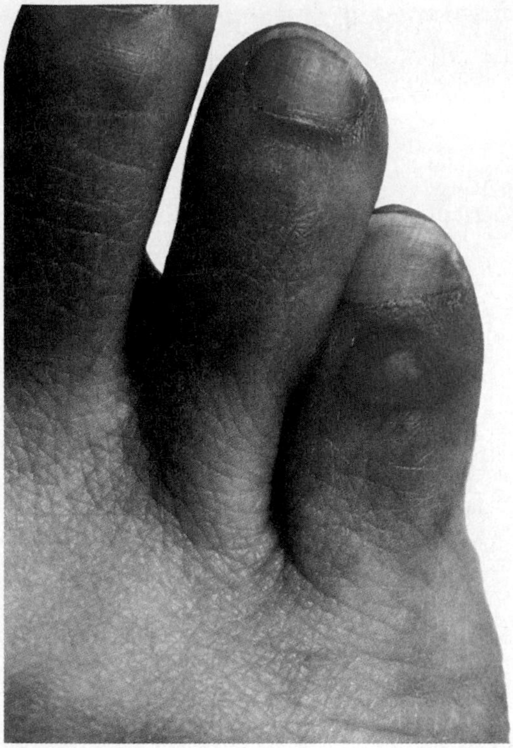

FIGURE 9-10 Friction blister (closed).

Rubbing—as between a sock and a foot—causes stress on the skin's surface because the underlying supporting tissue remains stationary. The stress separates the skin into two layers, and the resulting space fills with fluid. The fluid may collect under or within the skin's outer layer, the epidermis. Because of differences in skin, blister formation varies considerably from person to person.

When caring for a friction blister, try to (1) avoid the risk of infection, (2) minimize the person's pain and discomfort, (3) limit the blister's enlargement when resting is not an option, and (4) promote fast skin healing. The best care for a blister is determined mainly by its size and location.

Refer to **FLOWCHART 9-3** for additional information regarding the care of friction blisters.

What to Look For	What to Do
Hot spot (painful, red area caused by rubbing)	1. Depending upon availability and the location of the blister, relieve pressure on the area by applying one of the following: ▪ Blister bandage (Blist-O-Ban) ▪ Surgical tape (Micropore paper tape) ▪ Elastic tape (Elastikon) 2. Trim and round the edges of the tape to prevent it from peeling off.
Blister that is closed and not very painful	Depending upon availability and the location of the blister, use the most appropriate method previously discussed.
Blister that is closed and very painful	1. Clean the blister and a needle with an alcohol pad. 2. Make several small holes at the base of the blister with the needle **FIGURE 9-11**. **DO NOT** make one large hole. Gently press the fluid out. **DO NOT** remove the blister roof unless it is torn. 3. Apply paper tape to protect the blister roof from being torn away when other overlying tape is removed. 4. Cover paper tape with elastic or adhesive tape. 5. Trim and round the edges of the tape to prevent it from peeling off. 6. Watch for signs of an infection.
Blister that is very painful and open or torn	1. Use scissors to carefully trim off the dead skin. 2. Place a blister pad (Spenco 2nd Skin) over the raw skin. 3. Cover the blister pad with paper tape. 4. Cover paper tape with elastic or adhesive tape. Trim and round the edges of the tape to prevent it from peeling off. 5. Watch for signs of an infection.

FYI

Moleskin for Blisters?

Moleskin has been a fixture in the first aid kits of hikers for decades. Applying a doughnut-shaped moleskin patch around a hot spot or blister places friction and pressure on the surrounding area rather than on the affected area. Large or open heel blisters may benefit from being surrounded by moleskin or molefoam; however, these products have a high failure rate and are difficult to anchor. Additionally, the size of the product in a well-fitted shoe may cause more blisters on the toes or elsewhere.

Data from Lipman GS, Scheer BV. Blisters: the enemy of the feet. *Wilderness Environ Med*. 2015;26(2):275–276.

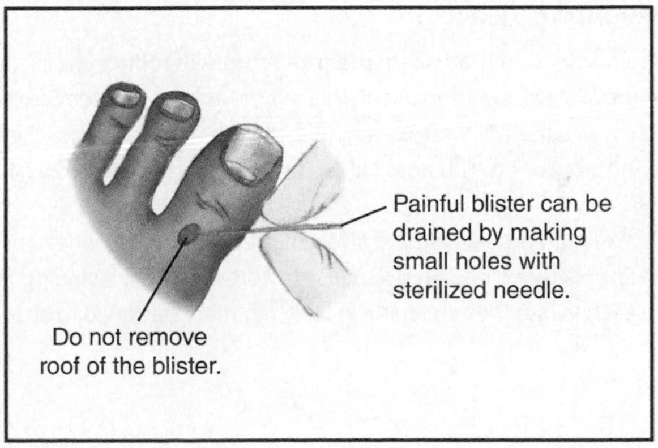

Painful blister can be drained by making small holes with sterilized needle.
Do not remove roof of the blister.

FIGURE 9-11 Blister care.

Flowchart 9-3 Friction Blisters

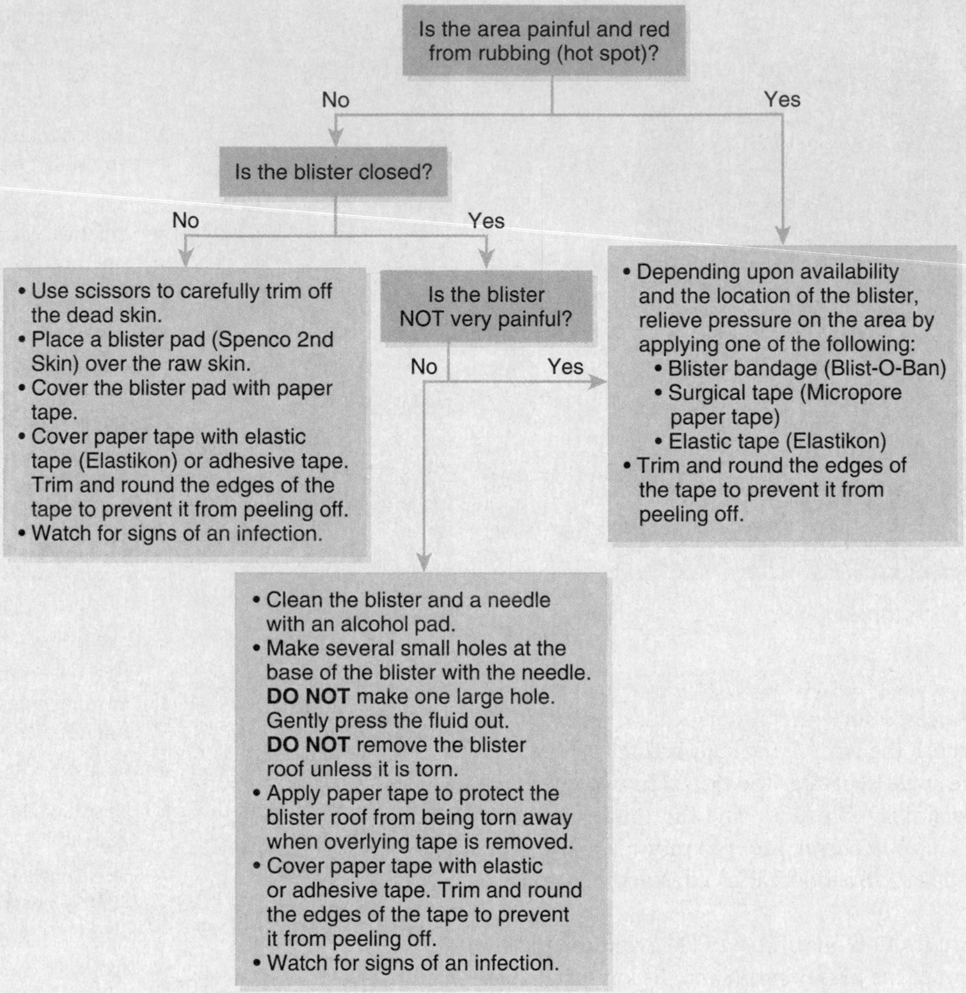
Is the area painful and red from rubbing (hot spot)?
No
Yes
Is the blister closed?
No
Yes
• Use scissors to carefully trim off the dead skin.
• Place a blister pad (Spenco 2nd Skin) over the raw skin.
• Cover the blister pad with paper tape.
• Cover paper tape with elastic tape (Elastikon) or adhesive tape. Trim and round the edges of the tape to prevent it from peeling off.
• Watch for signs of an infection.
Is the blister NOT very painful?
No
Yes
• Depending upon availability and the location of the blister, relieve pressure on the area by applying one of the following:
• Blister bandage (Blist-O-Ban)
• Surgical tape (Micropore paper tape)
• Elastic tape (Elastikon)
• Trim and round the edges of the tape to prevent it from peeling off.
• Clean the blister and a needle with an alcohol pad.
• Make several small holes at the base of the blister with the needle. DO NOT make one large hole. Gently press the fluid out. DO NOT remove the blister roof unless it is torn.
• Apply paper tape to protect the blister roof from being torn away when overlying tape is removed.
• Cover paper tape with elastic or adhesive tape. Trim and round the edges of the tape to prevent it from peeling off.
• Watch for signs of an infection.

FYI

Preventing Blisters

Keeping the skin lubricated and protected will reduce the potential for blister formation. Applying paper tape to problem areas, such as around a big toe, can help reduce blister formation by allowing the sock to rub against the tape instead of directly against the skin.

Wearing proper clothing also can prevent blisters. For example, acrylic socks are considered superior to cotton socks in avoiding foot blisters because they are made in layers that are designed to absorb friction. Synthetic socks such as acrylic wick better than cotton. Avoid tube socks made of any material because their less precise fit tends to cause more friction than regular, fitted socks. Wear gloves to protect the skin on your hands.

Anything that can be done to keep the skin dry can also reduce blister formation. Moist skin is more susceptible to blisters than either very dry or very wet skin. One method is to wear socks that wick moisture from the skin. The application of antiperspirants to the feet has been shown to reduce the formation of serious blisters.

Flowchart 9-4 Impaled (Embedded) Objects

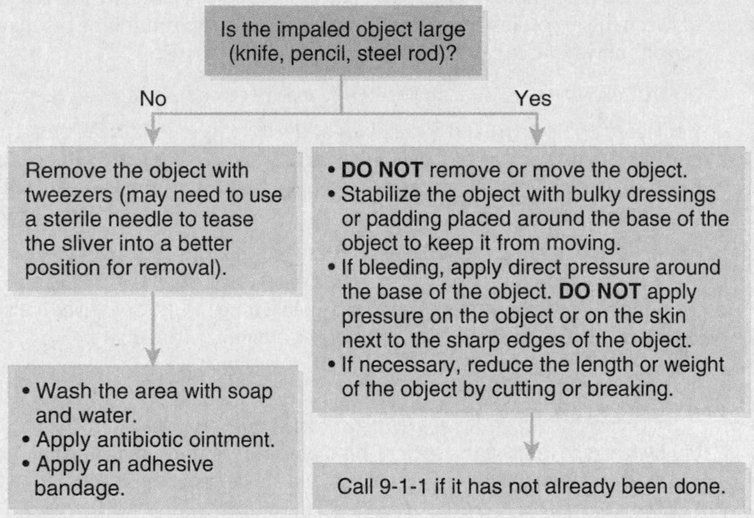
Is the impaled object large (knife, pencil, steel rod)?
No
Yes
Remove the object with tweezers (may need to use a sterile needle to tease the sliver into a better position for removal).
• Wash the area with soap and water.
• Apply antibiotic ointment.
• Apply an adhesive bandage.
• DO NOT remove or move the object.
• Stabilize the object with bulky dressings or padding placed around the base of the object to keep it from moving.
• If bleeding, apply direct pressure around the base of the object. DO NOT apply pressure on the object or on the skin next to the sharp edges of the object.
• If necessary, reduce the length or weight of the object by cutting or breaking.
Call 9-1-1 if it has not already been done.

Impaled (Embedded) Objects

Impaled objects come in all shapes and sizes, from pencils and screwdrivers to knives, glass, steel rods, and fence posts **FIGURE 9-12**. Proper first aid requires that the impaled object be stabilized because there can be significant internal damage.

Refer to **FLOWCHART 9-4** for additional information regarding the care of impaled (embedded) objects.

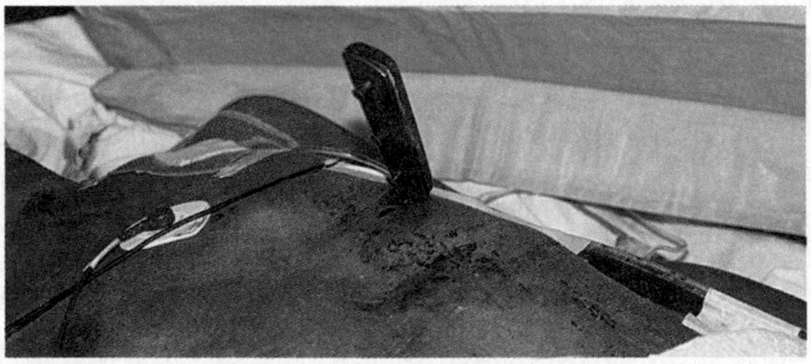

FIGURE 9-12 Impaled object.

What to Look For	What to Do
Sliver (also referred to as a splinter)	**1.** Remove with tweezers (may need to use a sterile needle to tease the sliver into a better position for removal). **2.** Wash the area with soap and water. **3.** Apply antibiotic ointment. **4.** Apply an adhesive bandage.
Large object (such as a knife, pencil, steel rod)	**1.** **DO NOT** remove or move the object. **2.** Stabilize the object with bulky dressings or padding placed around the base of the object to keep it from moving. **3.** If bleeding, apply direct pressure around the base of the object. **DO NOT** apply pressure on the object or on the skin next to the sharp edges of the object. **4.** If necessary, reduce the length or weight of the object by cutting or breaking it. **5.** Call 9-1-1.
Impaled object in the cheek	**1.** Examine the injury inside the mouth. If the object extends through the cheek and you are more than 1 hour from medical help, consider removing it.

What to Look For	What to Do
	2. To remove the object, place two fingers next to the object, straddling it; then gently pull it back through the cheek in the direction from which it entered. If it cannot be removed easily, leave it in place and secure it with bulky dressings. **3.** Control the bleeding. After you have removed the object, place dressings over the wound inside the mouth between the cheek and the teeth. The dressings will help control the bleeding and will not interfere with the person's airway. Also place a dressing on the outside wound.
Impaled object in the eye	**1.** **DO NOT** exert any pressure against the eyeball because fluid can be forced out of it, worsening the injury. **2.** Stabilize the object. Use bulky dressings or clean cloths to stabilize a long, protruding object. You can place a protective paper cup or cardboard folded into a cone over the affected eye to prevent bumping of the object. For short objects, surround the eye—without touching the object—with a doughnut-shaped (ring) pad held in place with a roller or cravat bandage. **3.** Cover the undamaged eye. Most experts suggest that the undamaged eye be covered to prevent sympathetic eye movement (ie, movement of the injured eye when the undamaged eye moves, thus aggravating the injury). Remember that the person is unable to see when both eyes are covered and may be very anxious. Make sure you explain to the person everything you are doing. **4.** Call 9-1-1.
Cactus spines	Use one of the following methods to remove cactus spines: **1.** Use tweezers to remove the spines. This method is easy but time consuming because the spines usually are acquired in groupings, are difficult to see, and are designed by nature to resist removal. **2.** Coat the area with a thin layer of white woodworking glue or rubber cement and allow it to dry for at least 30 minutes. Slowly roll up the dried glue from the margins. Applying the glue in strips rather than puddles will make the rolling procedure go more smoothly. A single layer of gauze gently pressed onto the still-damp glue helps to remove it after it has dried. The combination of using tweezers and glue will remove most of the spines. **3.** Use adhesive tape, duct tape, or cellophane tape. Although this method is quick and easy, it removes only about 30% of the spines, even after multiple attempts. **4.** **DO NOT** use super glue (or other similar products) to remove cactus spines. Not only does it fail to roll up when applied to the skin, but it also welds the spines to the skin. In addition, there is the risk that the skin will permanently bond to anything it touches.
Fishhooks	**1.** Tape an embedded fishhook in place and do not try to remove it if injury to a nearby body part (such as the eye or an underlying structure such as a blood vessel or nerve) is possible or if the person (such as a young child) is uncooperative **FIGURE 9-13**. **2.** If the point of a fishhook has penetrated the skin but the barb has not, remove the fishhook by backing it out. Then treat the wound like a puncture wound. Seek medical advice for a possible tetanus shot. **3.** If the hook's barb has entered the skin, follow these procedures: ▪ If professional medical care is near, transport the person and have a physician remove the hook. ▪ If you are in a remote area, far from professional medical care, remove the hook using either the pliers method or the string-jerk method. *To remove a hook using the pliers method:* **1.** Use pliers with tempered jaws that can cut through a hook **FIGURE 9-14**. (Test the pliers by first cutting a similar fishhook.) **2.** Use an ice pack or use hard pressure around the hook to provide temporary numbness. **3.** Push the embedded hook farther in, in a shallow curve, until the point and the barb come out through the skin. (Use extreme care; pushing the hook into blood vessels, nerves, or tendons can result in severe injury.) **4.** Cut off the barb, then back the hook out the way it came in. **5.** After removing the hook, treat the wound and seek professional medical attention for a possible tetanus shot. *To remove a hook using the string-jerk method:* **1.** Loop a piece of fishing line over the bend or curve of the embedded hook **FIGURE 9-15**. **2.** Stabilize the part of the person's body in which the hook is embedded. **3.** Use an ice pack or use hard pressure around the hook to provide temporary numbness. **4.** With one hand, press down on the hook's shank and eye while the other hand sharply jerks the fishing line that is over the hook's bend or curve. The jerk movement should be parallel to the skin's surface. The hook will neatly come out of the same hole it entered, causing little pain. **5.** After removing the hook, care for the wound and seek professional medical care for a possible tetanus shot.

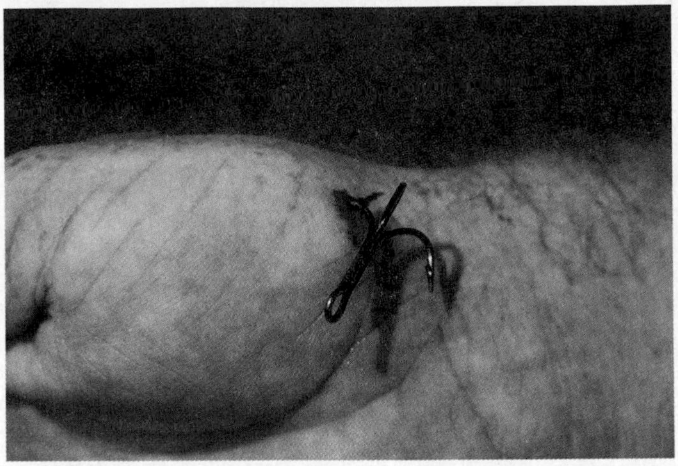

FIGURE 9-13 Fishhook.

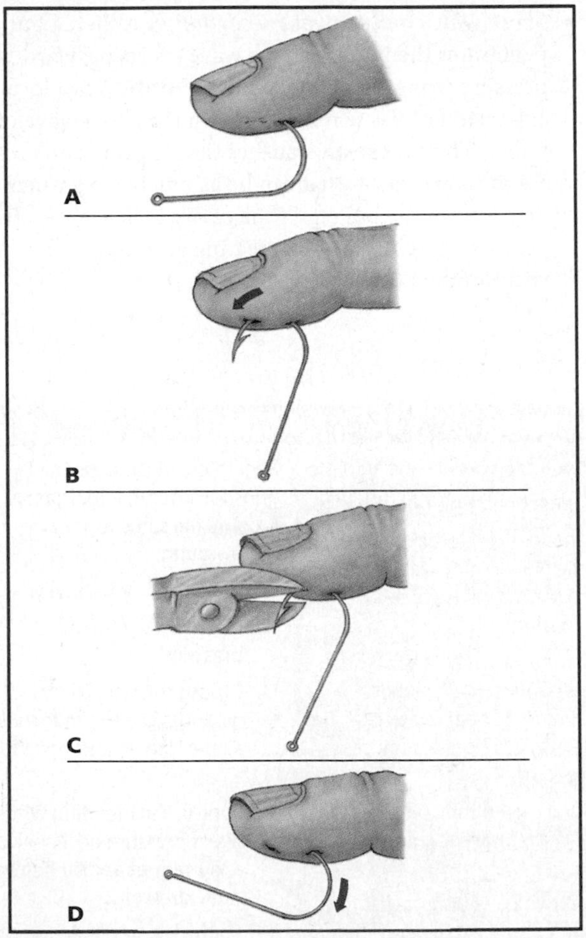

FIGURE 9-14 **A**. The pliers method can be used to remove a fishhook embedded in the skin. **B**. Push the embedded hook farther in until the barb comes out through the skin. **C**. Cut off the barb. **D**. Back the hook out the way it came in.

Closed Wounds

A closed wound happens when a blunt object strikes the body. The skin is not broken, but tissue and blood vessels beneath the skin's surface are crushed, causing bleeding inside the body.

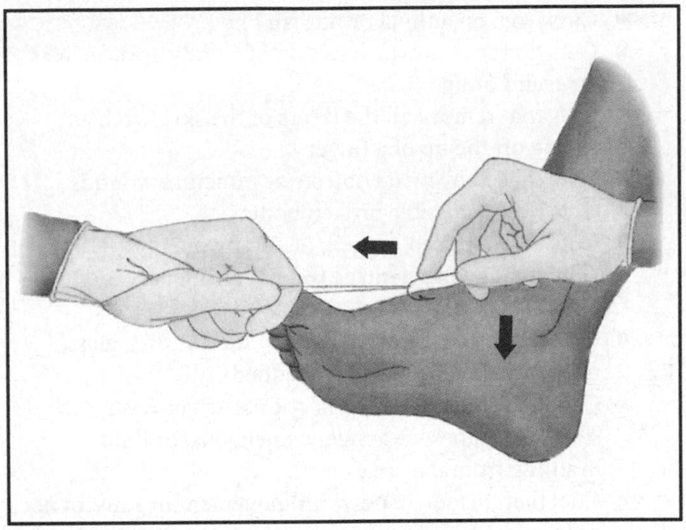

FIGURE 9-15 Fishhook removal: string-jerk method.

What to Look For	What to Do
There are three types of closed wounds: **1.** With a bruise (contusion), blood is dispersed within the tissues. Blood collects under the skin in the injured area. The person will experience pain and swelling (immediately or within 24 to 48 hours). As blood accumulates, a black-and-blue mark may appear. **2.** Hematomas contain a pool of blood—as much as a pint or more—surrounding a major bone fracture or any injury to a large blood vessel. There may be a lump with blue discoloration. **3.** Crush injuries are caused by extreme forces, which can injure vital organs and bones without breaking open the skin. Crush injuries may indicate an underlying condition such as a fracture. Signs and symptoms include discoloration, swelling, pain, and loss of use.	**1.** Control bleeding by applying an ice pack over the area for no more than 20 minutes. Place a cloth between the ice pack and the skin to prevent frostbite or frostnip. Wait at least 20 minutes before applying the ice pack again. Apply for 10 minutes if the person cannot tolerate the cold. **2.** If the injury involves a limb, apply an elastic bandage for compression. A splint may help make the person more comfortable. See Chapter 10, *Bandaging Wounds*. **3.** Check for a possible fracture. **4.** Elevate an injured extremity above the person's heart level to decrease pain and swelling unless doing so causes pain.

Wounds Requiring Professional Medical Care

At some point, you will probably have to decide whether professional medical care is needed for a wounded person. As a guideline, seek professional medical care for the following conditions, as offered by the American College of Emergency Physicians:

- Long or deep cuts that need stitches
- Cuts over a joint

- Cuts from an animal or human bite
- Cuts that may impair function of a body area, such as an eyelid or lip
- Cuts that remove all the layers of the skin, such as slicing off the tip of a finger
- Cuts caused by metal objects or puncture wounds
- Cuts over a possible broken bone
- Cuts that are deep, jagged, or gaping open
- Cuts that involve damage to underlying nerves, tendons, or joints
- Cuts in which foreign materials, such as dirt, glass, metal, or chemicals, are embedded
- Cuts that show signs of infection, such as fever, swelling, redness, a pungent smell, pus, or fluid draining from the area
- Cuts that include issues with movement or sensation, or increased pain

Call 9-1-1 immediately if the following are observed:

- Bleeding from a cut does not slow during the first 5 to 10 minutes of steady pressure
- Signs of shock occur
- Breathing is difficult because of a cut to the neck or chest
- A deep cut to the abdomen causes moderate to severe pain
- A cut occurs to the eyeball
- A cut amputates or partially amputates an extremity

Sutures

If sutures (stitches) are needed, they usually should be placed by a physician or physician assistant within 24 hours of the injury. Suturing wounds allows faster healing, reduces infection, and lessens scarring. Some wounds do not usually require sutures, including the following:

- Wounds in which the skin's cut edges tend to fall together
- Shallow cuts less than 1 inch (3 cm) long

Rather than close a gaping wound with butterfly bandages or elastic skin closures, cover the wound with sterile gauze. Closing the wound might trap bacteria inside, resulting in an infection. In most cases, a physician or physician assistant can be reached in time for sutures to be placed; if not, a wound without sutures will still heal but with scars. Scar tissue can be attended to later by a plastic surgeon.

Gunshot Wounds

Guns are abundant in the United States; it is estimated that about one-half of all American homes have a firearm. Shootings, stabbings, and other penetrating injuries that result from violence represent a major challenge to a first aid provider. Rescuers sometimes take greater than normal risks to help people who have been shot or stabbed. If you are at the scene of an active shooter, you should "run, hide, fight." Run when it is safe to run, hide where it is safe to hide, and fight if you or others around you have no other options.

There are two general types of firearms: low velocity, such as most civilian firearms, and high velocity, such as many tactical and hunting rifles. Shotguns have low velocity but create severe tissue damage.

A bullet causes injury in the following ways, depending on its velocity, or speed:

- *Laceration and crushing.* When the bullet penetrates the body, it crushes tissue and forces it apart. That is the main effect of low-velocity bullets. The crushing and laceration caused by the passage of the bullet usually are not life threatening unless vital organs or major blood vessels are injured. The bullet damages only the tissues that it contacts directly, and the wound is comparable to that caused by weapons such as knives.
- *Shock waves and temporary cavitation.* When a bullet penetrates the body, a shock wave exerts outward pressure from the bullet's path. **Cavitation** is a localized expansion of tissue resulting from the shockwave of a bullet. The shock wave pushes tissues away and creates a temporary cavity that can be as much as 30 times the diameter of the bullet. As the cavity forms, a negative pressure develops inside, creating a vacuum. The vacuum then draws debris in with it.

What to Look For	What to Do
Penetrating wound, indicated by: ▪ A bullet entry point but no exit ▪ Little or no external bleeding (the person may still bleed to death because of internal bleeding) ▪ Signs and symptoms of shock (ie, diminishing alertness, fainting, or near fainting) if the person has significant internal bleeding Perforating wound, indicated by both entry and exit points: ▪ The exit wound of a high-velocity bullet is usually larger than the entrance wound. ▪ The exit wound from a low-velocity bullet is about the same size as the entry wound **FIGURE 9-16**. ▪ If the bullet was fired at very close range, the entrance wound may be larger than the exit wound because the gases from the gun's muzzle contribute to the surface-tissue damage.	Regardless of the type of gunshot wound, initial care is roughly the same as for any other wound. **1.** Call 9-1-1 immediately. **2.** Monitor the person's breathing. **3.** Expose the wound or wounds. Make sure to look at all the skin, including hidden areas. **4.** Control the bleeding with direct pressure or, if needed, a tourniquet and/or hemostatic dressing. **5.** Apply dry, sterile dressings to the wound or wounds, and bandage them securely in place. **6.** Treat the person for shock. **7.** Keep the person calm and quiet.

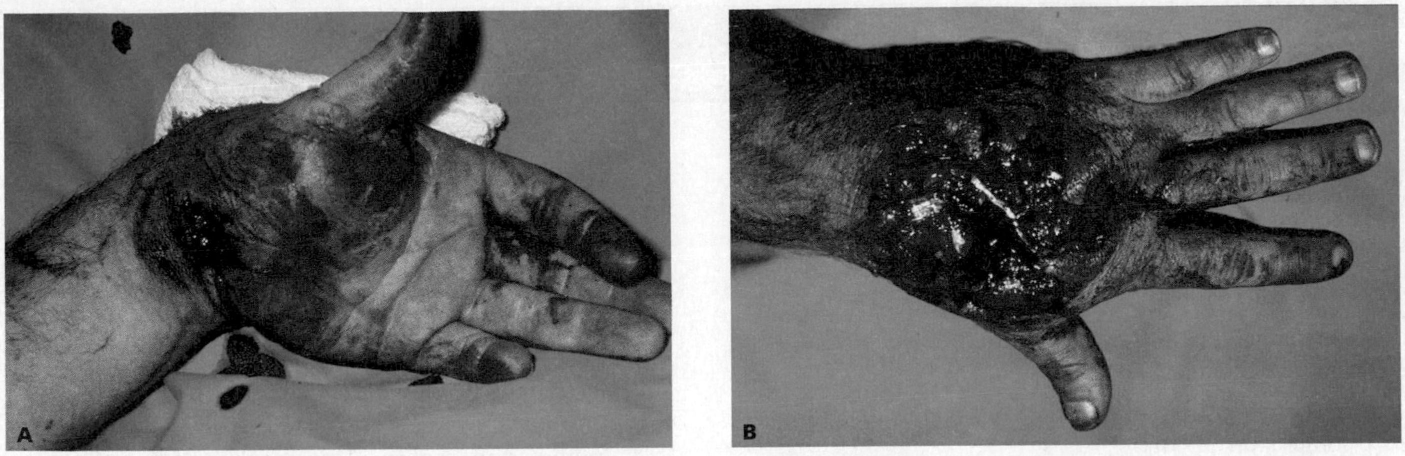

FIGURE 9-16 Gunshot wounds. **A**. An entrance wound from a gunshot may have burns around the edges. **B**. An exit wound is sometimes larger and results in greater damage to soft tissues.

Temporary cavitation occurs only with high-velocity firearms and is the main reason for their immensely destructive effect. The cavitation lasts only a millisecond but can damage muscles, nerves, blood vessels, and bone.

Bullets sometimes hit hard tissue such as bones and may bounce around in the body cavities, causing a great deal of damage to tissue and organs. Moreover, bone chips can ricochet to other body areas and cause damage. Because a split or misshapen bullet tumbles and exerts its force over a larger area, it does more damage than does a smooth bullet going in a straight line.

Legal Implications of Gunshot Wounds

Because interactions with people with gunshot wounds will involve contact with law enforcement agencies and will possibly require you to testify in court, carefully observe the scene and the person. Keep an accurate record of your observations. Do not touch or move anything unless absolutely necessary to treat the person. All gunshot wounds must be reported to the police regardless of whether they are intentional (suicide, assault, murder, self-defense) or unintentional.

Q&A

How do the physical characteristics of the bullet affect injury to the person?

- The larger the size of the bullet, the greater the size of the wound (eg, .22 [small] versus .45 [larger] caliber).
- A hollow-point bullet widens when it hits tissues, causing a wider path of destruction.
- A bullet that tumbles around damages more tissue.
- Soft-nose bullets or bullets with vertical cuts in the nose break apart on impact, spreading fragments in a wider path and causing more tissue and organ damage. A shotgun blast also causes fragmentation.

CAUTION

DO NOT try to remove material from a gunshot wound. The hospital emergency department personnel will clean the wound.

PREP KIT

Ready for Review

- An open wound is a break in the skin's surface resulting in external bleeding.
- Knowing what type of open wound the person has will help you in providing first aid.
- In many cases, an amputated extremity can be successfully replanted.
- A blister is a collection of fluid in a bubble under the outer layer of skin.
- Proper first aid of an impaled object requires that the object be stabilized, because significant internal damage can occur.
- A closed wound happens when a blunt object strikes the body. Although the skin remains unbroken, the tissue and blood vessels beneath the skin's surface are crushed, causing bleeding inside the body.
- Wounds that require professional medical care include the following:
  - Long or deep cuts that need stitches
  - Cuts over a joint
  - Cuts from an animal or human bite
  - Cuts that may impair function of a body area, such as an eyelid or lip
  - Cuts that remove all the layers of the skin, such as slicing off the tip of a finger
  - Cuts caused by metal objects or puncture wounds
  - Cuts over a possible broken bone
  - Cuts that are deep, jagged, or gaping open
  - Cuts that involve damage to underlying nerves, tendons, or joints
  - Cuts in which foreign materials, such as dirt, glass, metal, or chemicals, are embedded
  - Cuts that show signs of infection, such as fever, swelling, redness, a pungent smell, pus, or fluid draining from the area
  - Cuts that include issues with movement or sensation, or increased pain
- Call 9-1-1 immediately if the following situations are present:
  - Bleeding from a cut does not slow during the first 15 minutes of steady pressure
  - Signs of shock occur
  - Breathing is difficult because of a cut to the neck or chest
  - A deep cut to the abdomen causes moderate to severe pain
  - A cut occurs to the eyeball
  - A cut amputates or partially amputates an extremity
- Regardless of the type of gunshot wound, initial care is roughly the same as for any other wound.

Vital Vocabulary

abrasion An injury in which a portion of the skin is removed by rubbing or scraping on a hard, rough surface.

amputation An injury in which a body part is completely removed.

avulsion An injury that leaves a piece of skin or other tissue either partially or completely torn away from the body.

bandage A material used to cover a dressing to keep it in place on the wound and to apply pressure to help control bleeding.

cavitation A localized expansion of tissue resulting from the shock wave of a bullet.

clean amputation A clean-cut, complete detachment of an extremity.

crushing amputation An injury in which an extremity separates by being crushed or mashed off.

dressing A sterile gauze pad or clean cloth covering that is placed over an open wound.

incision A wound that is usually made deliberately in connection with surgery. The edges are cleanly cut as opposed to a laceration.

laceration A wound made by the tearing or cutting of body tissues.

puncture A deep, narrow wound in the skin and underlying organs.

PREP KIT continued

Assessment in Action

You are helping your mother prepare for a barbeque on a Saturday afternoon. She is slicing tomatoes with a very dull kitchen knife. She is startled by something and cuts into her finger. The wound is bleeding and you can see the bone in the wound.

Directions: Circle Yes if you agree with the statement; circle No if you disagree.

1. This type of wound is called an avulsion.
   YES **NO**
2. You should not be concerned about infection because she was using a clean knife.
   YES **NO**
3. You should cover the wound with a sterile dressing but should not close the wound with tape or butterfly bandages.
   YES **NO**
4. She may need sutures. Because you and your mother do not want to miss the barbeque, it will be okay to wait until the next day.
   YES **NO**

Check Your Knowledge

Directions: Circle Yes if you agree with the statement; circle No if you disagree.

1. An open wound may allow bacteria to enter the body, causing an infection.
   YES **NO**
2. A laceration is cut skin with smooth, straight edges.
   YES **NO**
3. A dressing is applied over a wound to control bleeding and prevent contamination.
   YES **NO**
4. A bandage is applied over a wound to hold a dressing in place.
   YES **NO**
5. Any wound can become infected.
   YES **NO**
6. The signs and symptoms of an infection include swelling and redness around the wound, throbbing pain, and a lack of fever.
   YES **NO**
7. A bite wound is more likely to become infected.
   YES **NO**
8. Impaled objects should be removed immediately.
   YES **NO**
9. Tetanus is communicable from one person to another.
   YES **NO**
10. In many cases, an amputated extremity can be successfully reattached.
    YES **NO**

Chapter Opener: Courtesy of Rhonda Hunt.

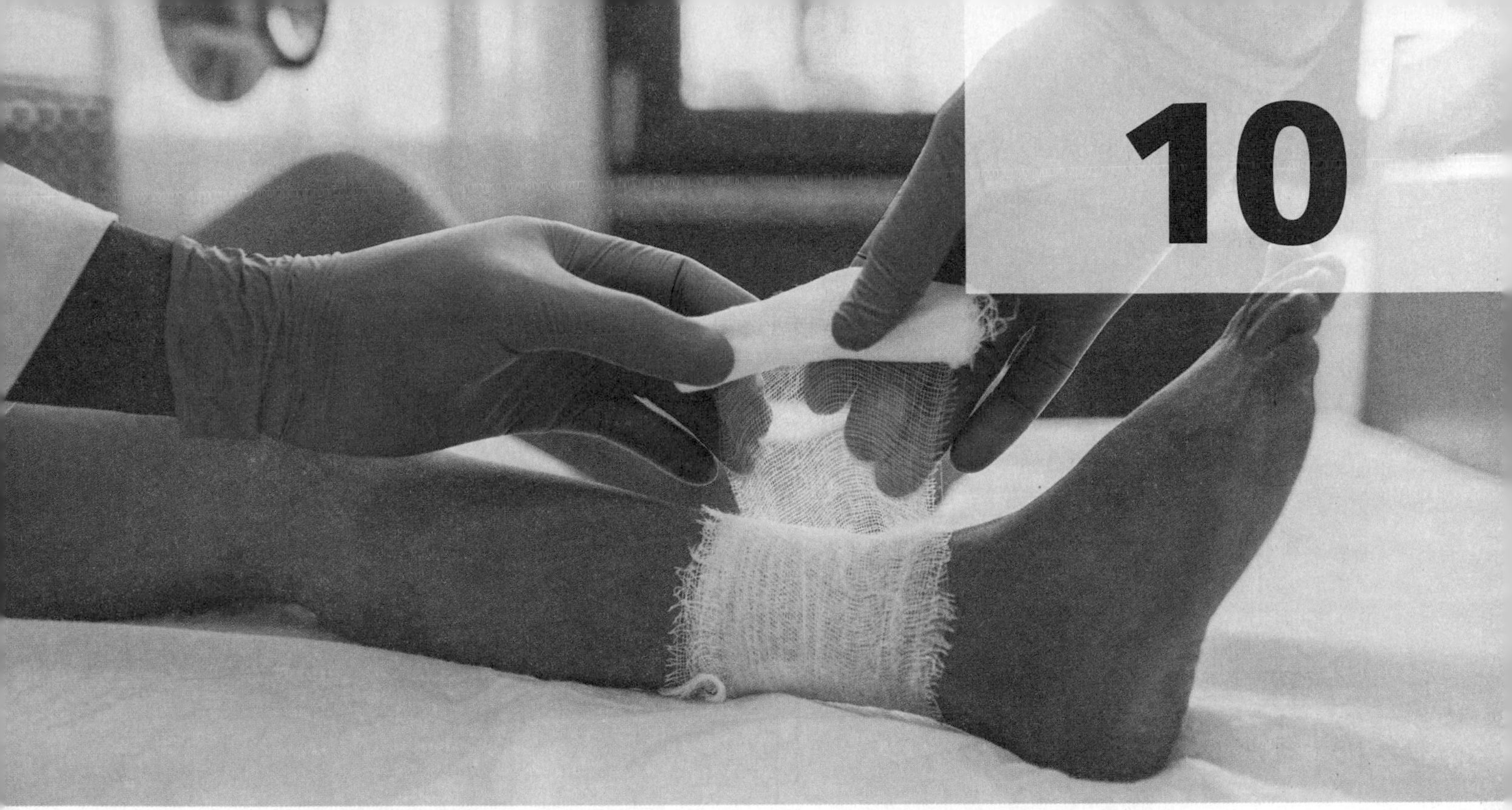

10

Bandaging Wounds

CHAPTER AT A GLANCE

- Dressings
- Bandages

Dressings

A dressing covers an open wound; it touches the wound. Whenever possible, a dressing should have the following characteristics:

- *Sterile*. If a sterile dressing is not available, use a clean cloth, handkerchief, washcloth, or towel.
- *Larger than the wound*.
- *Thick, soft, and compressible*. This allows pressure to be evenly distributed over the wound.
- *Lint free*.

The purposes of using a dressing are as follows:

- Control bleeding.
- Prevent infection and contamination.
- Absorb blood and wound drainage.
- Protect the wound from further injury.

Types of Dressings

Use commercial dressings whenever possible. Dressings used in most first aid situations are commercially prepared, but you may sometimes need to improvise dressings. The following describes types of dressings:

- **Gauze pads** are used for small wounds. They come in separately wrapped packages of various sizes

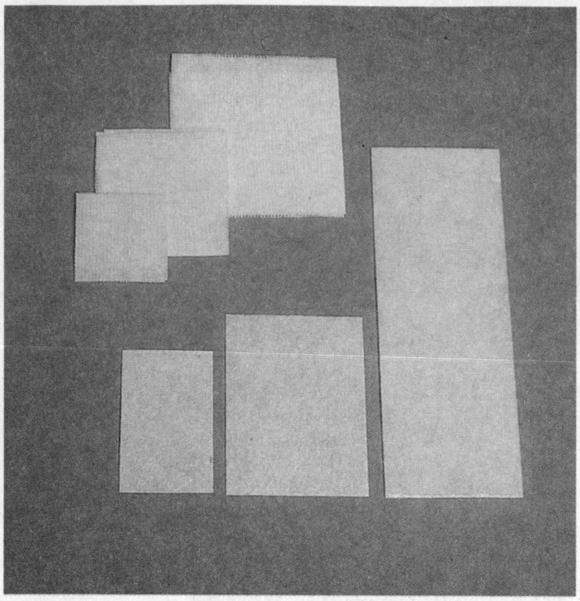

FIGURE 10-1 Gauze pads.

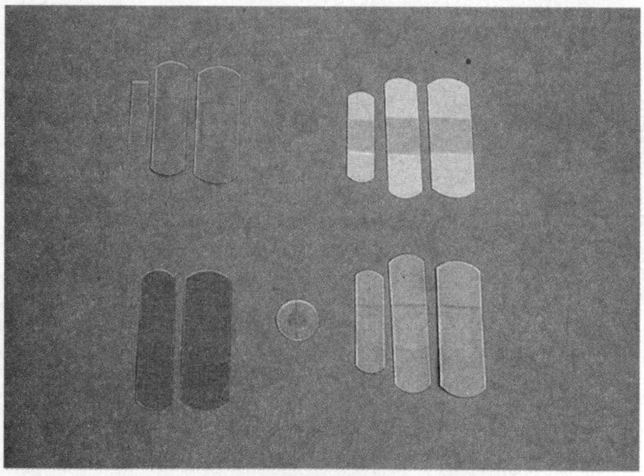

FIGURE 10-2 Adhesive bandages.

(eg, 2-inch × 2-inch [5-cm × 5-cm] squares; 4-inch × 4-inch [10-cm × 10-cm] squares) and are sterile, unless the package is broken. Some gauze pads have a special coating to keep them from sticking to the wound and are especially helpful for burns or wounds that are secreting fluids **FIGURE 10-1**.

- **Adhesive bandages** are used for small cuts and abrasions and are a combination of a sterile dressing and a bandage **FIGURE 10-2**.
- **Trauma dressings** are made of large, thick, absorbent, sterile materials. Individually wrapped sanitary napkins can serve as a dressing because of their bulk and absorbency, but they usually are not sterile **FIGURE 10-3**.
- When commercial sterile dressings are not available, an improvised dressing should be as clean, absorbent, soft, and as free of lint as possible (eg, a handkerchief or a towel). Use the cleanest cloth available, or, in some conditions and if time allows, sterilize a cloth by ironing it for several minutes.

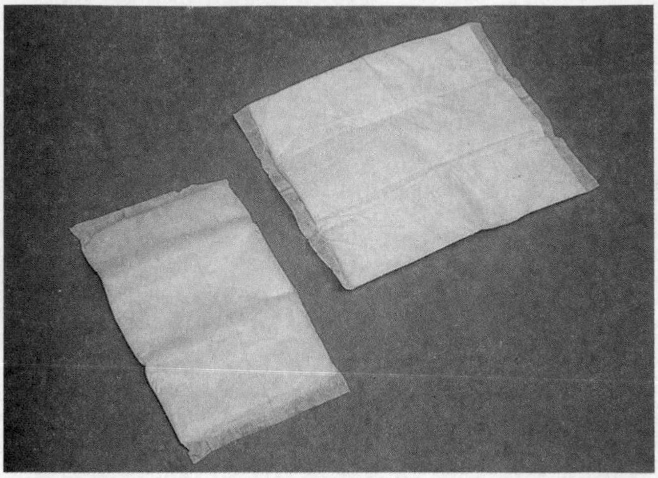

FIGURE 10-3 Trauma dressings.

CAUTION

DO NOT use fluffy cotton or cotton balls as a dressing. Cotton fibers can get in the wound and become difficult to remove.

DO NOT pull off a dressing stuck to a wound. If it needs to be removed, soak it off in warm water.

Applying a Sterile Dressing

1. Whenever possible, wash your hands and wear disposable medical exam gloves.
2. Use a dressing large enough to extend beyond the edges of the wound. Hold the dressing by a corner. Place the dressing directly over the wound. **DO NOT** slide it on; doing so can cause pain and dislodge blood clots.
3. Cover the dressing with one of the types of bandages.

CAUTION

DO NOT touch any part of the wound or any part of the dressing that will be in contact with the wound.

Bandages

A bandage should be clean but need not be sterile. A bandage can be used as follows:

- Hold a dressing in place over an open wound.
- Apply direct pressure over a dressing to control bleeding.

- Prevent or reduce swelling.
- Provide support and stability for an extremity or joint.

Remember, bandages should be applied firmly enough to keep dressings and splints in place but not so tightly that they will reinjure the body part or impede blood circulation. The signs that a bandage is too tight include the following:

- Blue tinge of the fingernails or toenails
- Skin looks blue or pale
- Tingling or loss of sensation
- Coldness of the extremity
- Swelling
- Inability to move the fingers or toes
- A slow capillary refill using the capillary refill test (see page 54).

A square knot is preferred because it is neat, holds well, and can be easily untied. If the knot or the bandage is likely to cause the person discomfort, a pad should be placed between the knot or bandage and the body.

CAUTION

DO NOT apply a bandage directly over a wound. Put a sterile dressing on first.

DO NOT bandage so tightly as to restrict blood circulation.

DO NOT bandage so loosely that the dressing will slip. This is the most common bandaging error. Bandages tend to stretch after a short time.

DO NOT leave loose ends. They might get caught on something or loosen.

DO NOT cover the person's fingers or toes unless they are injured. They need to be observed for color changes that would indicate impaired circulation.

DO NOT use elastic bandages over a wound. There is a tendency to apply them too tightly.

DO NOT apply a circular bandage around a person's neck; strangulation may occur.

DO NOT start a roller bandage above the wound.

DO NOT wrap roller bandage down an extremity (wrapping away from the heart).

Types of Bandages

The following are the basic types of bandages:

- **Roller bandages** come in various widths, lengths, and types of material. For best results, use different widths for different body areas:
  - 1-inch (3-cm) width for fingers
  - 2-inch (5-cm) width for wrists, hands, and feet
  - 3-inch (7-cm) width for ankles, elbows, and arms
  - 4-inch (10-cm) width for knees and legs
- **Self-adhering, conforming bandages** (eg, Kerlix) **FIGURE 10-4** come as rolls of slightly elastic, gauzelike material in various widths. Their self-adherent quality makes them easy to use.
- **Gauze rollers** are cotton and nonelastic. They come in various widths (1, 2, and 3 inches [3, 5, and 7 cm]) and usually are 10 yards (9 m) long. When commercial roller bandages are unavailable, you can improvise bandages from belts, neckties, or strips of cloth torn from a sheet or other similar material.
- **Elastic roller bandages** (eg, Ace bandages) **FIGURE 10-5** are used for compression on sprains, strains, and contusions and come in various widths. Elastic bandages are not usually applied over dressings covering a wound.

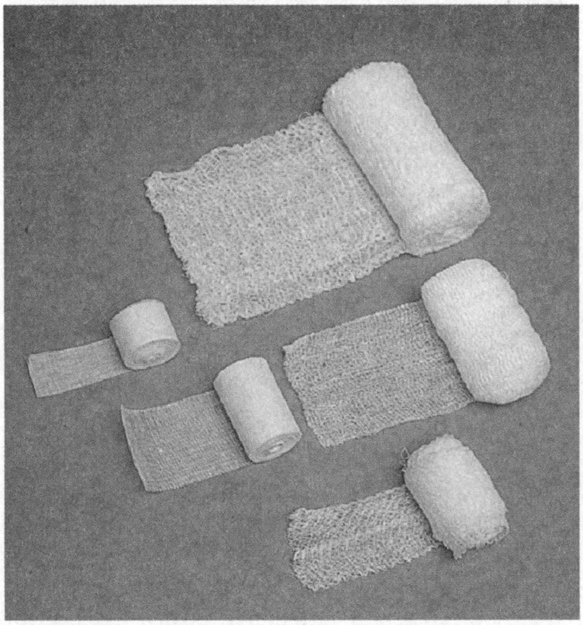

FIGURE 10-4 Self-adhering, conforming bandages and gauze bandages of various sizes.

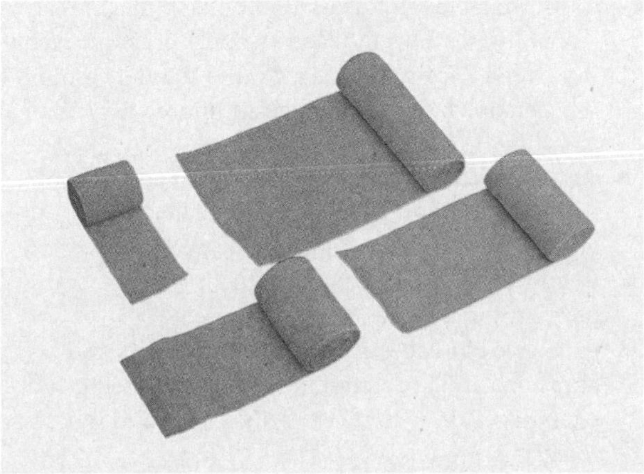

FIGURE 10-5 Elastic roller bandages of various sizes.

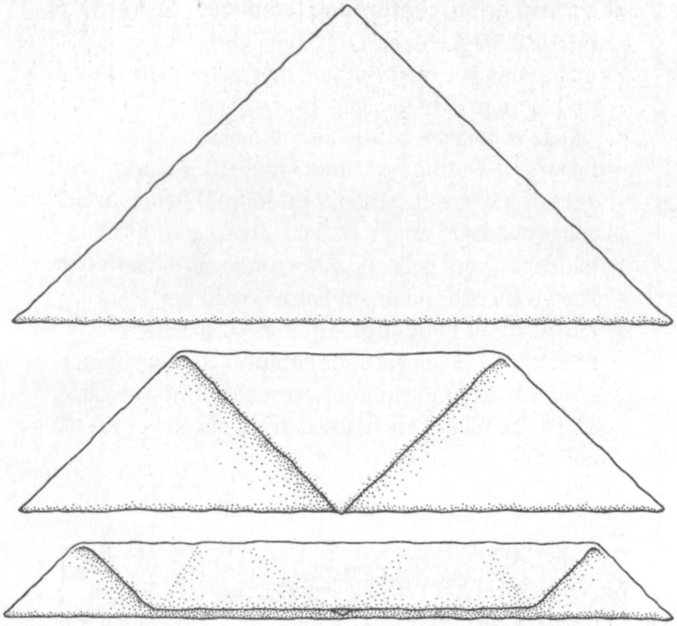

FIGURE 10-6 A triangular bandage folded into a cravat.

- **Triangular bandages FIGURE 10-6** are available commercially or can be made from a square piece of preshrunk cotton muslin measuring 36 to 40 inches (230 to 260 cm) along each side of the square. Cut the material diagonally from corner to corner to produce two triangular pieces of cloth. The longest side is called the base; the corner directly across from the base is the point; and the other two corners are called ends. A triangular bandage may be applied two ways:
  - *Fully opened* (*not folded*). Best used for an arm sling. When used to hold dressings in place, fully opened triangular bandages do not apply sufficient pressure on the wound.
  - **Cravat** (*folded triangular bandage*). The point is folded to the center of the base and then the fabric is folded in half again from the top to the base to form a cravat. It is used to hold splints in place, to hold dressings in place, to apply pressure evenly over a dressing, or as a swathe (binder) around the person's body to stabilize an injured arm in an arm sling.
- **Adhesive tape** comes in rolls and in a variety of widths. It is often used to secure roller bandages and small dressings in place. For people allergic to adhesive tape, use paper tape or special dermatologic tape.
- Adhesive bandages are used for small cuts and abrasions and are a combination of a dressing and a bandage. They come in various sizes and types of materials.

FYI

Removing Adhesive Tape

- When you first apply the tape, fold over one end (sticky sides together) to make a tab. When it comes time to remove the tape, you can grasp the starter tab. With this approach, there is no need to pick at the tape (and the person's skin) to get the strip started.
- To remove adhesive tape from the skin, gently lift the tape with one hand as you gently push the skin down and away from the tape with the other hand.
- Lift a corner of the tape and dab the adhesive with an alcohol wipe. The alcohol dissolves the adhesive as the tape is peeled off.
- When peeling off tape from hairy skin, pull in the direction in which the ends of the hair are naturally pointing.
- Firmly hold the skin from which the tape is pulled away.
- Older people often have very thin skin that can be torn when removing adhesive tape. When possible, use paper tape rather than other types of adhesive tape on older people.
- Save time and reduce frustration by leaving a tab on the end of the roll of tape for quick access the next time you need it.

Applying a Cravat Bandage

A cravat bandage can be applied on the head, forehead, ear, eyes, arm, leg, or hand (see Figure 10-6). For an injured eye, cover both eyes to prevent the injured eye from moving. Follow the steps in **SKILL SHEET 10-1** to apply a cravat bandage to the head, forehead, ear, or eyes using the cravat method. To apply a cravat bandage to the arm or leg using the cravat method, follow the steps in **SKILL SHEET 10-2**. To apply a cravat bandage to the palm of the hand using the cravat method, follow the steps in **SKILL SHEET 10-3**. To secure a cravat bandage, follow the steps in **SKILL SHEET 10-4**.

Applying a Roller Bandage

With a little ingenuity, you can apply a roller bandage to almost any body part. Self-adhering, conforming roller bandages eliminate the need for many of the complicated bandaging techniques that standard gauze roller, cravat, and triangular bandages require.

Spiral Method

This method employs a 2- or 3-inch (5- or 7-cm) roller bandage for the arm or a 4-inch (10-cm) bandage for the leg. To apply a bandage to the arm or leg using the spiral method, follow the steps in **SKILL SHEET 10-5**

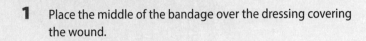

SKILL SHEET 10-1 Cravat Method of Bandaging the Head, Forehead, Ear, or Eyes

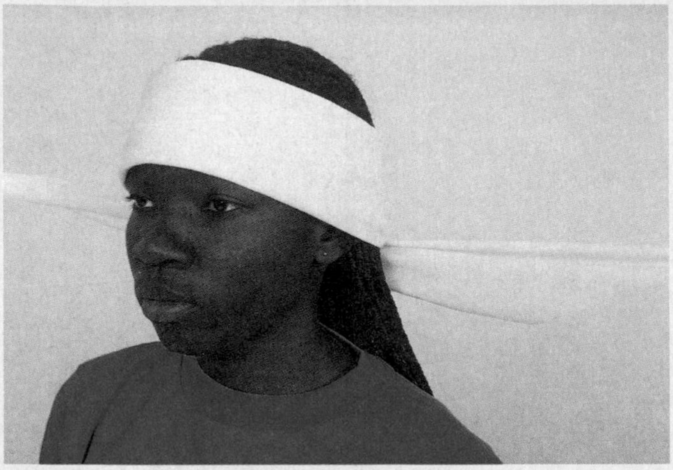

1 Place the middle of the bandage over the dressing covering the wound.

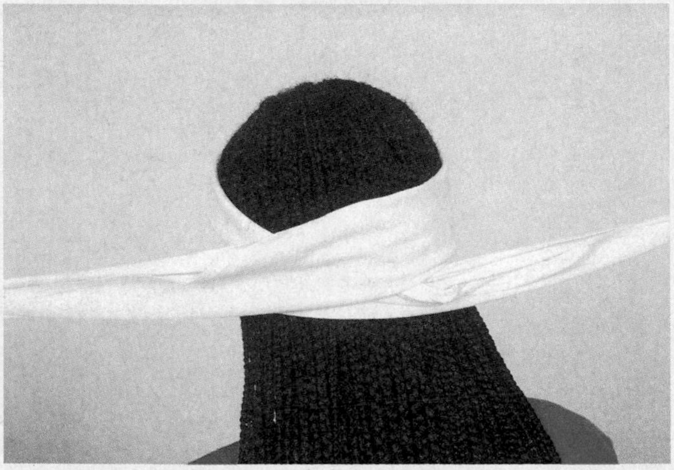

2 Cross the two ends snugly over each other.

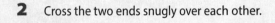

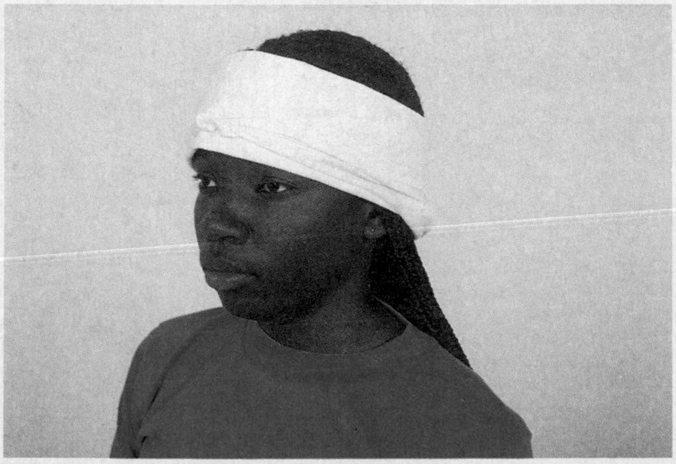

3 Bring the ends back around to where the dressing is and tie the ends in a knot over the wound. When wrapping a roller bandage around the head, keep the bandage near the eyebrows and low on the back of the head to prevent the bandage from slipping.

SKILL SHEET 10-2 Cravat Method of Bandaging the Arm or Leg

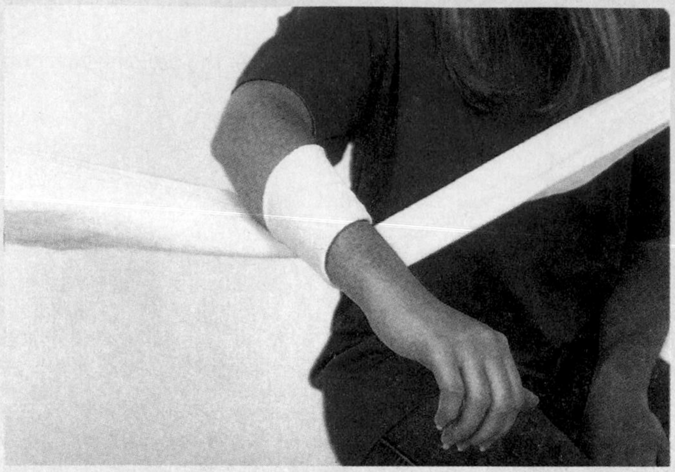

1 Wrap the bandage over the dressing.

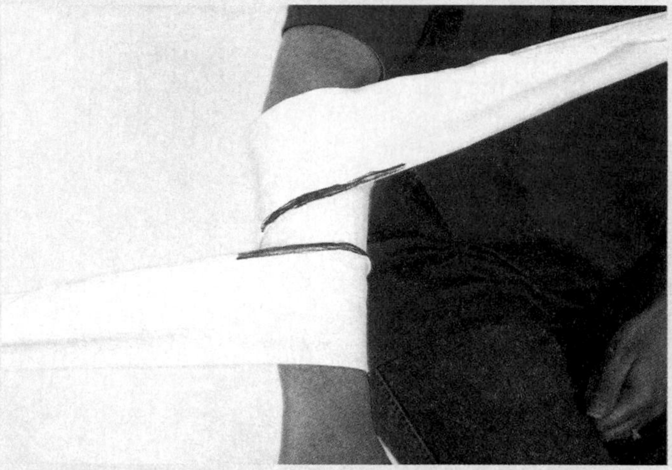

2 With one end, make one turn going up the extremity and another turn going down.

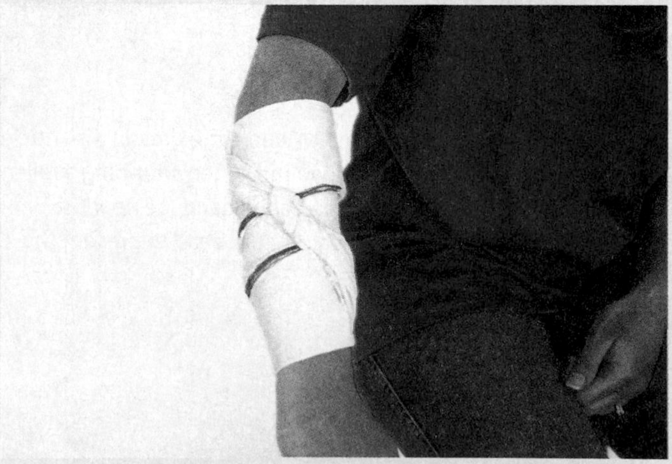

3 Tie the bandage over the dressing.

SKILL SHEET 10-3 Cravat Method for Applying a Bandage to the Palm of the Hand

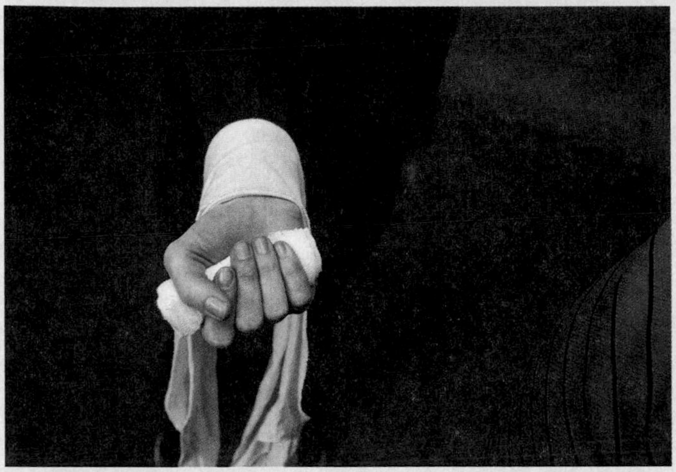

© Jones & Bartlett Learning.

1 Fill the palm with a bulky dressing or pad and close the fingers over it. Drape a cravat bandage over the upturned wrist.

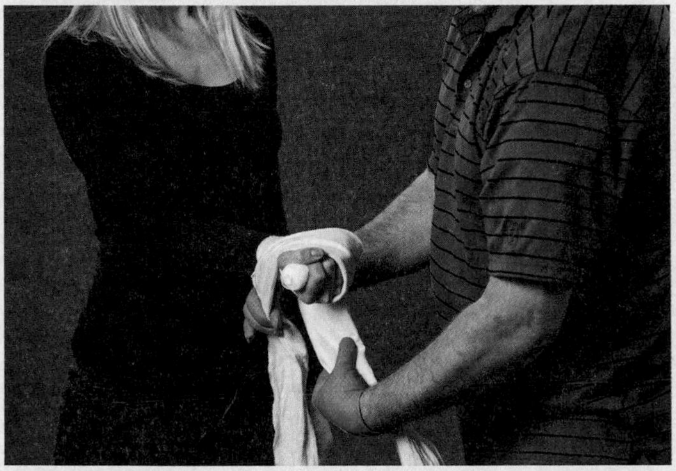

© Jones & Bartlett Learning.

2 Wrap one end of the bandage around several fingers and the other end around the thumb and remaining fingers.

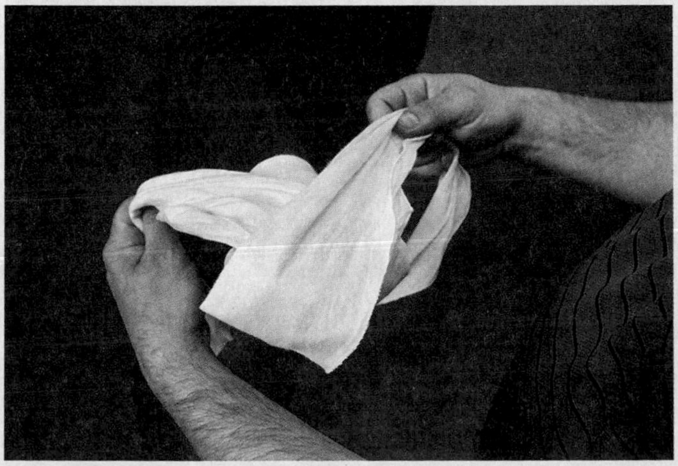

© Jones & Bartlett Learning.

3 Wrap the bandage crossing over the fingers and around the wrist.

Continues

SKILL SHEET 10-3 Cravat Method for Applying a Bandage to the Palm of the Hand (*Continued*)

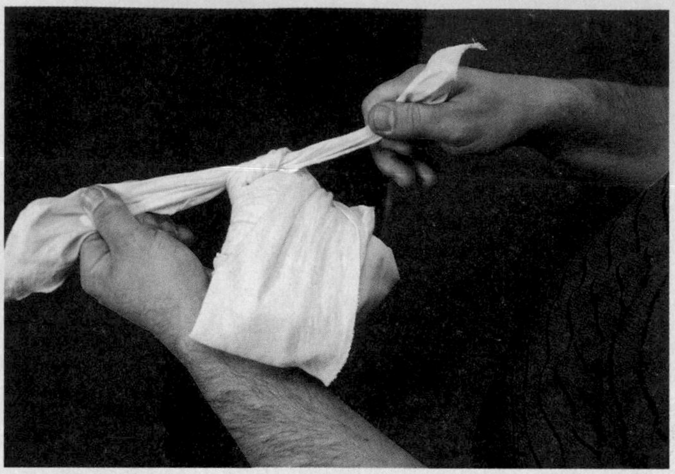

4 Tie the bandage at the wrist.

SKILL SHEET 10-4 Securing a Cravat Bandage With a Square Knot

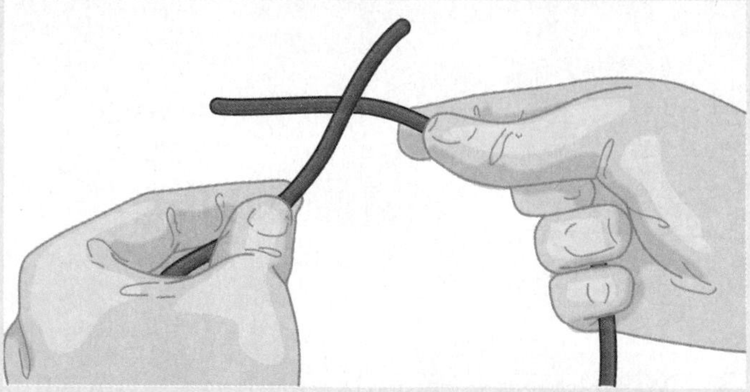

1 Take the left end of the bandage and cross it over the right end so it is now on top.

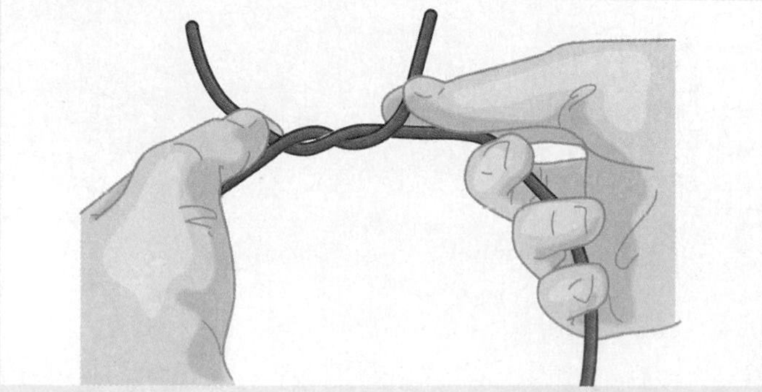

2 With that same end of bandage (the end that is now on top), wrap it under and around the bottom end.

SKILL SHEET 10-4 Securing a Cravat Bandage With a Square Knot (*Continued*)

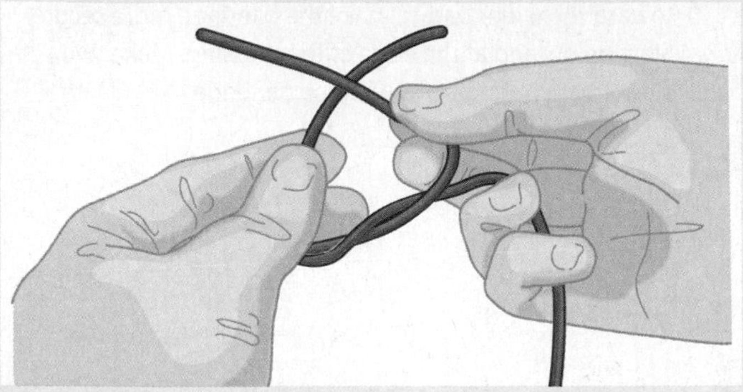

© Jones & Bartlett Learning.

3 Now do the same thing on the other side: Cross the right side over the left so that it is now on top . . .

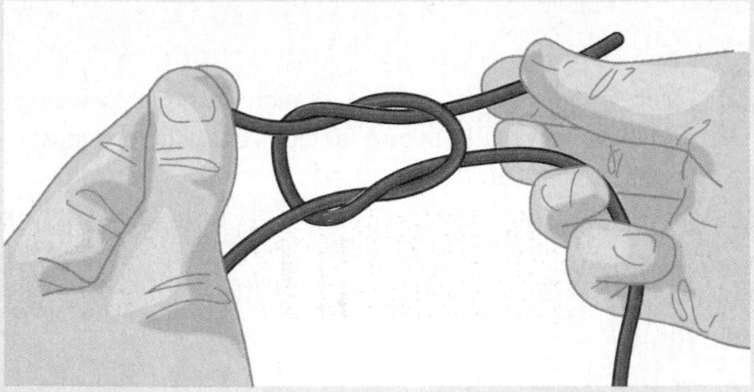

© Jones & Bartlett Learning.

4 . . . and wrap it around the other end.

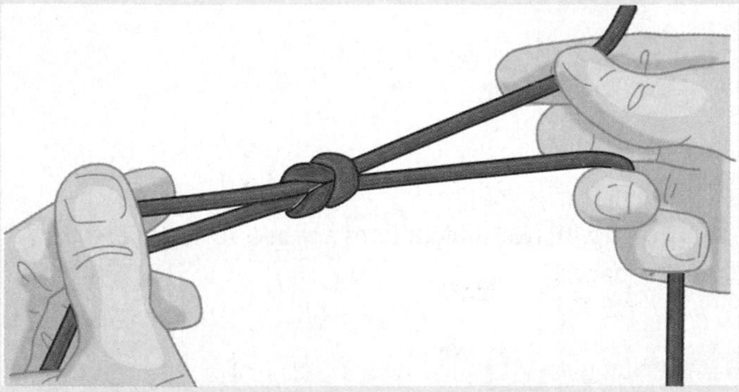

© Jones & Bartlett Learning.

5 Pull the ends in the opposite direction to tighten.

Figure-Eight Method

Use this method of applying a roller bandage to hold dressings or to provide compression at or near a joint such as the ankle. The figure-eight method involves continuous spiral loops of bandage, one up and one down, crossing each other to form an 8. To apply a 4- or 6-inch (10- or 15-cm) roller bandage to the elbow or knee using the figure-eight method, follow the steps in **SKILL SHEET 10-6**. To apply a roller bandage to the hand using the figure-eight method, follow the steps in **SKILL SHEET 10-7**. This method uses a 2- or 3-inch (5- or 7-cm) roller bandage.

To wrap an ankle or foot using the figure-eight method, follow the steps in **SKILL SHEET 10-8**. This wrapping will hold a dressing or apply pressure to treat a sprained ankle. It should not be used to support the ankle and foot during sports activity; that type of bandaging involves additional maneuvers. Either 2- or 3-inch (5- or 7-cm) roller bandages can be used.

SKILL SHEET 10-5 Spiral Method of Bandaging a Forearm

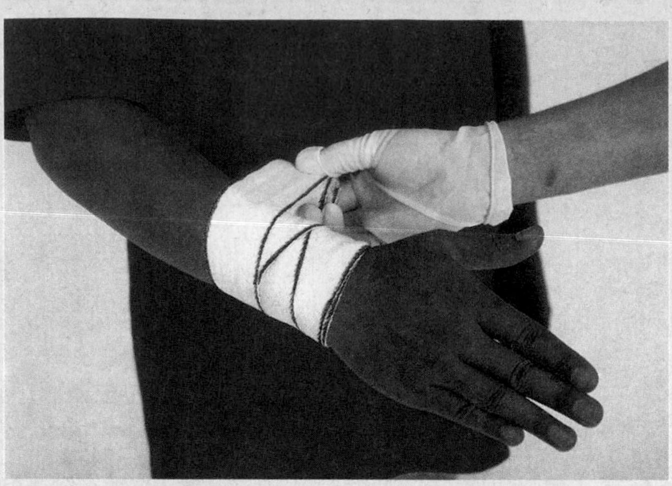

1 Start at the narrow part of an arm or leg and wrap upward toward the wider part to make the bandage more secure. Start below and at the edge of the dressing. Make two straight anchoring turns with the bandage.

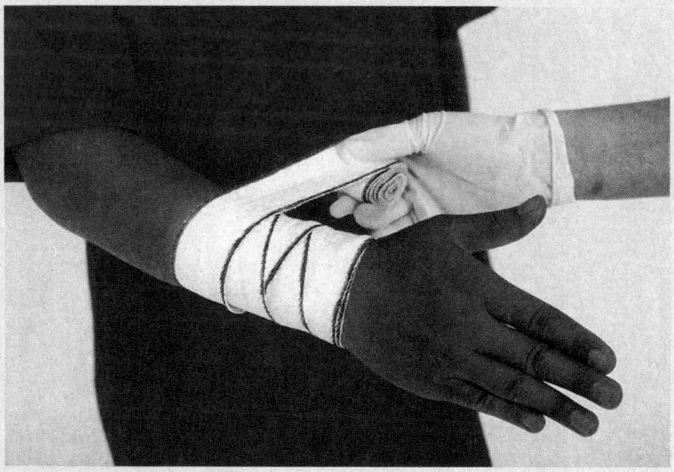

2 Make a series of crisscross (figure-eight) turns, progressing up the arm or leg. Each turn should overlap the previous wrap by about 50%.

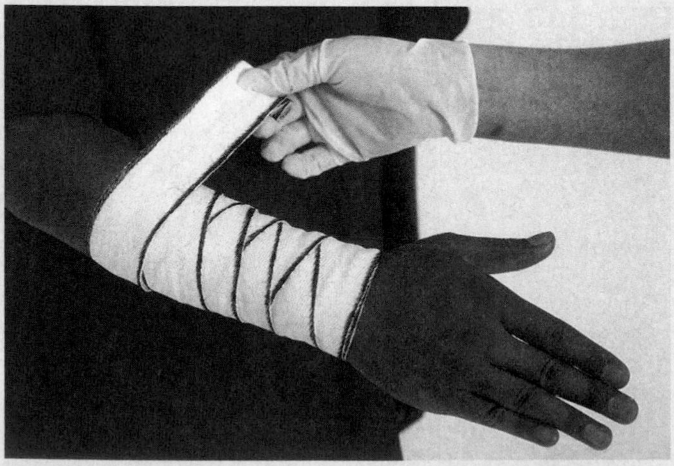

3 Finish with two straight turns and secure (ie, tape) the bandage.

SKILL SHEET 10-6 Figure-Eight Method of Bandaging a Knee or Elbow

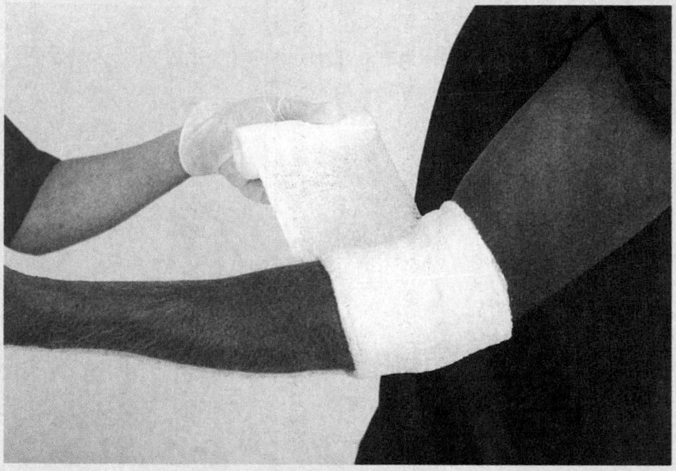

1 Bend the elbow or knee slightly and make two straight anchoring turns with the bandage over the elbow point or knee cap.

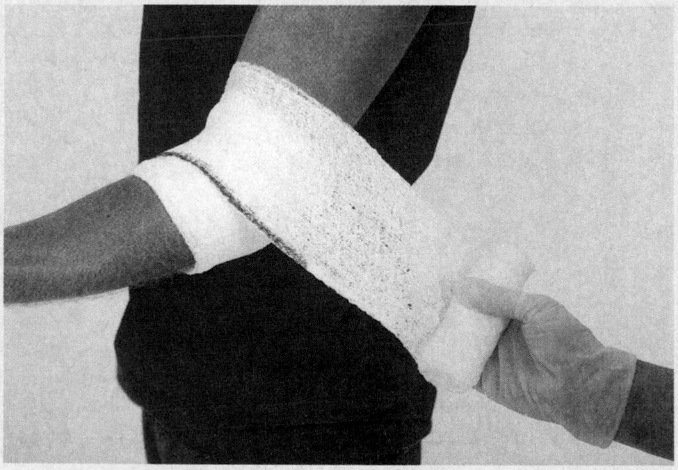

2 Bring the bandage above the joint to the upper arm or leg and make one turn, covering one-half to three-fourths of the bandage from the first turn.

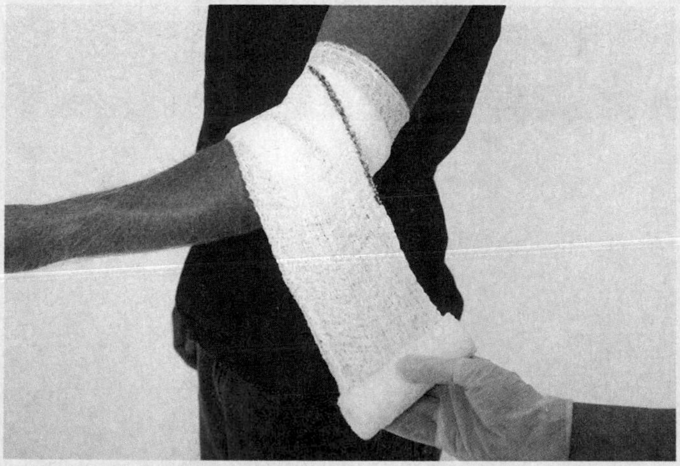

3 Bring the bandage just under the joint and make one turn around the lower arm or leg, covering one-half to three-fourths of the first straight turn.

Continues

SKILL SHEET 10-6 Figure-Eight Method of Bandaging a Knee or Elbow (*Continued*)

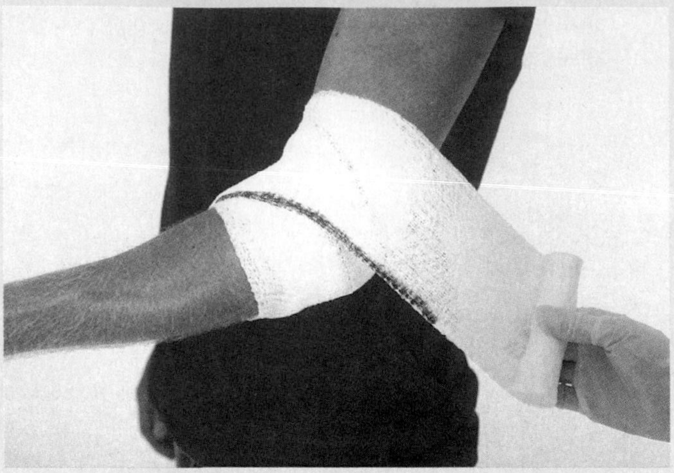

4 Continue alternating the turns in a figure-eight maneuver by covering the previous layers.

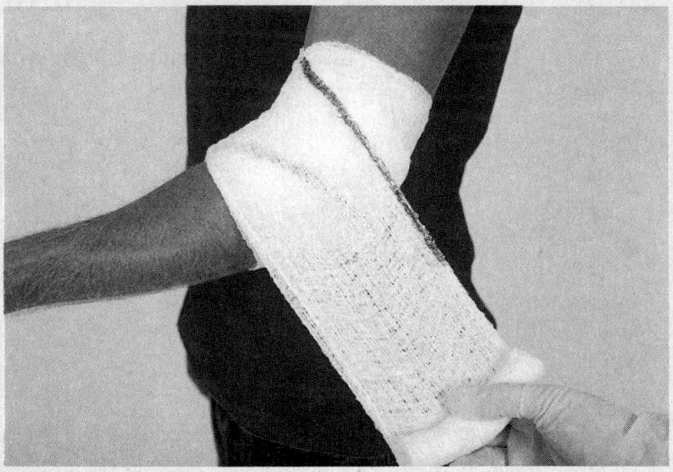

5 Alternate turns above and below the point or tip of the elbow or knee. Finish by making two straight turns, and secure the end.

SKILL SHEET 10-7 Figure-Eight Method of Bandaging a Hand

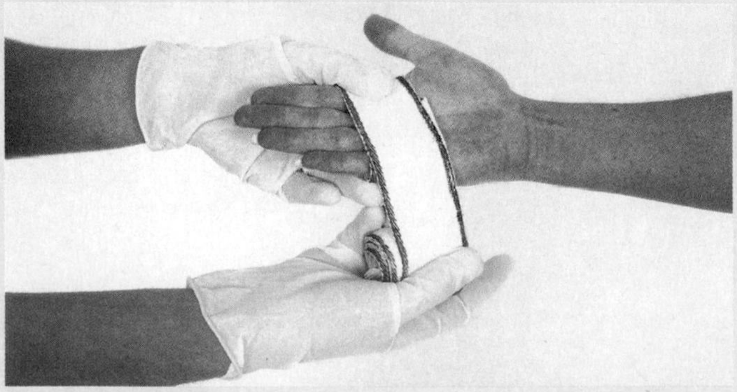

1 Anchor the bandage with one or two turns around the palm of the hand.

SKILL SHEET 10-7 Figure-Eight Method of Bandaging a Hand (*Continued*)

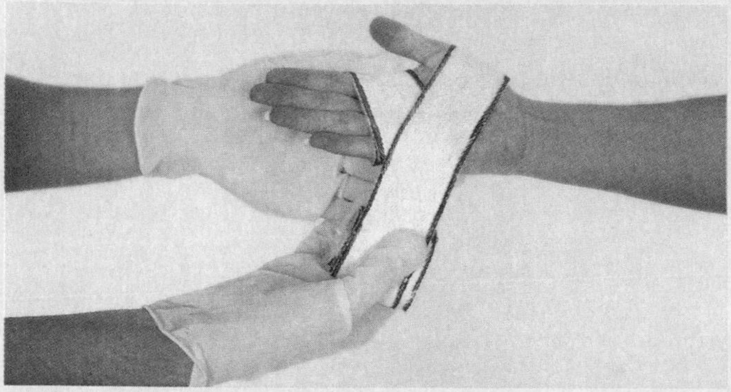

2 Carry the bandage diagonally across the back of the hand and then around the wrist.

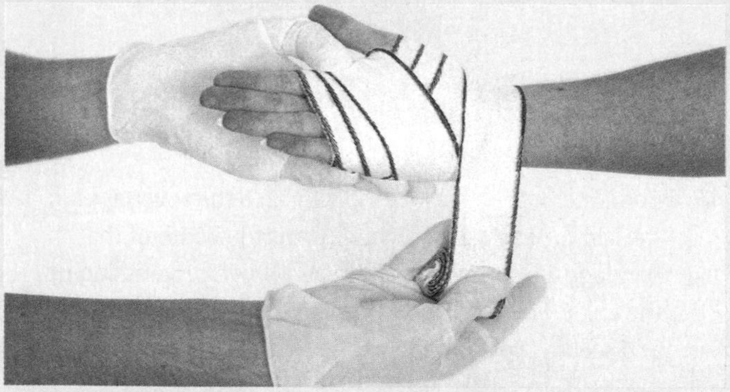

3 Repeat the figure-eight maneuver as many times as necessary to cover the dressing, overlapping wraps to "stair-step" up the hand.

Make two straight turns around the wrist, and secure the bandage.

SKILL SHEET 10-8 Figure-Eight Method of Bandaging an Ankle or Foot

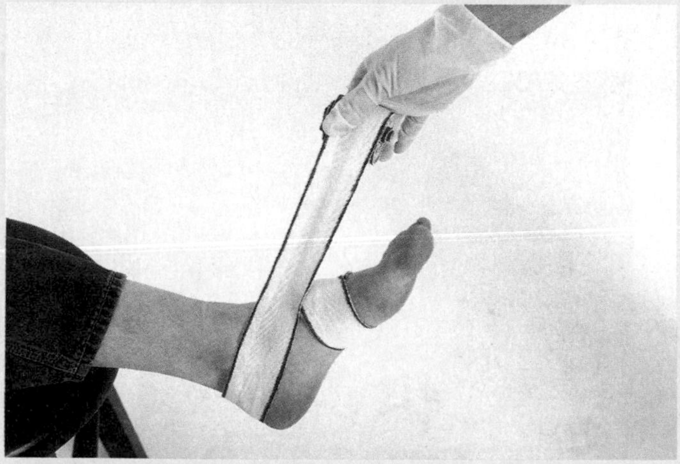

1 Anchor the bandage with one or two turns around the foot. Make a figure-right turn by taking the bandage diagonally across the top of the foot and around the back of the ankle.

Continues

SKILL SHEET 10-8 Figure-Eight Method of Bandaging an Ankle or Foot (*Continued*)

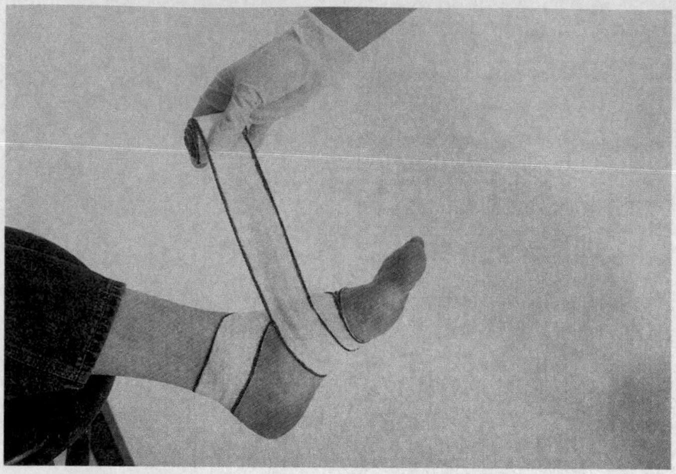

© American Academy of Orthopaedic Surgeons.

2 Continue to bandage across the top of the foot and underneath the arch of the foot.

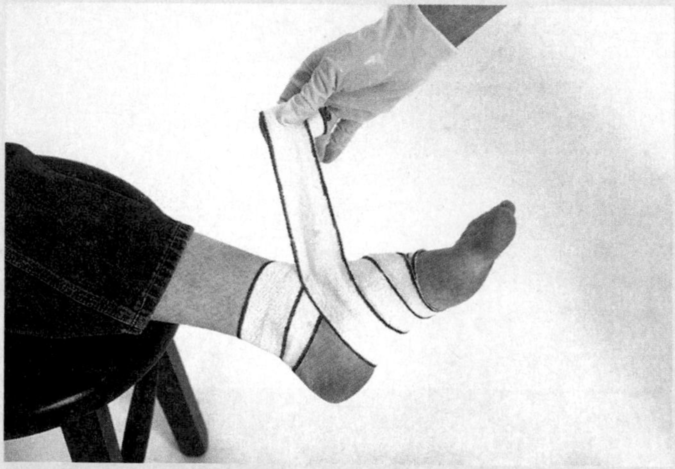

© American Academy of Orthopaedic Surgeons.

3 Continue figure-eight turns, with each turn overlapping the last turn by about three-fourths the width of the bandage. Be sure to cover the heel while progressing up the ankle. Finish with two straight turns around the leg, and secure the bandage.

Securing a Roller Bandage

To securely fasten a roller bandage, you can:

- Apply adhesive tape to secure the bandage **FIGURE 10-7**.
- Use safety pins to secure the bandage **FIGURE 10-8**. Be very careful with people who may have decreased sensation.
- Use the special clips provided with elastic bandages **FIGURE 10-9**.

You can also use either the loop or split-tail methods. To perform the loop method, follow the steps in **SKILL SHEET 10-9**. To perform the split-tail method of securing a bandage, follow the steps in **SKILL SHEET 10-10**.

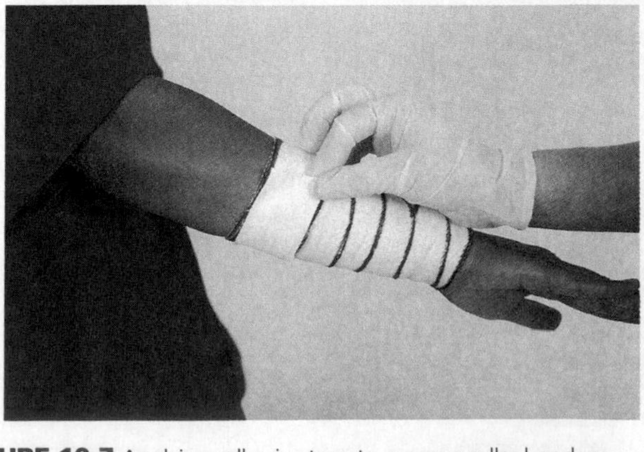

FIGURE 10-7 Applying adhesive tape to secure a roller bandage.
© American Academy of Orthopaedic Surgeons.

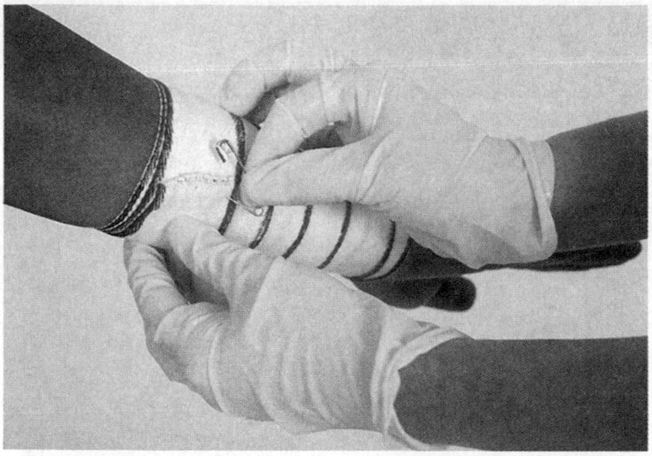

FIGURE 10-8 Using safety pins to secure a roller bandage. If available, cover the secured safety pins with tape to avoid snagging.

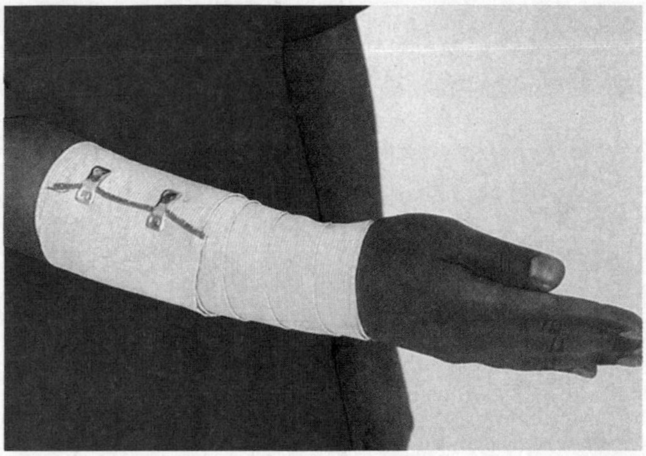

FIGURE 10-9 Using special clips to secure an elastic roller bandage. If available, cover the secured clips with tape to avoid snagging.

SKILL SHEET 10-9 Loop Method of Securing Bandages

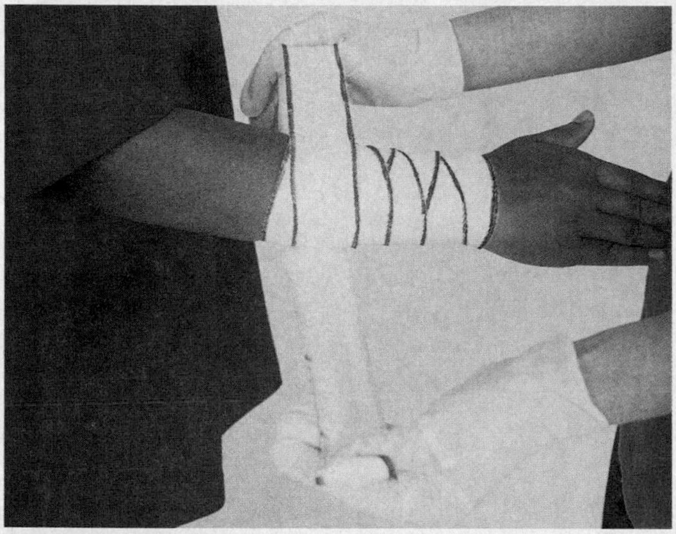

1 Reverse the direction of the bandage by looping it around a thumb or finger and continue back to the opposite side of the body part.

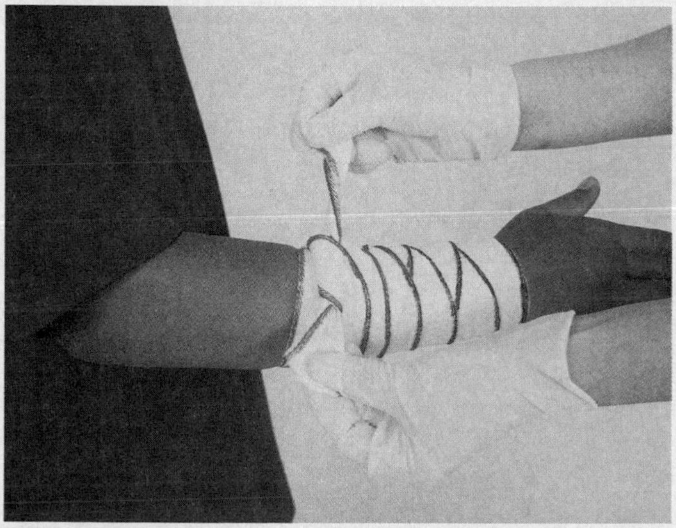

2 Encircle the part with the looped end and the free end and tie them together.

SKILL SHEET 10-10 Split-Tail Method of Securing Bandages

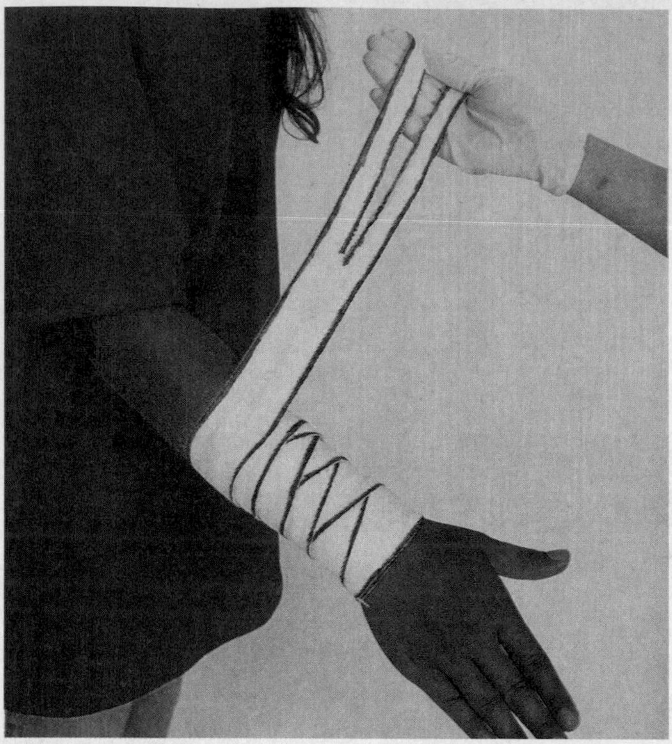

© American Academy of Orthopaedic Surgeons.

1 Split the end of the bandage lengthwise for about 12 inches (30 cm), then tie a knot to prevent further splitting.

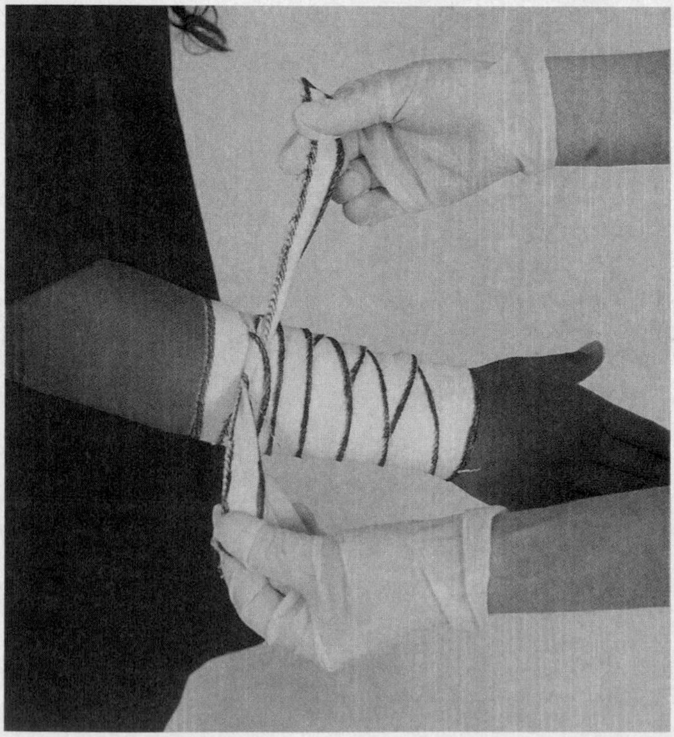

© American Academy of Orthopaedic Surgeons.

2 Pass the ends in opposite directions around the body part and tie.

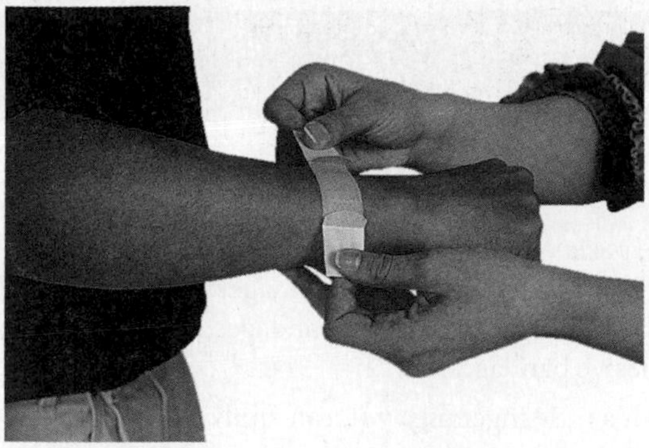

FIGURE 10-10 Applying an adhesive dressing.

FYI

Adhesive Bandage

To make an adhesive bandage snug on a chin, knee, or elbow, first cut the adhesive parts of the bandage lengthwise, but do not cut into the pad. Place the pad horizontally over the cut or wound. Then bring the bottom strips of the adhesive bandage up and smooth them on the skin. Bring the top parts of the adhesive bandage down and smooth them on the skin. Result: An adhesive bandage that contours to the wound.

Applying an Adhesive Bandage

Follow these steps to apply an adhesive bandage:

1. Remove the wrapping and hold the dressing, pad-side down, by the protective strips **FIGURE 10-10**.
2. Peel back, but do not remove, the protective strips. Without touching the dressing pad, place it directly onto the wound.
3. Carefully pull away the protective strips. Press the ends and edges down.

PREP KIT

Ready for Review

- A dressing covers an open wound; it touches the wound.
- Dressings used in most first aid situations are commercially prepared, but dressings may need to be improvised.
- A bandage should be clean but need not be sterile.
- The basic types of bandages are roller bandages; self-adhering, conforming bandages; gauze rollers; elastic roller bandages; triangular bandages; adhesive tape; and adhesive bandages.
- With a little ingenuity, you can apply a roller bandage to almost any body part.

Vital Vocabulary

adhesive bandage A combination of both a sterile dressing and a bandage.

adhesive tape Tape used to secure bandages and dressings; available in rolls and in a variety of widths.

cravat A folded triangular bandage used to hold splints and dressings in place, to apply pressure evenly over a dressing, or as a swathe (binder) for an injured arm in an arm sling.

elastic roller bandage A type of bandage used for compression on sprains, strains, and contusions; available in various widths.

gauze pad A type of sterile dressing used for small wounds; available in separately wrapped packages of various sizes. Some have a special coating to keep them from sticking to the wound.

gauze roller A type of bandage that is cotton and nonelastic, and used to wrap or bind various body parts; available in various widths.

roller bandage A type of bandage used to wrap or bind various body parts; available in various widths, lengths, and types of material.

self-adhering, conforming bandage A type of bandage that bonds to itself as it is wrapped, helping to secure itself in place; available as rolls of slightly elastic, gauzelike material in various widths.

trauma dressing A type of dressing made of large, thick, absorbent, sterile materials.

triangular bandage A type of bandage available commercially or that can be made from a square piece of preshrunk cotton muslin measuring 36 to 40 inches (230 to 260 cm) along each side of the square.

Assessment in Action

You are enjoying a fly-fishing trip along a popular trout fishing river. It is a Saturday and there are several others fishing the same area. You and your friend decide to descend a steep riverbank to access a less crowded spot. Your friend slips down the riverbank. You hurry down the bank and find her clutching her arm, which is bleeding. Another bystander arrives with a first aid kit.

Directions: Circle Yes if you agree with the statement; circle No if you disagree.

1. You should wash your hands with sanitizer and apply medical exam gloves from the first aid kit.

   YES **NO**

2. A dressing goes directly on the wound.

   YES **NO**

3. You can apply a roller bandage on the arm using spiral turns.

   YES **NO**

4. You should start bandaging from the upper part of the arm and progress down to the wrist.

   YES **NO**

5. After applying the bandage, you see that your friend's fingers look blue. This is a sign that the bandage is too tight.

   YES **NO**

PREP KIT continued

Check Your Knowledge

Directions: Circle Yes if you agree with the statement; circle No if you disagree.

1. A dressing does not touch an open wound.
   YES NO
2. Adhesive bandages are used for small cuts and abrasions.
   YES NO
3. A bandage should be clean but need not be sterile.
   YES NO
4. Roller bandages come in only one size.
   YES NO
5. Roller bandages can be used only on the arm.
   YES NO
6. A square knot is the preferred knot for bandages.
   YES NO
7. Check the person's lips for signs a bandage is too tight.
   YES NO
8. If the person can wiggle their fingers, the bandage is not on correctly.
   YES NO
9. Elastic roller bandages are used for compression on sprains, strains, and contusions.
   YES NO
10. The figure-eight method is used to apply a roller bandage to hold dressings or to provide compression at or near a joint.
    YES NO

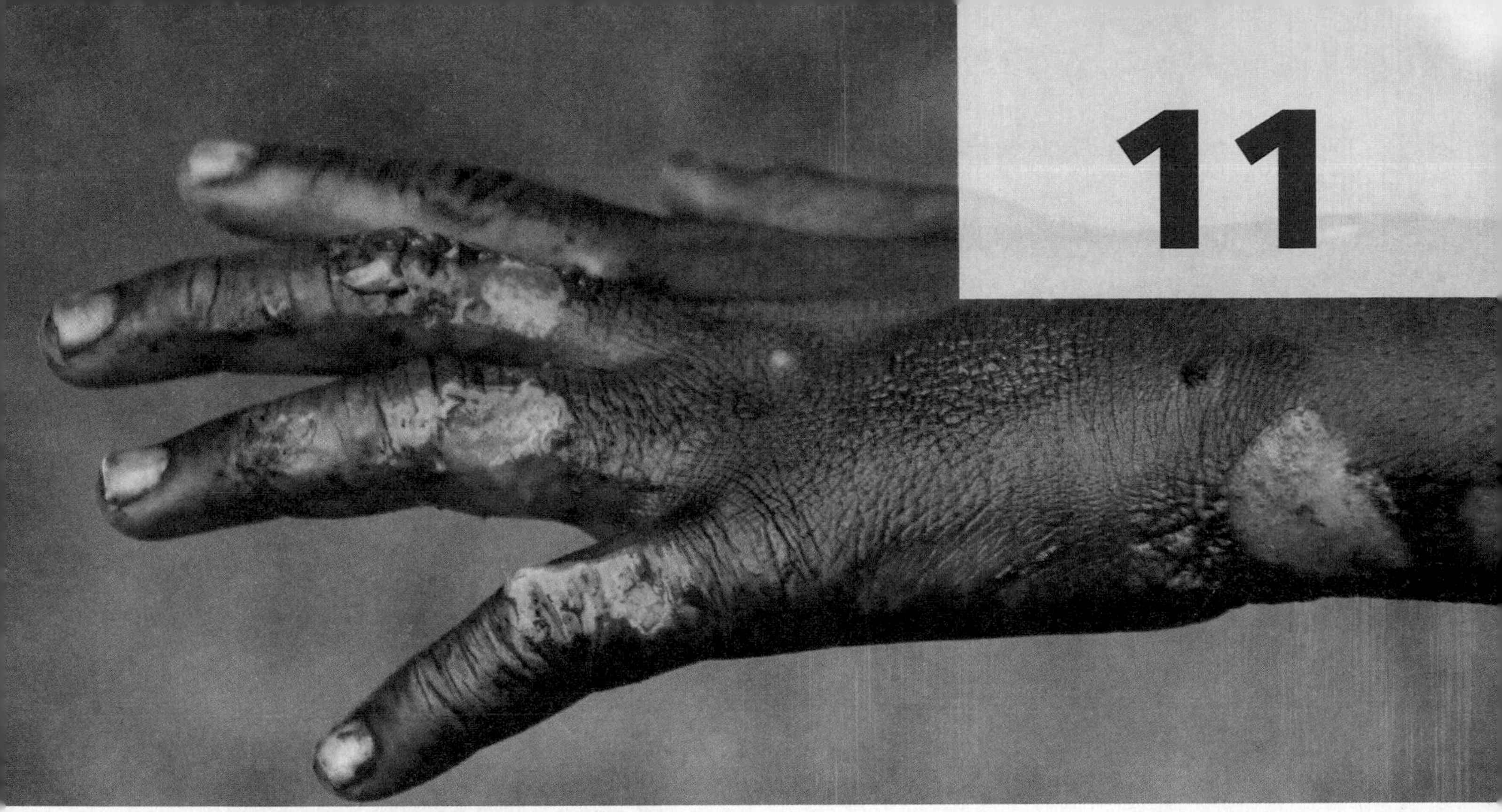

11

Burns

CHAPTER AT A GLANCE

Burns

A **burn** is an injury in which soft tissue absorbs more energy than it can dissipate from thermal heat, chemicals, or electricity. Burns occur in every age group, across all socioeconomic levels, at home and in the workplace, and in urban, suburban, and rural settings. It has been estimated that about 80% of all burn injuries occur in the home, with house fires responsible for the majority of fire deaths. Most people with burns are injured as a result of their own actions.

The highest-risk age groups for burn injuries are children younger than 5 years and adults older than 55 years. Both groups may have limited ability to recognize and escape from a fire or burn incident. In addition, their relatively thinner skin predisposes them to more serious injuries. Death and complications increase dramatically for people older than 55 years owing to the likelihood of preexisting health conditions and their immune systems' decreased ability to fight infection.

Skin death and injury occur as the applied heat exceeds the body's ability to disperse the heat; that point starts at about 113°F (45°C). The amount and depth of skin damage depend on the heat's intensity, the duration of contact, and the skin's thickness.

Burn injuries can be classified as thermal (heat), chemical, or electrical.

- **Thermal (heat) burns**. Not all thermal burns are caused by flames. Contact with hot objects, flammable vapor that ignites and causes a flash or an explosion, and steam and hot liquid are other common causes of burns. Just 3 seconds of exposure to water at 140°F (60°C) can cause a full-thickness (third-degree) burn in an adult. At 156°F (69°C), the same burn occurs in 1 second.
- **Chemical burns**. A wide range of chemical agents can cause tissue damage and death on contact with the skin. As with thermal burns, the amount of tissue damage depends on the duration of contact, the skin thickness in the area of exposure, and the strength of the chemical agent. Chemicals will continue to cause tissue destruction until the chemical agent is removed. Three types of chemicals—acids, alkalis, and organic compounds—are responsible for most chemical burns. Alkalis produce deeper, more extensive burns than do acids.
- **Electrical burns**. The injury severity from contact with electric current depends on the type of current (direct or alternating), the voltage, the area of the body exposed, and the duration of contact. Electricity can induce ventricular fibrillation (a cause of cardiac arrest), cause respiratory arrest, or "freeze" the person to the electrical contact point with powerful muscle spasms that increase the length of exposure. People with low-voltage electrical injuries may have no skin burns at all but might still experience cardiac or respiratory arrest.

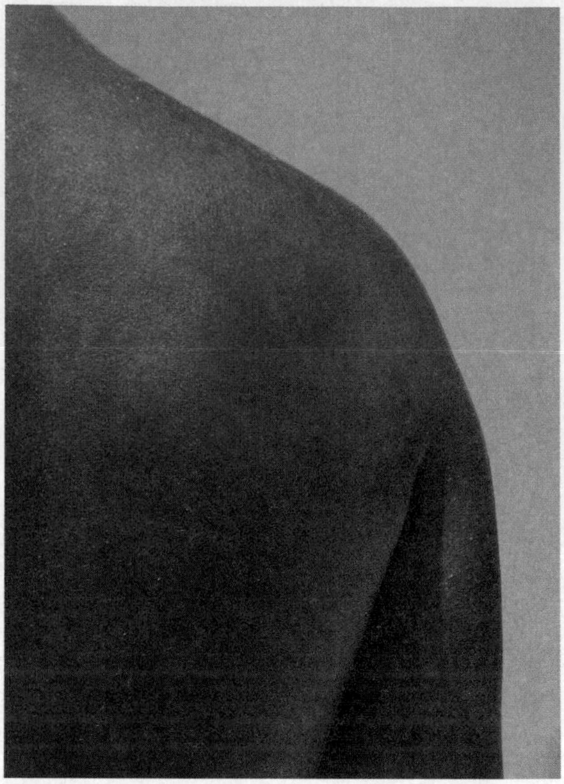

FIGURE 11-1 First-degree burn.

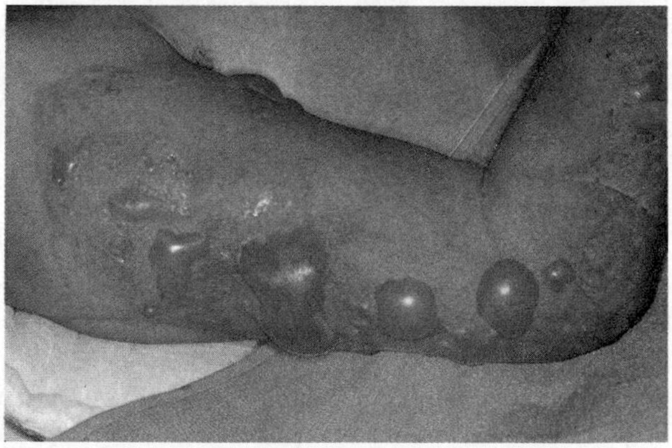

FIGURE 11-2 Second-degree burn blisters.

Thermal Burns

Evaluate a thermal burn using the following steps. Each step provides valuable information about the type and severity of injury the person has sustained. Insights gained can determine the immediate action you must take in caring for the person. Taken together, the steps will prepare you to effectively determine the burn's severity, which is the basis for treatment of thermal burns.

1. *Determine the depth (degree) of the burn.* Historically, burns have been described as first-degree, second-degree, and third-degree injuries. The terms *superficial, partial thickness*, and *full thickness* are often used by burn-care professionals because they are more descriptive of the tissue damage.
   - **First-degree (superficial) burns** affect the skin's outer layer (epidermis) **FIGURE 11-1**. Signs and symptoms include redness, mild swelling, tenderness, and pain. Healing occurs without scarring, usually within 1 week. The outer edges of deeper burns often are first-degree burns.
   - **Second-degree (partial-thickness) burns** extend through the entire outer layer and into the inner skin layer **FIGURE 11-2**. Signs and symptoms include blisters, swelling, weeping of fluids, and severe pain. The signs occur because the capillary blood vessels in the dermis are damaged and give up fluid into surrounding tissues. Intact blisters provide a sterile, waterproof covering. Once a blister breaks, a weeping wound results, and the risk of infection increases.
   - **Third-degree (full-thickness) burns** are severe burns that penetrate all the skin layers into the underlying fat and muscle **FIGURE 11-3**. Signs and symptoms include leathery, waxy, or pearly gray skin that is sometimes charred. The skin has a dry appearance because capillary blood vessels have been destroyed and no more fluid is brought

to the area. The skin does not blanch after being pressed because the area is dead. The person feels no pain from a third-degree burn because the nerve endings have been damaged or destroyed. Any pain felt is from surrounding burns of lesser degrees. A third-degree burn requires professional medical care and the removal of dead tissue and often a skin graft to heal properly.

2. *Determine the extent of the burn.* Skin will not ignite unless heated to thousands of degrees. However, if clothing ignites or skin is kept in contact with a heat source, such as scalding water, large areas of the skin will be injured. Determining the extent of a burn means estimating how much body surface area the burn covers.

   A rough guide known as the rule of nines assigns a percentage value of total body surface area (TBSA) to each part of an adult's body **FIGURE 11-4**. The entire head is 9%, one complete arm is 9%, the front torso is 18%, the complete back is 18%, and each leg is 18%. The rule of nines must be modified for small children to take into account the different proportions of their bodies. In small children and infants, the head accounts for 18%, and each leg is 14%.

   For small or scattered burns, use the rule of the hand **FIGURE 11-5**. The person's whole hand, which must include the fingers and the thumb held together, represents about 1% of their TBSA. For a very large burn, estimate the unburned area in number of hands and subtract from 100%. Although the exact percentage is nearly impossible to accurately determine at the scene, attempt to get as close as possible.

3. *Determine which parts of the body are burned.* Burns on the face, hands, feet, and genitals are more severe than those on other body parts. A circumferential burn (one that goes around a finger, toe, arm, leg, neck, or chest) is considered more severe than a noncircumferential one because of the possible constriction and tourniquet effect on circulation and, in some cases, breathing. All circumferential burns require professional medical care.

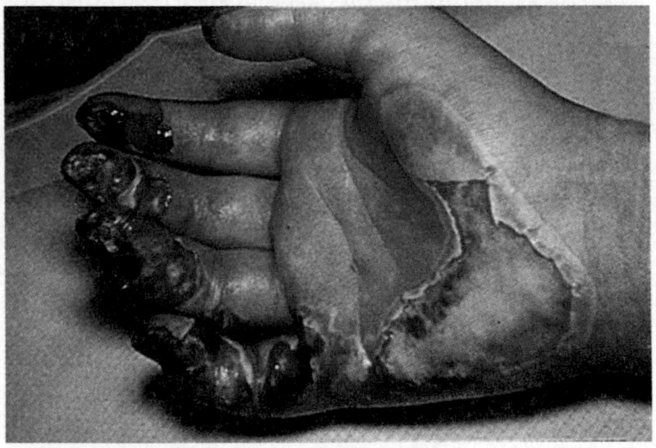

FIGURE 11-3 Third-degree burn.

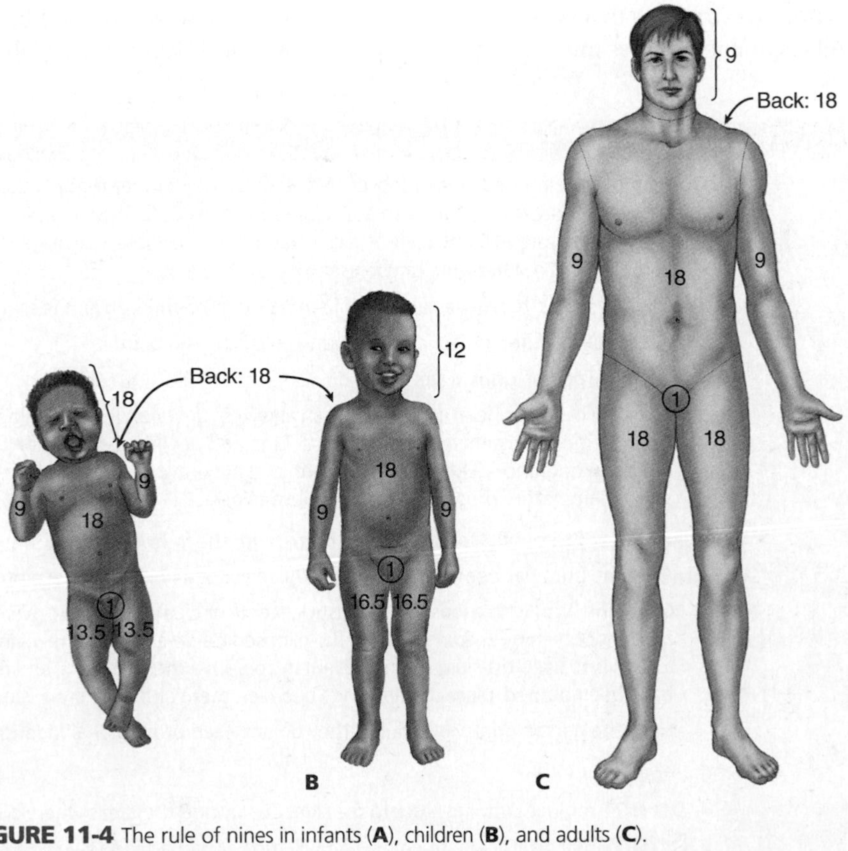

FIGURE 11-4 The rule of nines in infants (**A**), children (**B**), and adults (**C**).

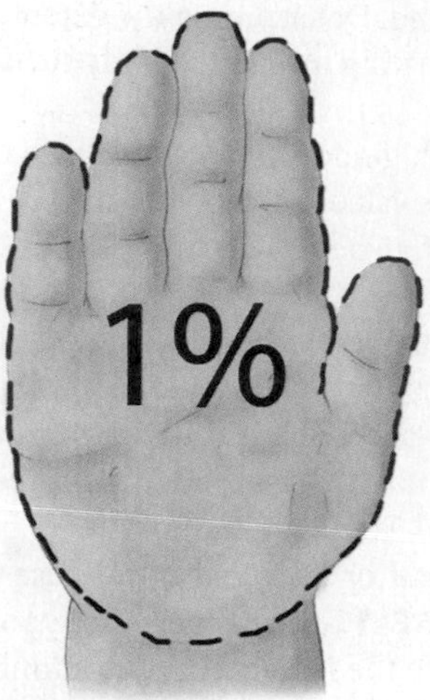

FIGURE 11-5 Rule of the hand.

4. *Determine respiratory involvement.* Respiratory tract damage caused by heat associated with a burn can cause death after a person is hospitalized. Respiratory damage may result from breathing heat or the products of combustion, from being burned by a flame while in a closed space, or from being in an explosion. In these cases, even with no burn injury to the skin, there may be respiratory damage. Super-heated air is absorbed by the upper respiratory tract (the area from the nose to the trachea), resulting in inflammation. Swelling occurs in 2 to 24 hours, restricting or completely shutting off the airway so that air cannot reach the lungs. All respiratory injuries must receive professional medical care. The following are signs and symptoms of respiratory injury:
   - Burns around the nose or mouth
   - Breathing difficulty
   - Hoarseness, wheezing, coughing
   - Coughing that expels sooty substance
   - Soot on face
   - Swollen nostrils or throat
   - A person who is rescued from a burning building
5. *Determine whether other injuries or preexisting medical conditions exist or whether the person is older than 55 years or younger than 5 years.* Having a medical condition or being in one of the sensitive age groups increases a burn's severity. Burns can aggravate existing medical conditions such as diabetes, heart disease, and lung disease, as well as other medical conditions. Concurrent injuries such as fractures, internal injuries, and open wounds increase the severity of a burn.
6. *Determine the burn's severity.* How you care for the burned person depends on the burn's severity. Most burns are minor, occur at home, and can be managed outside a medical setting. Seek professional medical care for any of the following conditions:
   - The person has difficulty breathing.
   - Other injuries exist.
   - Chemical burns.
   - An electrical injury exists, including lightning strike injuries.
   - The face, hands, feet, or genitals are burned.
   - Child abuse is suspected.
   - Large second-degree burn (partial thickness).
   - Third-degree burn (full thickness).

What to Look For	What to Do
First-degree (superficial) burn **FIGURE 11-6**, indicated by: ▪ Redness ▪ Mild swelling ▪ Tenderness ▪ Pain	**1.** Immerse the burned area in cool or cold water, place it under running cold water, or apply a wet, cool or cold compress for up to 30 minutes for burns <5% TBSA and at least 10 minutes for large burns as soon as possible **FIGURE 11-7**. If cold water is unavailable, use any available cold liquid. A clean, cool pad, but not freezing, can be useful for cooling a burn. **2.** Give ibuprofen to relieve pain and inflammation. (For children and teenagers, give acetaminophen.) **3.** Keep a burned arm or leg raised to reduce swelling and pain. **4.** Have the person drink water. **5.** After the burn has been cooled, apply an aloe vera gel or an inexpensive skin moisturizer lotion to keep the skin moistened and to reduce itching and peeling. Use a lotion that does not have alcohols or strong fragrances. Lotions with glycerin and mineral oil are best. Aloe vera has antimicrobial and anti-inflammatory properties and is a mild analgesic.
Small (<20% TBSA) second-degree (partial-thickness) burn, indicated by: ▪ Blisters ▪ Swelling ▪ Weeping of fluids ▪ Severe pain	Follow Steps 1 through 3 for first-degree burns, with the following additions: **1.** After the burn has been cooled, apply a thin layer of an antibacterial ointment. **2.** Cover the burn with a loose, dry, nonstick, sterile or clean dressing. Covering the burn reduces the amount of pain by keeping air from the exposed nerve endings. The main purpose of a dressing over a burn is to keep the burn clean, prevent evaporative moisture loss, and reduce pain. If fingers or toes have been burned, place dry dressings between them and seek professional medical care. **3.** Have the person drink water only if they do not need professional medical care. Caution ▪ **DO NOT** remove clothing stuck to the skin. Cut around the areas where clothing sticks to the skin. ▪ **DO NOT** pull on stuck clothing; pulling will further damage the skin.

What to Look For	What to Do
Large (>20% TBSA) second-degree (partial-thickness) burn	Follow Steps 1 through 3 for first-degree burns, with the following additions: **1.** Apply cold, but monitor the person for cold stress, which could lead to hypothermia. **2.** Call 9-1-1.
Third-degree (full-thickness) burn, indicated by: ▪ Dry, leathery, gray-colored, or charred skin	**1.** Cover the burn with a dry, nonstick, sterile or clean dressing. **2.** Call 9-1-1.

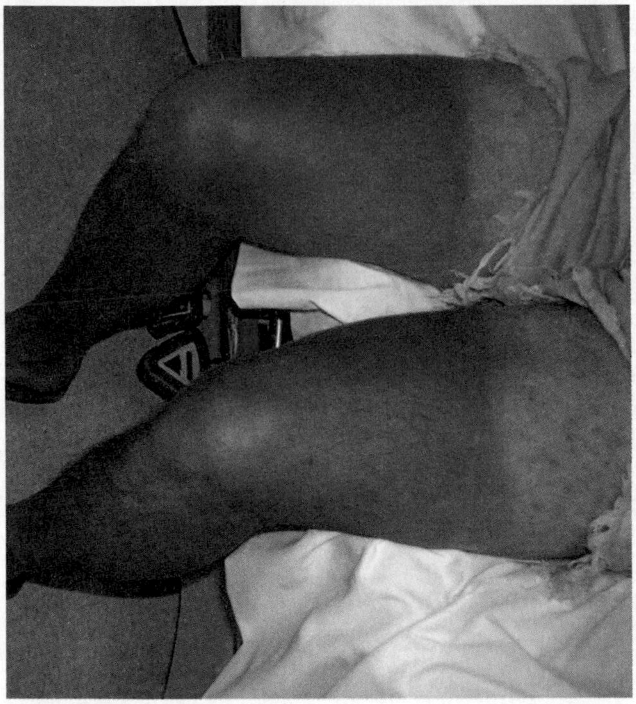

FIGURE 11-6 Sunburn.

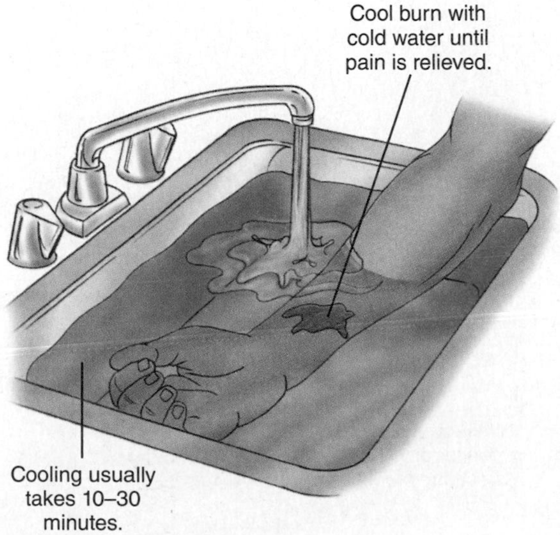
Cool burn with cold water until pain is relieved.
Cooling usually takes 10–30 minutes.

FIGURE 11-7 Immerse the burn. Cool the burn with cold water until pain is relieved but no longer than 30 minutes.

CAUTION

DO NOT apply cold over a large burn for a prolonged time because it can produce hypothermia.

DO NOT use an ice pack or ice water unless it is the only source of cold available. If you must use it, apply it for only 10 to 15 minutes.

DO NOT apply grease, butter, cream, or a home remedy. Such coatings are unsterile and can lead to infection. They also can seal in heat, causing further damage.

DO NOT cover a first-degree burn.

DO NOT break any blisters. Intact blisters serve as excellent burn dressings. Cover a ruptured blister with an antibiotic ointment and a dry, sterile dressing.

DO NOT use plastic as a dressing because it will trap moisture and provide a good place for bacteria to grow. (Its only advantage is that it will not stick to the burn.)

Later Care for Thermal Burns

For thermal burn care, follow a physician's recommendations, if a physician has been consulted (many burns are never seen by a physician). The following suggestions may apply:

- Wash hands thoroughly before changing any dressing.
- Leave unbroken blisters intact.
- Change dressings once or twice per day unless a physician instructs otherwise.

To change a dressing:

1. Remove the old dressing. If a dressing sticks, soak it off with cool, clean water.
2. Cleanse the area gently with mild soap and water.
3. Pat the area dry with a clean cloth.
4. Apply a thin layer of antibiotic ointment to the burn.
5. Apply a nonstick sterile dressing.

Watch for signs of infection. Call a physician if any of the following appear:

- Increased redness, pain, tenderness, swelling, or red streaks near the burn
- Pus
- Elevated temperature (fever)

Keep the area and dressing as clean and dry as possible. Elevate the burned area, if possible, for the first 24 hours. Give over-the-counter (OTC) pain medication, if necessary.

Refer to **FLOWCHART 11-1** for additional information regarding the care of thermal burns.

FYI

Burned Tongue

A few grains of sugar sprinkled on the tongue can relieve the misery of a tongue burned by hot food or drink. Repeat as often as needed. Sucking on ice chips or a popsicle can cool the burn.

CAUTION

DO NOT use topical OTC burn ointments or sprays or anesthetic sprays because:

- Some products may cause allergic reactions.
- Most do not contain enough benzocaine or lidocaine to suppress pain.
- The duration of any possible relief is relatively short (30 to 40 minutes). More than three or four applications per day of products containing local anesthetics is discouraged because toxic effects can occur if the agents are used too frequently.
- They seal in the heat.
- They are expensive.

Flowchart 11-1 Thermal Burns

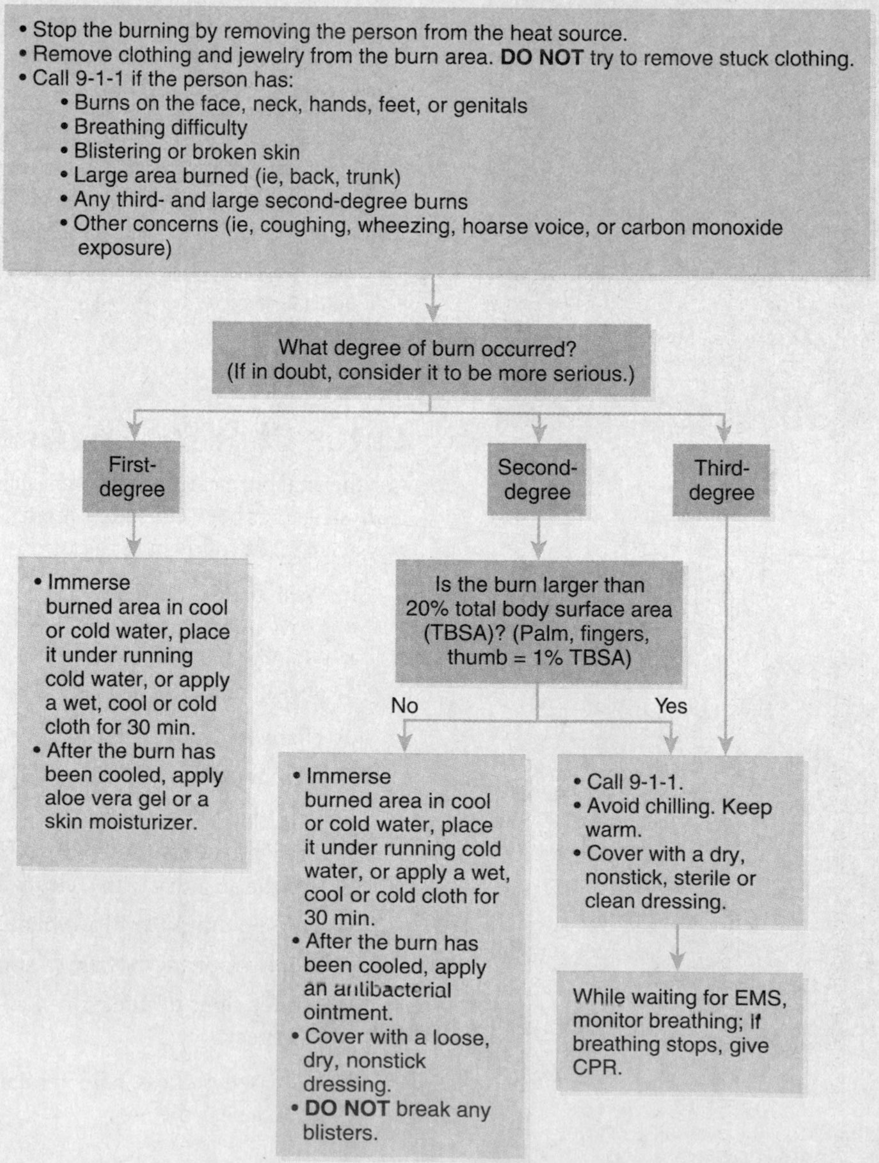

• Stop the burning by removing the person from the heat source.
• Remove clothing and jewelry from the burn area. DO NOT try to remove stuck clothing.
• Call 9-1-1 if the person has:
• Burns on the face, neck, hands, feet, or genitals
• Breathing difficulty
• Blistering or broken skin
• Large area burned (ie, back, trunk)
• Any third- and large second-degree burns
• Other concerns (ie, coughing, wheezing, hoarse voice, or carbon monoxide exposure)
What degree of burn occurred? (If in doubt, consider it to be more serious.)
First-degree
Second-degree
Third-degree
• Immerse burned area in cool or cold water, place it under running cold water, or apply a wet, cool or cold cloth for 30 min.
• After the burn has been cooled, apply aloe vera gel or a skin moisturizer.
Is the burn larger than 20% total body surface area (TBSA)? (Palm, fingers, thumb = 1% TBSA)
No
Yes
• Immerse burned area in cool or cold water, place it under running cold water, or apply a wet, cool or cold cloth for 30 min.
• After the burn has been cooled, apply an antibacterial ointment.
• Cover with a loose, dry, nonstick dressing.
• DO NOT break any blisters.
• Call 9-1-1.
• Avoid chilling. Keep warm.
• Cover with a dry, nonstick, sterile or clean dressing.
While waiting for EMS, monitor breathing; if breathing stops, give CPR.

Chemical Burns

A chemical burn is the result of an acid or an alkali substance touching the skin **FIGURE 11-8**. Because chemicals continue to burn as long as they are in contact with the skin, they should be removed from the person as rapidly as possible.

First aid is the same for all chemical burns. Alkalis, such as drain cleaners, cause more serious burns than acids, such as battery acid, because they penetrate deeper and remain active longer. Organic compounds, such as petroleum products, are also capable of burning.

If the burn occurred at a workplace, send someone to check the **safety data sheet (SDS)** for the hazardous materials used at the worksite. SDSs include first aid procedures. The Occupational Safety and Health Administration (OSHA) requires employers to identify chemical hazards using labels **FIGURE 11-9**.

Refer to **FLOWCHART 11-2** for additional information regarding the care of chemical burns.

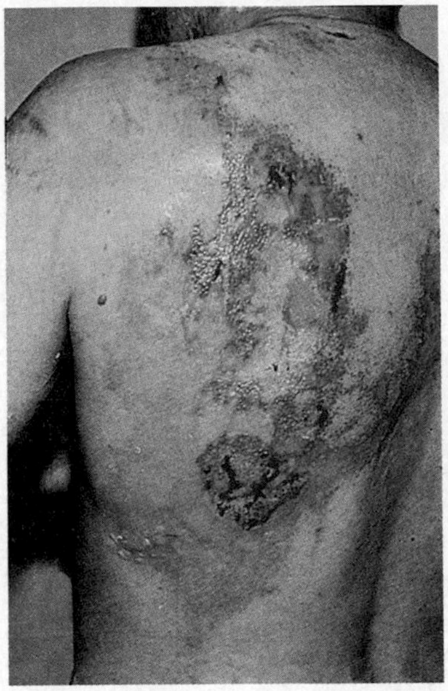

FIGURE 11-8 Chemical burn from sulfuric acid.

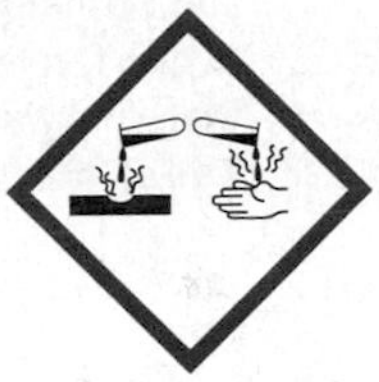

FIGURE 11-9 This pictogram is displayed on the packaging of corrosive chemicals.

Flowchart 11-2 Chemical Burns

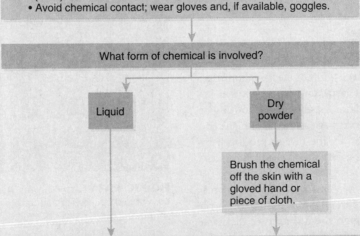

- Call 9-1-1.
- If at a workplace, send someone to check the safety data sheet (SDS) for the hazardous materials used at the worksite.
- Avoid chemical contact; wear gloves and, if available, goggles.

↓

What form of chemical is involved?

↓

Liquid → (go to final step)

Dry powder → Brush the chemical off the skin with a gloved hand or piece of cloth.

↓

- Remove clothing and jewelry, and immediately flush the burn with large amounts of cool running water for at least 20 min. or until EMS arrives.
- **DO NOT** use high-pressure water.
- **DO NOT** try to neutralize the chemical.
- For chemical in an eye:
  - Tip the head so the affected eye is below the nose, and wash the eye with warm water from nose out to side of face for at least 20 min.

What to Look For	What to Do
▪ Pain ▪ Burning ▪ Breathing difficulty ▪ Eye pain or vision changes	First aid is the same for most chemical burns. Once the area is safe: 1. Brush a dry or powder chemical off the skin with a gloved hand or piece of cloth before flushing with water. 2. Flush the burn immediately with large amounts of cool running water for at least 20 minutes or until EMS arrives **FIGURE 11-10**. Clothing and jewelry can be removed while flushing. 3. Call 9-1-1 immediately for all chemical burns. 4. For a chemical in an eye: Tip the head so the affected eye is below the nose, and wash the eye with warm water (which is tolerated in the eye better than cold water) from nose out to side of face for at least 20 minutes.

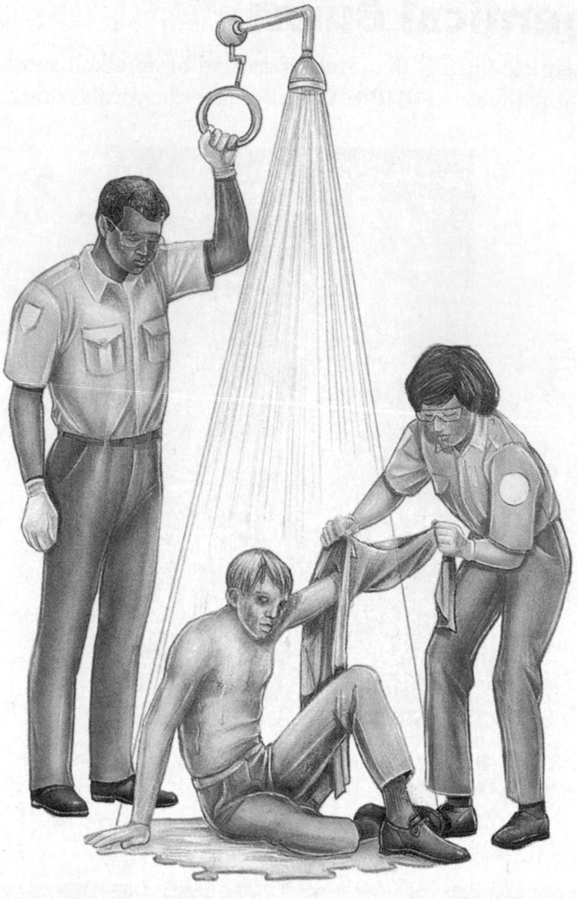

FIGURE 11-10 Flushing a chemical burn.

CAUTION

DO NOT waste time! A chemical burn is an emergency!

DO NOT apply water under high pressure; it will drive the chemical deeper into the tissue.

DO NOT try to neutralize a chemical even if you know which chemical is involved; heat may be produced, resulting in more damage. Some product labels for neutralizing may be wrong. Save the container or the label for the chemical's name.

Electrical Burns

Even a mild electrical shock can cause serious internal injuries **FIGURE 11-11**. There are three types of electrical injuries: thermal burn (flame), arc burn (flash), and true electrical injury (contact). A thermal burn (flame) results when clothing or objects in direct contact with the skin are ignited by an electric current. These injuries are caused by the flames produced by the electric current and not by the passage of the electric current or arc.

An arc burn (flash) occurs when electricity jumps, or arcs, from one spot to another and not from the passage of an electric current through the body. Although the duration of the flash may be brief, it usually causes extensive superficial injuries.

A true electrical injury (contact) happens when an electric current passes directly through the body. This type of injury is characterized by an entrance wound and an exit wound. The important factor with this type of injury is that the surface injury may be just the tip of the iceberg. High-voltage electric currents passing through the body may disrupt the normal heart rhythm and cause cardiac arrest, internal burns, and other injuries.

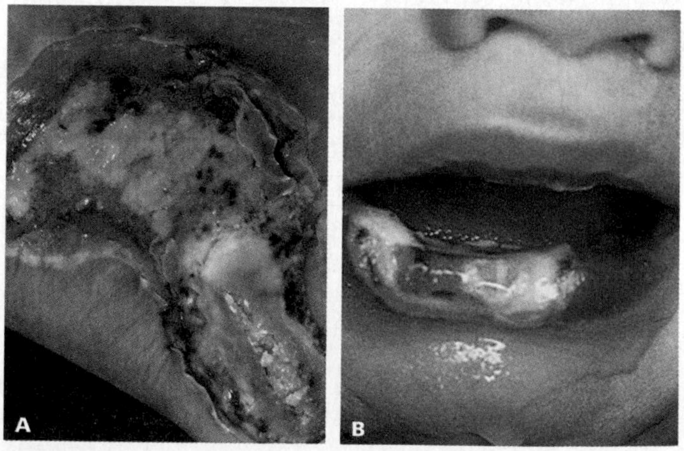

FIGURE 11-11 Electrical burns. **A**. Exit wound on a foot. **B**. Electrical burn caused by chewing through an electrical cord.

During an electrical shock, electricity enters the body at the point of contact and travels along the path of least resistance (nerves and blood vessels). Although the entrance burn may appear small, major damage may occur inside the body. Usually, the electricity exits where the body is touching a surface or is in contact with a ground (eg, a metal object). The exit wound can be extensive. Sometimes, a person has more than one exit site.

If . . .	Then . . .
Electrical shock is from contact with a downed powerline.	▪ The power must be turned off before anyone approaches a person who may be in contact with the wire. ▪ **DO NOT** attempt to move downed wires off a person. Wait until trained personnel with the proper equipment can cut the wires or disconnect them.
Power line falls across a vehicle containing a person.	Tell the person to stay in the vehicle until the power can be shut off.
Power line falls across a vehicle containing a person and a fire threatens the vehicle.	Tell the person to jump out of the vehicle without making contact with the vehicle or the wire. This will be a very difficult maneuver for most people.
You feel a tingling sensation in your legs and lower body as you approach a person. The sensation signals that you are on energized ground and that an electric current is entering through one foot, passing through your lower body, and leaving through the other foot.	Stop where you are. Raise one foot off the ground, turn around, and hop to a safe place.
You can safely reach the person.	**DO NOT** attempt to move any wires, even with wooden poles, tools with wood handles, or tree branches. Wood can conduct electricity and the rescuer will be electrocuted.

Contact With an Outdoor Power Line

When the area becomes safe and the electrocuted person has been rescued:

- Check breathing of any unresponsive person and, if absent, begin CPR.
- Most electrical burns are third-degree burns, so cover all burn wounds with sterile dressings.
- All persons who have been electrocuted should receive professional medical care.

Contact Inside Buildings

Most electrical burns that occur indoors are caused by faulty electrical equipment or careless use of electrical appliances. Turn off the electricity at the circuit breaker, fuse box, or outside switch box, or unplug the appliance if the plug is undamaged. Do not touch the appliance or the person until the current is off.

Once there is no danger to first aid providers, first aid can begin. Electric current flows quickly into the body's tissues and then exits. The surface injuries of the skin involve small surface areas (entrance and exit points); the major damage occurs deep under the skin **FIGURE 11-12**. See Chapter 24, *Wilderness First Aid*, for lightning burns and their care.

Refer to **FLOWCHART 11-3** for additional information regarding the care of electrical burns.

What to Look For	What to Do
▪ Burn wound, which might appear small ▪ Entrance and exit wounds (Usually, the electricity exits where the body is touching a surface or is in contact with a ground [ie, a metal object]; this is often the hand or foot.) ▪ Multiple burns (Most electrical burns are third-degree burns.) ▪ Absent breathing/pulse (Electricity can cause a person's breathing or heart to stop.)	Once the area is safe: 1. Check breathing of any unresponsive person and, if absent, begin CPR. 2. Call 9-1-1 immediately. Every person who has been electrocuted needs professional medical care. 3. If the person fell, check for broken bones and spinal injury. 4. Most electrical burns are third-degree burns, so cover all burn wounds with dry, sterile dressing.

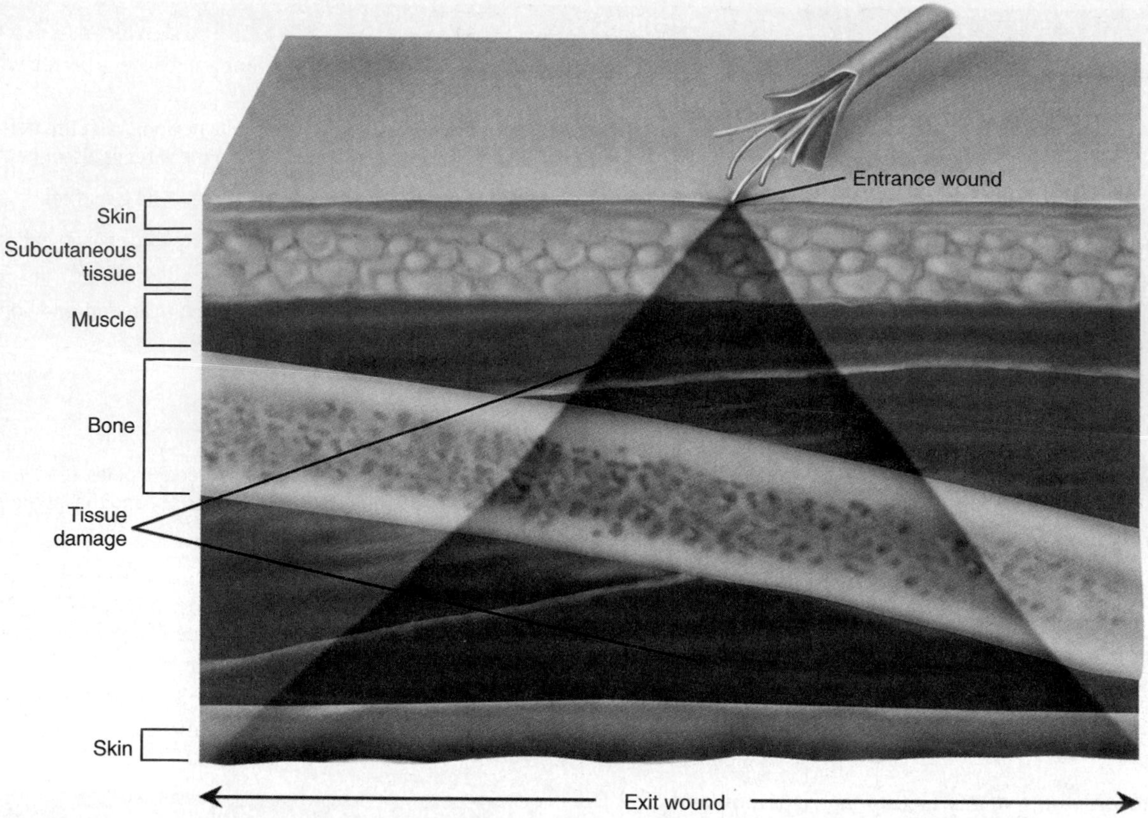

FIGURE 11-12 The external signs of an electrical burn may be deceiving. The entrance wound may be a small burn, while the damage to deeper tissue may be massive.

Flowchart 11-3 Electrical Burns

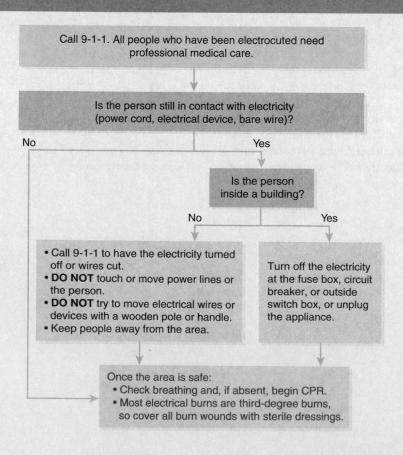

Call 9-1-1. All people who have been electrocuted need professional medical care.

↓

Is the person still in contact with electricity (power cord, electrical device, bare wire)?

No → go to "Once the area is safe"

Yes → Is the person inside a building?

- **No**:
  - Call 9-1-1 to have the electricity turned off or wires cut.
  - **DO NOT** touch or move power lines or the person.
  - **DO NOT** try to move electrical wires or devices with a wooden pole or handle.
  - Keep people away from the area.
- **Yes**: Turn off the electricity at the fuse box, circuit breaker, or outside switch box, or unplug the appliance.

↓

Once the area is safe:
- Check breathing and, if absent, begin CPR.
- Most electrical burns are third-degree burns, so cover all burn wounds with sterile dressings.

PREP KIT

Ready for Review

- Burns occur in every age group, across all socioeconomic levels, at home and in the workplace, and in urban, suburban, and rural settings.
- Burn injuries can be classified as thermal, chemical, or electrical.
- Treatment depends on the size and depth of burns.
- A chemical burn is the result of a caustic or corrosive substance touching the skin.
- There are three types of electrical injuries: thermal burn (flame), arc burn (flash), and true electrical injury (contact).

Vital Vocabulary

burn An injury in which soft tissue absorbs more energy than it can dissipate from thermal heat, chemicals, or electricity.

chemical burn An injury to the skin caused by contact with chemicals.

electrical burn An injury to the skin and the inside of the body caused by contact with electric current.

first-degree (superficial) burn A burn affecting only the epidermis; characterized by skin that is red but not blistered or burned through.

safety data sheet (SDS) A form, provided by manufacturers and distributors of chemicals, containing information about chemical composition, physical and chemical properties, health and safety hazards, first aid procedures, and handling and storage of a specific chemical.

second-degree (partial-thickness) burn A burn affecting the epidermis and some portion of the dermis but not the subcutaneous tissue; characterized by blisters and skin that is white to red and moist.

thermal (heat) burn Damage to the skin caused by contact with hot objects, flammable vapor, steam, hot liquid, or flames.

third-degree (full-thickness) burn A burn that affects all skin layers and possibly the subcutaneous layers, muscle, bone, and internal organs, leaving the area dry, leathery, and white, dark brown, or charred.

Assessment in Action

After a long, hot day at the water park, your friend reports a severe sunburn on their back and shoulders. They failed to apply sunscreen while at the water park. Blisters have formed, and your friend refuses to sit up in a chair and reports severe pain.

Directions: Circle Yes if you agree with the statement; circle No if you disagree.

1. The blisters and pain are signs that this is a first-degree burn.
   YES NO
2. You should break the blisters to relieve pressure and clean the burn.
   YES NO
3. Cool compresses can be used to relieve pain.
   YES NO
4. You can apply antibiotic ointment and aloe vera to keep the skin moist.
   YES NO
5. This person does not need professional medical care.
   YES NO

PREP KIT continued

Check Your Knowledge

Directions: Circle Yes if you agree with the statement; circle No if you disagree.

1. People with burns requiring professional medical care should not drink water.
   YES **NO**
2. Petroleum jelly can be applied over a burn.
   YES **NO**
3. The rule of the hand can help determine the size of a burned area.
   YES **NO**
4. Neutralize an acid on the skin by using baking soda.
   YES **NO**
5. Use a large amount of water to flush chemicals off the body.
   YES **NO**
6. Brush a dry chemical off the skin before flushing with water.
   YES **NO**
7. When someone gets electrocuted, there can be two burn wounds: entrance and exit.
   YES **NO**
8. When a person is in contact with a power line, use a tree branch to remove the wires.
   YES **NO**
9. Ibuprofen helps relieve pain and swelling.
   YES **NO**
10. Cold water can be used, in moderation, on any burn of any size.
    YES **NO**

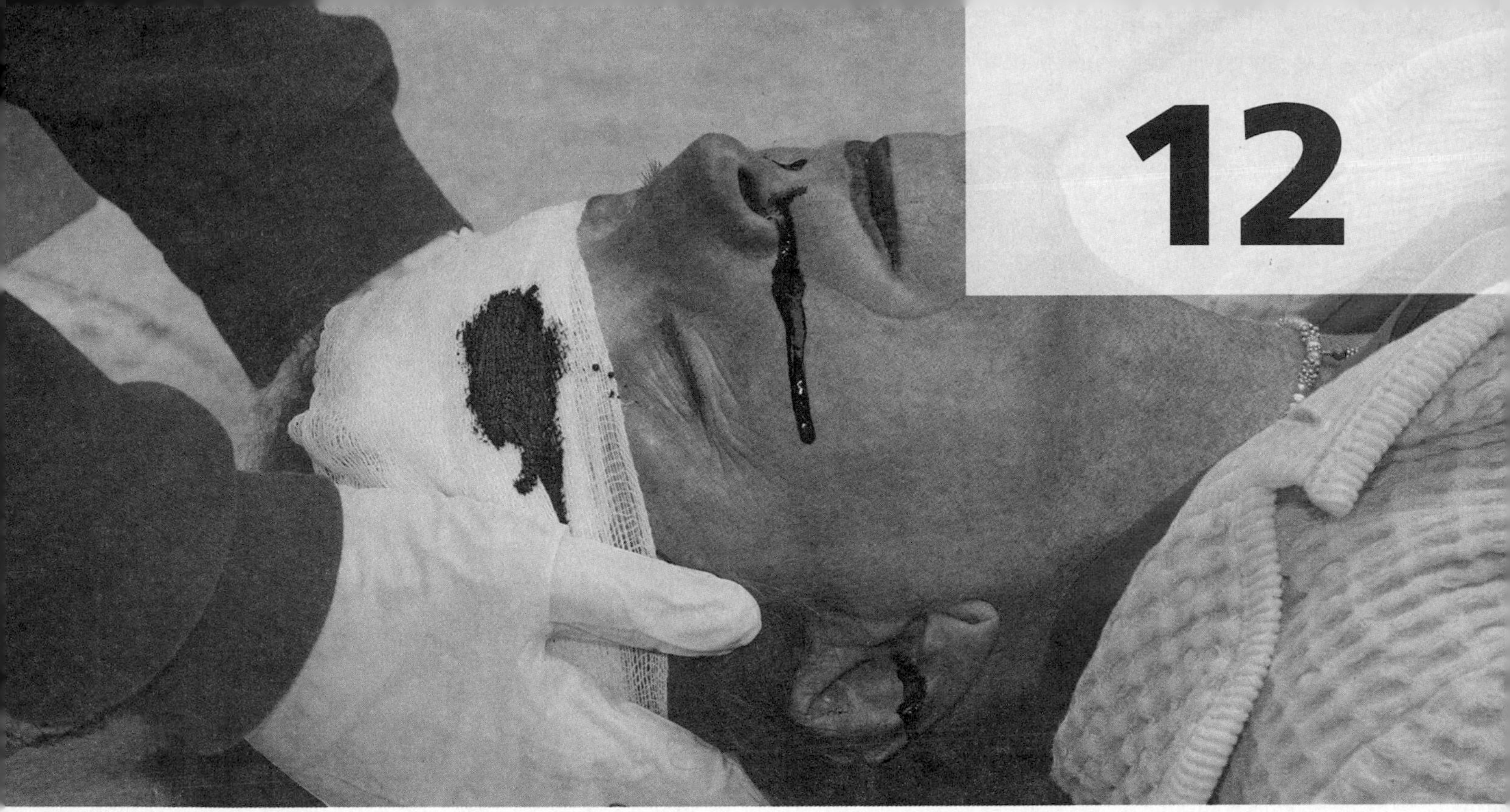

12

Head and Spinal Injuries

CHAPTER AT A GLANCE

Head Injuries

Any head injury is potentially serious. If not properly treated, injuries that seem minor could become life threatening. Head injuries include scalp wounds, skull fractures, and brain injuries. Spinal injuries (ie, neck and back injuries) can also be present in people with a head injury.

Scalp Wounds

Scalp wounds bleed profusely because the scalp has many blood vessels. A bleeding scalp wound does not affect the blood supply to the brain. The brain obtains its blood supply from arteries in the neck, not the scalp. A concussion, skull fracture, impaled object, brain injury, or spinal injury may accompany a severe scalp wound.

What to Look For	What to Do
Scalp wound	1. Control bleeding by pressing on the wound **FIGURE 12-1**. Replace any skin flap to its original position and apply pressure. Another option is applying an ice pack or instant cold pack to control bleeding. 2. If you suspect a skull fracture, **DO NOT** apply excessive pressure; doing so may push bone pieces into the brain. Press on the edges of the wound to help control bleeding **FIGURE 12-2**.

Continues

Continued

What to Look For	What to Do
	3. Apply a dry, sterile or clean dressing. 4. Keep the head and shoulders raised if no spinal injury is suspected. 5. If bleeding continues, remove the first blood-soaked dressing and apply well-aimed direct pressure with a new dressing. 6. Call 9-1-1 if the following occur: ▪ The wound is extensive. ▪ There is significant facial damage. ▪ Signs of concussion occur (eg, nausea and vomiting, headache, drowsiness).

Skull Fracture

A **skull fracture** is a break or a crack in the cranium (bony case surrounding the brain). Skull fractures may be open (with an accompanying scalp laceration) or closed (without an accompanying scalp laceration).

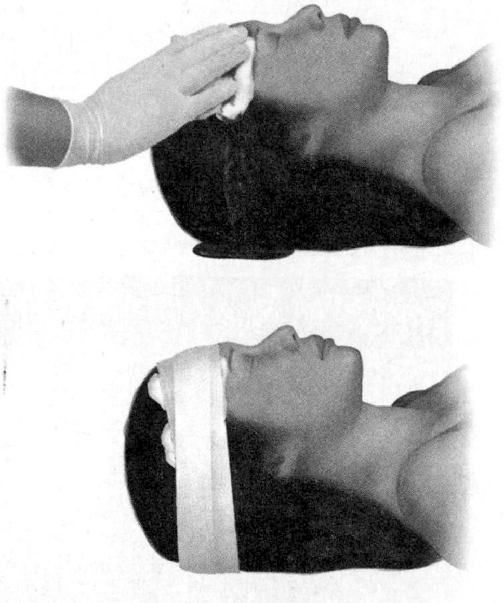

FIGURE 12-1 Apply direct pressure with a dry, sterile dressing to control the bleeding.

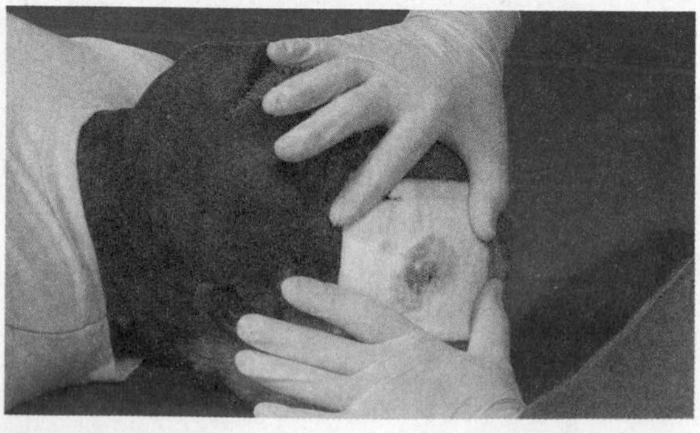

FIGURE 12-2 Apply pressure around the edges of the wound to control bleeding from a suspected skull fracture.

What to Look For	What to Do
▪ Pain ▪ Skull deformity ▪ Bleeding from an ear or the nose ▪ Leakage of **cerebrospinal fluid (CSF)** (clear or pink-tinged, watery fluid from an ear or the nose) ▪ Discoloration around the eyes **FIGURE 12-3** or behind the ears, known as **Battle sign FIGURE 12-4**, that appears several hours after the injury ▪ Unequal-size pupils of the eye ▪ Heavy scalp bleeding (skull and/or brain tissue may be exposed) ▪ Penetrating or impaled object	1. Apply a sterile or clean dressing over the wound and hold it in place with gentle pressure. 2. Control bleeding by pressing on the edges of the wound and gently on the center of it to avoid pressing bone pieces in the brain. A doughnut-shaped pad is useful in applying pressure around the edges of a suspected skull fracture **FIGURE 12-5**. 3. Call 9-1-1.

CAUTION

DO NOT stop the flow of blood or CSF from an ear or nose. Blocking the flow could increase pressure within the skull.

DO NOT remove an impaled object from the head. Stabilize it in place with bulky dressings.

DO NOT clean an open skull fracture; infection of the brain could result.

DO NOT press on the fractured area.

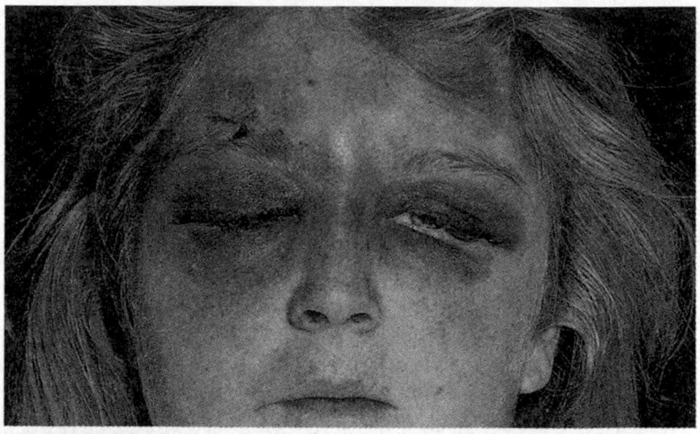

FIGURE 12-3 Discoloration around the eyes.

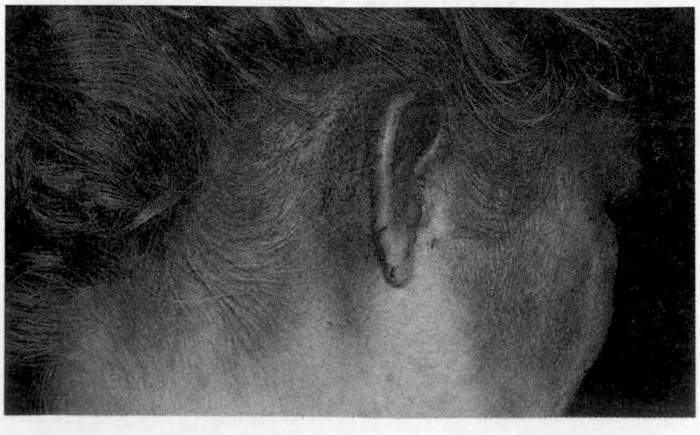

FIGURE 12-4 Battle sign.

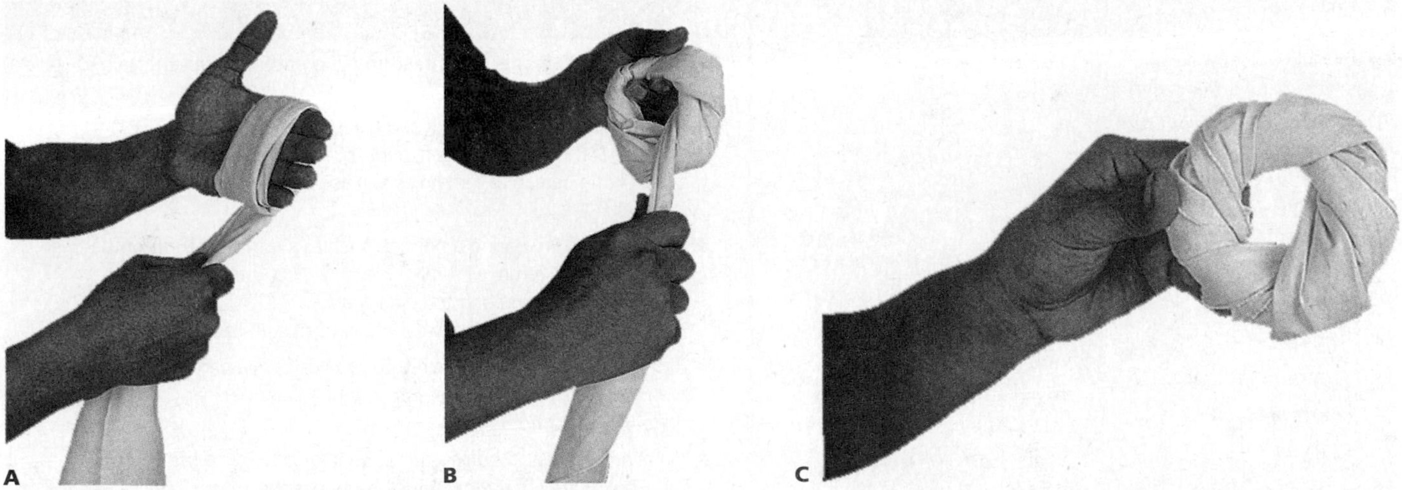

FIGURE 12-5 Make a doughnut for skull fracture–related bleeding and to surround an eye for protection when a short object is embedded in an eye. **A**. Using a cravat bandage or strip of cloth, wrap about half the length into a circle large enough to surround the injured area. **B**. Pass the tail thorough the hole repeatedly to form a circle. **C**. The completed dressing should have a hole large enough to surround the injury.

Traumatic Brain Injuries

It is not injury to the head, per se, that causes most short- and long-term conditions, but injuries to the brain itself. Most head injuries are a result of motor vehicle crashes, sports injuries, and falls. While many of these injuries are minor—shallow lacerations or localized bruising and swelling—others can be traumatic and cause permanent damage.

The brain is a delicate organ. When the head is struck with sufficient force, the brain bounces against the inside of the skull. Brain injuries can be serious and difficult first aid emergencies to handle. The person is often confused or unresponsive, making assessment difficult. Many brain injuries are life threatening. Mishandling a person with a brain injury could result in permanent damage or death.

The brain, like other body tissues, will swell from bleeding when it is injured. Unlike other tissues, however, the brain is confined in the skull, where there is little room for swelling. Any swelling of brain tissue or accumulation of blood inside the skull compresses the brain and increases the pressure inside the skull, which interferes with brain functioning. Furthermore, because the skull is hard, the brain and its surface blood vessels may be damaged if they strike the inside of the skull, which can occur when the head is struck directly or is rapidly accelerated or decelerated (such as in a vehicle crash). The phenomenon of a person "seeing stars" when struck on the back of the head results because the occipital lobe of the brain (the part that controls vision) strikes the back of the skull.

The nerve cells of the brain and the spinal cord, unlike most other cells in the body, are unable to regenerate. When those cells die, they are lost forever and cannot be replaced. Injuries to the brain can be caused by a penetrating foreign object, by bony fragments from a skull fracture, or by the brain striking the inside of the skull after a person's head has hit a stationary object such as the ground (a deceleration injury) or by being hit by something like a baseball bat or a teammate's knee—an acceleration injury. Sometimes there will be two points of injury: one at the point of impact and one where the brain rebounds off the skull on the opposite side; this is referred to as coup-contrecoup.

All brain injuries are unique. The brain can sustain several types of injuries depending on the type and amount of force that impacts the head. The type of injury may affect just one functional area of the brain, various areas, or even the entire brain.

The following sections on traumatic brain injury are adapted from the Centers for Disease Control and Prevention.

Concussion

A **concussion** is considered a mild traumatic brain injury (MTBI) and occurs when a blow to the head alters the function of the brain.

Most concussions (80% to 90%) resolve within 7 to 10 days, but some people take much longer to recover. Children, adolescents, and older adults tend to take longer to recover than do younger and middle-aged adults. A person with a concussion who has experienced previous concussions may need increased recovery time as well. Although most people with a concussion make a full recovery, it is possible for people to experience postconcussion syndrome, in which concussion symptoms last longer than 3 months.

FYI

Suspect a Concussion (MTBI)

- High-speed activities (motor vehicle crashes, skiing, bike riding, skateboarding)
- Sports and recreation activities
- Falls (including those among older adults), especially from a significant distance (eg, off a ladder, from a tree)
- Suspected child maltreatment (eg, shaking, hitting, throwing)
- Exposure to blasts (including military personnel returning from war zones)
- Injuries to the external parts of the head and/or scalp (eg, lacerations) and orthopedic injuries (eg, fractures, dislocations)

Data from: Centers for Disease Control and Prevention, U.S. Department of Health and Human Services. *Heads up: Facts for physicians about mild traumatic brain injury (MTBI)*. http://www.brainlinemilitary.org/concussion_course/course_content/pdfs/mtbi.pdf. Accessed January 1, 2021.

What to Look For	What to Do
Signs of concussion or mild traumatic brain injury, which may worsen over minutes or hours: *Thinking/remembering symptoms*: ▪ Difficulty thinking clearly ▪ Feeling slowed down ▪ Difficulty concentrating ▪ Difficulty remembering new information *Physical symptoms*: ▪ Headache ▪ Fuzzy or blurred vision ▪ Nausea or vomiting (early on) ▪ Dizziness ▪ Sensitivity to noise or light ▪ Balance problems ▪ Feeling tired, having no energy *Emotional/mood symptoms*: ▪ Irritability ▪ Sadness ▪ More emotional ▪ Nervousness or anxiety *Sleep disturbance symptoms*: ▪ Sleeping more than usual ▪ Sleeping less than usual ▪ Trouble falling asleep	**1.** If unresponsive, check for breathing. If breathing is absent, call 9-1-1 and give CPR. **2.** If a neck injury is suspected, or if the person is unresponsive: ▪ **DO NOT** move the head, neck, or spine. ▪ Tell the person to remain as still as possible. ▪ Call 9-1-1. **3.** If the person is wearing a helmet, such as a motorcycle or football helmet, **DO NOT** remove it unless: ▪ You suspect an obstructed airway. ▪ The helmet is so loose that you cannot stabilize the spine. If the helmet must be removed to provide life-saving care of an airway condition, make sure to stabilize the head and neck as the helmet is carefully removed. **4.** Seek professional medical care as soon as possible if the person: ▪ Looks very drowsy or cannot be awakened ▪ Has one pupil (the black part in the middle of the eye) that is larger than the other ▪ Has a seizure ▪ Cannot recognize people or places ▪ Becomes more and more confused, restless, or agitated ▪ Exhibits unusual behavior ▪ Becomes unresponsive ▪ Has a headache that gets worse and/or does not go away ▪ Has repeated vomiting or nausea ▪ Has slurred speech **5.** Following the injury, the person should: ▪ Get plenty of sleep at night and rest during the day. ▪ Avoid visual and sensory stimuli (eg, video games and loud music). ▪ Ease into normal activities slowly, not all at once. ▪ Avoid strenuous physical activities that increase the heart rate or require a lot of concentration. ▪ Avoid driving, cycling, operating machinery, or playing sports until assessed by a health care provider. ▪ Avoid anything that could cause another blow to the head or body. ▪ **DO NOT** use aspirin or anti-inflammatory medications such as ibuprofen or naproxen because of the risk of bleeding. Acetaminophen can be used for postconcussion headaches.

Other Traumatic Brain Injuries

Other types of traumatic brain injuries include the following:

- **Contusion**. A direct blow to the head can cause a bruise to the brain.
- **Coup-contrecoup**. In this injury, a blow to the head is strong enough to cause a contusion at the site of impact, as well as move the brain, causing it to hit the opposite side of the skull. This second hit causes a second contusion.
- **Diffuse axonal**. Shaking or strong rotation of the head causes this tearing injury. One example of diffuse axonal injury is shaken baby syndrome.
- *Penetration*. In this injury, an object such as a bullet, knife, or other sharp object enters the brain. The wound is then contaminated by hair, skin, bone, and pieces of the penetrating object. These contaminants may not be retrievable.

Q&A

How does blunt head trauma cause death?

Blunt trauma can cause bleeding into or around the brain, or it can lead to swelling of the brain (called edema). Bleeding in or around the brain causes a rapid rise of pressure within the rigid skull. The only escape route for this excess pressure is through the foramen magnum, an opening at the base of the skull through which the brainstem and spinal cord exit. The pushing of brain material through this opening compresses the brainstem, resulting in the cessation of breathing, followed by death.

Further Care of Head Injury

Several signs appearing within 48 hours of a head injury indicate the need to seek professional medical care. A person who has a concussion and experiences any of the following signs and symptoms may have a blood clot that is pushing the brain against the skull:

- *Headache.* Expect a headache. If it lasts more than 1 or 2 days or increases in severity, seek medical advice.
- *Nausea, vomiting.* If nausea lasts more than 2 hours, seek medical advice. Vomiting once or twice, especially in children, may be expected after a head injury. Vomiting does not indicate the severity of the injury. However, if vomiting begins again hours after the initial episodes have ceased, seek professional medical care.
- *Drowsiness.* Allow the person to sleep, but wake the person at least every 2 hours to check the state of consciousness and sense of orientation by asking their name and testing information-processing skills (eg, "Recite the months of the year backward."). If the person cannot respond or appears confused or disoriented, seek medical advice.
- *Vision impairment.* If the person "sees double," if the eyes do not move together, or if one pupil appears to be larger than the other, seek medical advice.
- *Mobility impairment.* If the person cannot use their arms or legs as well as previously or is unsteady when walking, seek professional medical care.
- *Speech impairment.* If the person has slurred speech or is unable to talk, seek professional medical care.
- *Seizures (convulsions).* If the person has a violent involuntary contraction (spasm) or series of contractions of the skeletal muscles, seek professional medical care.

Refer to **FLOWCHART 12-1** for additional information regarding the care of head injuries.

Flowchart 12-1 Head Injuries

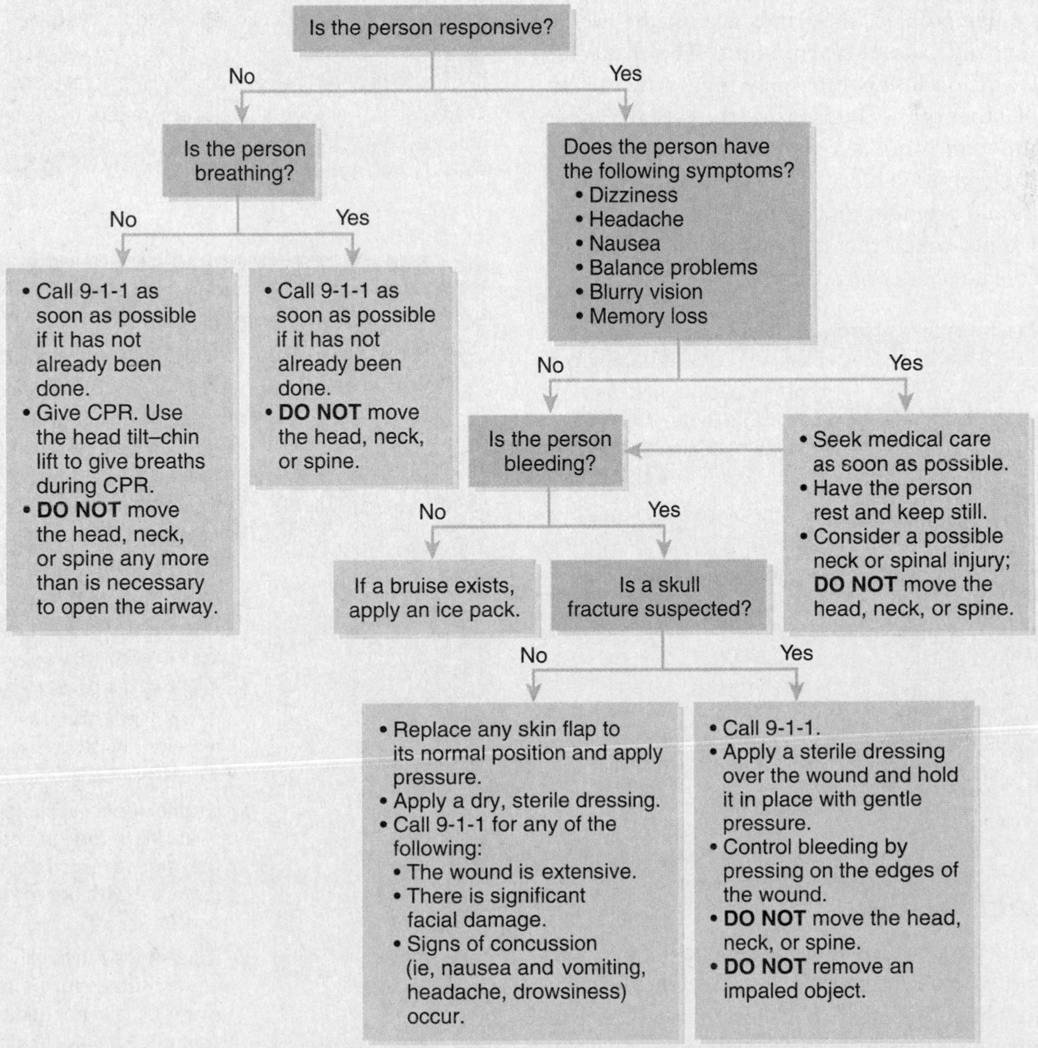

Is the person responsive?
No
Yes
Is the person breathing?
No
Yes
• Call 9-1-1 as soon as possible if it has not already been done.
• Give CPR. Use the head tilt–chin lift to give breaths during CPR.
• DO NOT move the head, neck, or spine any more than is necessary to open the airway.
• Call 9-1-1 as soon as possible if it has not already been done.
• DO NOT move the head, neck, or spine.
Does the person have the following symptoms?
• Dizziness
• Headache
• Nausea
• Balance problems
• Blurry vision
• Memory loss
No
Yes
Is the person bleeding?
• Seek medical care as soon as possible.
• Have the person rest and keep still.
• Consider a possible neck or spinal injury; DO NOT move the head, neck, or spine.
No
Yes
If a bruise exists, apply an ice pack.
Is a skull fracture suspected?
No
Yes
• Replace any skin flap to its normal position and apply pressure.
• Apply a dry, sterile dressing.
• Call 9-1-1 for any of the following:
• The wound is extensive.
• There is significant facial damage.
• Signs of concussion (ie, nausea and vomiting, headache, drowsiness) occur.
• Call 9-1-1.
• Apply a sterile dressing over the wound and hold it in place with gentle pressure.
• Control bleeding by pressing on the edges of the wound.
• DO NOT move the head, neck, or spine.
• DO NOT remove an impaled object.

Eye Injuries

Significant eye injuries are rare. However, of all the parts of the human body, an injured eye probably causes the most anxiety and concern in a person. The eyes—arguably the most important human sense organs—are easily damaged by trauma. For example, the slightest penetration by a metal fragment means hospitalization. Professional medical care may include surgery; despite technical advances, blindness or the loss of an eye remains a possibility whenever there is an eye injury. Have an ophthalmologist or other physician examine the eye as soon as possible, even if an injury seems minor at first.

CAUTION

DO NOT assume that any eye injury is minor. When in doubt, seek professional medical care immediately.

DO NOT remove an object stuck in the eye or try to wash out an object with water.

DO NOT exert pressure on an injured eyeball or a penetrating object.

Blows to the Eye

A direct blow or a flying object that lands against the eye or pierces it can potentially cause a severe injury. The chance of partial or complete vision loss is especially high if the injury involves leakage of either of the fluids inside the eyeball. These fluids, vitreous humor and aqueous humor, give the eyeball its shape and grapelike compressibility. When injured, it may be difficult for the first aid provider to determine whether the eye fluid is leaking. Do not touch the area to find out. The fluid could be the result of an allergy or infection.

What to Look For	What to Do
Blow to the eye (ranging in severity from minor to sight threatening), indicated by: ▪ A shiner, or black eye, occurring when some of the many delicate blood vessels around the eye rupture **FIGURE 12-6** ▪ Person reports being hit by a fist, ball, or other blunt object ▪ Broken bone around the eyeball indicated by double vision and the inability to look upward	1. Apply ice pack around the eye for 15 minutes. **DO NOT** place ice pack directly on the eye or put pressure on eye. 2. Have the person keep the eyes closed. 3. Seek professional medical care.

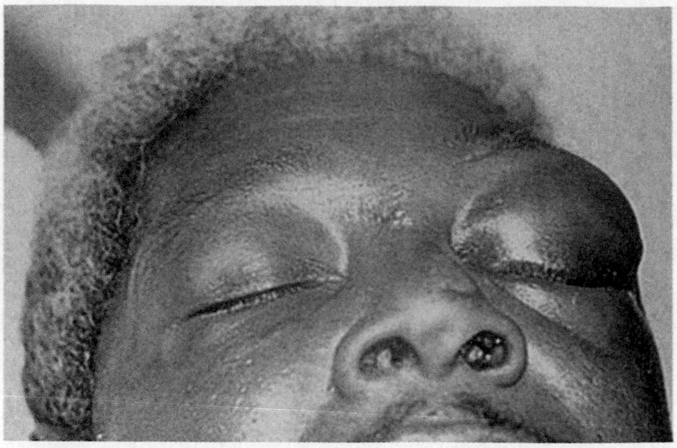

FIGURE 12-6 Blow to the eye.

Q&A

What causes a black eye?

A black eye is a bruise (contusion) caused by the leakage of blood from the small capillary blood vessels that have been injured. The extent of a blue-black discoloration depends on how much blood seeps from the damaged vessels, and it varies in different areas of the body. The tissues around the eyes have a lot of blood vessels. As a result, they bruise easily. The discoloration appearing in this area is more pronounced and prolonged than a contusion of the leg or arm.

Loose Object in Eye

Loose objects, whether an eyelash or a shard of glass, can cause pain and discomfort when they enter the eye. It can be difficult for the person who is hurt to remove the object themselves, so it is important to know how to help someone with a loose object in the eye.

What to Look For	What to Do
Loose object in the eye, indicated by: ▪ Severe pain ▪ Tearing (the body's way of trying to remove the object)	Try, in order, each of the following methods: 1. Have the person blink the eye several times. 2. Using the eyelashes, pull the upper eyelid out and over the lower lid. This allows the lower lashes to brush the object off the inside of the upper lid. Have the person blink a few times and let the eye move the object out. 3. Gently irrigate the eye with clean, warm water. Hold the eyelid open and tell the person to move the eye as it is rinsed. 4. Examine the lower lid by pulling it down gently. If you see the object, remove it with a moistened gauze pad **FIGURE 12-7**. 5. Lift the upper eyelid up and over a cotton swab. Many foreign bodies lodge under the upper eyelid; if the object is seen, remove it with the corner of a wet gauze pad. 6. If any of the previously discussed methods are successful, professional medical care is usually not needed unless there is continued pain or itching to the eye.

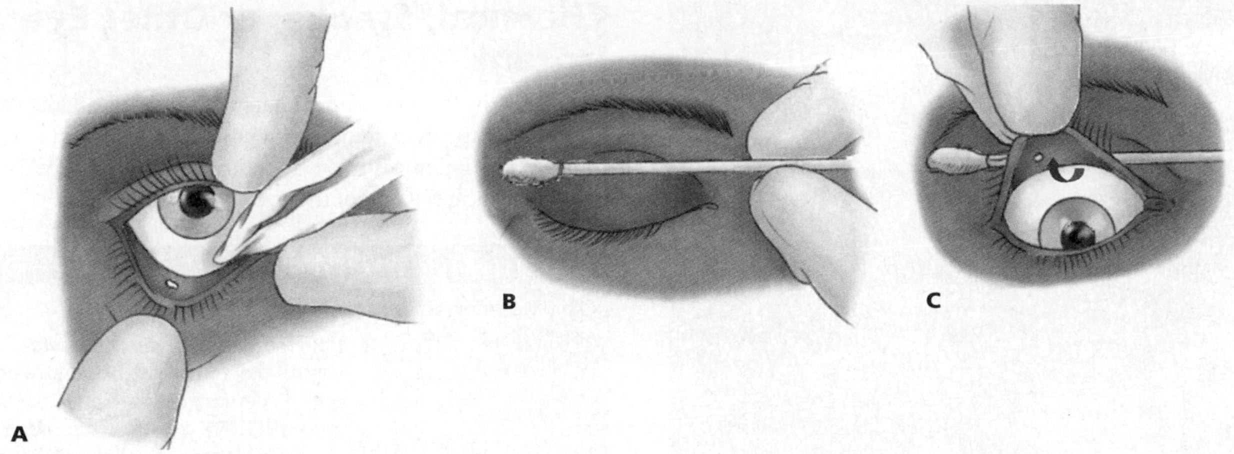

FIGURE 12-7 Removing loose objects from the eye. **A**. If tears or gentle flushing do not remove the object, gently pull down the lower lid. Remove an object by gently flushing with lukewarm water or by using wet, sterile gauze. **B**. If unsuccessful, tell the person to look down. Pull gently downward on the upper eyelashes. Lay a swab or matchstick across the top of the lid. **C**. Next, fold the lid over the swab or matchstick. Remove an object by gently flushing with lukewarm water or by using wet, sterile gauze.

Cut or Scratch on Eyeball or Eyelid

There are a range of objects that can scratch the cornea, the clear front part of the eye. This includes dust, dirt, and sand as well as wood shavings and metal particles. The sclera (white part of eye) and the eyelid can also be damaged. It is important to seek professional medical care for this type of eye injury.

What to Look For	What to Do
Cut on the eyeball **FIGURE 12-8**, indicated by: ▪ Cut appearance of the cornea (clear part of the eye) or sclera (white part of eye) ▪ Inner liquid filling of the eye coming out through the wound ▪ Cut lid	1. **DO NOT** apply pressure to the eye. 2. Cover both eyes with gauze pads, and lightly wrap a bandage around the head to hold the pads in place. 3. Call 9-1-1 or drive the person to a medical facility as soon as possible.
Scratch on the eyeball: ▪ Symptoms are similar to those of a loose object in the eye. ▪ A severe scratch or abrasion may be visible. ▪ Person reports changes in vision.	1. Treat as a loose object in the eye. 2. Try sunglasses to soothe the eye. 3. Use over-the-counter (OTC) pain medication (eg, acetaminophen) according to package directions. A damp cloth over the eyes can provide some relief. 4. If pain persists, patch the eye until symptoms improve. 5. If pain or visual changes last beyond 48 hours, signs of infection develop (such as pus), or a visible ulcer develops on the eye, seek professional medical care.
Cut eyelid	1. If only the eyelid is cut, apply a soft, sterile or clean dressing with gentle pressure, and lightly wrap a bandage around the head to hold the pad in place. 2. Seek professional medical care for sutures. If not sutured, the eyelid may be permanently droopy or partially closed.

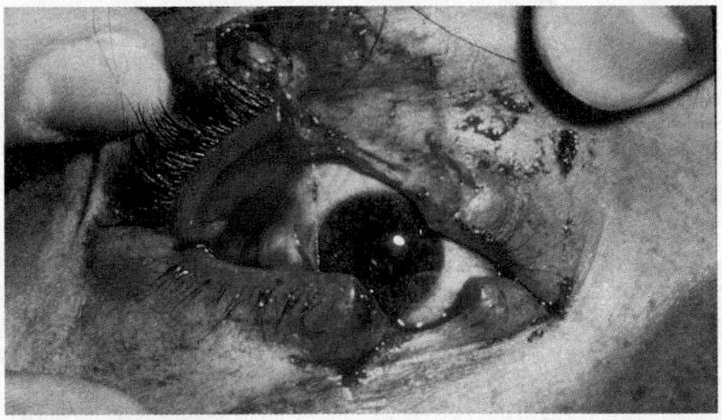

FIGURE 12-8 Lacerated eyelid.

Penetrating Eye Injury

One type of severe eye injury is a penetrating injury, which occurs when there is something protruding from the eye. It is important to not remove the object and to stabilize it if possible. Seek immediate professional medical care for this type of eye injury.

What to Look For	What to Do
Penetrating eye injury, indicated by lid laceration or cut	1. **DO NOT** remove the object. 2. For a long object, place padding around the object to stabilize against movement, and place a paper cup or similar object over the object for protection **FIGURE 12-9**. 3. For a short object, place a doughnut-shaped pad (formed from a roller gauze bandage or a cravat bandage made from a triangular bandage) around the eye without touching the object, and wrap a bandage around the head to hold the pad in place. 4. Cover both eyes; movement of the uninjured eye will cause movement of the injured eye. 5. Keep the person flat on their back. 6. Call 9-1-1.

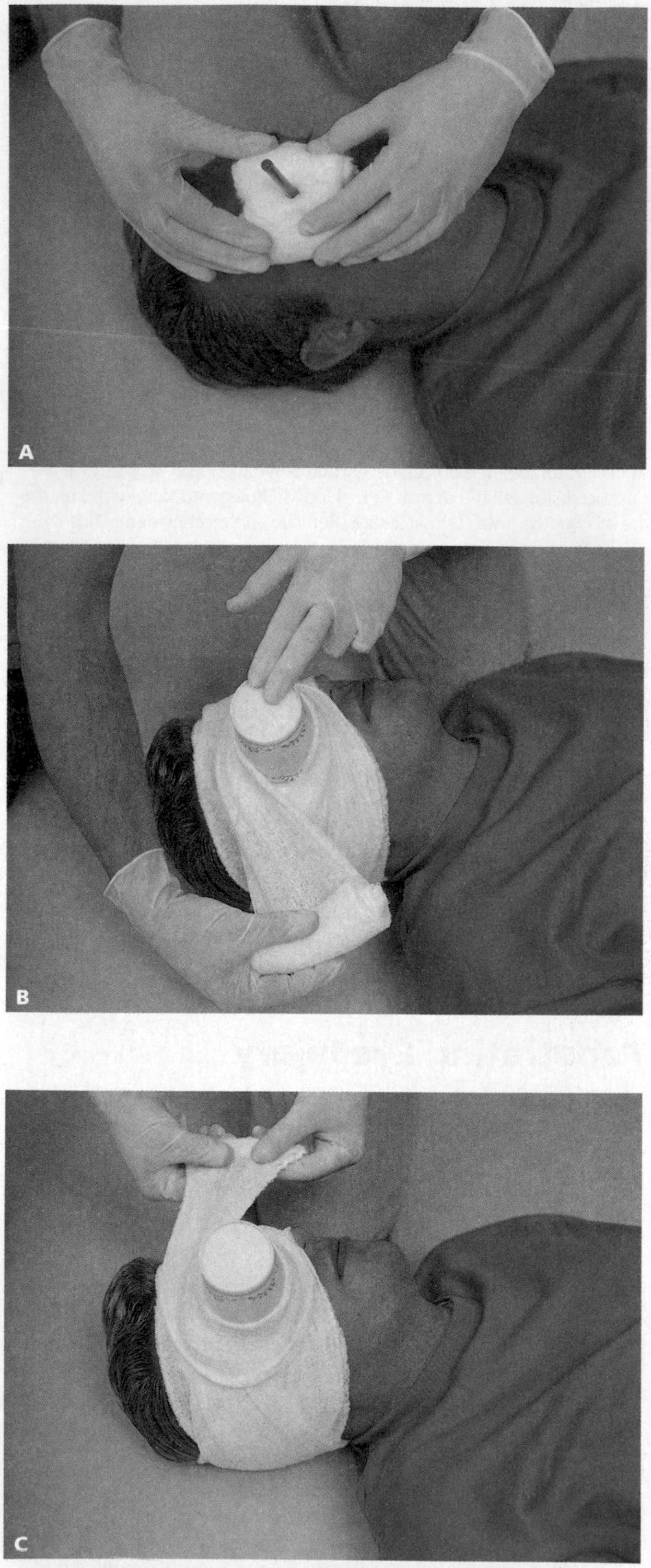

FIGURE 12-9 Stabilize a long penetrating object against movement. **A**. Place padding around the object. **B**. Place a shield (ie, paper cup or similar object) over, but not touching, the penetrating object to protect the object from being hit. **C**. Cover both eyes to prevent the uninjured eye from moving with the injured eye.

Chemical, Smoke, or Other Eye Irritant

Chemicals in the eyes can threaten sight, with alkalis causing greater damage than acids. Because damage can occur in 1 to 5 minutes, the chemical must be removed immediately. First aid may determine the fate of the eye and vision.

What to Look For	What to Do
Chemical, smoke, or other irritant in eye	Act immediately: **1.** Hold the eye wide open; flush with warm water for at least 15 minutes or until emergency medical services (EMS) arrive **FIGURE 12-10**. If tap water is not available, normal saline or other eye irrigation solution may be used. ▪ Irrigate from the nose side of the eye toward the outside to avoid flushing the material into the other eye. ▪ Tell the person to roll the eye as much as possible to help wash out the eye. **2.** Loosely bandage the eye or eyes, if necessary. **3.** For a chemical eye injury, contact the poison control center (1-800-222-1222). If not available, seek professional medical care as soon as possible or call 9-1-1.

CAUTION

DO NOT try to neutralize a chemical in the eye. Water usually is readily available for eye irrigation.
DO NOT use an eye cup for a chemical burn.
DO NOT bandage an eye tightly.
DO NOT try to remove an object stuck in the eye.
DO NOT allow the person to rub an injured eye.
DO NOT try to remove an embedded foreign object in the eye.
DO NOT use dry cotton (cotton balls or cotton-tipped swabs) or instruments such as tweezers to remove an object from the surface of an eye.

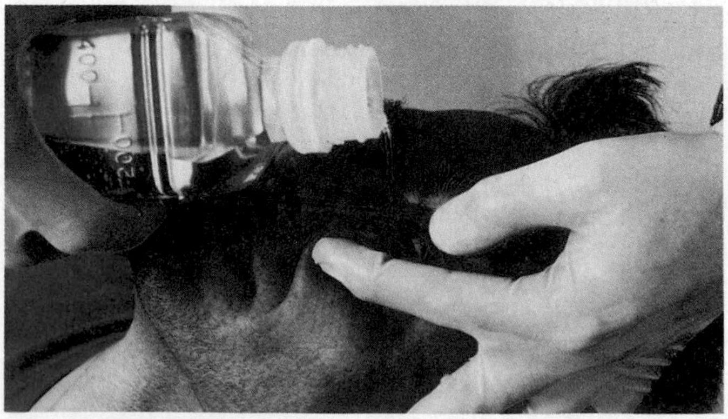

FIGURE 12-10 Flushing the eye to treat a chemical burn.

Eye Avulsion

Another traumatic eye injury is an eye avulsion, which occurs when the eyeball is knocked out of its socket.

What to Look For	What to Do
Eye avulsion, indicated by: ▪ Eye knocked out from its socket	1. Cover the eye loosely with a sterile or clean dressing that has been moistened with clean water. Do not try to push the eyeball back into the socket. 2. Protect the injured eye with a paper cup, a piece of cardboard folded into a cone, or a doughnut-shaped pad made from a roller gauze bandage or a cravat bandage. 3. Cover the undamaged eye with a patch to stop movement of the damaged eye. 4. Call 9-1-1.

Eye Burns

Searing pain can be an indication of eye burn. This occurs when the eye has been exposed to bright, damaging light.

What to Look For	What to Do
Burns caused by light, indicated by: ▪ Person reports looking at a source of ultraviolet light, such as sunlight, arc welding, bright snow, or tanning lamps ▪ Severe pain occurring 1 to 6 hours after exposure	1. Cover both eyes with moist, cool cloths. 2. Give OTC pain medication, if needed. 3. Seek medical advice.

Dry Eye

Dry eye is caused by increased tear evaporation, usually in very dry climates, windy conditions, or dusty or smoky environments.

What to Look For	What to Do
▪ Person complains about an eye being itchy, scratchy, stinging, or tired ▪ Pain and redness ▪ Impaired vision over time	1. Have the person blink more often and rest the eyes. 2. Twice an hour, have the person close their eyes and then move the eyeballs around underneath the closed lids as you count slowly to 10. 3. **DO NOT** rub the eyes, which can further irritate them. 4. Apply artificial tears one to two times every hour, which can provide temporary relief. ▪ Liquid drops are fine for mild or intermittent dryness. A gel product lasts longer. Longer lasting than liquid drops or gel are OTC lubricating ointments used every few hours; note that ointments may cause blurry vision so it is best to try them at bedtime. 5. Drink lots of water. 6. Avoid environments that might exacerbate the condition. 7. Wearing wraparound eyeglasses can help reduce the drying effects of wind. 8. If eye dryness does not improve, consult an ophthalmologist (physician specializing in eye care).

Conjunctival Problems

One of the most common causes off a red eye is conjunctivitis, or "pinkeye." The conjunctiva is a thin, clear membrane that lines the inner part of the eyelids and sclera (white part of the eye). Conjunctivitis means "inflammation of the conjunctiva." It is known as pinkeye because the blood vessels in the sclera dilate and redden. It seldom affects vision. Conjunctivitis is caused by allergies (e.g., pollen, animal dander, dust), viral infections, and bacterial infections. Viral infection is the most common cause of conjunctivitis and is often associated with an upper respiratory infection. Foreign bodies in the eye and infection may have a similar appearance. If you suspect infection, also look for foreign objects.

What to Look For	What to Do
Conjunctivitis, indicated by: ▪ Redness in the sclera (white part of the eye) ▪ Itching or gritty sensation in the eye ▪ Oozing discharge ▪ Excessive tearing ▪ Swollen eyelids ▪ Dried crusts that form during sleep may bind the eyelids together. ▪ Discomfort caused by bright lights	**If allergic conjunctivitis is suspected:** 1. Apply cool compresses to the eye. 2. Apply artificial tears to dilute the offending allergen and relieve some of the itching. Antihistamine drops may also be considered for relieving symptoms but should not be used for more than 2 or 3 days. 3. Seek professional medical care if signs and symptoms do not improve after 3 or 4 days of treatment, especially if fever, increased pain, or changes in vision develop.
	It is difficult to distinguish between viral and bacterial conjunctivitis. If either is suspected: 1. Soak a clean cloth in warm water, wring out the excess water, and apply it to the eye. 2. Apply artificial tears as needed to provide comfort. 3. Seek professional medical care for prescription antibiotic eye drops.

Continues

Continued

What to Look For	What to Do
	4. Apply antibiotic eye drops four times per day. This treats a bacterial infection and, in the case of a viral infection, prevents a secondary infection from developing. 5. Avoid spreading an infection to other people. The person, their close contacts, and the first aid provider should wash their hands frequently to prevent the infection from spreading. 6. Seek professional medical care if signs and symptoms do not improve after 3 or 4 days of treatment, especially if fever, increased pain, or changes in vision develop.
Subconjunctival hemorrhage (bleeding under the conjunctiva) ▪ Affects only one eye ▪ Appears as a red patch or large area of redness in the sclera (white part of eye); appearance differs from conjunctivitis in that the redness is uniform, has distinct borders, and completely conceals the area of the sclera it covers ▪ Does not cause pain, visual changes, tearing, irritation, itching, or discharge from the eye ▪ Sometimes occurs in people who have had an eye injury or sneezed violently; can also occur during bowel movement or while lifting a heavy weight ▪ Occurs more often in people known to use drugs that help prevent blood from clotting (eg, aspirin or warfarin) ▪ Causes eye pain	1. Treatment is not required. Depending on size, subconjunctival hemorrhage usually clears up on its own within 2 weeks. 2. **DO NOT** use OTC eye drops that aim to eliminate redness. 3. Reassure the person that it is safe to continue activities. 4. If the eye is injured and hyphema is suspected, seek professional medical attention immediately.

Hyphema

Hyphema is bleeding in the eye. It appears as a collection of blood in front of the iris (the colored portion of the eye). Hyphema only affects one eye.

What to Look For	What to Do
▪ Visible pool of blood in front of the iris of the eye **FIGURE 12-11** ▪ Impaired vision ▪ Pain in eye	1. Keep physical activity to a minimum. 2. Tell the person to keep both eyes closed and cover the affected eye with an eye patch. **DO NOT** apply pressure on the eyeball because further damage can occur. 3. Apply an eye shield (eg, paper or plastic cup) over the eye patch to protect the eye from being struck. 4. Keep the person's head in an elevated and upright position. 5. Seek professional medical care immediately.

Refer to **FLOWCHART 12-2** for additional information regarding the care of eye injuries.

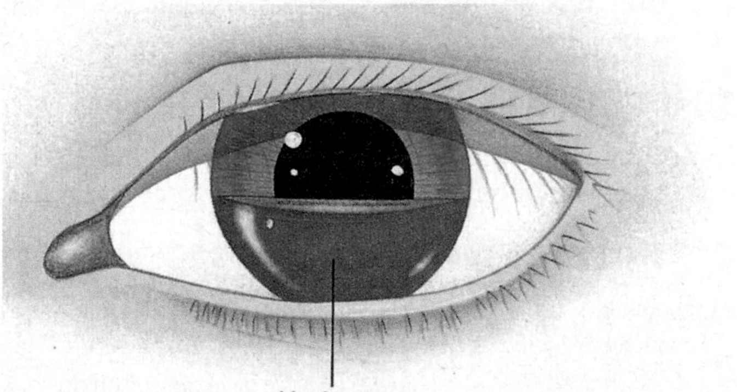

FIGURE 12-11 Hyphema.

Flowchart 12-2 Eye Injuries

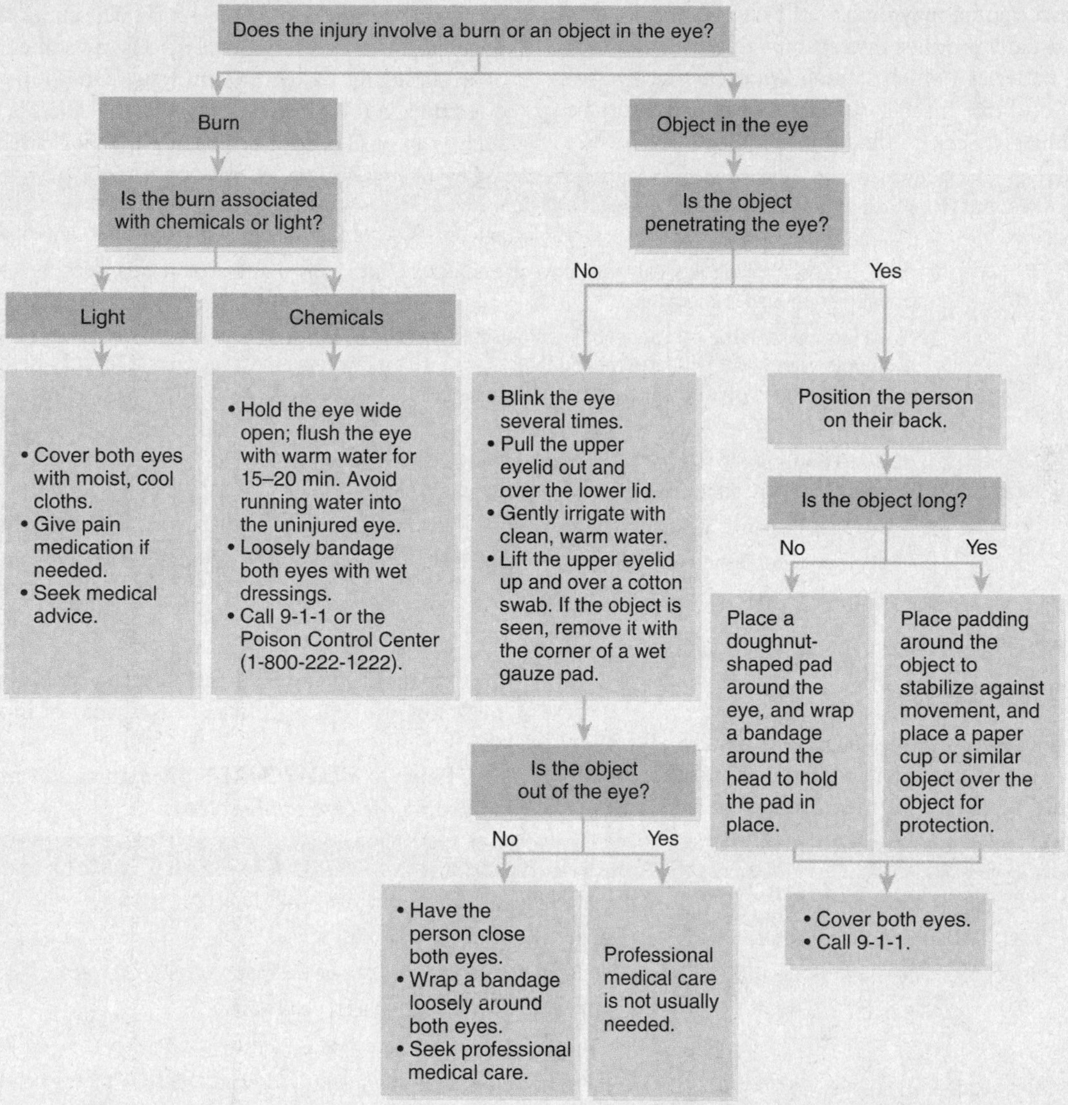
Does the injury involve a burn or an object in the eye?
Burn
Object in the eye
Is the burn associated with chemicals or light?
Is the object penetrating the eye?
No
Yes
Light
Chemicals
• Cover both eyes with moist, cool cloths.
• Give pain medication if needed.
• Seek medical advice.
• Hold the eye wide open; flush the eye with warm water for 15–20 min. Avoid running water into the uninjured eye.
• Loosely bandage both eyes with wet dressings.
• Call 9-1-1 or the Poison Control Center (1-800-222-1222).
• Blink the eye several times.
• Pull the upper eyelid out and over the lower lid.
• Gently irrigate with clean, warm water.
• Lift the upper eyelid up and over a cotton swab. If the object is seen, remove it with the corner of a wet gauze pad.
Position the person on their back.
Is the object long?
No
Yes
Place a doughnut-shaped pad around the eye, and wrap a bandage around the head to hold the pad in place.
Place padding around the object to stabilize against movement, and place a paper cup or similar object over the object for protection.
Is the object out of the eye?
No
Yes
• Have the person close both eyes.
• Wrap a bandage loosely around both eyes.
• Seek professional medical care.
Professional medical care is not usually needed.
• Cover both eyes.
• Call 9-1-1.

FYI

Sympathetic Eye Movement

Eyes move in the same direction together, focusing on the same object. This is known as sympathetic eye movement. Therefore, when the uninjured eye moves, the injured eye moves as well. This movement may aggravate an injury.

To lessen movement in an injured eye:

- Tell the person to keep the uninjured eye closed.
- Cover the undamaged eye with a cravat or roller bandage.

The person may become very anxious if both eyes are covered and they cannot see. Help overcome anxiety by explaining everything that you are doing and why.

FYI

An Unresponsive Person's Eyes

An unconscious person may lose the reflexes that protect the eye, such as blinking. If the eyes do not stay closed, keep them closed by covering them with moist dressings.

FYI

Contact Lenses

Determine whether a person is wearing contact lenses by asking, by checking a driver's license, or by looking for them on the eyeball, using a light shining on the eye from the side. In cases of chemicals in the eye, lenses should be removed immediately. Usually the person can remove the lenses.

Ear Injuries

Most ear conditions are not life threatening. Fast action may be needed, however, to relieve pain and to prevent or reverse hearing loss. Head trauma may involve the ear. Foreign bodies in the ear canal usually produce overzealous removal attempts. Except for disk batteries (which damage moist tissue by creating a current) and live insects, few foreign bodies must be extracted immediately. Seek professional medical care for the person; attempts to remove a foreign body from the ear can rupture the eardrum or lacerate the ear canal.

Children insert all sorts of things into their ears that may be impossible for you to remove safely. If the object is visible near the ear canal opening and you feel it is safe, cautiously try to remove the object with tweezers. Small objects can sometimes be removed by irrigating the ear with warm water. Do not try irrigation if the object blocks the entire ear canal or if the object is vegetable matter such as a kernel of corn or a bean, which will swell when wet.

What to Look For	What to Do
Objects stuck in an ear	1. **DO NOT** use tweezers or try to pry an object out unless the object can be seen near the ear canal opening. 2. Seek professional medical care to remove the object. Except for disk batteries and live insects, few foreign bodies must be removed immediately. 3. For a live insect in the ear canal, shine a small light into the ear. The insect may crawl out toward the light; if it does not, pour warm water into the ear and then drain it. This may drown the insect; regardless of whether it is dead or alive, it should wash out. When draining the water, turn the head to the side. If the insect cannot be removed, seek professional medical care.
Fluids coming from the ear (Blood or clear fluid draining from the ear may indicate a skull fracture.)	1. **DO NOT** attempt to stop bleeding or clear fluid (CSF) with or without blood coming from an ear. Doing so could increase pressure on the brain, causing permanent damage. 2. Place a sterile gauze dressing over the ear and loosely bandage it in place to prevent bacteria getting into the brain. 3. Stabilize the head and neck against movement. Tell the person to remain as still as possible. 4. Call 9-1-1.

Nose Injuries

A severe nose injury frightens the injured person and often challenges the first aid provider's skill. Most nosebleeds are self-limiting and do not require medical attention. In cases of accompanying head or neck injuries, stabilize the head and neck for protection. In some cases, loss of blood could cause shock.

Refer to **FLOWCHART 12-3** for additional information regarding the care of nosebleeds.

What to Look For	What to Do
Broken nose, indicated by: ▪ Pain, swelling, and a possible crooked appearance ▪ Bleeding and difficulty breathing through the nostrils ▪ Black eyes appearing 1 to 2 days after the injury	1. If bleeding, provide care as you would for a nosebleed. 2. Apply ice pack for 15 minutes. 3. Professional medical care can be delayed. 4. **DO NOT** try to straighten a crooked nose.
Nosebleed ▪ The **anterior nosebleed** (front of nose) is the most common type (90%). Blood flows from the nose through one nostril. ▪ The **posterior nosebleed** (back of nose) may involve massive bleeding, usually backward into the mouth or down the back of the throat. A posterior nosebleed is serious and requires professional medical care.	1. If the nose was hit, suspect a broken nose. 2. Have the person sit leaning slightly forward. **DO NOT** tilt the head back or lie the person down. 3. Pinch the nostrils shut constantly for 10 minutes **FIGURE 12-12**. Tell the person to breathe through the mouth and not swallow any blood. 4. If bleeding has not stopped, have the person gently sniff or blow their nose to get rid of ineffective blood clots. Pinch the nostrils shut again for 10 minutes. 5. If bleeding continues, try other methods in addition to nose pinching, such as spraying nasal decongestant spray into the nostrils. 6. Professional medical care is not usually needed unless bleeding continues, a foreign object is in the nose, or the nose is broken. 7. After a nosebleed has stopped, suggest that the person: ▪ Sneeze through an open mouth, if they need to sneeze. ▪ Avoid bending over and participating in too much physical exertion. ▪ Elevate the head with two pillows when lying down. ▪ Keep the nostrils moist by applying a little petroleum jelly just inside the nostril for 1 week; increase the humidity in the bedroom during the winter months by using a cold-mist humidifier. ▪ Avoid picking or rubbing the nose.
Foreign object in the nose (a medical condition mainly occurring to small children, who often put peanuts, beans, raisins, and other similar objects into their nostrils)	Try one or more of the following methods to remove the object: 1. Have the person gently blow their nose while compressing the opposite nostril. 2. If an object is visible, pull it out with tweezers. **DO NOT** push the object deeper. 3. Seek professional medical care if the object cannot be removed.

Flowchart 12-3 Nosebleeds

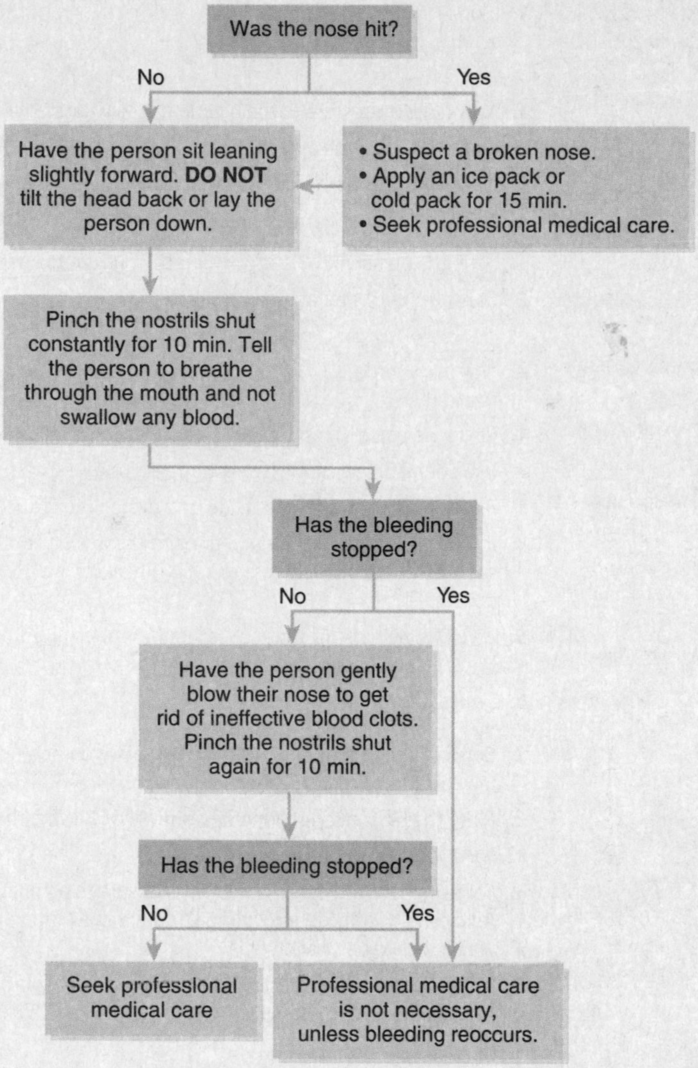
Was the nose hit?
No
Yes
Have the person sit leaning slightly forward. DO NOT tilt the head back or lay the person down.
• Suspect a broken nose.
• Apply an ice pack or cold pack for 15 min.
• Seek professional medical care.
Pinch the nostrils shut constantly for 10 min. Tell the person to breathe through the mouth and not swallow any blood.
Has the bleeding stopped?
No
Yes
Have the person gently blow their nose to get rid of ineffective blood clots. Pinch the nostrils shut again for 10 min.
Has the bleeding stopped?
No
Yes
Seek professional medical care
Professional medical care is not necessary, unless bleeding reoccurs.

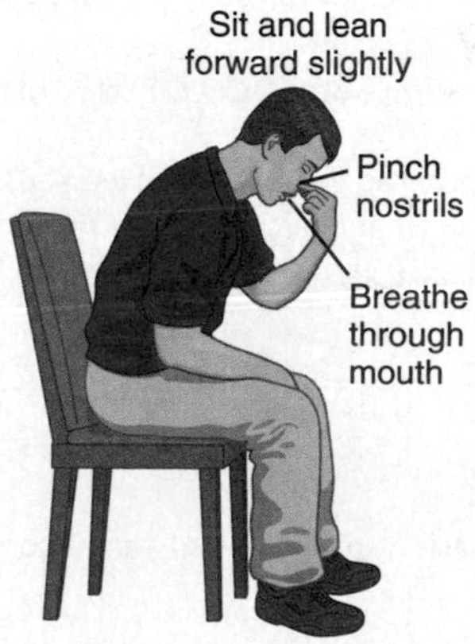
Sit and lean forward slightly
Pinch nostrils
Breathe through mouth

FIGURE 12-12 Control bleeding from the nose by pinching the nostrils together.

CAUTION

DO NOT allow the person to tilt the head backward.

DO NOT probe the nose with a cotton-tipped swab.

DO NOT move the person's head and neck if a spinal injury is suspected.

Tooth Injuries

Because dental emergencies generally cause considerable pain and anxiety, managing them promptly can provide great relief to the person. Seek dental care for all dental injuries—in most cases, as soon as possible.

What to Look For	What to Do
Object caught between teeth, indicated by: ▪ Person reports that something is caught between their teeth ▪ An object that may or may not be seen (Even with the use of a flashlight, it is still difficult to see a small object.)	1. Try to remove the object with dental floss. Guide the floss carefully to avoid cutting the gums. 2. **DO NOT** try to remove the object with a sharp or pointed instrument. 3. If unsuccessful, seek dental care.
Bitten lip or tongue, indicated by: ▪ Immediate pain ▪ Bleeding ▪ Swelling	1. Apply direct pressure to the bleeding area with sterile gauze or a clean cloth. 2. Clean the area with a cloth. 3. If swelling is present, apply an ice pack or have the person suck on a Popsicle or ice chips. 4. If the bleeding does not stop, seek professional medical care.
Loosened tooth ▪ Apply pressure on either side of each tooth with the fingers to determine looseness. ▪ Any tooth movement, even if it is barely felt, indicates a possibly loose tooth.	1. Have the person bite down on a piece of gauze to keep the tooth in place. 2. Consult a dentist or an oral surgeon.
Toothache, indicated by: ▪ Person reports pain limited to one area of the mouth (although it can be more widespread); pain can also affect the ear, eye, neck, or even the opposite side of the jaw. ▪ Person reports a tooth that is sensitive to heat and cold. ▪ Dental decay (identified by tapping the area with a spoon handle or similar object; a diseased tooth will hurt).	1. Rinse the person's mouth with warm water. Be sure they don't swallow the water. 2. Use dental floss to remove any trapped food. 3. Place an ice pack on the outside of the cheek to reduce swelling. 4. If available, use a cotton swab to paint the aching tooth with oil of cloves (eugenol) to help suppress the pain. Take care to keep the oil off the gums, lips, and inside surfaces of the cheeks. 5. Give OTC pain medication (eg, acetaminophen, ibuprofen) according to package directions. **DO NOT** place aspirin on the aching tooth or gum tissue. 6. Seek a dentist.
Broken tooth **FIGURE 12-13**	1. Collect all the tooth or teeth fragments. Depending upon the severity of injury, a dentist may be able to reattach them. 2. Rinse the person's mouth with warm water. Be sure they don't swallow the water. 3. For swelling over the injured area, place an ice pack on the outside of the cheek. 4. For pain, have the person keep air exposure to a minimum by keeping the mouth closed. Additionally, consider providing OTC pain medication according to package directions, which should be swallowed. 5. If a jaw fracture is suspected, stabilize the jaw by wrapping a bandage under the chin and over the top of the head. **DO NOT** tie the mouth closed. Be sure to allow space for fluids to drain. 6. Seek a dentist as soon as possible. 7. Transport the fragments as you would a knocked-out tooth (see next section).
Knocked-out (avulsed) tooth **FIGURE 12-14**	1. Attempt to reimplant the tooth (only if it is a permanent [adult] tooth and unable to see a dentist within 1 hour of the injury): ▪ Hold the tooth by the crown (tooth part normally seen when looking into a mouth). **DO NOT** touch the root. ▪ If the tooth is dirty, rinse it in a bowl of warm water. **DO NOT** scrub or remove any of the attached tissue fragments. ▪ Gently push the tooth down into the socket so the top is even with adjacent teeth. The person can bite down gently on gauze or a handkerchief placed between the teeth. 2. If unable to reimplant the tooth, keep the knocked-out tooth viable by storing it in a solution (listed in order of preference): ▪ Hank's Balanced Salt Solution ▪ Egg white ▪ Coconut water ▪ Cow's milk ▪ If none of these is available, have the person spit saliva into a small container into which the tooth can be placed. 3. Seek a dentist as soon as possible.

Continues

What to Look For	What to Do
Infected or abscessed tooth, indicated by: ▪ Swelling of the gums around the affected tooth ▪ Foul breath ▪ Pain that is increased by tapping the tooth on the top with something metal (eg, spoon handle)	1. Have the person rinse their mouth several times per day with warm water. Remind them not to swallow the water. 2. Give OTC pain medication according to package directions. **DO NOT** have the person suck an aspirin, and **DO NOT** place an aspirin on the tooth or gum tissue. 3. An ice pack on the cheek may help. 4. Use dental floss to remove any trapped food. 5. Seek a dentist.
Cavity, caused by decay or lost filling, indicated by: ▪ Sensitivity to heat, cold, or sweets ▪ Sensitivity to touch (Tap the tooth gently with something metal [eg, spoon handle] on the top and side. This increases the pain in the affected tooth.)	1. Have the person rinse their mouth with warm water. Be sure they don't swallow the water. 2. Apply oil of cloves (eugenol) with a cotton swab to the cavity to deaden the pain. **DO NOT** apply any on the gums or lips, or inside the cheeks. 3. If available, apply a temporary filling with cavity dental filling paste. Other options include sugarless chewing gum, candle wax, or ski wax. 4. Seek a dentist.
Bleeding from mouth	1. Allow blood to drain out of the mouth. 2. For a bleeding tongue, put a dressing on the wound and apply pressure. 3. For a cut through a lip, place a rolled dressing between the lip and gum and press another dressing against the outer lip. 4. Seek professional medical care.

CAUTION

DO NOT touch the root of a knocked-out tooth.

DO NOT handle a knocked-out tooth roughly.

DO NOT put a knocked-out tooth in water, mouthwash, alcohol, or povidone iodine (Betadine).

DO NOT put a knocked-out tooth in reconstituted powdered milk or milk by-products such as yogurt.

DO NOT rinse a knocked-out tooth unless you are reinserting it in the socket.

DO NOT place a knocked-out tooth in anything that can dry or crush the outside of the tooth.

DO NOT scrub a knocked-out tooth or remove any attached tissue fragments.

DO NOT remove a partially extracted tooth. Push it back into place and seek a dentist so the loose tooth can be stabilized.

DO NOT place pain medication (such as aspirin, acetaminophen, or ibuprofen) on the aching tooth or gum tissues or allow them to dissolve in the mouth. A serious acid burn can result.

DO NOT cover a cavity with cotton if there is any pus discharge or facial swelling. See a dentist immediately.

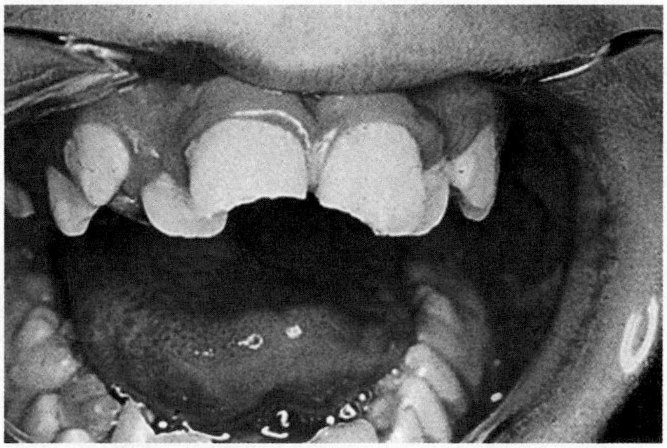

FIGURE 12-13 Broken teeth.

FYI

Dental First Aid

If you are in a remote area with no dentist nearby, you can make a temporary cap from melted candle wax or paraffin. When the wax begins to harden but can still be molded, press a wad of it onto the tooth. Other improvisations include using ski wax or chewing gum (preferably sugarless).

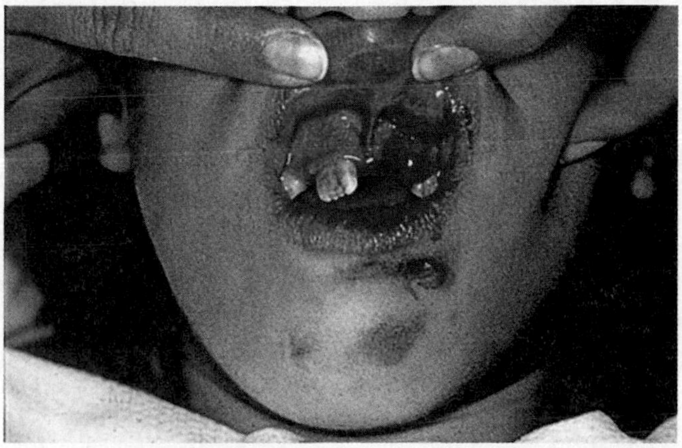

FIGURE 12-14 Knocked-out tooth.

Flowchart 12-4 Tooth Injuries

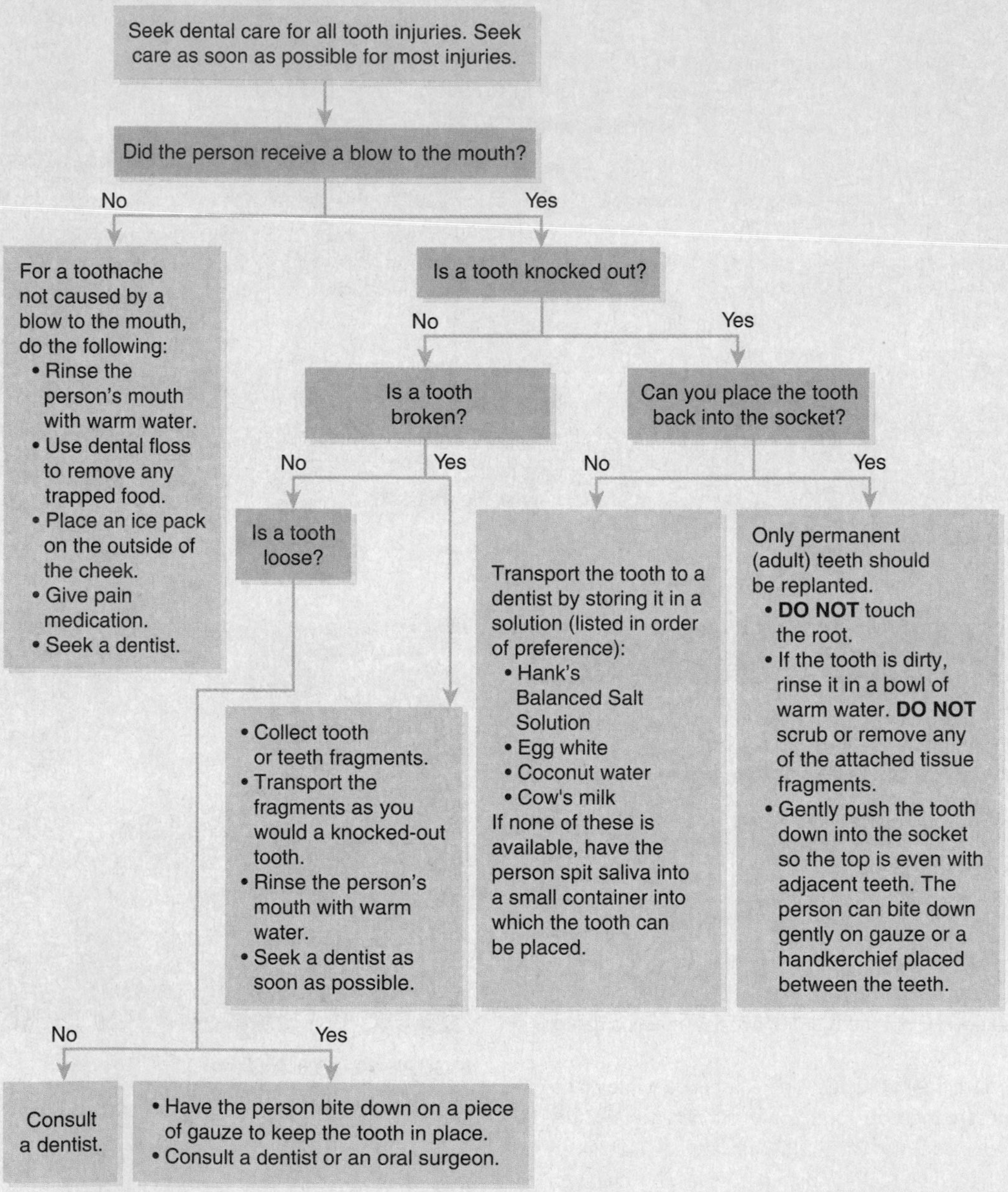

Seek dental care for all tooth injuries. Seek care as soon as possible for most injuries.
Did the person receive a blow to the mouth?
No
Yes
For a toothache not caused by a blow to the mouth, do the following:
• Rinse the person's mouth with warm water.
• Use dental floss to remove any trapped food.
• Place an ice pack on the outside of the cheek.
• Give pain medication.
• Seek a dentist.
Is a tooth knocked out?
No
Yes
Is a tooth broken?
Can you place the tooth back into the socket?
No
Yes
No
Yes
Is a tooth loose?
• Collect tooth or teeth fragments.
• Transport the fragments as you would a knocked-out tooth.
• Rinse the person's mouth with warm water.
• Seek a dentist as soon as possible.
Transport the tooth to a dentist by storing it in a solution (listed in order of preference):
• Hank's Balanced Salt Solution
• Egg white
• Coconut water
• Cow's milk
If none of these is available, have the person spit saliva into a small container into which the tooth can be placed.
Only permanent (adult) teeth should be replanted.
• DO NOT touch the root.
• If the tooth is dirty, rinse it in a bowl of warm water. DO NOT scrub or remove any of the attached tissue fragments.
• Gently push the tooth down into the socket so the top is even with adjacent teeth. The person can bite down gently on gauze or a handkerchief placed between the teeth.
No
Yes
Consult a dentist.
• Have the person bite down on a piece of gauze to keep the tooth in place.
• Consult a dentist or an oral surgeon.

Refer to **FLOWCHART 12-4** for additional information regarding the care of tooth injuries.

Spinal Injuries

The spine is a column of **vertebrae** stacked on one another from the tailbone to the base of the skull. Each vertebra has a hollow center through which the spinal cord passes. The spinal cord consists of long tracts of nerves that join the brain with all other body organs and parts.

If a broken vertebra pinches spinal nerves, paralysis can result. All unresponsive people with an injury should be treated as though they have a spinal injury. Suspect a possible spinal injury any time one of the following are encountered **FIGURE 12-15**:

- Motor vehicle crashes (includes motorcycles, snowmobiles, and all-terrain vehicles) involving a rollover, ejection, or high speeds
- Pedestrian–motor vehicle crashes
- Falls greater than the person's standing height, especially in older persons
- A hit to the head, neck, or back
- Violent assaults and direct blows

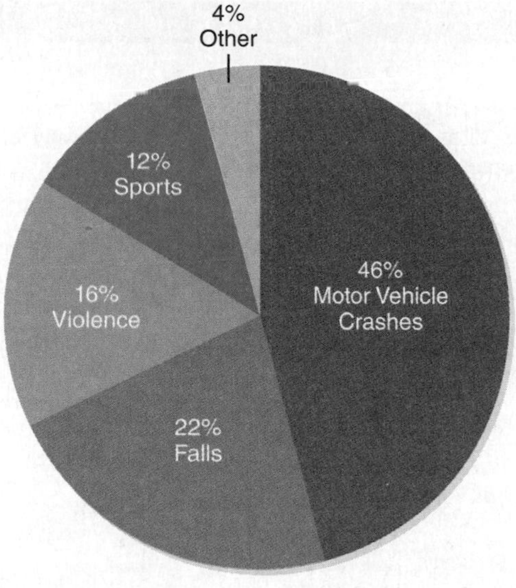

FIGURE 12-15 Common causes of spinal cord injury.

Reproduced from National Spinal Cord Injury Statistical Center, Facts and Figures at a Glance. Birmingham, AL: University of Alabama at Birmingham, 2016.

- Dives into shallow water
- Sports injuries
- Bicycle or skateboard crash

A mistake in the handling of a person with a spinal injury could mean a lifetime of paralysis for the person. Suspect a spinal injury whenever a significant cause of injury occurs.

Spinal cord injuries result in paralysis or loss of function. Paralysis occurs when the neural connections between the brain and the extremities are severed or damaged. **Paraplegia** refers to spinal damage that paralyzes just the legs, while **quadriplegia** affects the arms and the legs. Most people who suffer total loss of sensation and function above the third cervical vertebra (C3) die before professional medical care can be provided.

In cases in which spinal injury is suspected, it is important not to move the person and to encourage the person to be still. Wait for EMS to arrive. In the unusual event that a life is threatened, such as from a fire or imminent explosion, use good judgment about whether to move the person.

Refer to **FLOWCHART 12-5** for additional information regarding the care of spinal injuries.

Flowchart 12-5 Suspected Spinal Injuries

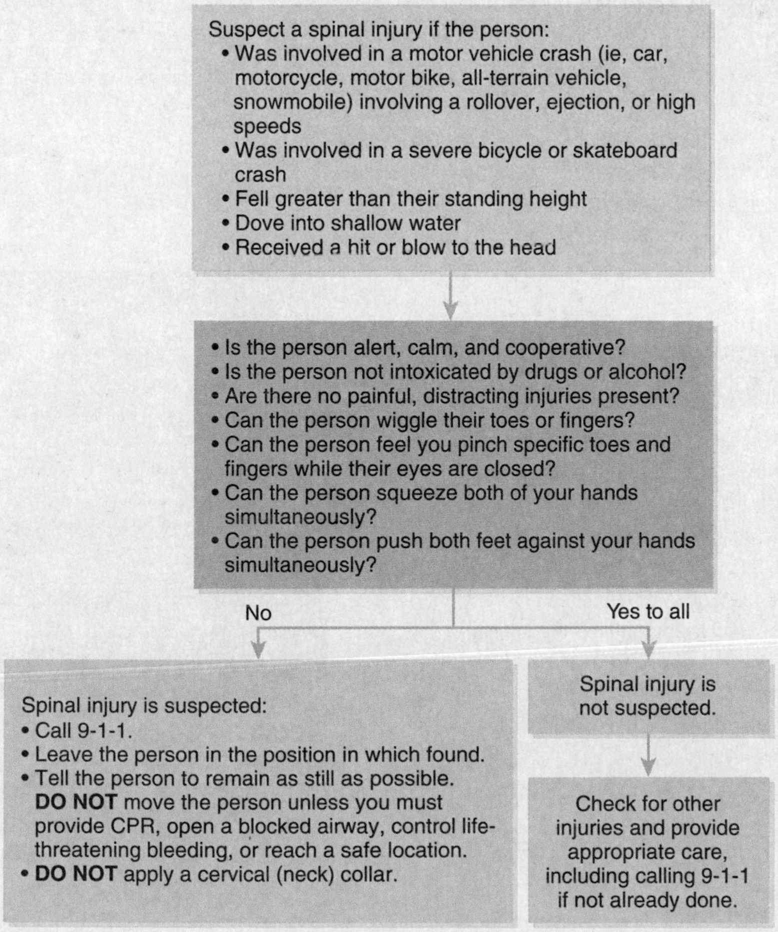
Suspect a spinal injury if the person:
• Was involved in a motor vehicle crash (ie, car, motorcycle, motor bike, all-terrain vehicle, snowmobile) involving a rollover, ejection, or high speeds
• Was involved in a severe bicycle or skateboard crash
• Fell greater than their standing height
• Dove into shallow water
• Received a hit or blow to the head
• Is the person alert, calm, and cooperative?
• Is the person not intoxicated by drugs or alcohol?
• Are there no painful, distracting injuries present?
• Can the person wiggle their toes or fingers?
• Can the person feel you pinch specific toes and fingers while their eyes are closed?
• Can the person squeeze both of your hands simultaneously?
• Can the person push both feet against your hands simultaneously?
No
Yes to all
Spinal injury is suspected:
• Call 9-1-1.
• Leave the person in the position in which found.
• Tell the person to remain as still as possible. DO NOT move the person unless you must provide CPR, open a blocked airway, control life-threatening bleeding, or reach a safe location.
• DO NOT apply a cervical (neck) collar.
Spinal injury is not suspected.
Check for other injuries and provide appropriate care, including calling 9-1-1 if not already done.

What to Look For	What to Do

A reliable (alert, calm, cooperative, lacking distracting injuries, not intoxicated by drugs or alcohol) person with signs of spinal injury **SKILL SHEET 12-1**, indicated by:
▪ Reports of back pain and leg numbness and tingling
▪ Failure of the following tests for sensation and movement (test all four extremities):
  ▪ Upper body:
    ▪ Pinch several fingers while the person has their eyes closed, and ask, "Can you feel this?" and "Which finger am I touching?"
    ▪ Ask, "Can you wiggle your fingers?"
    ▪ Have the person squeeze your hand.
  ▪ Lower body:
    ▪ Pinch toes while the person has their eyes closed, and ask, "Can you feel this?" and "Which toes am I touching?"
    ▪ Ask, "Can you wiggle your toes?"
    ▪ Have the person push and pull a foot against your hand.
	1. Call 9-1-1.
	2. **DO NOT** attempt to move the person. Leave the person in the position in which found. Tell the person to remain as still as possible. Consider moving a person only for the following: to provide CPR, to open a blocked airway, to control life-threatening bleeding, or to reach a safe location.
	3. **DO NOT** apply a cervical (neck) collar **FIGURE 12-16**.
	4. Cover to prevent heat loss.

A reliable person without signs of a spinal injury, indicated by: ▪ Alert, not intoxicated, and no distracting injuries ▪ No report of neck pain or neurologic symptoms (eg, tingling, numbness) ▪ No loss of sensation when fingers and toes are pinched, and able to move the fingers and toes	1. Spinal injury is not suspected. 2. Treat other injuries (eg, wounds, bruises, fractures).
An unreliable person (altered mental status, intoxicated by drugs or alcohol, combative, confused, painful distracting injury) with signs of a spinal injury	1. Assume a spinal injury exists. 2. Use the methods previously discussed for a reliable person.

CAUTION

DO NOT move a person with a suspected spinal injury, even if the person is in water, unless the person's location puts them in additional danger. During an emergency when the spine may be injured, move the person so that the spine stays in a straight line. This is done by pulling or dragging to keep the spine in line. See Chapter 25. (For a water-related rescue, manually stabilize the person while keeping the injured person floating on the water's surface. Only perform a water rescue if you are properly trained.) Wait for EMS personnel to arrive; they have the proper training and equipment to safely move the injured person.

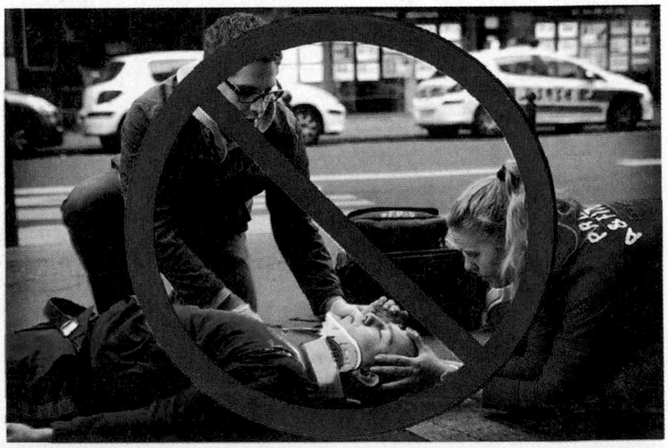

FIGURE 12-16 Do not place a cervical (neck) collar on a person with a suspected spinal injury.

SKILL SHEET 12-1 Checking for Spinal Injuries in a Responsive Person

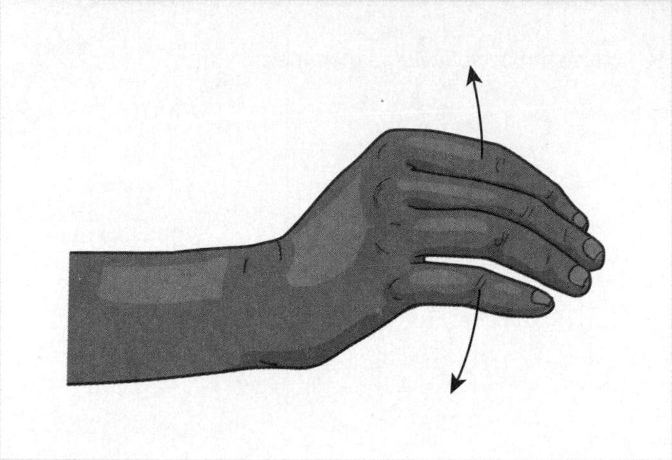

1 Have the person wiggle their fingers while they have their eyes closed.

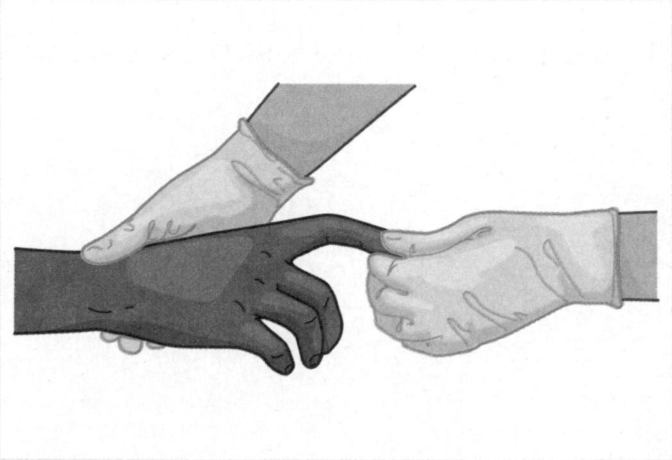

2 Squeeze the person's fingers.

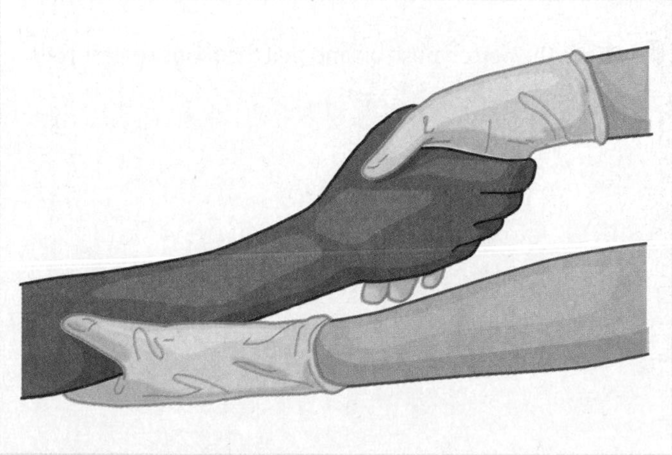

3 Have the person squeeze your hand.

Continues

SKILL SHEET 12-1 Checking for Spinal Injuries in a Responsive Person (*Continued*)

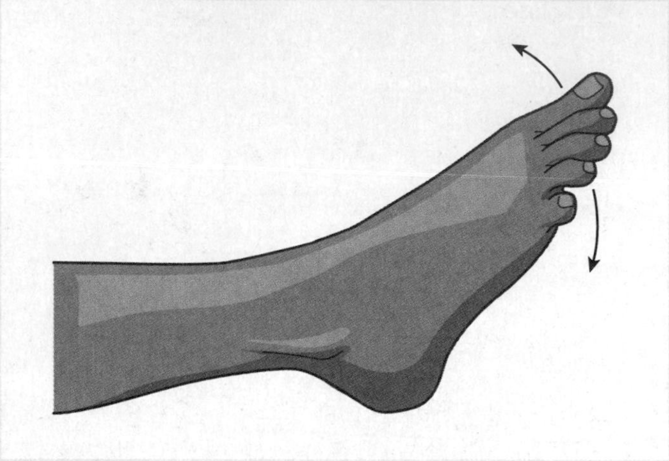

4 Have the person wiggle their toes.

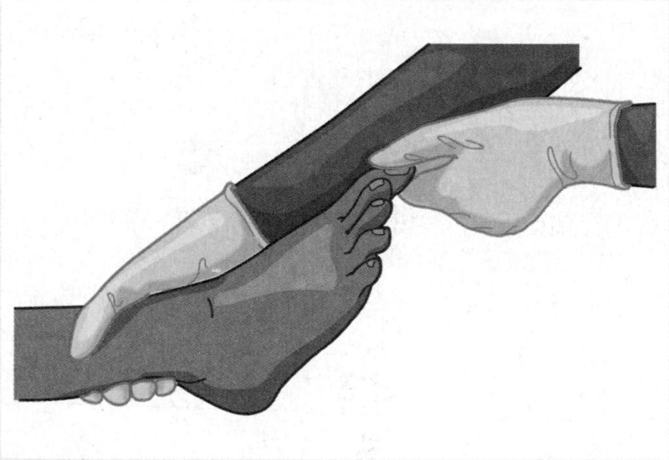

5 Squeeze the person's toes while they have their eyes closed.

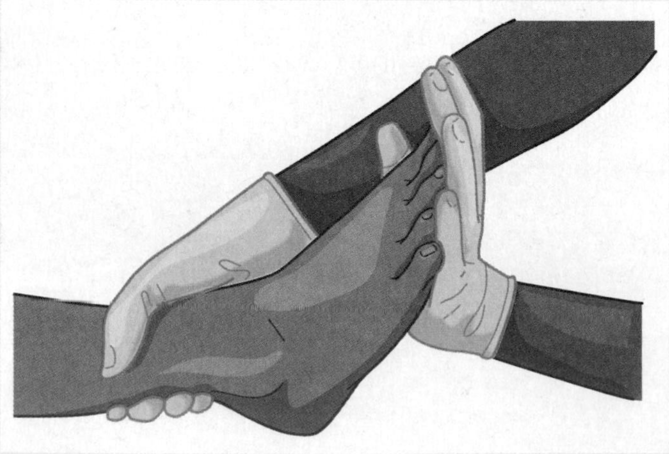

6 Have the person push on and pull their foot against your hand.

PREP KIT

Ready for Review

- Any head injury is potentially serious. If not properly treated, injuries that seem minor could become life threatening.
- Scalp wounds bleed profusely because the scalp has a rich supply of blood.
- A skull fracture is a break or crack in the cranium. Skull fractures may be open or closed.
- Injuries to the brain cause short- and long-term conditions.
- An injured eye probably causes the most anxiety and concern in a person.
- Penetrating eye injuries are severe injuries that result when a sharp object penetrates the eye.
- Blows to the eye can range in severity from minor to sight threatening.
- Cuts of the eye or lid require professional medical care.
- Chemicals in the eyes can threaten sight.
- A blow to the eye can knock it from its socket.
- Loose objects in the eye are the most frequent eye injury and can be very painful.
- Burns to the eye can result if a person looks at a source of ultraviolet light.
- Most ear injuries are not life threatening, but fast action may be needed to relieve pain or to prevent or reverse hearing loss.
- Most nosebleeds are self-limiting and seldom require medical attention.
- A foreign object in the nose is a condition mainly among small children who put small objects up their nostrils.
- Because dental emergencies generally cause considerable pain and anxiety, managing them promptly can provide great relief to the person.
- Trauma can cause teeth to become loosened in their sockets.
- A knocked-out tooth is a dental emergency.
- The front teeth are frequently broken by falls or direct blows.
- The most common reason for toothaches is dental decay.
- A mistake in the handling of a person with a spinal injury could mean a lifetime of paralysis for the person.

Vital Vocabulary

anterior nosebleed Bleeding from the front of the nose.

Battle sign A contusion on the mastoid area of either ear; sign of a basilar skull fracture.

cerebrospinal fluid (CSF) A clear, watery solution similar to blood plasma.

concussion A temporary disturbance of brain activity caused by a blow to the head; also known as mild traumatic brain injury.

contusion A bruise; an injury that causes bleeding under the skin

coup-contrecoup Dual impacts of the brain into the skull; coup injury occurs at the site of impact; contrecoup injury occurs on the opposite side of impact, as the brain rebounds.

diffuse axonal Tearing brain injury caused by shaking or strong rotation of the head.

paraplegia Paralysis of the legs caused by damage to the spine.

posterior nosebleed Bleeding from the back of the nose, which may flow out of the nostrils and into the mouth or throat.

quadriplegia Paralysis of the arms and legs caused by damage to the spine.

skull fracture A break or a crack in the cranium (bony case surrounding the brain).

vertebrae The 33 bones that make up the spinal column.

Assessment in Action

While working at a construction site, you witness a fellow worker fall to the ground after being struck by a piece of wood thrown by a table saw. He was not wearing his safety glasses and you see a cut to his eyeball and eyelid.

Directions: Circle Yes if you agree with the statement; circle No if you disagree.

1. Apply pressure immediately to the injured eyeball.
   YES **NO**
2. Tell the person to keep both eyes closed. Both eyes can be covered with a cravat or roller bandage.
   YES **NO**
3. Position the person with his head elevated.
   YES **NO**
4. Professional medical care is not necessary in this case.
   YES **NO**

PREP KIT continued

Check Your Knowledge

Directions: Circle Yes if you agree with the statement; circle No if you disagree.

1. Remove objects embedded in an eyeball.
   YES **NO**
2. Scalp wounds produce very little bleeding.
   YES **NO**
3. Scrub and rinse the roots of a knocked-out tooth.
   YES **NO**
4. After a blow to the area around an eye, apply a cold pack.
   YES **NO**
5. Tears are sufficient to flush a chemical from the eye.
   YES **NO**
6. Use clean, damp gauze to remove an object from the eyelid's surface.
   YES **NO**
7. Preserve a knocked-out tooth in mouthwash.
   YES **NO**
8. Do not move a person with a suspected spinal injury.
   YES **NO**
9. Inability to move the hands or feet, or both, may indicate a spinal injury.
   YES **NO**
10. To care for a nosebleed, have the injured person sit down and tilt their head back.
    YES **NO**

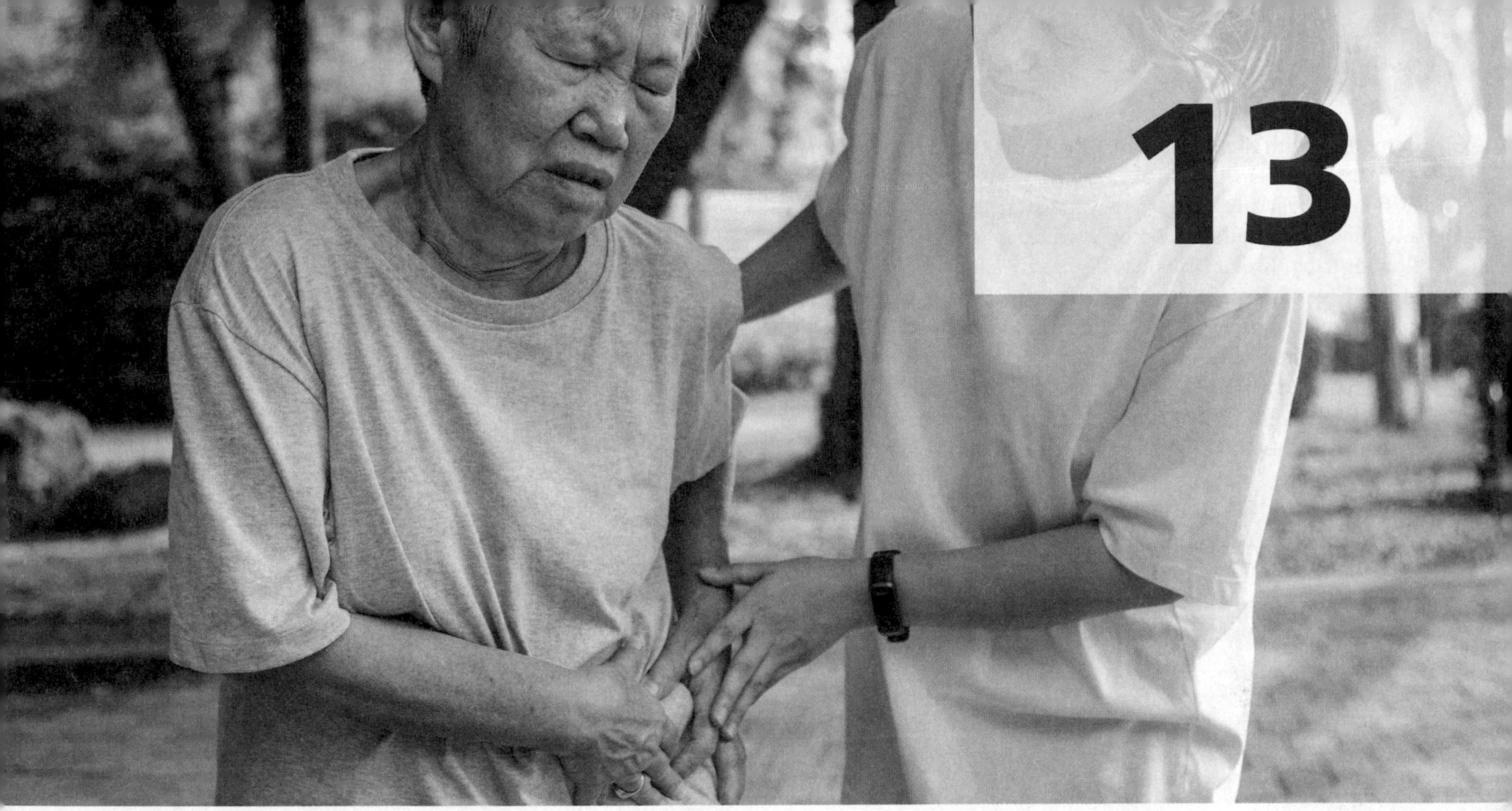

13

Chest, Abdominal, and Pelvic Injuries

CHAPTER AT A GLANCE

Chest Injuries

Chest injuries fall into two categories: open or closed. In an open chest injury, the chest wall is penetrated by some object (eg, knife, bullet). In a closed chest injury, the skin is not broken. The injury is caused by blunt trauma (eg, falling object, motor vehicle crash, sports injury, struck during an assault).

Check and recheck the airway, breathing, and circulation of all people with chest injuries. A responsive person with a chest injury should usually sit up in a comfortable position or, if the injury is on a side, be placed with the injured side down. This position prevents blood inside the chest cavity from seeping into the uninjured side and allows the uninjured side to expand.

Closed Chest Injuries

As mentioned, in a **closed chest injury**, the skin is not broken. Closed chest injuries include rib fractures and flail chest.

Rib Fractures

The upper four ribs are rarely fractured because they are protected by the collarbone and the shoulder blades. The upper four ribs are so enmeshed with the muscles that they rarely need to be splinted or realigned like other broken bones. The lower two ribs are difficult to fracture because they are attached on only one end and have the freedom to move, which is why they are called floating ribs. Broken ribs usually occur along the side of the chest. The main symptom of a rib fracture is pain at the injured rib site; pain when the person breathes, coughs, or moves; or pain when the area is touched.

Fractured ribs are a common injury and most frequently occur between ribs 4 and 10. The location for most fractures is on the sides of the body. The first three pairs of ribs are protected by the clavicles, whereas the last two pairs move freely and give with impact. Little can be done to assist the healing of broken ribs. Tightly binding the chest limits breathing, and because inhalation is inadequate, fluid accumulates in the air sacs (alveoli) and can result in pneumonia. This relationship between broken ribs and fluid accumulation in the lungs often explains pneumonia deaths.

What to Look For	What to Do
▪ Sharp pain when the person takes deep breaths, coughs, or moves ▪ Guarding (tensing the muscles around the injury to help to protect the area) ▪ Tenderness ▪ Shallow breathing due to pain that occurs from normal or deep breathing ▪ Bruising of skin over the injury (usually occurs along the side of the chest)	1. Help the person find a comfortable position. 2. Stabilize the chest **FIGURE 13-1** by: ▪ Having the person hold a pillow or other similarly soft material against the area, *or* ▪ Placing the arm on the injured side in a sling and binder (swathe) if necessary to control pain. 3. **DO NOT** apply tight bandages around the chest. 4. Give over-the-counter pain medication according to package directions. 5. Tell the person to take very deep, slow breaths every few breaths to prevent pneumonia. 6. Call 9-1-1.

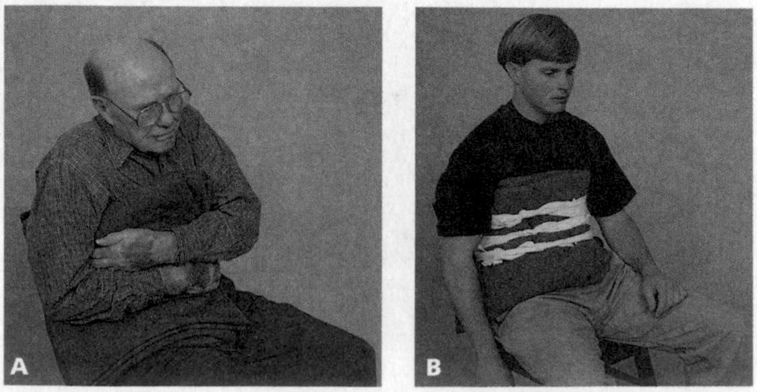

FIGURE 13-1 Stabilize the ribs by holding (**A**) or tying in place (**B**) a soft object such as a pillow, coat, or blanket. Tell the person to take very deep, slow breaths every few breaths.

Q&A

How could broken ribs become life threatening?

A rib fracture is extremely painful, especially because it cannot be stabilized while it heals. Inhaling air causes the muscles between the ribs to expand the chest and move the fractured rib, making inhalation a painful process. In an attempt to avoid the pain, a person may develop shallow breathing, which does not fully inflate the small air sacs (alveoli) in the lungs. As a result, fluid may accumulate in the alveoli, leading to pneumonia.

The pain is usually localized to the area of the fracture. If the sharp end of the broken rib protrudes into the chest cavity, it may puncture the lung, causing it to collapse and allow air between the lung and the chest wall (known as a **pneumothorax**). A life-threatening condition known as tension pneumothorax occurs when air progressively accumulates in the space between the venae cavae lung and the chest wall (known as the pleural space) during inhalation and cannot escape during exhalation. This accumulation compresses the heart, uninjured lung, aorta, and vena cava, causing a decrease in blood return to the heart and thereby decreasing cardiac output.

Flail Chest

A **flail chest** is a serious injury that involves several ribs in the same area broken in more than one place creating a free-floating segment. The area over the injury may move in a direction opposite to that of the rest of the chest wall during breathing (known as **paradoxical movement**). This injury is very painful and makes breathing difficult.

What to Look For	What to Do
▪ Area over the injury moving in a direction opposite to that of the rest of the chest wall during breathing ▪ Very painful and difficult breathing ▪ Bruising of skin over the injury ▪ Same signs as for rib fractures	1. **DO NOT** apply tight bandages around the chest. 2. Stabilize the chest by: ▪ Placing a pillow or similar soft material against area or wrapping the arm on the injured person. ▪ Placing the person on their injured side with a blanket or similar soft material underneath the person. ▪ Give the person a blanket to hug. 3. Call 9-1-1.

Open Chest Injuries

In an **open chest injury**, the skin has been broken and the chest wall is penetrated by an object such as a knife or bullet.

Sucking Chest Wound

A **sucking chest wound** results when a chest wound allows air to pass into and out of the chest with each breath. Bubbles may be seen at the wound during exhalations and a sucking sound heard during inhalations.

What to Look For	What to Do
▪ Blood bubbling out of a chest wound during exhalation ▪ Sucking sound heard during inhalation	**1.** Leave the wound exposed to air without a dressing or any airtight material. **2.** **DO NOT** cover an open chest wound unless using direct pressure and a dry gauze dressing to control bleeding. If the dressing becomes blood-soaked, replace it to avoid trapping air in the chest, which may result in death. **3.** Call 9-1-1.

Penetrating (Impaled, Embedded) Object in the Chest

If an object penetrates the chest wall, air and blood escape into the space between the lungs and the chest wall. The air and blood cause the lung to collapse. Lung collapse can lead to shock and death.

Refer to **FLOWCHART 13-1** for additional information regarding the care of chest injuries.

What to Look For	What to Do
An impaled object is usually easily recognized. However, in some cases the object may be below the skin surface and difficult to see. Carefully look at wounds that could be hiding the object that caused the damage.	**1.** Stabilize the object against movement by placing bulky dressings or padding around it. **DO NOT** remove the object. **2.** Call 9-1-1.

Abdominal Injuries

Injuries to the abdomen are either open or closed and can involve hollow and/or solid organs. A closed abdominal injury is one of the most frequently unrecognized injuries; when missed, it becomes one of the main causes of death. A hollow organ rupture (eg, of the stomach or intestines) spills the contents of the organ into the abdominal cavity, causing inflammation. Solid organ rupture (eg, of the liver or spleen) results in severe internal bleeding.

Flowchart 13-1 Chest Injuries

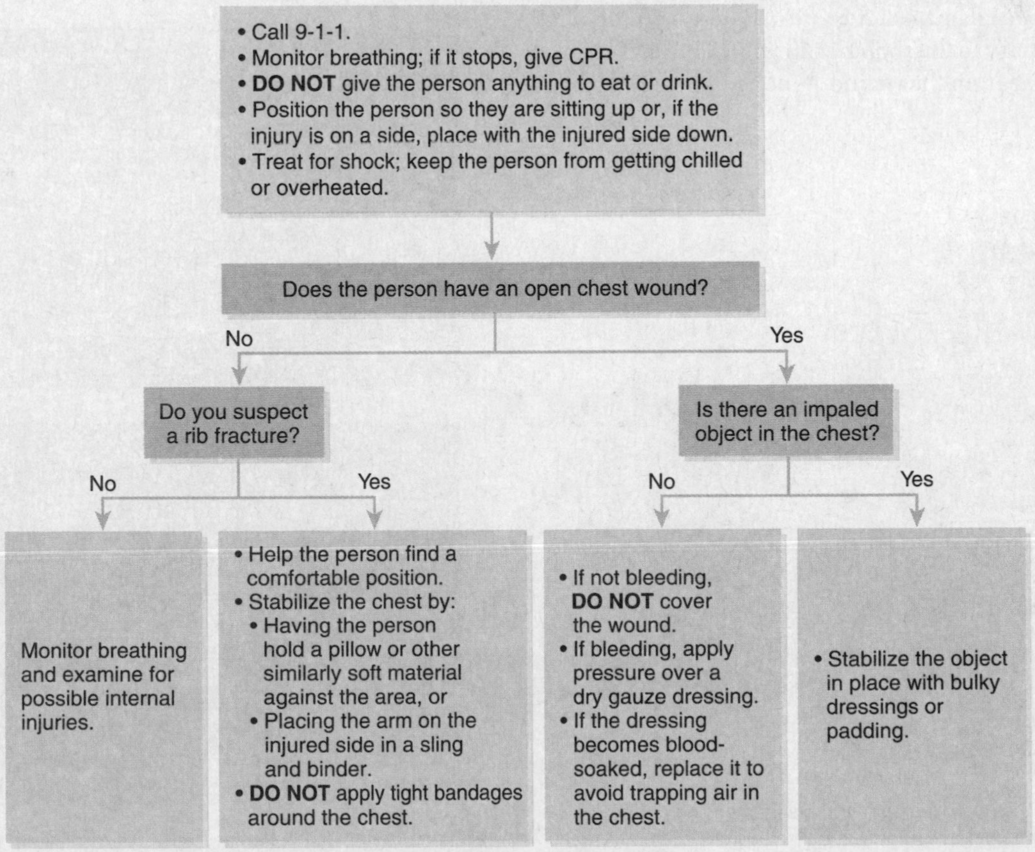

What to Look For	What to Do
▪ Bruises or other marks ▪ Pain, tenderness, muscle tightness, or rigidity ▪ Distention (swelling) ▪ Nausea and vomiting ▪ Blood in urine, stool, or vomit ▪ Increased breathing and pulse rates	1. Place the person in a comfortable, side-lying position with the legs slightly bent. Be prepared for vomiting. 2. Call 9-1-1.

Closed Abdominal Injury

Closed abdominal injuries occur when the internal abdominal tissues are damaged but the skin is unbroken. These are also known as blunt injuries. Such an injury might result from striking the handlebar of a bicycle or the steering wheel of a car, or from being struck by a board or baseball bat.

Bruising and damage to internal organs can result from a severe blow to the abdomen. Examine the abdomen by gently pressing all four quadrants of the abdomen with your fingertips **FIGURE 13-2**. A normal abdomen is soft and not tender when pressed.

Open Abdominal Injury

Open abdominal injuries are those in which the skin has been broken. These injuries are also known as penetrating injuries. Examples include stab wounds and gunshot wounds. It is difficult to know whether a penetrating injury involves more than just the abdominal wall. Always assume the worst—that internal organs have been damaged. A **protruding organ injury** refers to a severe injury to the abdomen in which internal organs escape or protrude from the wound. When removing clothing to help treat a gunshot wound, never cut through the bullet hole. Be sure to cut around it to help preserve the evidence.

Refer to **FLOWCHART 13-2** for additional information regarding the care of abdominal injuries.

What to Look For	What to Do
▪ Penetrating object such as a knife or other sharp object	1. If the penetrating object is still in place, stabilize the object against movement and control bleeding by placing bulky dressings or padding around it **FIGURE 13-3**. **DO NOT** remove the object. 2. Call 9-1-1.
▪ Internal organs escaping or protruding from the wound **FIGURE 13-4** ▪ Significant bleeding	1. Tell the person to stay lying down on their back with the legs pulled up toward the abdomen. 2. Cover the organs with a moist, clean dressing **FIGURE 13-5**. Place a loose plastic wrap or another layer of dressing, if available, over the moist dressing to prevent it from drying out. Loosely tape the plastic wrap or dressings in place. 3. Call 9-1-1.

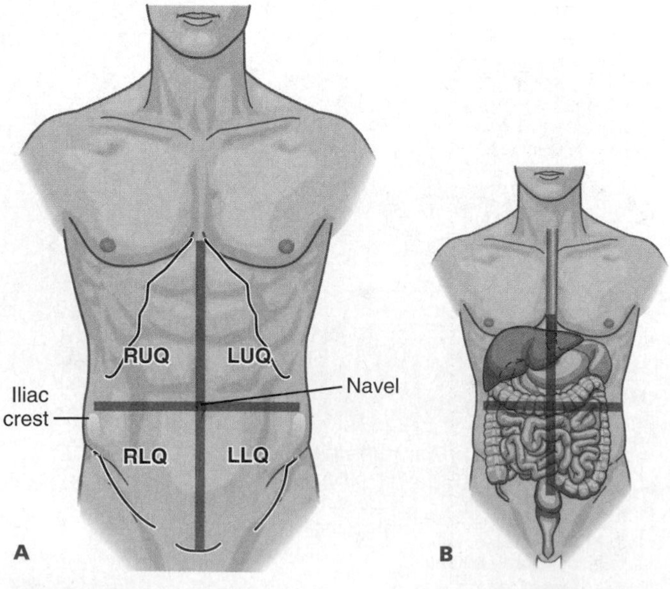

FIGURE 13-2 A. The four quadrants of the abdomen: left upper quadrant (LUQ), right upper quadrant (RUQ), right lower quadrant (RLQ), and left lower quadrant (LLQ). **B**. The abdominal organs.

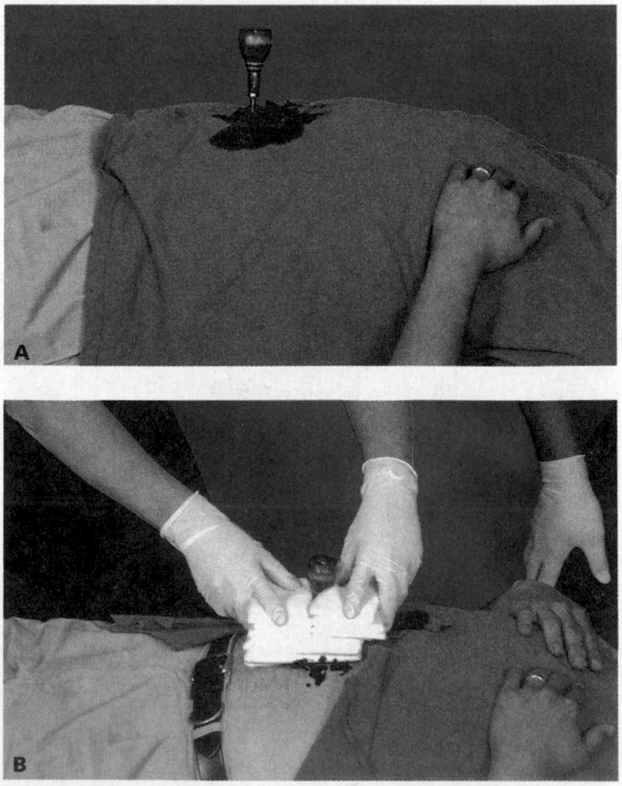

FIGURE 13-3 Stabilize a penetrating object against movement (**A**) and control bleeding by placing bulky dressings around it (**B**).

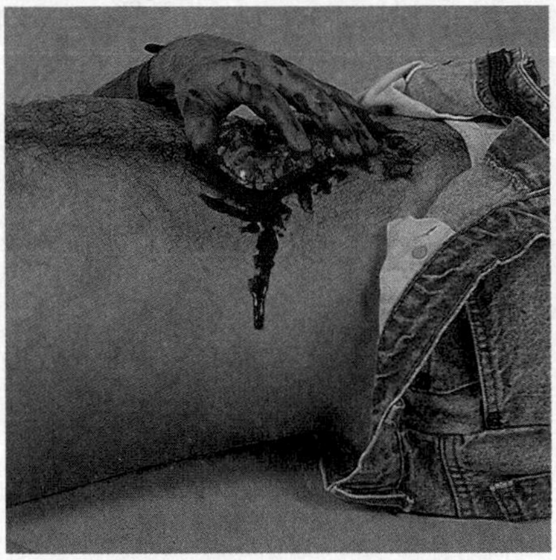

FIGURE 13-4 Protruding organs.

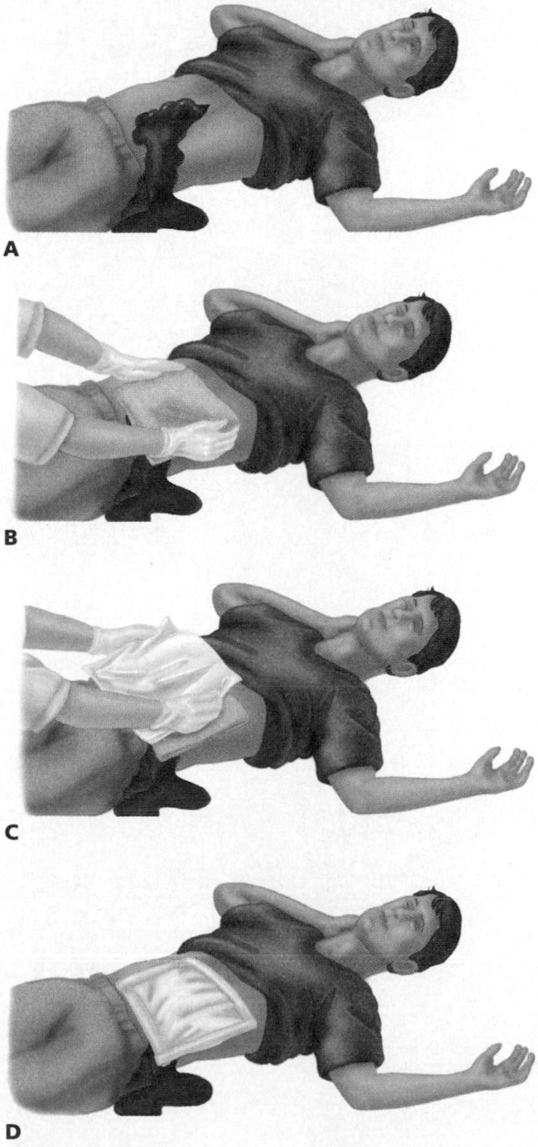

FIGURE 13-5 Open abdominal injuries. **A**. Severe injuries to the abdomen can result in protruding organs. **B**. Apply a large moist, sterile dressing over the wound. **C**. Place a loose plastic wrap or occlusive dressing, if available, over the dressing. **D**. Loosely tape the plastic wrap or occlusive dressing in place.

CAUTION

DO NOT try to reinsert protruding organs into the abdomen; you could introduce infection or damage the intestines.

DO NOT cover the organs tightly.

DO NOT cover the organs with any material that clings or disintegrates when wet.

DO NOT give anything by mouth.

DO NOT touch the organs.

Flowchart 13-2 Abdominal Injuries

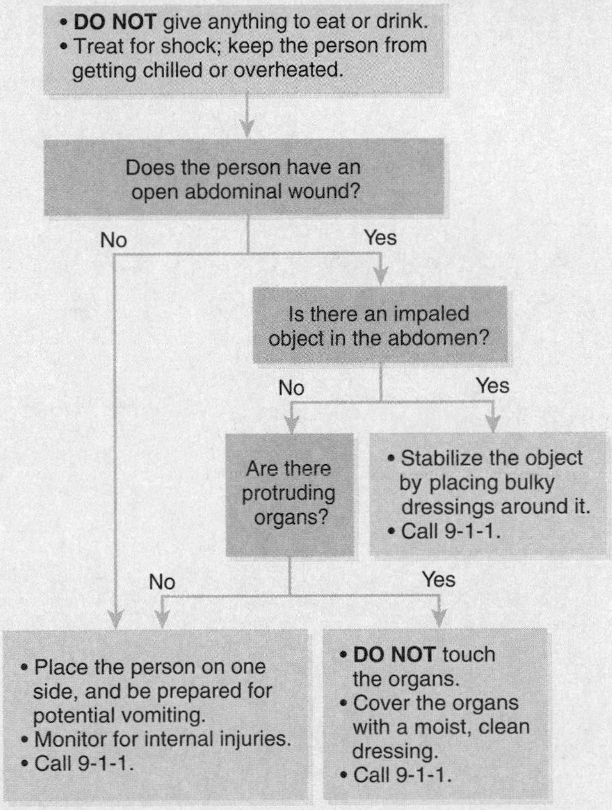

Pelvic Injuries

Pelvic fractures are usually caused by falling or a motor vehicle crash. A pelvic fracture should be suspected in anyone with pelvic pain on movement. Motor vehicle crashes, being struck by a motor vehicle, falls, and bicycle and motorcycle crashes are common causes of pelvic injury. It is important to suspect pelvic injuries because they can result in massive blood loss. Unstable pelvic bones can cause continued arterial and venous bleeding that can go unnoticed. This is made worse when a person has a full bladder, increasing the likelihood of bladder rupture spilling its contents into the pelvic cavity. Splinting is necessary. Laypeople should stabilize the person and wait for trained emergency medical services (EMS) personnel and their equipment to transport the person to a hospital emergency department.

What to Look For	What to Do
▪ Pain in the hip, groin, or back that increases with movement ▪ Inability to stand or walk ▪ Signs of shock	1. Call 9-1-1. 2. **DO NOT** move the person. 3. Keep the person lying flat. 4. Restrict pelvic motion.

CAUTION

DO NOT roll the person; additional internal damage could result.

DO NOT move the person. Whenever possible, wait for trained EMS personnel with their ambulance, backboard, and other specialized equipment.

PREP KIT

Ready for Review

- Chest injuries fall into two categories: open or closed.
- Closed chest injuries include rib fractures and flail chest.
- In an open chest injury, the skin has been broken and the chest wall is penetrated by an object such as a knife or bullet.
- Injuries to the abdomen are either open or closed and can involve hollow and/or solid organs.
- Closed abdominal injuries occur when the internal abdominal tissues are damaged but the skin is unbroken.
- Open abdominal injuries are those in which the skin has been broken and the abdominal wall penetrated.
- Pelvic fractures are usually caused by falling or a motor vehicle crash.

Vital Vocabulary

closed abdominal injury An injury to the abdomen that occurs as a result of a direct blow from a blunt object. There is no break in the skin.

closed chest injury An injury to the chest in which the skin is not broken; usually due to blunt trauma.

flail chest A condition that occurs when several ribs in the same area are broken in more than one place.

open abdominal injury An injury to the abdomen in which the skin is broken; can involve a penetrating wound or protruding organs.

open chest injury An injury to the chest in which the chest wall itself is penetrated by an external object such as a bullet or knife.

paradoxical movement The movement of the portion of the chest wall that is detached in a flail chest; the movement (in during inhalation, out during exhalation) is the opposite of normal chest wall movement during breathing.

pneumothorax Accumulation of air in the pleural space.

protruding organ injury A severe injury to the abdomen in which the internal organs escape or protrude from the wound; also known as evisceration.

sucking chest wound A chest wound that allows air to pass into the chest cavity with each breath.

Assessment in Action

You are on the first aid team at a local scout camp. The scout leaders are conducting a funny skit on a stage at the main lodge. One of the scouts in the skit jumps in the air and lands on his side. As he runs off the stage toward you, he is in obvious pain and is clutching his side. He lies down and a knife falls to the ground. You hear a sucking sound coming from the wound on his side whenever he inhales.

Directions: Circle Yes if you agree with the statement; circle No if you disagree.

1. You should check the person's breathing and treat accordingly.
   YES NO
2. Blood bubbling out of the wound during breathing is a sign of a sucking chest wound.
   YES NO
3. The wound should be covered tightly to prevent air from escaping.
   YES NO
4. If the person develops breathing difficulty, remove any dressing in order to allow trapped air to escape.
   YES NO
5. This is a medical emergency, and 9-1-1 should be called immediately.
   YES NO

Check Your Knowledge

Directions: Circle Yes if you agree with the statement; circle No if you disagree.

1. Stabilize a broken rib with a soft object, such as a pillow or blanket, tied to the chest.
   YES NO
2. For suspected rib fractures, apply tight bandages around the chest.
   YES NO

PREP KIT continued

3. Remove a penetrating or impaled object from the chest or the abdomen.

   YES **NO**

4. A flail chest refers to a single broken rib.

   YES **NO**

5. Keep the person with a broken pelvis still.

   YES **NO**

6. Sharp pain while breathing can be a sign of a rib fracture.

   YES **NO**

7. Rib fractures should be treated by tightly taping the chest.

   YES **NO**

8. Most people with abdominal injuries are more comfortable with their knees bent.

   YES **NO**

9. Leave a chest wound uncovered if you hear air being sucked in and out.

   YES **NO**

10. A broken pelvis can threaten life because of the large amount of blood loss.

    YES **NO**

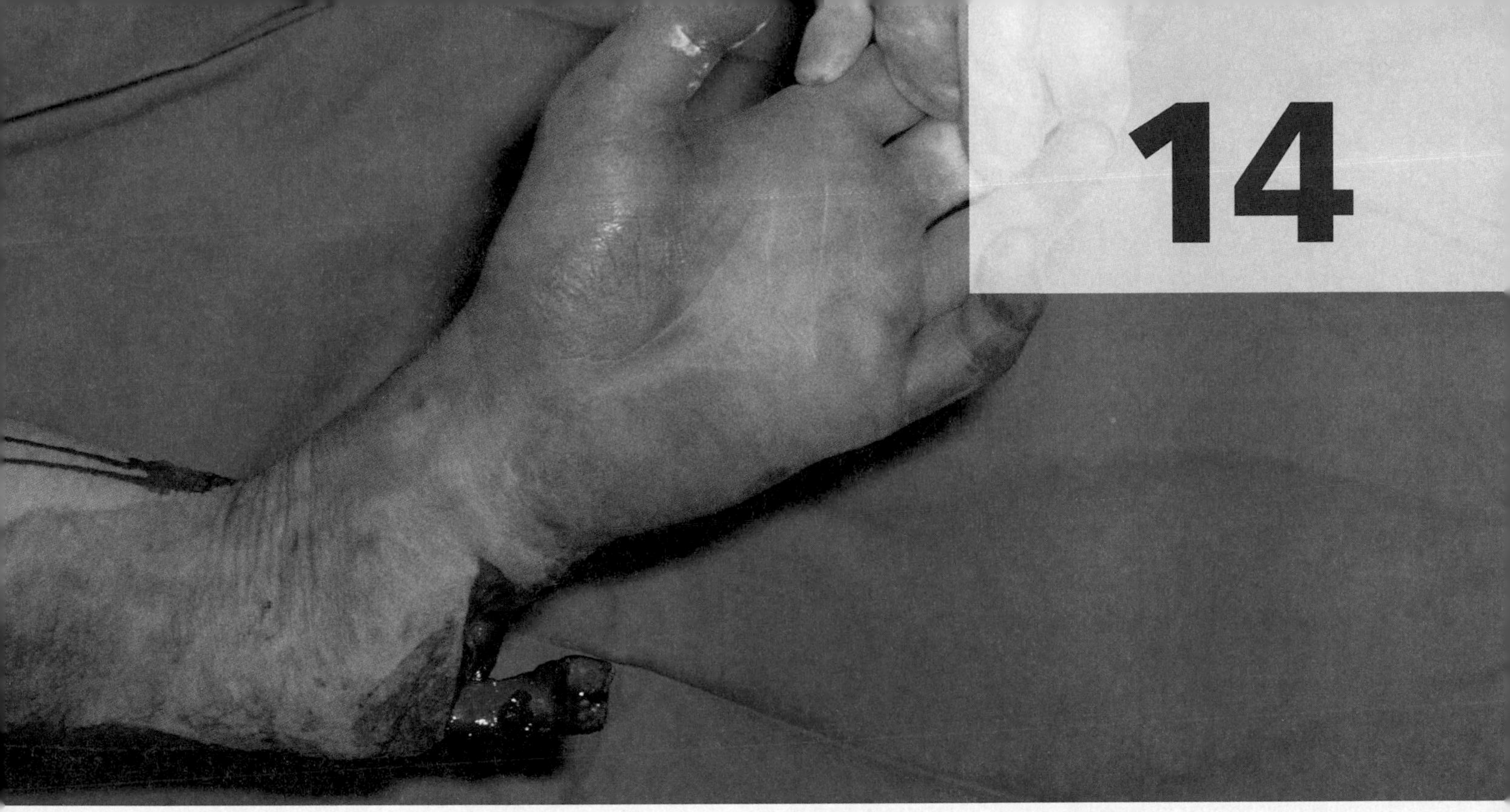

14

Bone, Joint, and Muscle Injuries

CHAPTER AT A GLANCE

- Bone Injuries
  - Fractures
- Joint Injuries
  - Dislocations
  - Sprains
- Muscle Injuries
  - Strains
  - Cramps
  - Contusions

Bone Injuries

Bone, joint, and muscle injuries are among the most common reasons for seeking professional medical care. They often result in short- or long-term disability. Significant extremity trauma resulting in orthopedic injuries can indicate that other significant injuries also exist. Of these orthopedic injuries, bone fractures and dislocations can be very distressing. They are typically associated with a forceful cause of injury and may present with obvious disfigurement. If not properly cared for, both at the time of injury and during the subsequent healing process, these injuries can result in long-term disability. As a first aid provider, your role is to help manage the person's pain and distress and to ensure no further damage is done before the person can receive professional medical care.

Fractures

The real issue is not the broken bones themselves but the potential injury to the vital organs next to them. People usually do not die of broken; rather, they die of airway obstruction, blood loss, and brain injury. However, broken bones can be painful and debilitating and can cause lifelong aggravation, disability, and deformity.

The terms **fracture** and broken bone have the same meaning: a break or crack in a bone. There are two categories of fractures **FIGURE 14-1**:

- **Closed fracture**. The skin is intact, and no wound exists anywhere near the fracture site. In many instances, you are dealing with suspected or potential factures, which may not be confirmed until the limb or joint is radiographed at a medical facility.
- **Open fracture**. The skin over the fracture has been broken. The wound may result from the bone protruding through the skin or from a direct blow that cut the skin at the time of the fracture. The bone may not always be visible in the wound.

It is not possible to determine the exact nature of a broken bone outside a medical facility. Nonetheless, it may be helpful for first aid providers to be familiar with the terminology that physicians use after a radiograph has been obtained to describe fractures **FIGURE 14-2**.

Greenstick fractures are incomplete fractures that commonly occur in children, whose bones (like green sticks) are pliable. A transverse fracture cuts across the bone at right angles to its long axis and is often caused by direct injury. The fracture line of an oblique fracture crosses the bone in a slanting direction (or at an oblique angle, thus the name). A comminuted fracture is one in which the bone is fragmented into more than two pieces (ie, splintered or crushed). In an impacted fracture, the broken ends of the bone are jammed together and the bone may function as if no fracture were present. A spiral fracture usually results from a twisting injury, and the fracture line has the appearance of a spring.

It may be difficult to tell if a bone is broken **FIGURE 14-3.** When in doubt, treat the injury as a suspected fracture. A quick check for circulation, sensation, and movement (CSM; see Skill Sheets 14-1 and 14-2 later) is extremely important. The most serious complication of a fracture is inadequate blood flow in an extremity. The major blood vessels of an extremity tend to run close to the bones, which means that any time a bone is broken, the adjacent blood vessels are at risk of being torn by bone fragments or pinched off between the ends of the broken bone. The tissues of the arms and legs cannot survive for more than about 3 hours without a continuing blood supply. If you note any disruption in the nerve or blood supply, seek immediate professional medical care. Major nerve pathways also travel close to bones and may be torn or pinched off between the ends of the broken bone.

Refer to **FLOWCHART 14-1** for additional information regarding the care of bone injuries.

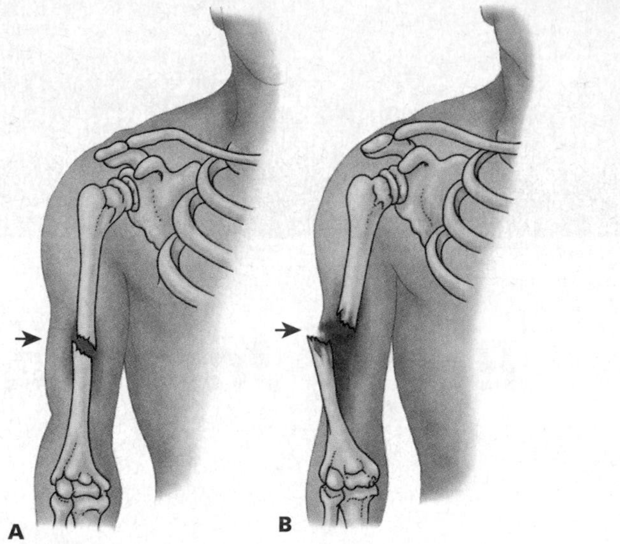

FIGURE 14-1 A. Closed fracture. **B**. Open fracture.

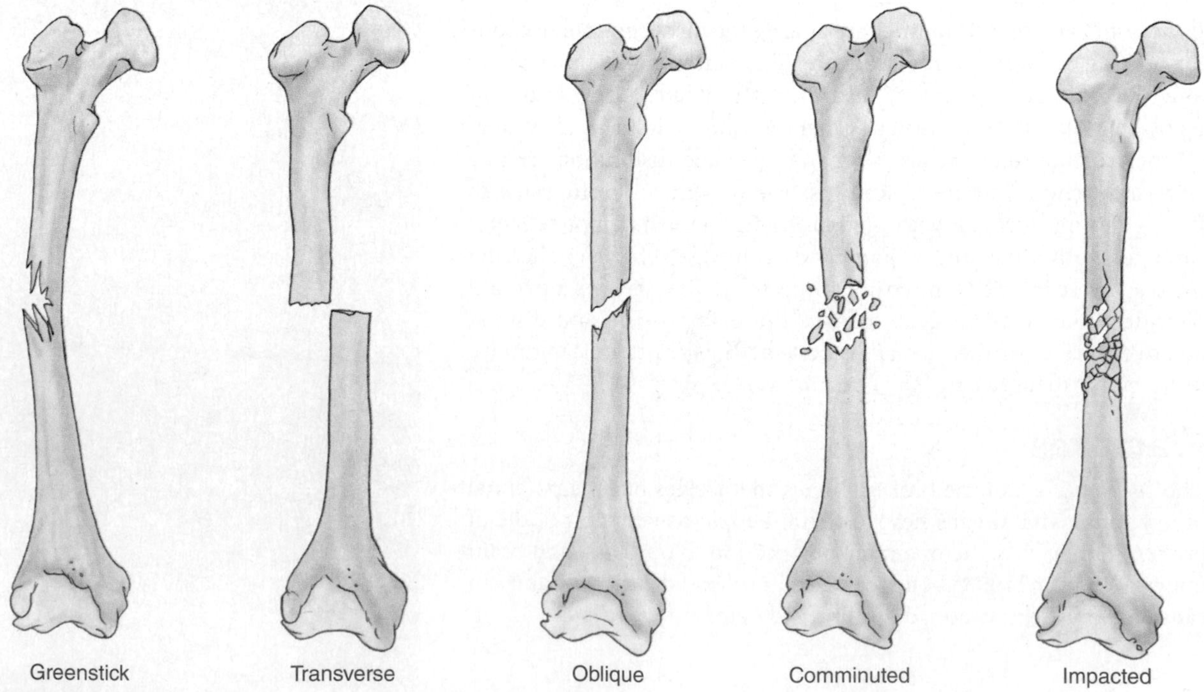

FIGURE 14-2 Types of fractures.

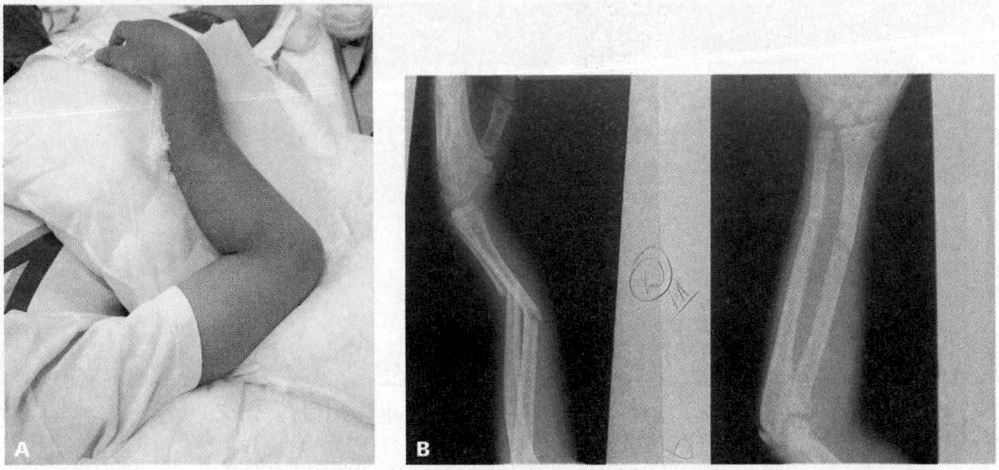
A
B

FIGURE 14-3 **A**. Forearm fracture. **B**. Radiographs of a forearm fracture before and after setting.

Flowchart 14-1 Bone Injuries

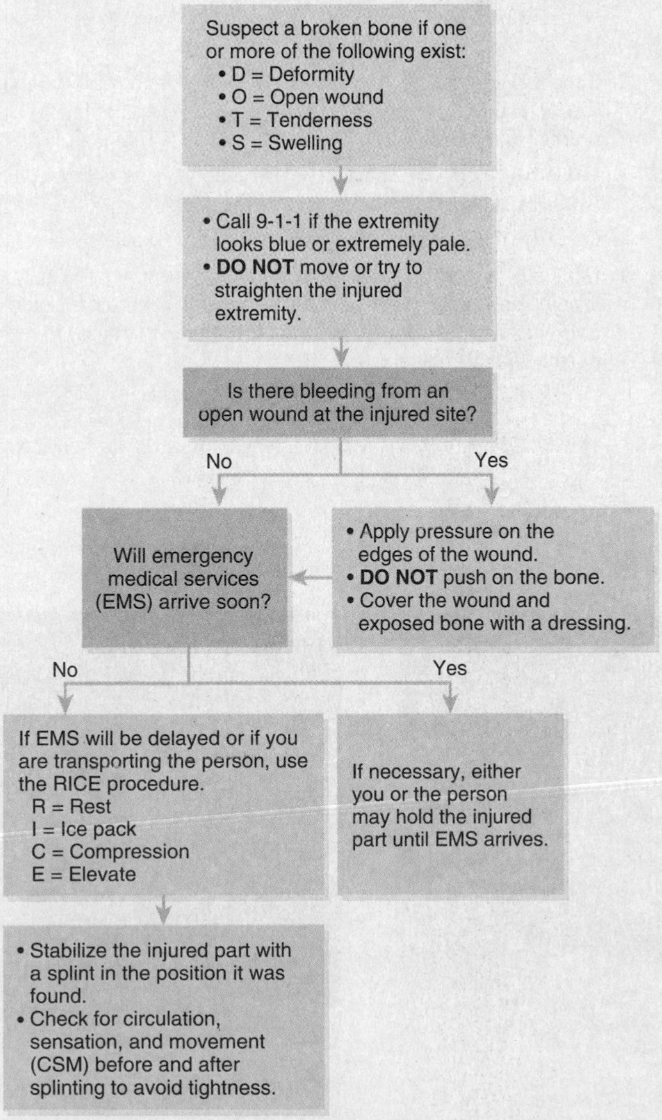
Suspect a broken bone if one or more of the following exist:
• D = Deformity
• O = Open wound
• T = Tenderness
• S = Swelling
• Call 9-1-1 if the extremity looks blue or extremely pale.
• DO NOT move or try to straighten the injured extremity.
Is there bleeding from an open wound at the injured site?
No
Yes
Will emergency medical services (EMS) arrive soon?
• Apply pressure on the edges of the wound.
• DO NOT push on the bone.
• Cover the wound and exposed bone with a dressing.
No
Yes
If EMS will be delayed or if you are transporting the person, use the RICE procedure.
R = Rest
I = Ice pack
C = Compression
E = Elevate
If necessary, either you or the person may hold the injured part until EMS arrives.
• Stabilize the injured part with a splint in the position it was found.
• Check for circulation, sensation, and movement (CSM) before and after splinting to avoid tightness.

Q&A

How strong is bone?

Bone is one of the strongest materials found in nature. One cubic inch of bone can withstand loads of at least 19,000 pounds (8,618 kg), which is about the weight of five standard-size pickup trucks. This is roughly four times the strength of concrete. Bone's resistance to load is equal to that of aluminum and light steel. Ounce for ounce, bone is actually stronger than steel and reinforced concrete, because steel bars of comparable size would weigh four or five times as much as bone.

What to Look For	What to Do
Use the mnemonic DOTS to assess for an injury: **D**eformity, such as: ▪ Shortening or severe deformity (angulation) between the joints or deformity around the joints ▪ Shortening of the extremity ▪ Rotation of the extremity when compared with the opposite extremity **O**pen wound. Lacerations or small puncture wounds near the site of a bone fracture are considered open fractures. **T**enderness and pain when pressed. **S**welling that happens rapidly Additional signs and symptoms include: ▪ Loss of function of the injured part. ▪ Guarding (The person refuses to use the injured part when motion produces pain.) ▪ **Crepitus** (a grating sensation felt and sometimes even heard when the ends of a broken bone rub together); **DO NOT** move the injured extremity in an attempt to detect crepitus. ▪ Extremity is blue or extremely pale.	**1.** Check for life-threatening conditions. A fracture, even an open fracture, seldom presents an immediate threat to life unless it has severed an artery or large vein. Only when all life-threatening conditions have been dealt with is it appropriate to identify and stabilize fractures. **2.** After receiving consent, gently remove clothing covering the injured body part. Cut away clothing at the seams if necessary. **3.** Examine the area by looking for and asking about DOTS. **4.** Check for CSM. Follow the steps in **SKILL SHEET 14-1** for checking CSM in an upper extremity and **SKILL SHEET 14-2** for a lower extremity. **5.** Allow the injured person to stabilize the injured part in a position of comfort. ▪ If EMS will arrive soon, allow the injured person to stabilize the injured part with their hands until they arrive. ▪ If EMS will be delayed or if you are transporting the person to professional medical care, stabilize the injured part with a splint. **6.** If the injury is an open fracture, **DO NOT** push on any protruding bones **FIGURE 14-4**. Cover the wound and exposed bones with a dressing. Place rolls of gauze around the bone, applying pressure on the wound's edges and bandage the injury without applying pressure on the bone. **7.** Call 9-1-1 for any open fractures or large-bone (ie, femur) fractures or when transporting the person would be difficult or would aggravate the injury. **8.** Call 9-1-1 if the extremity looks blue or extremely pale. **9.** Generally, first aid providers should not move or straighten an injured extremity. However, if there is no pulse in an extremity and the person is in a remote location or wilderness setting distant from EMS, you may need to gently realign the injured extremity to restore blood flow or to transport the person. In this situation: ▪ Use the RICE (Rest, Ice pack, Compression, Elevate) procedure. See pages 206–209. An ice pack helps reduce swelling and pain. ▪ Stabilize the part against movement. Doing so limits pain and reduces the chance for further injury.

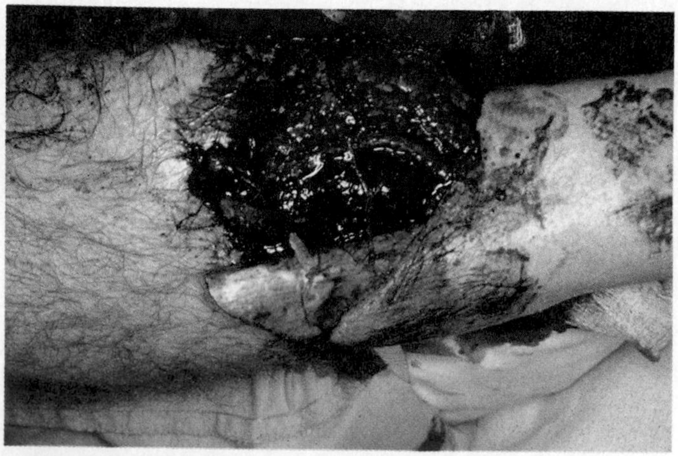

FIGURE 14-4 Open tibia, fibula fracture of the leg.

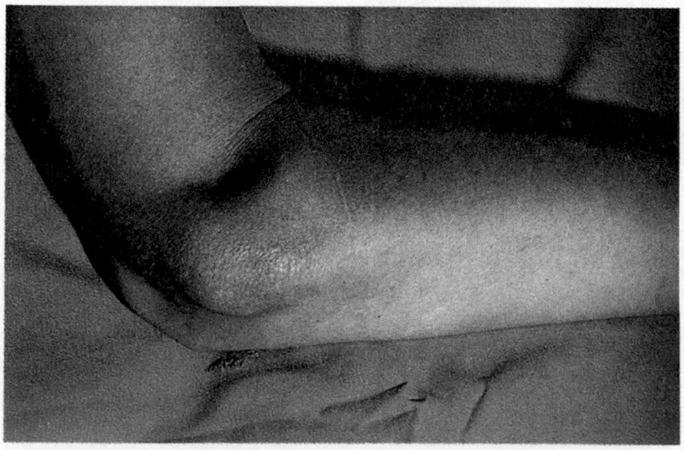

FIGURE 14-5 Dislocation of the elbow.

SKILL SHEET 14-1 Checking CSM in an Upper Extremity

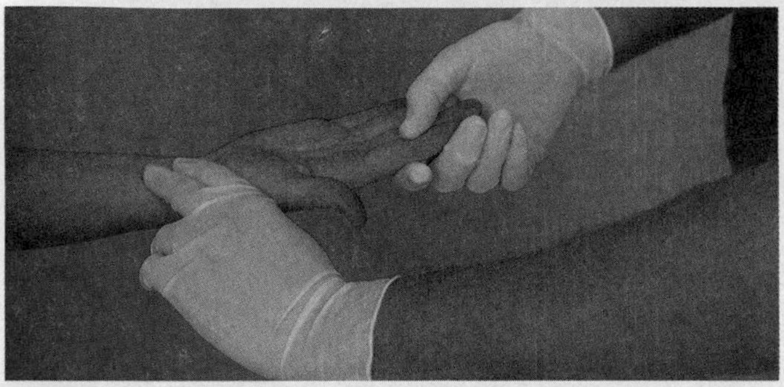

1 *Circulation.* Check an upper extremity for circulation using the radial pulse (located on the thumb side of the wrist).

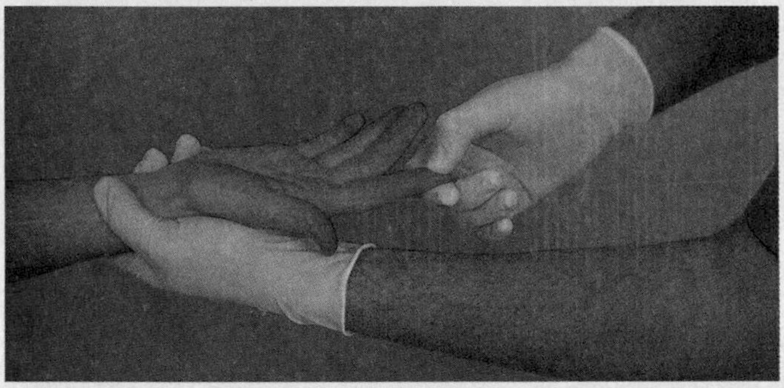

2 *Sensation.* Lightly touch or squeeze one of the person's fingers while their eyes are closed, and ask the person which finger they feel being squeezed.

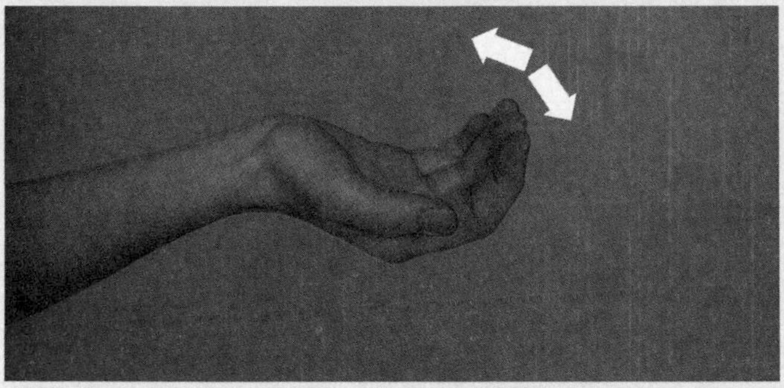

3 *Movement.* Ask the person to wiggle the fingers.

SKILL SHEET 14-2 Checking CSM in a Lower Extremity

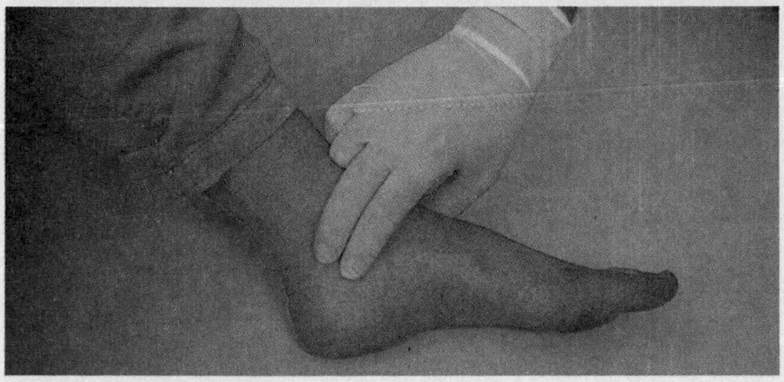

1 *Circulation.* Check a lower extremity for circulation using the posterior tibial pulse (located between the inside ankle bone and the Achilles tendon).

Continues

SKILL SHEET 14-2 Checking CSM in a Lower Extremity (*Continued*)

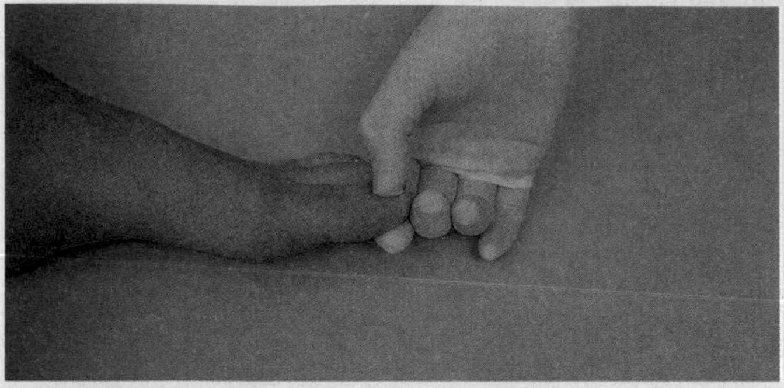

2 *Sensation.* Lightly touch or squeeze one of the person's toes while their eyes are closed, and ask the person which toe they feel being squeezed.

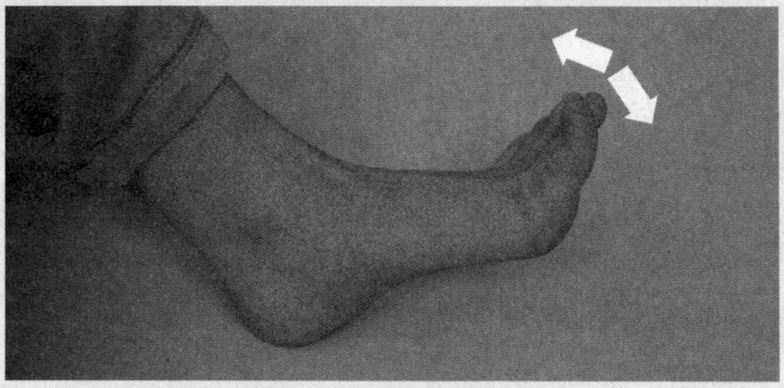

3 *Movement.* Ask the person to wiggle the toes.

Joint Injuries

A joint is where two or more bones come together.

Dislocations

A **dislocation** occurs when a joint comes apart and stays apart, with the bone ends no longer in contact. The shoulders, elbows, fingers, hips, kneecaps (patellae), and ankles are the joints most frequently affected.

Dislocations cause signs and symptoms similar to those of fractures: deformity, severe pain, swelling, and inability of the person to move the injured joint. The main sign of a dislocation is deformity. Its appearance will be different from that of an uninjured joint **FIGURE 14-5**.

Sprains

A **sprain** occurs when a joint is twisted or stretched beyond its normal range of motion. Bones are held together at joints by tough bands of tissue called ligaments. When a joint is sprained, the ligaments are either partially or completely torn. There are different degrees of sprains, but it is difficult for a first aid or EMS provider to classify the degree of a sprain **FIGURE 14-6**. Sprains most often occur in the knee and the ankle, but can occur in any joint.

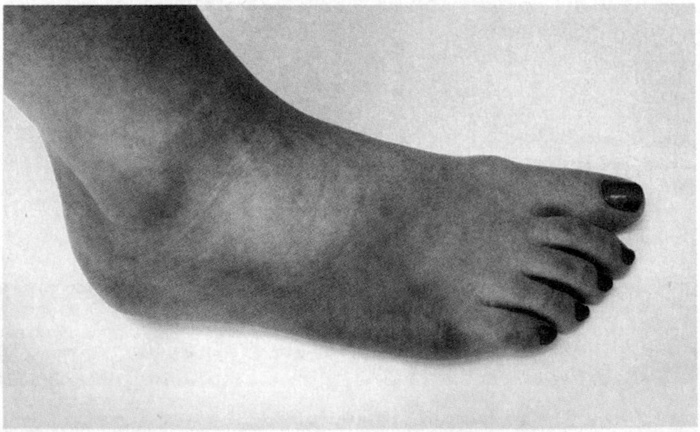

FIGURE 14-6 Sprained ankle.

Ankle sprains most often occur when the foot turns inward and stress is placed on the outside (lateral side) of the ankle. A severe lateral ankle sprain, if not correctly treated, can result in a chronically unstable ankle that is prone to sprains. Any ligament or bone injury on the inner side of the ankle usually represents a serious condition and requires professional medical care.

What to Look For	What to Do
▪ Obvious deformity compared with the opposite, uninjured joint ▪ Tenderness ▪ Severe pain ▪ Swelling ▪ Inability to move the injured part ▪ Numbness or impaired circulation of the extremity	1. Call 9-1-1 for the following: ▪ Extremity looks blue or extremely pale, an open wound, or a deformed or bent part. ▪ Transport of the person would be difficult or might aggravate the injury. 2. Check CSM, as previously described. If the end of the dislocated bone is pressing on nerves or blood vessels, numbness or paralysis may exist below the dislocation. If there is no pulse in the injured extremity, transport the person to a medical facility immediately. 3. If EMS has been called and will arrive soon, either you or the person may hold the injured part to stabilize it against movement until EMS arrives. 4. If EMS will be delayed or you are transporting the person to distant professional medical care, use the RICE procedure (see pages 208–210), but apply a splint (eg, pillow, wood board, or adjacent body part) before elevating. 5. **DO NOT** try to reduce a dislocation by putting the displaced part back into its normal position because nerve and blood vessel damage could result. Wilderness medical experts have identified easy and safe ways to reduce kneecap, finger, and anterior shoulder dislocations when medical help is more than 1 hour away. (See Chapter 24, *Wilderness First Aid.*) 6. **DO NOT** move or try to straighten an injured extremity. 7. If a wound is bleeding: ▪ Control the bleeding by applying pressure on the wound edges. ▪ Cover the exposed bone with a sterile dressing. **DO NOT** push on the bone.

Refer to **FLOWCHART 14-2** for additional information regarding the care of joint injuries.

Muscle Injuries

Although muscle injuries pose no real emergency, first aid providers have ample opportunities to care for them.

What to Look For	What to Do
It is often difficult to distinguish between a severe sprain and a fracture without a radiograph because their signs and symptoms are similar: ▪ Severe pain, which may prevent the person from moving or using the joint ▪ Swelling ▪ Discolored skin around the joint resulting from bleeding from torn blood vessels	1. Most sprains do not require professional medical care. If recuperation seems long, consult a physician. 2. Use the RICE procedure: ▪ *Rest*. Remove weight from and avoid movement of the injured joint. ▪ *Ice*. Apply an ice pack for about 20 minutes; an elastic bandage can be applied to keep the ice pack in place. ▪ *Compression*. After the 20 minutes, apply compression with an elastic bandage for 3 to 4 hours. ▪ Repeat the cycles of an ice pack for 20 minutes and compression for 3 to 4 hours. ▪ *Elevate*. Raise the injured part to reduce swelling.

Strains

A muscle **strain**, also known as a muscle pull, occurs when a muscle is torn as a result of stretching beyond its normal range of motion. There are different degrees of strains, but it is difficult for first aid and EMS providers to classify the degree of a strain without hospital testing such as an MRI (magnetic resonance imaging). When muscle fibers tear, fluid from nearby tissues leaks out and starts to build up near the injury. The area becomes inflamed, swollen, and tender. Inflammation begins immediately after an injury, but it can take 24 to 72 hours for enough tissue fluid to build up to cause pain and stiffness.

What to Look For	What to Do
▪ Occurs during physical activity ▪ Sharp pain ▪ Extreme tenderness ▪ Inability to use injured part ▪ Stiffness and pain when muscle is used	To care for strains, follow the RICE procedure.

Cramps

A **cramp** occurs when a muscle goes into an uncontrolled spasm and contraction. Although scientific literature has yet to confirm the causes of muscle cramps, several factors are associated with them. For example, muscle cramping is associated with certain diseases, such as diabetes and atherosclerosis (hardening of the arteries). Muscle cramps are often associated with physical activity. For the most part, muscle cramps can be divided into two categories: night cramps, which include any cramp occurring at night or while a person is at rest, and heat cramps, which are related to dehydration and electrolyte imbalance. (The electrolytes potassium and

Flowchart 14-2 Joint Injuries

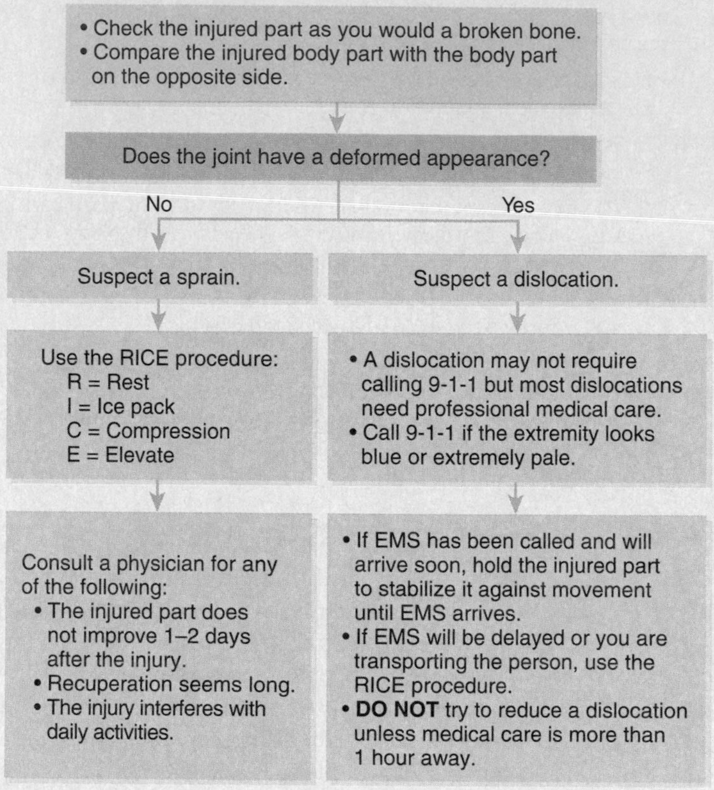
• Check the injured part as you would a broken bone.
• Compare the injured body part with the body part on the opposite side.
Does the joint have a deformed appearance?
No
Yes
Suspect a sprain.
Suspect a dislocation.
Use the RICE procedure:
R = Rest
I = Ice pack
C = Compression
E = Elevate
• A dislocation may not require calling 9-1-1 but most dislocations need professional medical care.
• Call 9-1-1 if the extremity looks blue or extremely pale.
Consult a physician for any of the following:
• The injured part does not improve 1–2 days after the injury.
• Recuperation seems long.
• The injury interferes with daily activities.
• If EMS has been called and will arrive soon, hold the injured part to stabilize it against movement until EMS arrives.
• If EMS will be delayed or you are transporting the person, use the RICE procedure.
• DO NOT try to reduce a dislocation unless medical care is more than 1 hour away.

sodium carry an electric charge that helps trigger muscles to contract and relax.)

What to Look For	What to Do
▪ Sudden severe muscle pain ▪ A muscle, often the calf muscle, that feels hard because of muscle contraction ▪ Residual discomfort, which may last for a few hours	Try one or more of these methods to relax the muscle: **1.** Have the person gently stretch the affected muscle. Because the muscle cramp is an uncontrolled muscle contraction or spasm, a gradual extension of the muscle may help lengthen the muscle fibers and relieve the cramp. **2.** Relax the muscle by pressing and massaging it. **3.** Apply an ice pack (unless in a cold environment). **4.** If cramping occurs during exertion in a hot environment, drink lightly salted cool water (one-fourth teaspoon [1.25 mL] salt in 1 quart [about 1 L] of water) or a commercial sports drink.

Contusions

A muscle **contusion**, or bruise, results from a blow to the muscle.

Refer to **FLOWCHART 14-3** for additional information regarding the care of muscle injuries.

What to Look For	What to Do
▪ Person reports receiving blow to a muscle ▪ Swelling ▪ Tenderness and pain ▪ Black and blue mark appearing hours later	**1.** Use the RICE procedure. **2.** Seek professional medical care for any contusion larger than the person's palm.

Flowchart 14-3 Muscle Injuries

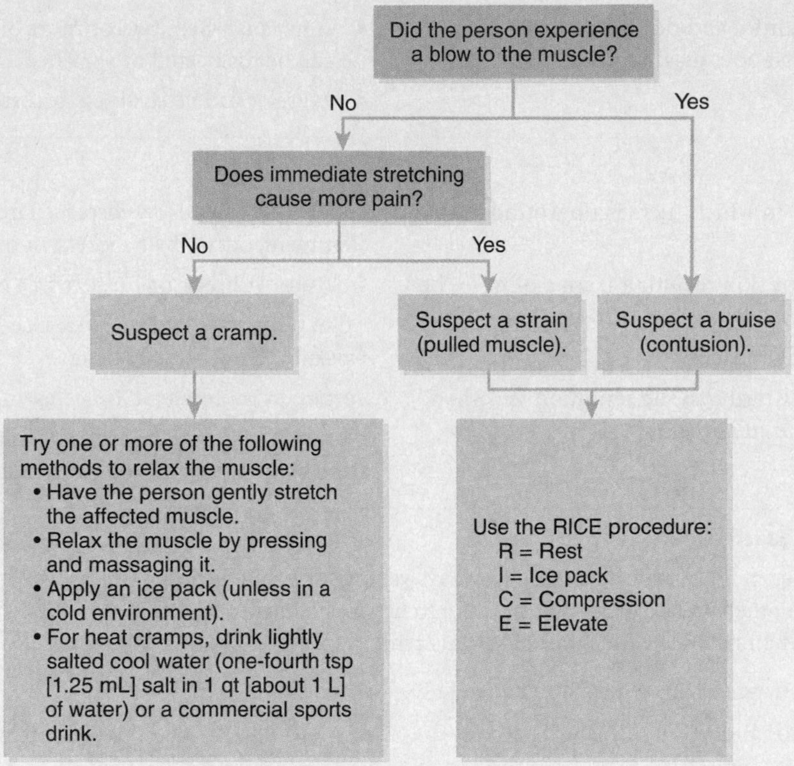

PREP KIT

Ready for Review

- Broken bones can be painful and debilitating and can cause lifelong aggravation, disability, and deformity.
- A joint is where two or more bones come together. Joints can be dislocated or sprained.
- Muscles can be strained, bruised, or cramped.

Vital Vocabulary

closed fracture A fracture in which there is no wound in the overlying skin.

contusion Injured tissue or skin resulting from a blow to the muscle in which blood vessels rupture; a bruise.

cramp A painful spasm of a muscle.

crepitus A grating sound heard and the sensation felt when the fractured ends of a bone rub together.

dislocation Bones are displaced from their normal joint alignment, out of their sockets, or out of their normal positions.

fracture A break or rupture in a bone.

open fracture A fracture exposed to the exterior; an open wound lies over the fracture.

sprain A trauma to a joint that injures the ligaments.

strain A tearing of muscle that occurs when the muscle is stretched beyond its normal range of motion.

Assessment in Action

While walking through your neighborhood, you see two boys yelling for help on the sidewalk. One is on the ground in pain and clutching his arm. The other boy explains that the injured boy lost control while skateboarding and crashed. The injured boy says he heard a snap when he crashed and landed on his arm.

Directions: Circle Yes if you agree with the statement; circle No if you disagree.

1. You should look for and ask about DOTS.
   YES **NO**
2. You notice a severe deformity on the boy's forearm but the skin is not broken. This is a closed fracture.
   YES **NO**
3. You should check the injured arm for CSM.
   YES **NO**
4. You should not splint the arm because of the deformity.
   YES **NO**
5. Applying ice helps reduce swelling.
   YES **NO**

Check Your Knowledge

Directions: Circle Yes if you agree with the statement; circle No if you disagree.

1. Apply cold on a suspected sprain.
   YES **NO**
2. The letters RICE stand for rest, ice pack, compression, and elevate.
   YES **NO**
3. DOTS stands for deformity, open wound, tenderness, and swelling.
   YES **NO**
4. Guarding occurs when motion produces pain.
   YES **NO**
5. Crepitus cannot be heard, but it can be felt by the person.
   YES **NO**
6. A dislocation is cared for much differently than a fracture.
   YES **NO**
7. Check a suspected fracture by having the person move the extremity.
   YES **NO**
8. Treat a muscle cramp by stretching the affected muscle.
   YES **NO**
9. CSM stands for cold, swelling, and motion.
   YES **NO**
10. Do not push on a protruding bone.
    YES **NO**

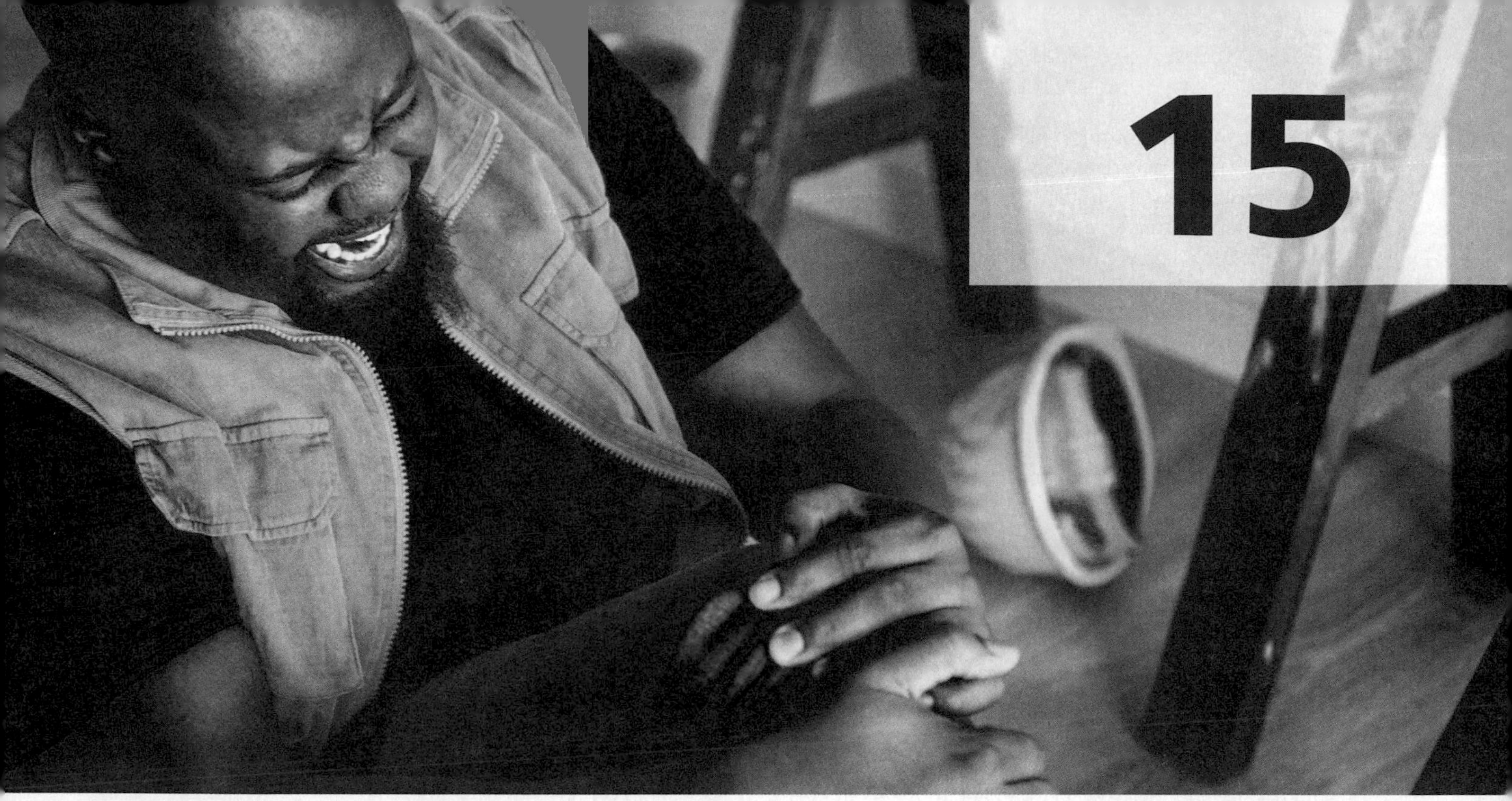

15

Extremity Injuries

CHAPTER AT A GLANCE

Extremity Injuries

Injuries to the extremitics are common, because people are involved in active lifestyles that include sports and wilderness activities. This chapter focuses on bone, joint, and muscle injuries of the extremities; bleeding, wounds, and other soft-tissue injuries are covered elsewhere. Most of the conditions discussed result from sudden trauma, although some chronic injuries that are incurred over time, such as tennis elbow, are included.

Assessment

Use these guidelines to assess injuries to the extremities:

1. Look for signs and symptoms of fractures and dislocations.
2. Examine the extremities, using the mnemonic DOTS (Deformity, Open wound, Tenderness, Swelling). Look at and ask about the extremity, starting with the distal end (fingers or toes) and working upward.
3. Compare one extremity with the other to determine size and shape differences.
4. Use the rule of thirds for extremity injuries. Imagine each long bone as being divided into thirds. If deformity, tenderness, or swelling is located in the upper or lower third of a long bone, assume that the nearest joint is injured.

5. Consider the cause of injury when evaluating the possibility of a fracture and its location. Forces that cause musculoskeletal injuries are direct forces (eg, a car bumper striking a pedestrian's leg), indirect forces along the long axis of bones (eg, a person falling onto an outstretched hand and fracturing the collarbone), and twisting forces (eg, a person's foot being fixed in one spot and the leg suddenly twisting).
6. Use the mnemonic CSM as a reminder to check the extremity for circulation, sensation, and movement of fingers or toes. If there is any CSM irregularity, then 9-1-1 should be called early. (See Skill Sheet 14-1 for CSM procedures.)

Types of Injuries

Types of injuries to the extremities range from simple contusions to complex open fractures:

1. **Contusions**, or bruising of the tissue
2. **Strains**, in which muscles are stretched or torn
3. **Sprains**, which involve the tearing or stretching of the joints, causing mild to severe damage to the ligaments and joint capsules
4. **Tendinitis**, which is inflammation of a tendon (cord that attaches muscle to bone) caused by overuse
5. **Dislocations**, in which bones are displaced from their normal joint alignment, out of their sockets, or out of their normal positions
6. **Fractures**, which are breaks in bones that may or may not be accompanied by open wounds

RICE Procedure for Bone, Joint, and Muscle Injuries

RICE is the acronym for rest, ice pack, compression, and elevation—the recommended immediate treatment for bone, joint, and muscle injuries. The steps taken during the first 48 to 72 hours after an injury can do a lot to relieve—even prevent—aches and pains. Treat all extremity bone, joint, and muscle injuries with the RICE procedure. In addition to RICE, fractures and dislocations should be splinted to stabilize the injured area.

R = Rest

Injuries heal faster if rested. *Rest* means the person does not use or move the injured part. Using any part of the body increases the blood circulation to that area, which can cause more swelling of an injured part. Crutches may be used to rest leg injuries.

I = Ice Pack

An ice pack should be applied to the injured area as soon as possible after the injury for about 20 minutes (or 10 minutes if uncomfortable) every 3 to 4 hours while awake, during the first 24 to 48 hours. Never apply an ice pack directly to the skin. Skin treated with cold passes through four stages: cold, burning, aching, and numbness. When the skin becomes numb, usually in 20 minutes, remove the ice pack. After removing the ice pack, compress the injured part with an elastic bandage and keep it elevated (the "C" and "E" of RICE).

Cold constricts the blood vessels to and within the injured area, which helps reduce the swelling and inflammation, and it dulls the pain and relieves muscle spasms. Cold should be applied as soon as possible after the injury; healing time often is directly related to the amount of swelling that occurs. Heat has the opposite effect when applied to fresh injuries: It increases circulation to the area and increases the swelling and the pain. Although it might be tempting, someone who has a bone, joint, or muscle injury should not initially apply heat attempt to relieve the pain.

Use either of the following methods to apply cold to an injury:

1. Put crushed ice (or cubes) into a double plastic bag or commercial ice bag, and place a layer of cloth between the bag of ice and the skin. Alternatively, a wet towel or cloth can be used to hold the ice. Secure the ice in place with an elastic bandage for about 20 minutes. Crushed ice offers the advantage of conforming to the body's contours.

CAUTION

DO NOT apply an ice pack for more than 20 minutes at a time. Frostbite or nerve damage can result.

DO NOT apply an ice pack on the back outside part of the knee. Nerve damage can occur.

DO NOT apply cold if the person has Raynaud disease (spasms in the arteries of the extremities that reduce circulation), abnormal sensitivity to cold, or if the injured part has been frostbitten previously.

DO NOT stop using an ice pack too soon. A common mistake is the early use of heat, which may result in swelling and pain. Use an ice pack three to four times a day for the first 24 hours, preferably up to 48 hours while awake, before applying any heat. For severe injuries, using ice on and off for up to 72 hours is recommended.

FYI

Heat and Cold: When to Use Which

Many people use heat devices or ice packs to speed recovery from sports injuries—but when is the right time to use each technique? Apply cold immediately after an acute injury, such as an ankle sprain. Icing reduces pain, swelling, and muscle spasm immediately after injury, but its use should be discontinued after 2 days for most injuries or 3 days for severe injuries. Heat applications (heat packs, radiant heat, or whirlpool baths) can then be used to reduce muscle spasms and pain. In addition, heat increases blood flow and joint flexibility. Use vigorous heat to treat chronic injuries, but mild heat to reduce muscle spasm. Heat is also effective for acute back pain, but ice massage is preferred if the back pain persists for 2 weeks or more.

Data: from Kaul MP, Herring SA. Superficial heat and cold. *Phys Sportsmed.* 1994;22(12):65–74.

FYI

Homemade Ice Packs

- Ice bags kept in a freezer freeze solid and cannot be shaped to fit the injured area. One part isopropyl (rubbing) alcohol to three parts water prevents freezing, and the ice bag can be easily molded. Bags can be reused for months.
- An unopened bag of frozen vegetables is inexpensive, keeps its basic shape (unlike ice chips, which melt), molds to the shape of the injured area, is reusable, and is packaged in a fairly puncture-resistant, watertight bag.
- For cold therapy over a fairly large area, soak a face towel in cold water, wring it out, fold it, and place it in a large self-sealing plastic bag. Store the bag in the freezer. To use the cold pack, wrap it in a light cotton towel and apply for 20 minutes, after which it can be refrozen. A washcloth in a smaller bag can be used to treat a smaller area.
- Fill a plastic bag with snow.
- Fill a polystyrene plastic cup with water and freeze it. When you need an ice pack, peel the cup to below ice level; the remaining part of the cup forms a cold-resistant handle. Rub the ice over the injured area (movement is necessary to prevent skin damage). These ice packs are inexpensive and convenient and take up little space.
- To make a funnel for filling an ice bag, push out the bottom of a paper cup and fit it into the neck of the ice bag. The ice will slide through the cup and into the bag.

2. Use a chemical cold pack, a sealed pouch that contains two chemical envelopes. Squeezing the pack mixes the chemicals, producing a chemical reaction that has a cooling effect. Although they do not cool as well as other methods, they are convenient to use when ice is not readily available. They lose their cooling power quickly, however, and can be used only once. Also, they may be impractical because they are expensive.

C = Compression

Compressing the injured area squeezes fluid out of the injury site. Compression limits the ability of the skin and other tissues to expand and reduces internal bleeding. When not applying ice packs, apply an elastic bandage to the injured area, especially the foot, ankle, knee, thigh, hand, or elbow. Fill the hollow areas with padding such as a sock or washcloth before applying the elastic bandage.

Elastic bandages come in various sizes for different body areas:

- 2-inch (5-cm) width for the wrist, hand, and foot
- 3-inch (8-cm) width for the elbow and arm
- 4-inch (10-cm) width for the ankle, knee, and leg

Start the elastic bandage several inches below the injury and wrap in an upward, overlapping (about one-half to three-fourths of the bandage's width) spiral, starting with even and somewhat tight pressure, then gradually wrapping more loosely above the injury. Stretch the elastic bandage no more than one third its ability to stretch.

Applying compression may be the most important step in preventing swelling. The person should wear the elastic bandage continuously for the first 18 to 24 hours (except when cold is applied). At night, have the person loosen but not remove the elastic bandage.

For an ankle injury, place a horseshoe-shaped pad around the ankle knob and secure it with the elastic bandage **FIGURE 15-1**. The pad can be made from various materials (eg, twisted washcloth, socks). The pad will compress the soft tissues and the bones. Wrap the bandage tightest nearest the toes and loosest above the ankle. It should be tight enough to decrease swelling but not tight enough to inhibit blood flow. For a contusion or a strain, place a pad between the injury and the elastic bandage.

E = Elevation

Gravity slows the return of blood to the heart from the lower parts of the body. Once fluids get to the hands or feet, they have nowhere else to go, and those parts of the body swell. Elevating the injured area, in combination with ice and compression, limits circulation to that area, which in turn helps limit internal bleeding and minimize swelling.

It is simple to prop up an injured leg or arm to limit bleeding. Whenever possible, elevate the injured part above the level

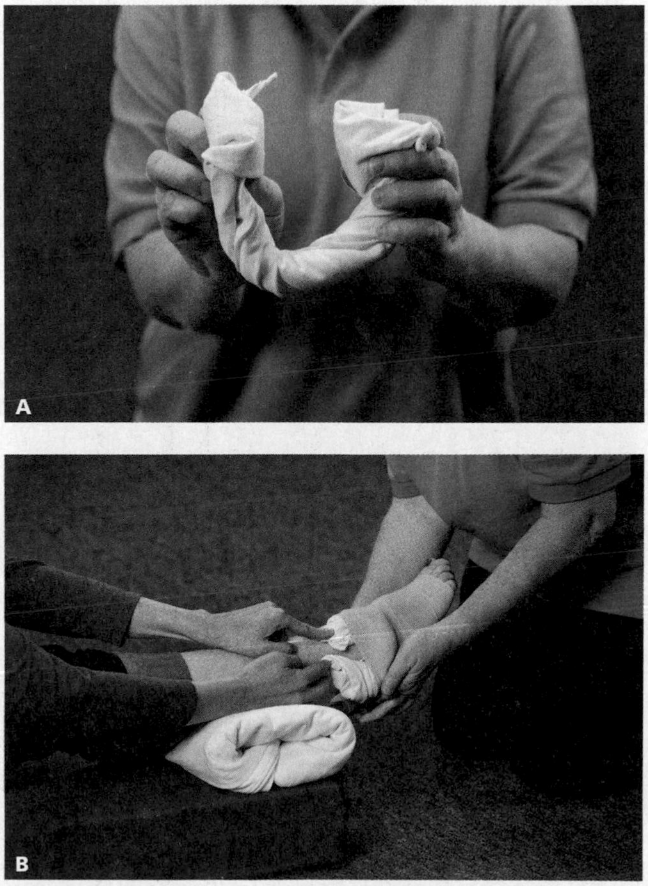

FIGURE 15-1 **A**. Place a horseshoe-shaped pad around the ankle knob. **B**. Secure the pad with an elastic bandage.

CAUTION

DO NOT apply an elastic bandage too tightly. If applied too tightly, elastic bandages will restrict circulation. Stretch a new elastic bandage to about one-third its maximum length for adequate compression. Leave fingers and toes exposed so possible color change can be easily observed. Compare the toes or fingers of the injured extremity with those on the uninjured one. Pale skin, pain, numbness, and tingling are signs that the bandage is too tight. If any of these symptoms appears, immediately remove the elastic bandage. Leave the elastic bandage off until all the symptoms disappear, then rewrap the area less tightly. Always wrap from below the injury and move toward the heart.

of the heart for the first 24 hours after an injury. If a fracture is suspected, do not elevate an extremity until it has been stabilized with a splint. Along with the use of the RICE procedure, fractures and dislocations can be splinted unless emergency medical services (EMS) will soon arrive. In this case, the person can hold the injured part.

To perform the RICE procedure, follow the steps in **SKILL SHEET 15-1**.

Shoulder Injuries

Shoulder Dislocation

Three bones come together at the shoulder: the **scapula** (shoulder blade), the **clavicle** (collarbone), and the **humerus** (upper arm bone). The shoulder is the most freely movable joint in the body. The extreme range of its possible movements makes the shoulder joint highly susceptible to dislocation (separation). A dislocation of the shoulder occurs when the bones of the shoulder come apart as a result of a blow or a particular movement. Shoulder dislocation is second in frequency only to finger dislocations.

What to Look For	What to Do
▪ Person holds the upper arm away from the body, supported by the uninjured arm (occurs in about 95% of shoulder dislocations; this position differentiates a dislocation from a fracture of the humerus, in which the person holds the arm against the chest) ▪ The dislocated arm cannot be brought across the chest wall to touch the opposite shoulder (ie, the sling position) ▪ Extreme pain in the shoulder area ▪ Shoulder looks squared off, rather than rounded **FIGURE 15-2** ▪ Complete loss of shoulder function ▪ Reported history of previous dislocations ▪ Numbness or paralysis in the arm from pressure, pinching blood vessels or nerves	1. **DO NOT** try to force, twist, or pull the shoulder back in place because doing so may cause bone, nerve, or blood vessel injury. 2. Place a folded or rolled blanket or a pillow between the upper arm and the chest to support the arm. 3. Apply an arm sling and swathe (binder) to stabilize and rest the arm. (See Chapter 16, *Splinting Extremities*, for more details.) 4. Apply an ice pack for 20 minutes. 5. Seek immediate professional medical care.

SKILL SHEET 15-1 RICE Procedure for Bone, Joint, and Muscle Injuries

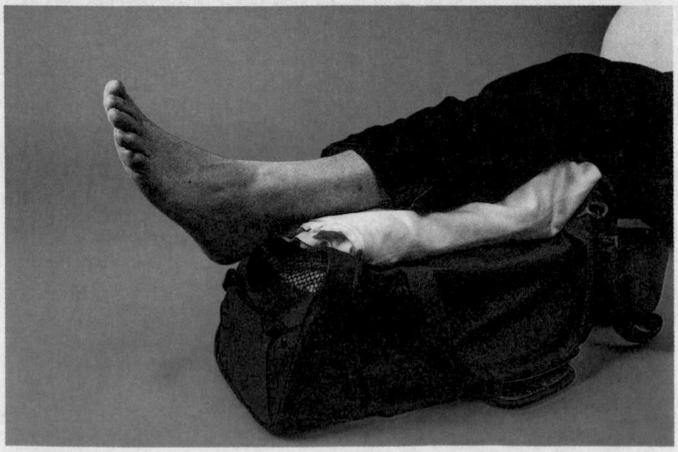

1 R = Rest

DO NOT use or move the body part.

SKILL SHEET 15-1 RICE Procedure for Bone, Joint, and Muscle Injuries (*Continued*)

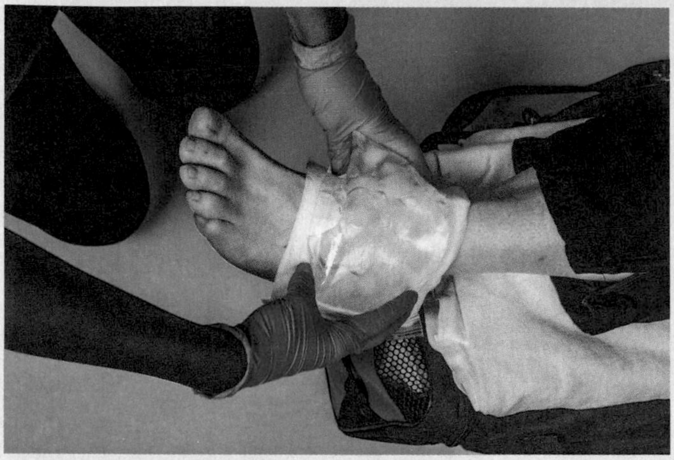

2 I = Ice Pack

Apply cold for 20 minutes (or 10 minutes if uncomfortable) every 3 to 4 hours during the first 24 to 48 hours. Put crushed or cubed ice in a plastic bag and place a paper towel or thin cloth between the ice pack and skin for protection, or wrap ice in a damp towel or cloth filled with a mixture of ice and water. An elastic bandage can be used to hold the ice pack in place.

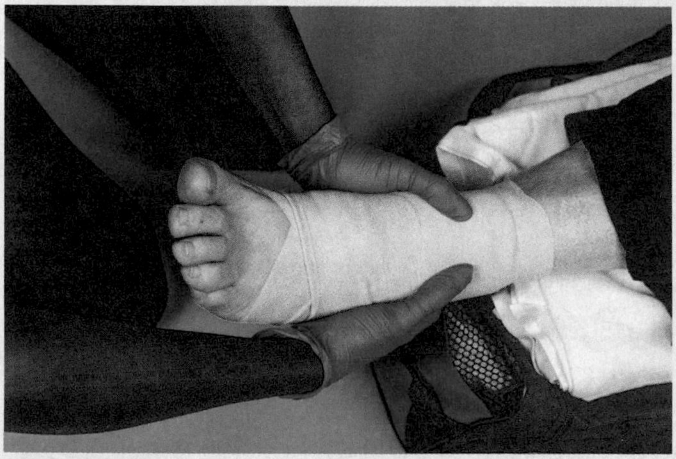

3 C = Compression

Apply an elastic bandage when not applying ice.

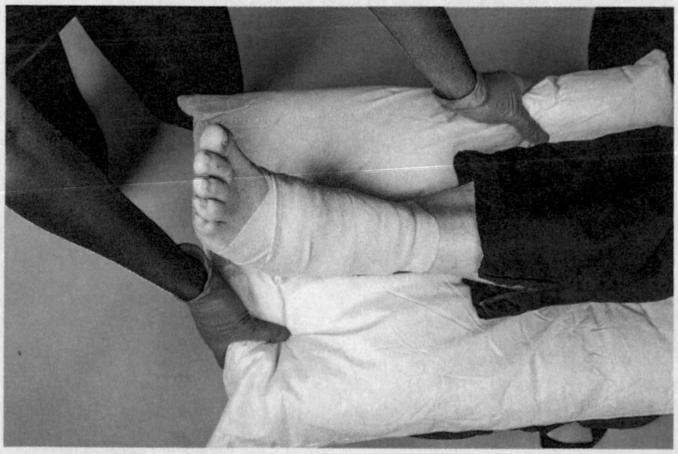

4 E = Elevation

When possible, keep the injured part raised higher than the heart as much as possible.

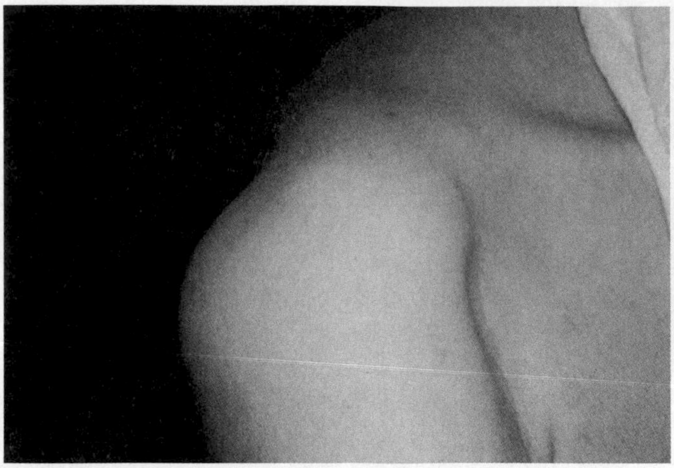

FIGURE 15-2 Shoulder dislocation. Note the absence of the normal rounded appearance of the shoulder.

What to Look For	What to Do
▪ Swelling ▪ Pain at the injury site ▪ Feeling of firmness when pressure is exerted on the shoulder ▪ Tenderness ▪ Discoloration under the skin (black and blue)	1. Apply an ice pack to the area for 20 minutes, three to four times during the first 24 hours. 2. Place the arm in a sling and swathe (binder) to stabilize and rest the arm.

Tendinitis

The general cause of tendinitis (inflammation) in the shoulder is continuous overuse or unusual use. Repeated arm movement often results in painful shoulders. These injuries are often seen in athletes engaged in the throwing sports (eg, baseball pitcher, football quarterback) and in other sports in which the shoulder is used extensively (eg, swimming).

What to Look For	What to Do
▪ Constant pain or pain with motion of the shoulder ▪ Limited motion of the shoulder ▪ Crackling sound when the joint is moved ▪ Tenderness over the area	1. Apply an ice pack for 10 minutes or an ice massage for 10 minutes after exercise. Fill a polystyrene cup with water and freeze. Tear a small amount of foam from the top so ice protrudes. Massage firmly over the injured area in a circle about the size of a baseball. 2. Use a sling and swathe (binder) to rest the shoulder. 3. Use over-the-counter (OTC) pain medication such as ibuprofen according to package directions. 4. Seek professional medical advice if needed.

Clavicle Fracture

Fractures of the clavicle (collarbone) are common and usually are the result of falling directly on the shoulder or on an outstretched arm. They can also be the result of a direct blow to the clavicle that occurs during a fall or a motor vehicle crash. Most clavicle fractures (80%) occur in the middle third of the bone.

What to Look For	What to Do
Person reports one of the following: ▪ Falling directly on the shoulder or on an outstretched arm ▪ Receiving a direct blow to the clavicle or shoulder ▪ Severe pain over the injured area ▪ Person holds the injured arm against the chest with the uninjured arm to stabilize the injury ▪ Person does not move the arm because of the pain ▪ Swelling ▪ Visible deformity ▪ Tenderness ▪ Dropped or drooped shoulder ▪ Bruising	1. Assess and treat for shock if indicated. 2. Apply an arm sling and swathe (binder) to stabilize and rest the arm. 3. Apply an ice pack to the area for 20 minutes, three to four times during the next 24 hours. 4. Seek immediate professional medical care.

Humerus Fracture

The shaft of the humerus (upper arm) can be felt throughout its entire length along the inner side of the upper arm. Gently pushing on the bone may reveal pain indicating a fracture.

What to Look For	What to Do

▪ The person reports having one of the following:
  ▪ Direct blow to the area
  ▪ Twist or fall on the outstretched arm
  ▪ Severe pain
▪ Swelling
  ▪ Visible deformity
  ▪ Tenderness if pressed or pushed
  ▪ Inability to move the arm
  ▪ Person holds the arm against the chest for comfort
	1. Assess and treat for shock if indicated.
	2. Apply an ice pack for 20 minutes.
	3. Stabilize the arm by applying one rigid splint on the part of the arm away from the body. Apply an arm sling and swathe (binder).
	4. Seek immediate professional medical care.

Contusions

Direct blows to the shoulder resulting in contusions, or bruises, are often called shoulder pointers. Contusions of this type may cause severe discomfort.

Elbow Injuries

Elbow Fractures and Dislocations

All elbow fractures and dislocations should be considered serious and treated with extreme care. Inappropriate care can result in injury to the nearby nerves and blood vessels.

What to Look For	What to Do
▪ Immediate swelling ▪ Severe pain ▪ Possible visible deformity; compare it with the uninjured elbow ▪ Restricted, painful motion ▪ Numbness or coldness of the hand and fingers below the elbow	1. **DO NOT** move the elbow. 2. Splint the elbow in the position found to prevent nerve and blood vessel damage: ▪ If straight, keep the splinted elbow straight. ▪ If bent, keep the elbow bent. 3. Apply an ice pack for 20 minutes. 4. Seek immediate professional medical care.

Tennis Elbow

Tennis elbow results from sharp, quick twists of the wrist. Despite its name, it does not occur exclusively from playing tennis. The muscles that bend the wrist back and straighten the fingers all begin in one spot, no bigger than a dime, on the outside bony prominence (protrusion) of the elbow. Tennis elbow, which is an inflammation of the tendons on this outer side of the elbow, can be very painful whenever the wrist and the elbow are used.

What to Look For	What to Do
▪ Pain that increases while using the arm ▪ Gradual grip weakness ▪ The injured elbow fatigues quicker than normal ▪ Very tender on outer protrusion of elbow	1. Apply heat before an activity; the person might wear a brace or rubber sleeve on the sore elbow. 2. Apply an ice pack for 20 minutes after completion of the activity. 3. Seek professional medical advice for an appropriate rehabilitation program.

Golfer's Elbow

Repetitive motion produces pain. Golfer's elbow is the equivalent of the more common tennis elbow but with pain on the inside of the elbow. It is tendinitis affecting the tendons attached to the bony protrusion on the inside of the elbow.

What to Look For	What to Do
▪ Pain that increases while using the arm ▪ Gradual grip weakness ▪ The injured elbow fatigues quicker than normal	1. Apply heat before an activity; the person might wear a brace or rubber sleeve on the tender elbow. 2. Apply an ice pack for 20 minutes after completion of an activity. 3. Seek medical advice for an appropriate rehabilitation program.

Radius and Ulna Fracture

There are two large bones (**radius** and **ulna**) in the forearm, and either or both bones may be broken. When only one bone is broken, the other acts as a splint and there may be little or no deformity. However, a marked deformity may be present in a fracture near the wrist. When both bones are broken, the arm usually appears deformed.

What to Look For	What to Do
Person reports having pain in the forearm or wrist from one of the following: ▪ A direct blow ▪ Falling on an outstretched hand ▪ Visible deformity ▪ Severe pain radiating up and down from the injury site ▪ An inability to move the wrist or pain when moving the wrist	1. Assess and treat for shock if indicated. 2. Apply an ice pack to the area for 20 minutes. 3. Do one of the following: ▪ Keeping the hand and fingers in the position of function (cupping shape as though holding a baseball) with extra padding in the palm, apply a rigid splint against the forearm. ▪ Apply two rigid splints on both sides of the arm from the tip of the elbow to the fingers. 4. Place the arm in a sling and swathe (binder) with the hand in a thumb-up position. 5. Seek professional medical care.

Wrist Fracture

The wrist usually is broken when the person falls with the arm and hand outstretched.

What to Look For	What to Do
▪ Injury to the wrist associated with a snapping or popping sensation within the wrist ▪ Pain in the wrist that is aggravated by movement ▪ Tenderness ▪ Swelling ▪ Inability or unwillingness to move the wrist ▪ Lumplike deformity on the back of the wrist	1. Use the RICE procedure (with the exception of compression). 2. Stabilize the wrist with a splint. 3. Seek professional medical care.

Hand Injuries

Crushed Hand

The hand may be fractured by a direct blow or by a crushing injury.

What to Look For	What to Do
▪ Pain ▪ Swelling ▪ Loss of motion ▪ Open wounds ▪ Broken bones	1. Control any bleeding. 2. Cover wounds with a dressing. 3. Depending upon the situation, apply an ice pack for no longer than 20 minutes; doing so should not delay seeking professional medical care. 4. Seek professional medical care. While transporting to medical care, prop the person's hand on a pillow or on their chest, or splint the person's hand as you would for a radius and ulna fracture.

Finger Injuries

The three bones that make up each finger are the most commonly broken bones in the body. Many of the tendons attached to the finger bones can tear with or without a fracture, and the three joints—the distal interphalangeal, the proximal interphalangeal, and the metacarpal phalangeal—can also be injured. A so-called finger sprain may be a complicated fracture or dislocation.

Finger Fracture

Contrary to popular belief, broken bones—especially the fingers—can move.

What to Look For	What to Do
The finger or thumb has: ▪ A visible deformity; finger has a twisted look ▪ Immediate pain; hurts with or without movement ▪ Numbness ▪ Swelling ▪ Pinpointed tenderness that usually indicates a fracture	1. Test for a finger fracture: ▪ If possible, straighten the fingers and place them on a hard surface. ▪ Tap the tip of the injured finger toward the hand. Pain lower down in the finger or into the hand can indicate a fracture. 2. **DO NOT** try to realign the finger. 3. Gently apply an ice pack. 4. Splint the finger using one of the following methods: ▪ Buddy tape the fractured finger to another for support. For a thumb, tape it with three to four figure-eight patterns around the joint. Monitor the finger for swelling and circulation issues. ▪ Keep the hand and fingers in the position of function (cupping shape as though holding a baseball) with extra padding in the palm. Secure the hand, fingers, and arm to a rigid splint. 5. Seek professional medical care.

Finger Dislocation

Finger dislocations are common. The same causes of fractured fingers can also cause a dislocated finger.

What to Look For	What to Do
▪ The finger or thumb has: ▪ A visible deformity **FIGURE 15-3** ▪ Immediate pain ▪ Swelling ▪ Shortening of the finger ▪ May be unable to bend the finger in the injured area; motion is impossible	1. **DO NOT** try to realign the dislocation. 2. Apply an ice pack for 20 minutes. 3. If possible, splint the finger using one of the following methods: ▪ Buddy tape the finger for support. For a thumb, tape it with three to four figure-eight patterns around the joint. Monitor the finger for swelling and circulation issues. ▪ Keep the hand and fingers in the position of function (cupping shape as though holding a baseball) with extra padding in the palm. Secure the hand, fingers, and arm to a rigid splint. 4. Seek professional medical care.

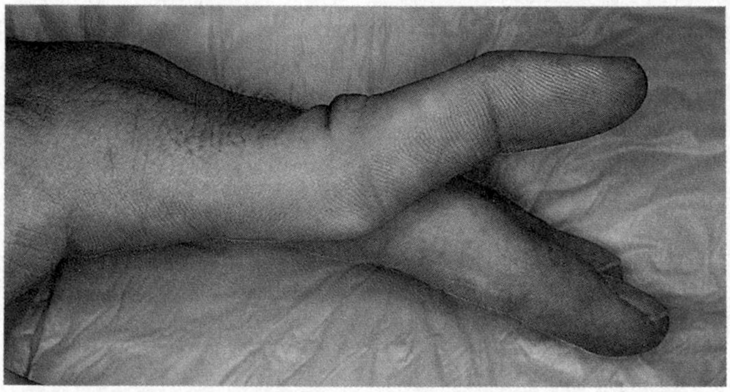

FIGURE 15-3 Finger dislocation.

Sprained Finger

The distal joints of the fingers have a ligament on each side of the joint.

What to Look For	What to Do
▪ The finger or thumb has been: ▪ Jammed or compressed ▪ Stepped on ▪ Forced or twisted sideways ▪ Pain and swelling over a joint (especially tenderness on both sides of a joint) ▪ Inability to make a fist ▪ Weakness while curling the injured finger alone ▪ Weakness or pain when gripping	1. Apply an ice pack for 20 minutes. 2. Reevaluate after the ice pack application and seek professional medical care if pain and weakness exist. 3. Tape fingers with buddy taping for support. Tape thumb with three to four figure-eight patterns around joint.

Nail Avulsion

A person may have had a blow to the nail, the nail may have been torn away by a piece of machinery, or a long toenail may have caught on a loop of carpet or other fixed object. An injury in which a nail is partly or completely torn loose is known as a nail avulsion **FIGURE 15-4**.

What to Look For	What to Do
The nail may be completely detached or partially held in place by the skin.	1. Secure the damaged nail in place with an adhesive bandage or tape. 2. **DO NOT** trim away the loose nail. 3. Consult a physician for further advice.

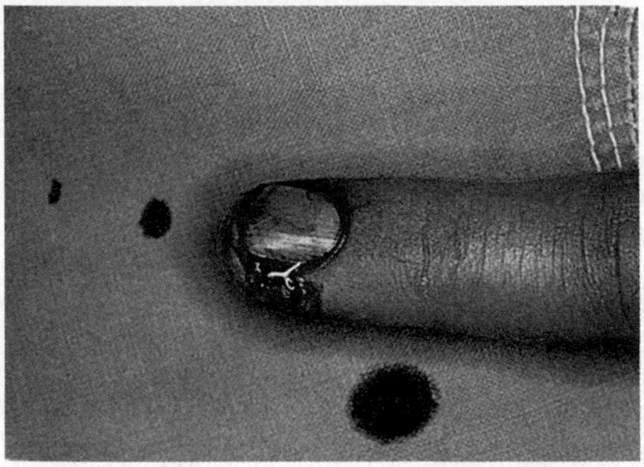

FIGURE 15-4 Relieve pain by releasing the blood under a nail.

Splinters

Sharp splinters (usually wooden) can be impaled into the skin or under a fingernail or toenail.

What to Look For	What to Do
▪ A small puncture wound ▪ The sliver may be seen	1. If embedded in the skin, use tweezers to remove it. In some cases, you may need to tease it out with a sterile needle until the end can be grasped with tweezers or fingers. Clean the wound with soap and water. 2. If the splinter is impaled under a fingernail or toenail and breaks off flush, cut a V-shaped notch in the nail to gain access to the splinter. Remove the embedded splinter by grasping its end with tweezers.

Blood Under a Nail

Blood collects under a fingernail when underlying tissues are bruised (eg, finger struck by a hammer or caught between a door and its frame).

What to Look For	What to Do
▪ Excruciating pain, because of the pressure of the blood pushing against the nail ▪ Pain that does not disappear until the collection of blood is drained	1. Immerse the finger in ice water or apply an ice pack with the hand elevated to reduce pain and swelling. 2. Relieve the pressure under the injured nail: ▪ Using a knife, sewing needle, or small drill bit (**DO NOT** use a drill), slowly and gently rotate the sharp point of the object through the nail. 3. Apply a dressing to absorb the draining blood and to protect the injured nail. 4. If necessary, seek professional medical care.

Ring Strangulation

Ring strangulation can be a serious condition if it cuts off the blood supply long enough. Permanent damage may result within 4 or 5 hours.

What to Look For	What to Do
The ring has become tight on the finger after an injury or after some other cause of swelling, such as a local reaction to a bee sting.	Try one or more of the following methods to remove a ring: 1. Lubricate the finger with soap and water, grease, oil, butter, petroleum jelly, or some other slippery substance, and then try to remove the ring. 2. Immerse the finger in cold water or apply an ice pack for several minutes to reduce the swelling. 3. Liberally spray window or glass cleaner onto the finger, and then try to slide off the ring. 4. Massage the finger from the tip toward the hand to move the swelling; lubricate the finger again and try removing the ring. 5. Wind thread around the finger, starting approximately 1 inch (2.5 cm) from the ring edge and going toward the ring, keeping each round of thread touching the next. Wind smoothly and tightly right up to the edge of the ring. This action will push the swelling toward the hand. Slip the end of the thread under the ring with a matchstick or toothpick, then slowly unwind the thread on the hand side of the ring. You should be able to twist the ring gently over the thread and off the finger **FIGURE 15-5**.

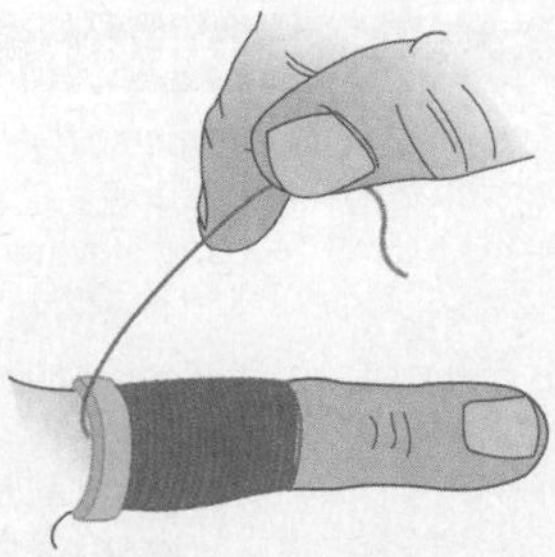

FIGURE 15-5 Removing a tight ring with thread.

FYI

Ring Removal From an Extremely Swollen Finger

Rings on swollen fingers are not uncommon, but they must be removed or serious conditions can result. Generally, the removal method is simply to cut the ring off the finger or to use one of several nondestructive removal methods using string or a rubber band. A simple method that eliminates the swelling and permits the removal of a ring involves wrapping the entire finger starting approximately 1 inch (2.5 cm) from the ring edge and wrapping toward the ring with a tight, elastic band, which reduces the swelling and frees the ring.

Data from Cresap CR. Removal of a hardened steel ring from an extremely swollen finger. *Am J Emerg Med.* 1995 May;13(3):318–320.

Hip Joint Injuries

Hip Dislocation

A hip can be dislocated by a fall, a blow to the thigh, or direct force to the foot or knee. The hip joint is a stable ball-and-socket joint that requires great force to dislocate. Often a hip is dislocated when the knee strikes the dashboard during a motor vehicle crash. It is difficult to differentiate a hip dislocation from a hip fracture.

What to Look For	What to Do
▪ Severe pain at the injury site ▪ Swelling at the injury site ▪ Hip flexed and knee bent and rotated inward toward the opposite hip ▪ Visible injury	1. Assess and treat for shock if indicated. 2. Stabilize the injury. 3. Check CSM. 4. Seek professional medical care. This injury is best transported by EMS personnel.

Hip Fracture

A hip fracture is a fracture of the upper end of the **femur** (thigh bone), not the pelvis. A fractured hip usually is caused by a fall. Older people, especially women, are susceptible to this type of injury because of brittle bones (osteoporosis). Occasionally, the bone actually fractures while the person is walking, resulting in a fall (rather than the fall causing the fracture).

What to Look For	What to Do
▪ Severe pain in the groin area ▪ Inability to lift the injured leg ▪ Leg may appear shortened and be rotated with the toes pointing abnormally outward or inward	1. Seek immediate professional medical care. This injury is best transported by EMS personnel. 2. Assess and treat for shock if indicated. 3. Stabilize the injured leg against movement. 4. Check CSM.

Thigh Injuries

Femur Fracture

Because the femur is the largest bone in the body, considerable force is required to break it. Femur injuries can occur in any part of the femur, from the hip to just above the knee joint. A fracture of the femur usually is caused by a fall or a direct blow.

Femur fractures often include open wounds, and external bleeding may be severe. If the blood vessels are damaged, the person may have 1 to 2 quarts (1 to 2 L) of blood loss into the thigh. There may be loss of blood circulation to the lower part of the extremity or nerve damage, especially with lower-third femur fractures.

What to Look For	What to Do
▪ Severe pain at the injury site ▪ Deformity; leg may appear shorter ▪ Swelling, resulting from severe damage to blood vessels ▪ Person reports having heard or felt a severe pop or snap at the time of injury	1. Call 9-1-1. This injury is best transported by EMS personnel. 2. Assess and treat for shock if indicated. 3. Cover a wound with a sterile dressing. 4. Stabilize the injured leg against movement. 5. Check CSM.

Muscle Contusion

The muscle group on the front of the thigh, the quadriceps group, often gets bruised. Depending on the force of impact and the muscles involved, the contusion may be of varying degrees of severity.

What to Look For	What to Do
The person received a direct hit producing: ▪ Swelling ▪ Pain and tenderness ▪ Tightness or firmness of the site when pressed ▪ Visible bruise that may appear hours later	1. Follow the RICE procedure. 2. Stretch the muscle by bending the knee toward the person's chest.

Muscle Strain

When a muscle is overstretched, it can result in a tear, called a strain. Different degrees of strains occur, but first aid providers will be unable to determine their degree.

What to Look For	What to Do
▪ Person reports feeling a pop or pulling sensation while running or jumping ▪ Tenderness ▪ Stiffness and pain during movement ▪ Swelling ▪ A visible bruise appearing days later	1. Follow the RICE procedure. 2. Stretch the muscle, but **DO NOT** force stretching.

Knee Injuries

Knee injuries, of which there are many types, are among the most serious joint injuries. Their severity is difficult to determine, thus professional medical care is necessary if the injury is from being hit or twisted and not from overuse. You probably have seen a physician or an athletic trainer performing stress tests on a player's knee on the sidelines at a football game. First aid providers should not perform such tests.

Knee Fracture

A fracture of the knee generally occurs as a result of a fall or a direct blow. Fractures about the knee may occur at the end of the femur, at the end of the **tibia**, or in the **patella** (kneecap).

What to Look For	What to Do
Determining whether a fracture exists is difficult. Some fractured knees may look like a dislocation. Other signs include: ▪ Deformity ▪ Tenderness ▪ Swelling	1. If CSM is absent in the ankle, immediately seek professional medical care. 2. If CSM exist with no deformity, splint the leg with the knee straight. 3. If CSM exist in the ankle with significant deformity, splint the knee in the position found. 4. Seek professional medical care.

Knee Dislocation

A knee dislocation is a serious injury. Do not confuse a knee dislocation with a patellar dislocation, which is a much less serious injury.

What to Look For	What to Do
▪ Excruciating pain ▪ Grotesque deformity ▪ Absent pulse in the ankle (posterior tibial)	1. Stabilize the knee in the position found. 2. Seek professional medical care immediately.

Patellar Dislocation

A dislocated patella can be a very painful injury and must be treated immediately. Some people have repeated kneecap dislocations, just as others have a tendency for shoulder dislocations. A dislocated patella most commonly occurs in teenagers and young adults who are engaged in athletic activities.

What to Look For	What to Do
▪ A blow or twisting causes the kneecap to be moved to the outside of the knee joint ▪ Possible swelling ▪ Inability to bend or straighten the knee ▪ Pain ▪ Deformity compared with the other kneecap **FIGURE 15-6**	1. Follow the RICE procedure (except compression). 2. **DO NOT** try to relocate a dislocated kneecap (sometimes the kneecap replaces itself). 3. Splint the knee in the position found. 4. Seek professional medical care.

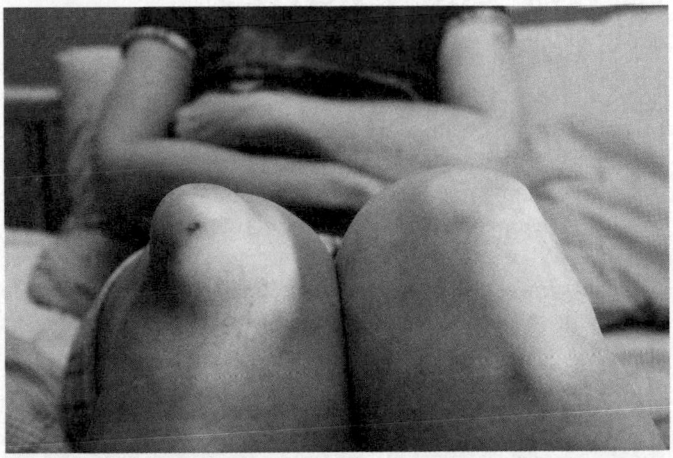

FIGURE 15-6 Patellar dislocation.

Knee Sprain

Ligament injuries occur most often in sports. The knee is very prone to ligament injury, ranging from mild sprains to complete tearing. The knee will be swollen and painful and usually cannot be used normally.

What to Look For	What to Do
At the time of injury, the following signs and symptoms may be present: ▪ Severe pain ▪ A pop or snap feeling ▪ A locking sensation ▪ Inability to walk without limping ▪ Inability to bend or straighten the knee Later, there may be: ▪ Swelling in the knee ▪ Bruising	1. Follow the RICE procedure. 2. Seek professional medical care.

Knee Contusion

Contusions of the knee are caused by a direct blow or by falling on the knee.

What to Look For	What to Do
After a direct blow to the kneecap, the person has: ▪ Pain ▪ Swelling ▪ Tenderness ▪ Bruise marks (black-and-blue discoloration)	Follow the RICE procedure.

Lower Leg Injuries

Tibia and Fibula Fractures

Tibia and **fibula** injuries can occur at any place between the knee joint and the ankle joint. When both bones are broken, there may be marked deformity of the leg. When only one bone is broken, the other acts as a splint, and little deformity may be present. Some people with a fibula fracture can walk on the injured leg. When the tibia is broken, an open fracture and severe deformity may exist. Injuries to the blood vessels, caused by the extreme deformity, are common with injuries of the tibia and the fibula, and the pain usually is severe.

What to Look For	What to Do
A direct blow or twisting force produces: ▪ Severe pain ▪ Swelling ▪ Visible deformity ▪ Tenderness when touched	1. Stabilize the leg using a splint, either improvised by tying the legs together or a rigid splint (two boards or two SAM splints—one on each side to prevent rotation of the lower leg bones). (See Chapter 16, *Splinting Extremities*.) 2. Apply an ice pack. 3. Seek professional medical care.

Tibia and Fibula Contusion

Many contusions simply cause a black-and-blue mark and some soreness, then clear up with little attention.

What to Look For	What to Do

▪ Person received a hit directly on the shin
▪ Tenderness when touched
▪ Sharp pain
▪ The following signs and symptoms appear later:
  ▪ Discoloration (black-and-blue mark)
  ▪ Difficulty moving ankle up and down
  ▪ Numbness or coldness in toes or foot
	1. Expose the injury.
	2. Follow the RICE procedure.
	3. If numbness or tingling exists, seek professional medical care.

Muscle Cramp

Muscle spasm or cramping usually occurs in the calf and sometimes in the thigh or hamstring. It is a temporary condition of little consequence.

What to Look For	What to Do

▪ Occurs during or after intense exercise sessions
▪ Painful, muscle contraction or spasm that disables the person
	1. There are many treatments for cramps. Try one or more of the following:
	  ▪ Have the person gently stretch the affected muscle. Because a muscle cramp is an uncontrolled muscle contraction or spasm, a gradual extension of the muscle may help lengthen the muscle fibers and relieve the cramp.
	  ▪ Relax the muscle by applying pressure to it.
	  ▪ Apply ice to the cramped muscle to make it relax (unless you are in a cold environment).
	  ▪ If the cramp is due to exertion in hot conditions, drink lightly salted, cool water (dissolve ¼ teaspoon [1.25 mL] salt in 1 quart [about 1 L] of water), or a commercial sports drink.

Shin Splints

Shin splints is a term that describes pain in the front of the lower leg, also called the shin. Shin splints are caused by repetitive stress in the leg, such as that caused by running and extensive walking.

What to Look For	What to Do
▪ Ache that occurs during activity but subsides significantly after activity stops ▪ Ache that is a result of an increase in the workout routine (eg, running longer, running on hills) ▪ Chronic condition that gets worse	1. Apply an ice pack before an activity. Heat can be applied later, when the person is well on the way to recovery. 2. Apply pressure with a 3-inch (8-cm) elastic bandage over the sorest point (start below the sore area and spiral wrap up and around the leg). 3. Apply an ice pack for 20 minutes after the activity. 4. Curtail activity until the shin is pain free. 5. OTC pain medications that are anti-inflammatory drugs may be taken according to package directions. Use ibuprofen or naproxen.

Ankle and Foot Injuries

The ankle and the foot frequently are injured, mainly by twisting, which stretches or tears the supporting ligaments. Incorrect treatment can have consequences that include lifelong disability. In some cases, the damage requires surgical correction. Most ankle injuries are sprains; about 85% of sprains involve the outside (lateral) ligaments and are caused by the ankle turning or twisting inward **FIGURE 15-7**.

What to Look For	What to Do
▪ Pain and/or a popping or tearing sensation that occurs at the time of the injury ▪ Swelling and complete loss of function of the ankle that develops minutes after the injury ▪ Tenderness or pain above, below, and to the sides of the injury when pressed	1. Take off the person's shoe and sock. **DO NOT** move the ankle. 2. Follow the RICE procedure. (**DO NOT** apply heat to the injury.) A horseshoe or "U"-shaped pad kept in place by an elastic bandage reduces fluid in the joint. 3. The amount of swelling and pain does not indicate the severity of the injury. If there is any question about the severity of the injury, splint and seek professional medical care.

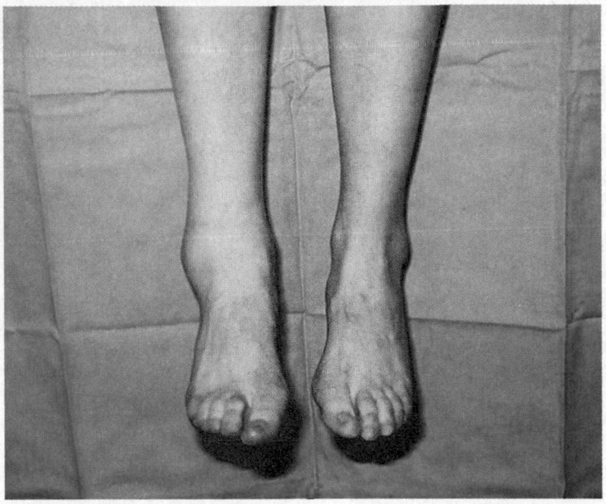

FIGURE 15-7 Sprained ankle.

FYI

Ankle and Foot Injuries: Is Something Broken?

Two symptoms were 95% accurate in predicting a broken ankle bone: (1) inability to bear weight and take four steps immediately after the injury and (2) tenderness at the back edge or tip of either malleolus bone (the projections on each side of the ankle). Similar symptoms predicted whether a foot bone was broken: (1) pain in the midfoot or tenderness at the base of the fifth metatarsal bone at the outer edge of the foot or at the navicular bone at the inner edge plus (2) inability to take four steps.

Data from Stiell IG, Greenberg GH, McKnight RD, et al. Implementation of the Ottawa ankle rules. *JAMA*. 1994;271(11):827–832.

Toe Injuries

The toes can be injured in various ways. The toes can be stepped on or the foot may kick a hard object, resulting in torn-off nails, hematoma (blood clot) formation under the nails, dislocations, or fractures.

What to Look For	What to Do
▪ Pain and swelling ▪ Deformity	For nail avulsions, splinters, blood under a nail, dislocations, and fractures, refer to the appropriate sections under finger injuries.

PREP KIT

Ready for Review

- Injuries to the extremities are common.
- There are many types of injuries to the extremities, ranging from simple contusions to complex open fractures.
- RICE is the acronym for Rest, Ice pack, Compression, and Elevation.
- Shoulder injuries include:
  - Shoulder dislocation
  - Clavicle fracture
  - Contusion
  - Tendinitis
- Elbow injuries include:
  - Elbow fracture and dislocation
  - Tennis elbow
  - Golfer's elbow
- Hand injuries include:
  - Crushed hand
- Finger injuries include:
  - Finger fracture
  - Finger dislocation
  - Sprained finger
  - Nail avulsion
  - Splinters
  - Blood under a nail
  - Ring strangulation
- Hip joint injuries include:
  - Hip dislocation
  - Hip fracture
- Thigh injuries include:
  - Femur fracture
  - Muscle contusion
  - Muscle strain
- Knee injuries include:
  - Knee fracture
  - Knee dislocation
  - Patella dislocation
  - Knee sprain
  - Knee contusion
- Lower leg injuries include:
  - Tibia and fibula fracture
  - Tibia and fibula contusion
  - Muscle cramp
  - Shin splints
  - Ankle and foot injuries
  - Toe injuries

Vital Vocabulary

clavicle The collarbone.

contusion A bruise; an injury that causes a hemorrhage in or beneath the skin but does not break the skin.

dislocation The displacement of a bone from its normal joint alignment, out of its socket, or out of its normal position.

femur The thigh bone; the longest and one of the strongest bones in the body.

fibula The smaller of the two bones of the lower leg.

fracture A break or crack in the bone.

humerus The supporting bone of the upper arm.

patella The kneecap; a specialized bone that lies within the tendon of the quadriceps muscle.

radius The bone on the thumb side of the forearm.

scapula The shoulder blade.

sprain A trauma to the joint that injures the ligaments.

strain An injury to a muscle caused by a violent contraction or an excessive, forcible stretching.

tendinitis Inflammation of a tendon caused by overuse.

tibia The shin bone; the larger of the two bones of the lower leg.

ulna The inner bone of the forearm, on the side opposite the thumb.

Assessment in Action

During a flag football game at a neighborhood park, your teammate is going back for a sure interception. He jumps for the ball, catches it, and comes down, twisting his ankle in a small hole on the field. Your teammate is in pain and is feeling nauseous.

Directions: Circle Yes if you agree with the statement; circle No if you disagree.

1. It is difficult to distinguish between a severely sprained ankle and a fractured ankle.

   YES **NO**

2. Use the RICE procedure, regardless of whether the ankle is sprained or fractured.

   YES **NO**

PREP KIT continued

3. Heat should be applied immediately to a sprained ankle to increase blood flow and decrease pain.

   YES **NO**

4. If you are unsure about the injury's severity, you should seek professional medical care.

   YES **NO**

Check Your Knowledge

Directions: Circle Yes if you agree with the statement; circle No if you disagree.

1. Injuries heal faster if rested.

   YES **NO**

2. Compression increases internal bleeding, helping the injury to heal faster.

   YES **NO**

3. Tennis elbow results from sharp, quick twists of the wrist.

   YES **NO**

4. The three bones in the fingers are very strong and do not break easily.

   YES **NO**

5. The hip joint is easily dislocated.

   YES **NO**

6. Considerable force is required to break the femur.

   YES **NO**

7. A strain is actually a tear in the muscle.

   YES **NO**

8. Knee injuries are not serious.

   YES **NO**

9. Shin splints are a pain that runs down the back of the leg.

   YES **NO**

10. Most ankle injuries are not fractures.

    YES **NO**

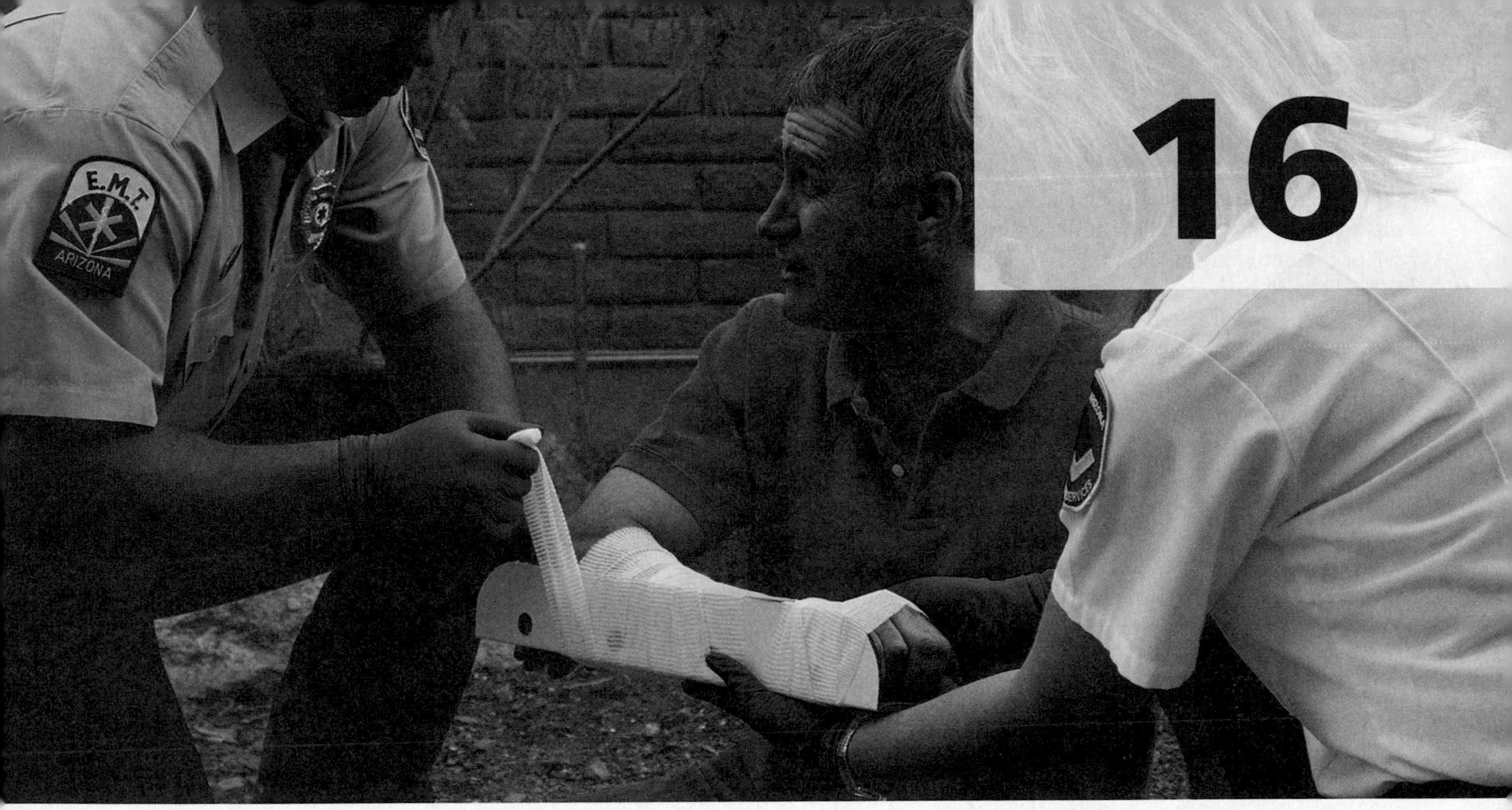

Splinting Extremities

CHAPTER AT A GLANCE

Splinting Extremities

First aid providers usually do not need to splint broken bones. The best first aid for most fractures, whether obvious or not, is nonmovement and comfort until emergency medical services (EMS) arrive; however, splinting is advantageous when EMS is delayed or the person is being transported by a first aid provider.

Injured extremities should be stabilized by splinting the extremity in the position in which it was found. To **stabilize** means to minimize further injury by holding a body part to prevent movement. All fractures should be stabilized before a person is moved. The reasons for splinting to stabilize an injured area are to:

- Reduce pain
- Prevent damage to muscles, nerves, and blood vessels
- Prevent a closed fracture from becoming an open fracture
- Reduce bleeding and swelling

All fractures are complicated to some degree by damage to the soft tissue and structures surrounding the bone. The major cause of tissue damage at a fracture site is movement by the end of the broken bone. The end of a broken bone is sharp, and it is important to prevent a fractured bone from moving into soft tissues.

Types of Splints

A **splint** is any device used to stabilize a fracture or a dislocation. Such a device can be improvised (eg, a folded newspaper), or it can be one of several commercially available splints (eg, padded aluminum splint such as a SAM splint). Lack of a commercial splint should never prevent you from properly stabilizing an injured extremity. Splinting sometimes requires improvisation.

A rigid splint is an inflexible device attached to an extremity to maintain stability. It can be a padded board, a piece of heavy cardboard, or a SAM splint molded to fit the extremity. Whatever its construction, a rigid splint must be long enough to be secured well above and below the fracture site.

A soft splint, such as a pillow, towel, or blanket tied with bandage materials (eg, cravat bandage), is useful mainly for stabilizing fractures of the lower leg or the forearm **FIGURE 16-1**.

A self-splint, also called an anatomic splint or buddy splint, is often available because it uses the body itself as the splint. A self-splint is one in which the injured extremity is tied to an uninjured part (eg, an injured finger to the adjacent finger, the legs together, or an injured arm to the chest).

Splinting Guidelines

All fractures and dislocations should be stabilized before the person is moved. When in doubt, apply a splint. To apply a splint:

1. Cover any open wounds with a sterile dressing before applying a splint.
2. Check the CSM (circulation, sensation, movement) before and after splinting Skill Sheet 14-1). If pulses are absent and medical help is hours away, gently line up a fracture or a dislocation to restore blood flow. Support the limb and move it gently to line up the parts. Joints may be left in a position of comfort. Line up the limb above and below the joint; however, **DO NOT** force anything into position. Any movement of a fracture is expected to cause pain; you should be aware of this and warn the person. You do not have to align the limb perfectly; just align it enough to allow the return of circulation.
3. Determine what to splint by using the **rule of thirds**. Imagine each long bone as being divided into thirds. If the injury is located in the upper or lower third of a bone, assume that the nearest joint is injured. Therefore, the splint should extend to stabilize the bones above and below the unstable joint. Stabilize or minimize movement of the bone ends and of the two adjacent joints. For example, for a fracture of the upper third of the tibia (shin bone), the splint must extend above the knee to include the upper leg, as well as the lower leg, because the knee is unstable. For a fracture of the middle third of a bone, stabilize the joints above and below the fracture (eg, the wrist and elbow for a fractured radius or ulna; the shoulder and elbow for a fractured humerus; the knee and ankle for a fractured tibia or fibula). In addition to splinting an upper extremity fracture, place the injured arm in an arm sling and a swathe (binder).
4. If two first aid providers are present, one should support the injury site and minimize movement of the extremity until splinting is completed.
5. When possible, place splint materials on both sides of the injured part, especially when two bones are involved, such as the radius and ulna in the lower arm or the tibia and fibula in the lower leg. This "sandwich splint" prevents the injured extremity from rotating and keeps the two bones from touching. With rigid splints, use extra padding in natural body hollows and around any deformities.

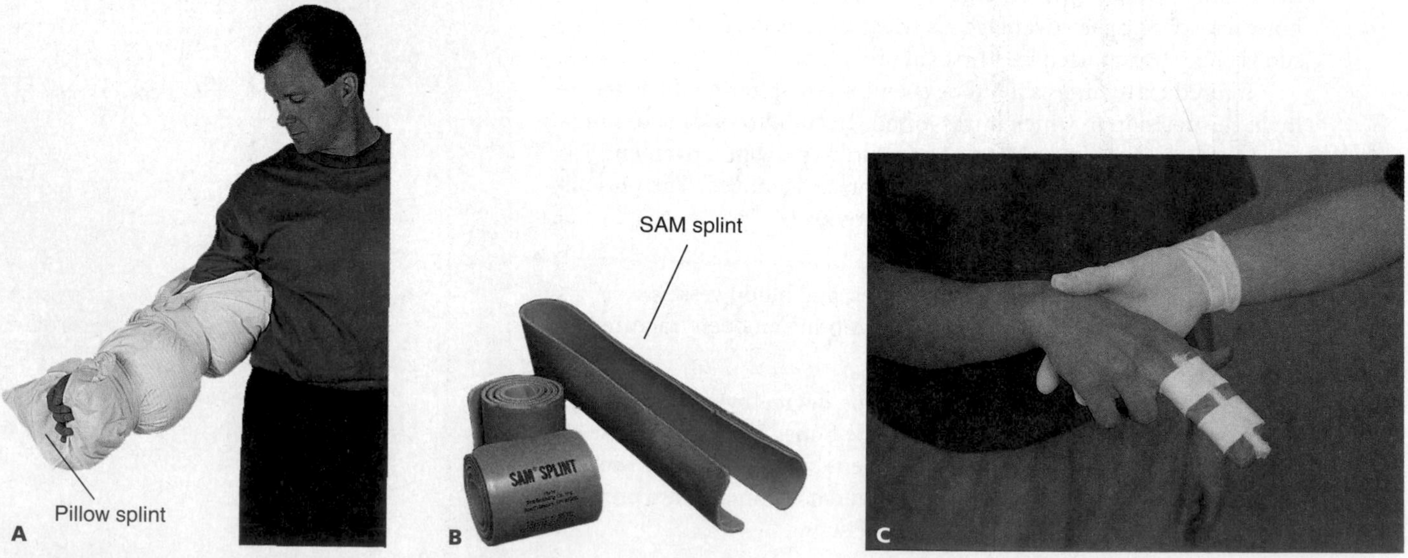

FIGURE 16-1 Examples of splints. **A**. Pillow splint. **B**. SAM® splint. **C**. Buddy splint.

6. Apply splints firmly but not so tightly that blood flow into an extremity is affected. Check the CSM before and periodically after the splint is applied. If the pulse disappears, loosen the splint enough so you can feel the pulse. Leave the fingers or toes exposed so the CSM can be checked easily.
7. Use the RICE (rest, ice pack, compression, and elevation) procedure on the injured part. When practical, elevate the injured extremity after it is stabilized to promote drainage and reduce swelling. **DO NOT**, however, apply ice packs if a pulse is absent.

If you suspect a spinal injury, have the person remain as still as possible. **DO NOT** apply a cervical collar. Wait for trained EMS providers to arrive with the proper equipment.

Most fractures do not require rapid transportation. An exception is an arm or a leg without a pulse, which means there is insufficient blood flow to the injured extremity. In that case, immediate professional medical care is necessary.

Seek professional medical care for the following injuries or situations:

- Any open fracture
- Any dislocation (injury that causes joint deformity)
- Any joint injury with moderate to severe swelling
- Any injury in which there is deformity, tenderness, or swelling over the bone
- If the person is unable to walk or bear weight after a lower extremity injury
- If a snap, crackle, or pop was heard at the time of injury
- If the injured area, especially a joint, becomes hot, tender, swollen, or painful
- If you are unsure whether a bone was broken
- If the injury does not improve rapidly, especially over the first few days

CAUTION

DO NOT straighten dislocations or fractures of the spine, elbow, wrist, hip, or knee because of the proximity of major nerves and arteries. Instead, if the distal CSM assessment findings are normal, splint joint injuries in the position in which you find them.

Slings

A **sling** is a triangular bandage applied around the neck to support an injured upper extremity. There are several types of slings:

- Regular/common
- Shoulder/clavicle
- Improvised—if materials are unavailable, you may need to improvise a sling **FIGURE 16-2**.

A folded triangular bandage, known as a cravat, can be used as a **swathe** (binder) in conjunction with a sling. A cravat can be used instead of a sling when splints on the arm are too large for a sling to fit. Loop the cravat around the wrist and around the neck to support the forearm. To apply a common arm sling to the upper arm, forearm, or hand/wrist injuries, follow the steps in **SKILL SHEET 16-1**. To apply a sling to the shoulder or clavicle, follow the steps in **SKILL SHEET 16-2**.

Splinting Specific Areas

Shoulder

Shoulder injuries involve the clavicle (collarbone), the scapula (shoulder blade), or the head of the humerus (upper arm). To stabilize the shoulder and upper arm against movement, apply a sling.

1. Check CSM and use the capillary refill test for signs of circulation loss.
2. The hand should be in a thumb-up position in the sling and slightly above the level of the elbow.

To further stabilize the arm, fold another triangular bandage to make a swathe that measures 3 to 4 inches (8 to 10 cm) wide. Tie the swathe (binder) around the upper arm and chest of the person. This stabilizes the clavicle (collarbone) and most shoulder injuries, as well as upper humerus (upper arm) fractures.

Most shoulder dislocations (approximately 95%) are anterior, meaning that the top of the humerus pops out in front of the shoulder joint. The person will hold the arm in a fixed position away from the chest wall. In these cases, the most comfortable splinting method is to place a pillow or rolled blanket between the involved arm and the chest. This fills the space created; you can then use cravats or a roller bandage to secure the arm against the chest. If the injury occurs in a remote setting (hours from professional medical care), use one of the methods described in Chapter 24, *Wilderness First Aid*, to reduce an anterior shoulder dislocation.

Humerus (Upper Arm)

Fractures of the humerus (upper arm) should be stabilized with a rigid splint. Extend the splint along the outside of the humerus. Then apply a sling and a swathe over the rigid splint, using the chest wall as an additional splint **SKILL SHEET 16-3**.

Elbow

An elbow must be stabilized in the position in which it is found—if bent, splint it bent; if straight, splint it straight. Be sure to assess CSM before and after splinting. If the injured elbow is straight, place a rigid splint along the inside of the arm from the hand to the armpit. Secure the splint with a roller bandage or several cravat bandages. For a bent elbow, apply a rigid splint diagonally, so that it extends from the humerus (near the armpit) to the wrist, to prevent motion of the elbow. Depending on how bent the elbow is, you can also use a sling and a swathe (binder) for a bent elbow.

To splint an elbow in the bent position, follow the steps in **SKILL SHEET 16-4**. To splint an elbow in the straight position, follow the steps in **SKILL SHEET 16-5**.

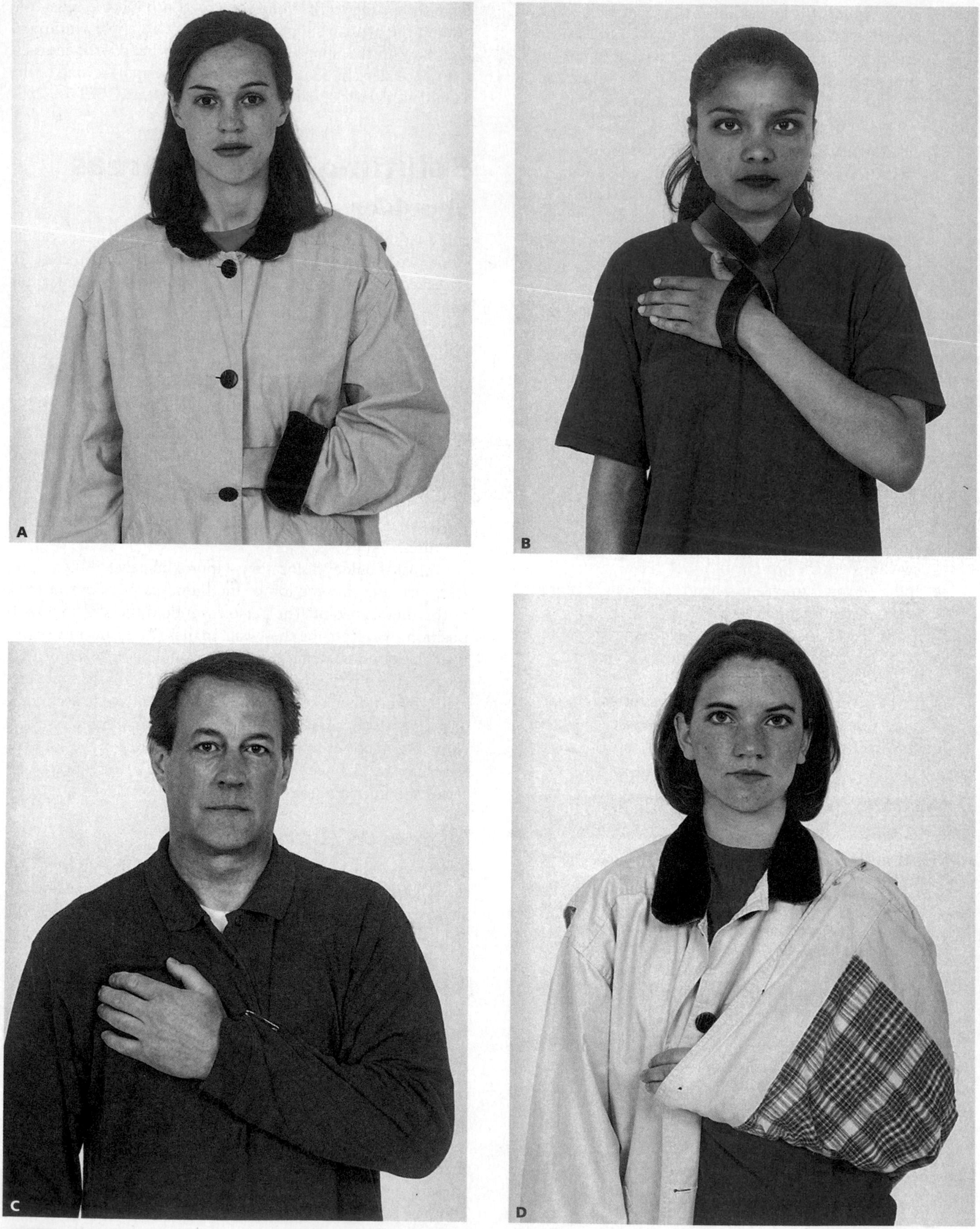

FIGURE 16-2 Improvised slings. **A**. A buttoned jacket. **B**. A belt, necktie, or other clothing item looped around the neck and the injured arm. **C**. Sleeve of the jacket or shirt pinned to the clothing. **D**. Lower edge of the person's jacket or shirt pinned up over the injured arm.

SKILL SHEET 16-1 Arm Sling for an Arm Injury

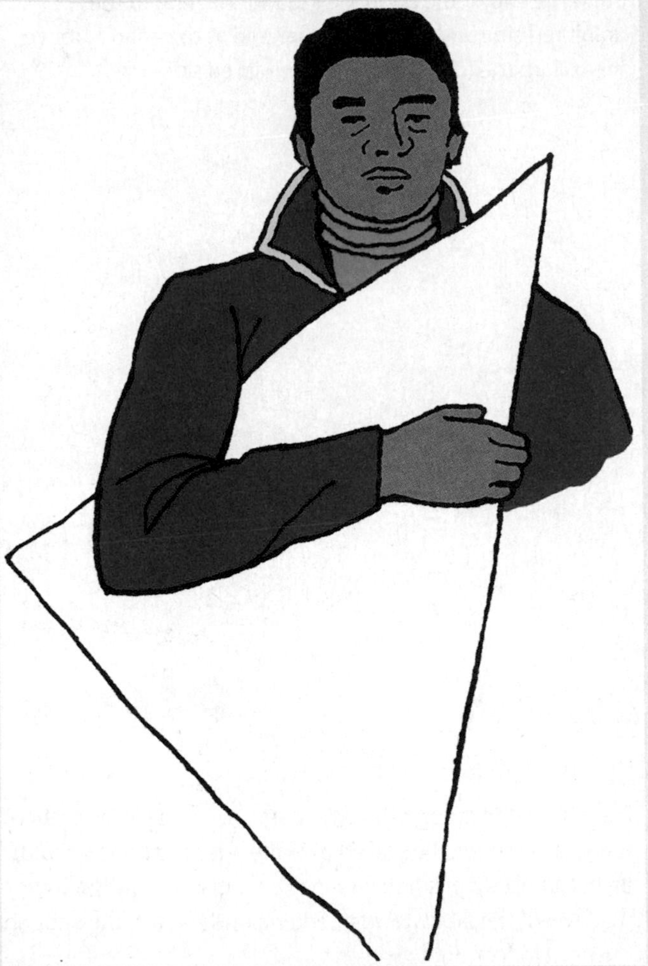

© Jones & Bartlett Learning.

1 Place the bandage between the forearm and the chest, with the point of the bandage toward the elbow of the injured arm, and stretch it beyond the elbow. Pull the upper end of the bandage over the uninjured shoulder.

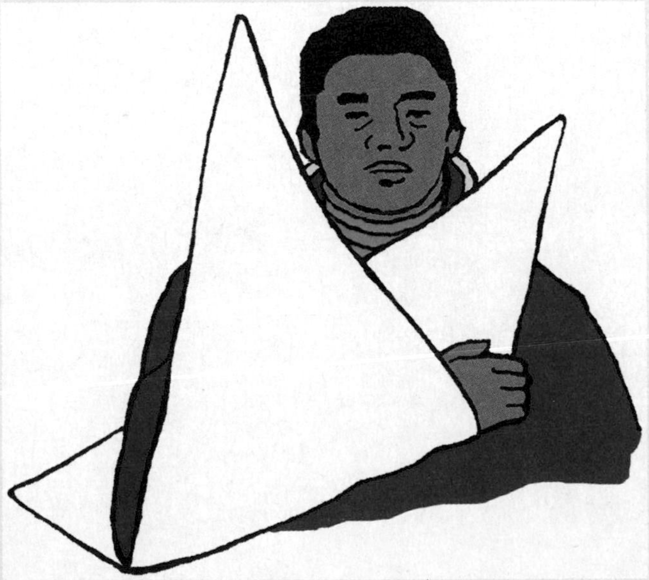

© Jones & Bartlett Learning.

2 Bring the lower end of the bandage over the forearm.

Continues

SKILL SHEET 16-1 Arm Sling for an Arm Injury (*Continued*)

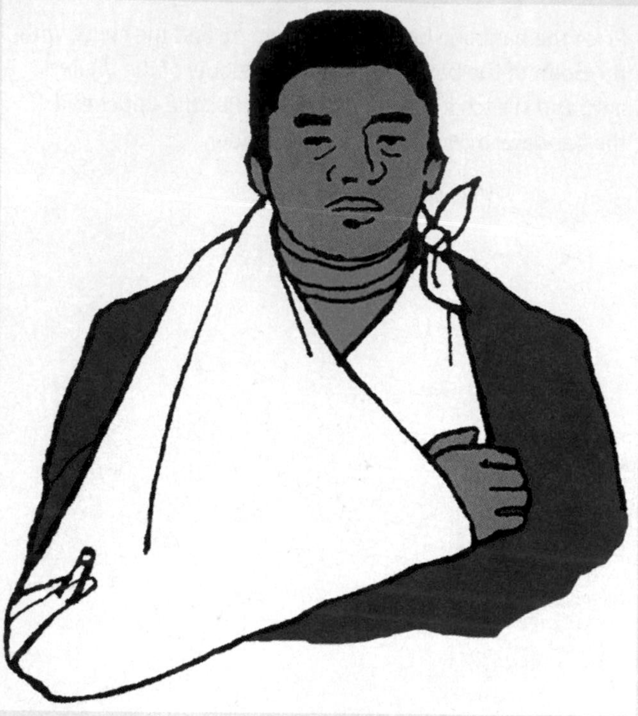

3 Bring the end of the bandage around the neck to the uninjured side and tie to the other end at the hollow above the collarbone (clavicle) on the uninjured side.

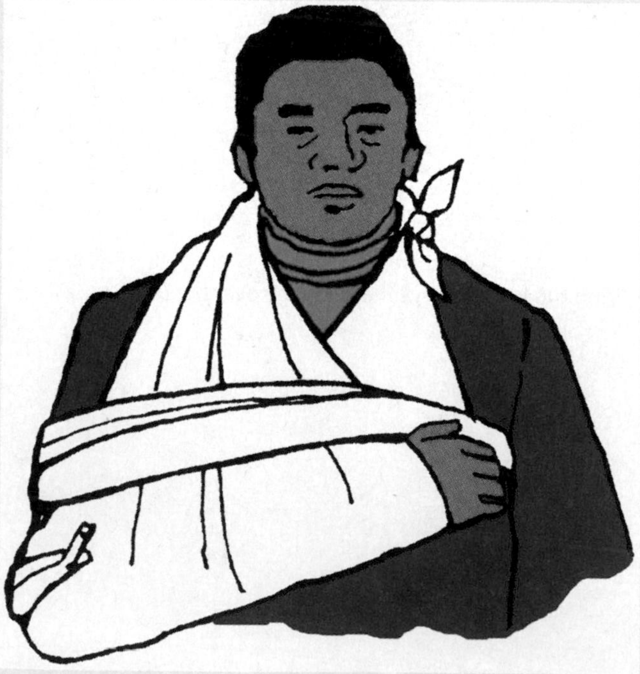

4 Place a swathe around the upper arm and body. The center of the swathe should be placed over the arm. The hand should be in thumb-up position within the sling and slightly above the level of the elbow. Place padding underneath the knot on the neck for comfort.

SKILL SHEET 16-2 Sling for Clavicle or Shoulder Injury

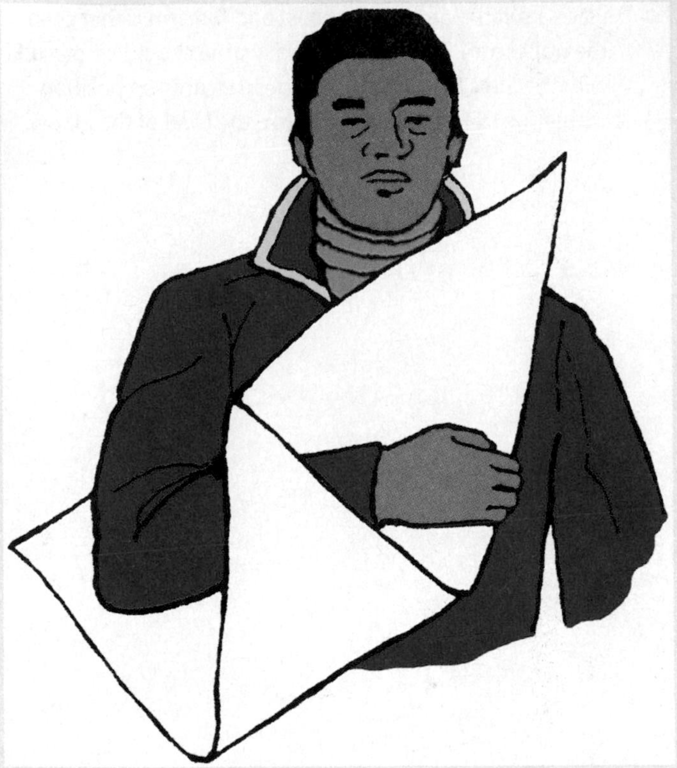

1 Place the bandage between the forearm and the chest, with the point of the bandage toward the elbow of the injured arm, and stretch it beyond the elbow. Pull the upper end of the bandage over the uninjured shoulder. Bring the other end out of the bandage over the forearm and tuck it under the armpit on the injured side.

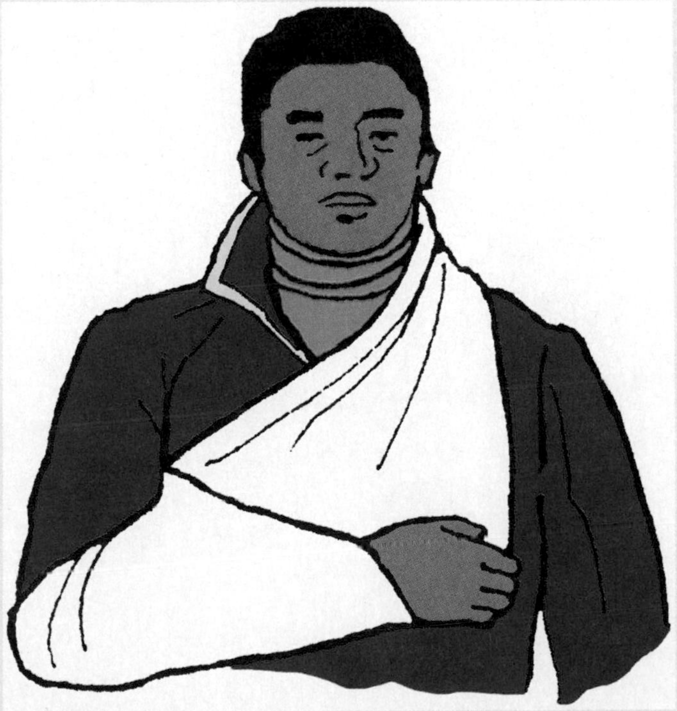

2 Continue bringing the lower end of the bandage around the victim's back and tie it to the upper end of the bandage.

Continues

SKILL SHEET 16-2 Sling for Clavicle or Shoulder Injury (*Continued*)

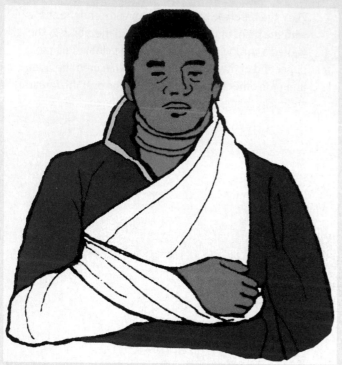

3 Place a swathe around the chest and forearm rather than the upper arm. The center of the swathe should be placed over the arm. The hand should be in thumb-up position within the sling and slightly above the level of the elbow.

4 Tie the swathe behind the person's back.

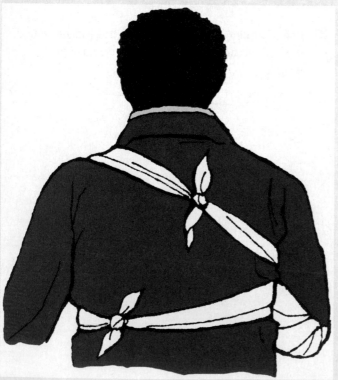

SKILL SHEET 16-3 Splinting Upper Arm (Humerus)

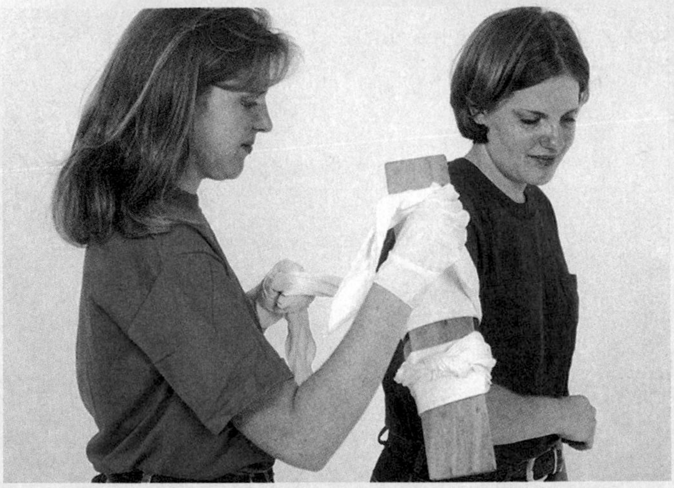

1 Assess CSM before splinting. Gently place the injured arm across the chest. If available, tie a rigid splint to the outside of the arm. If a rigid splint is not available, go to **Step 2**.

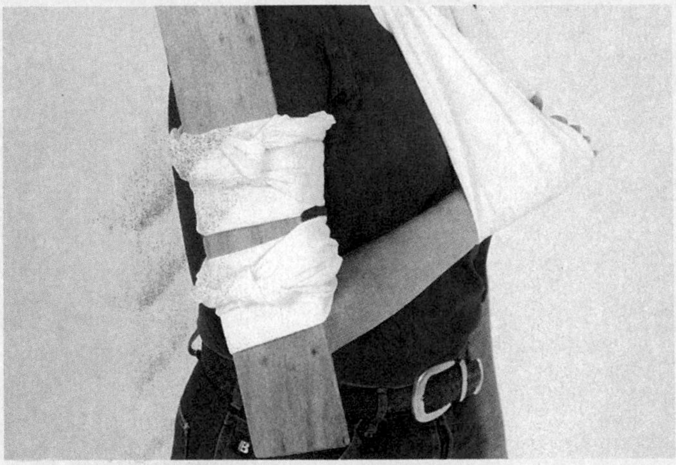

2 Loop a cravat or strap around the neck and wrist to allow the arm to hang in the sling position.

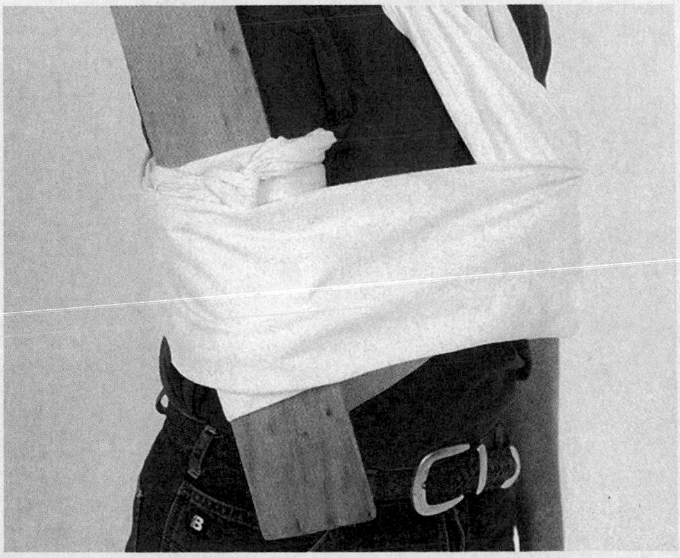

3 Secure the arm to the chest with a swathe (folded triangular bandage). Assess CSM after splinting.

SKILL SHEET 16-4 Splinting Elbow in Bent Position

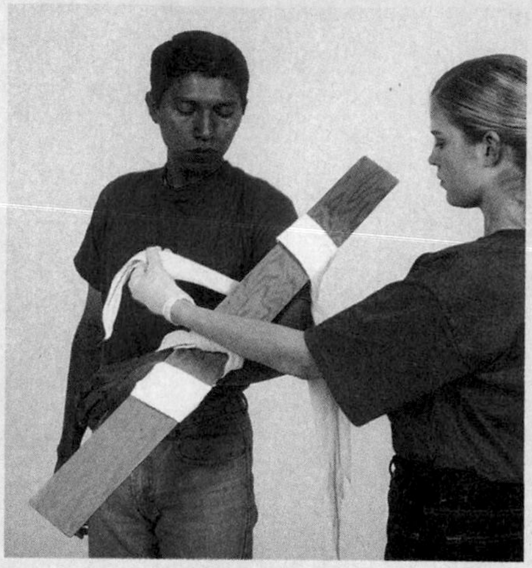

1 Assess CSM before splinting. If the injured elbow is bent, place a rigid splint or SAM splint from the upper arm to the wrist.

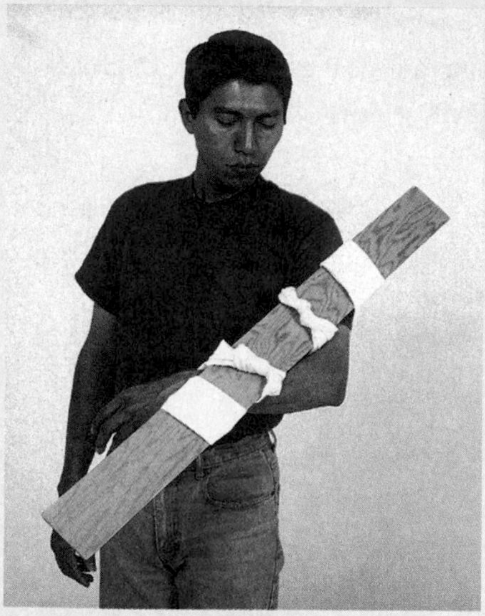

2 Tie a rigid splint or SAM splint onto the arm with cravat bandages.

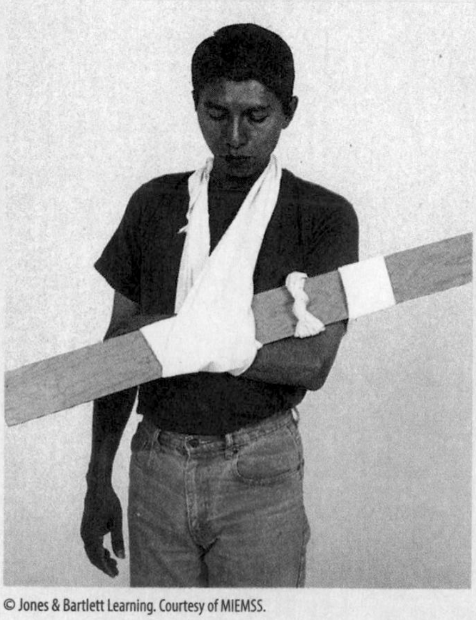

3 Place the arm in a sling, and assess CSM after splinting.

SKILL SHEET 16-5 Splinting Elbow in Straight Position

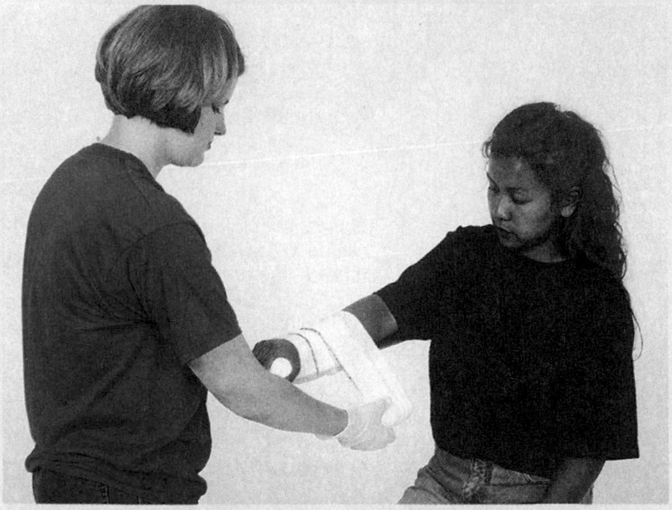

1 Assess CSM before splinting. If the injured elbow is straight, place a rigid splint along the inside of the arm from the hand to the armpit.

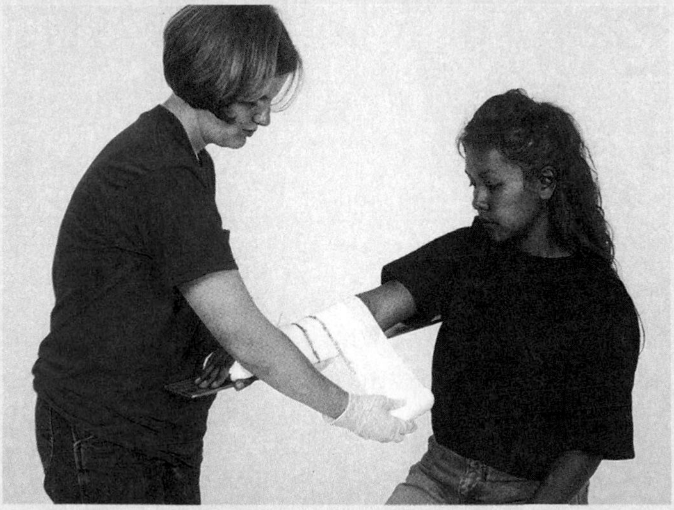

2 Secure with a roller bandage or several cravat bandages.

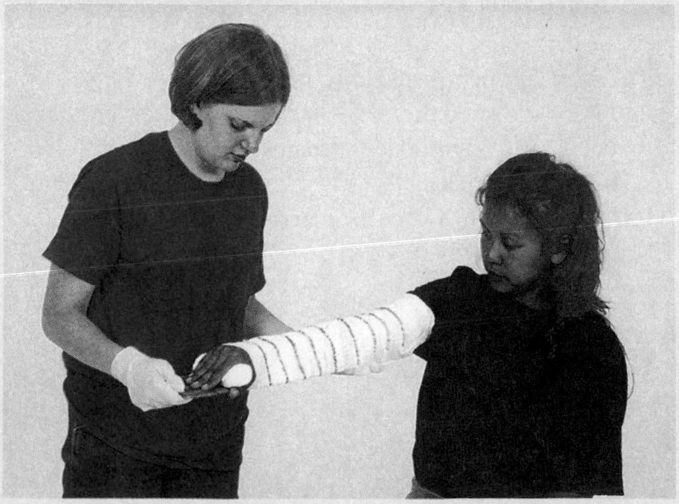

3 Assess CSM after splinting.

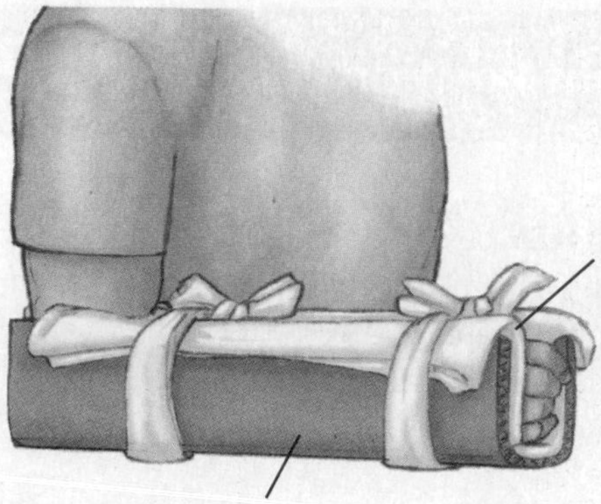
Keep thumb upright.
Rigid splint from palm out past elbow.
A

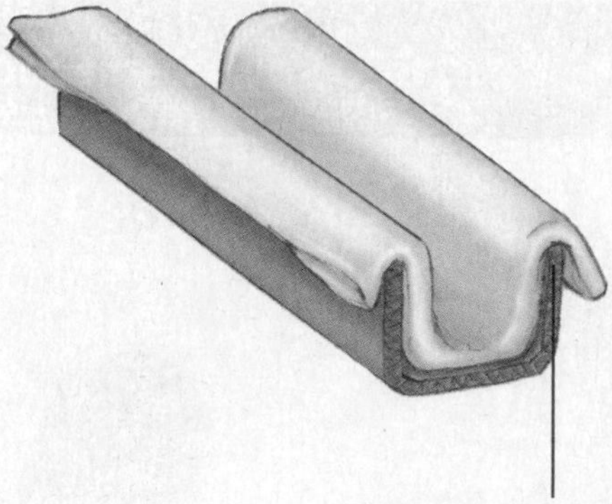
Splints should be on both sides to prevent rotation (shows use of cardboard).
B

FIGURE 16-3 Splinting a forearm fracture. **A**. Attach a rigid splint on both sides of the forearm that extends along the forearm. **B**. Place a rigid splint (eg, cardboard, wooden board, newspaper, magazine) under the forearm (see Skill Sheet 16-6 and Figure 16-5).

Forearm

To stabilize a forearm fracture, place the hand of the injured arm in the position of function (hand looks like it is holding a baseball) by placing a rolled pair of socks or a roller bandage in the palm. Then attach a rigid splint that extends past the tips of the fingers along the forearm and goes to or above the elbow. An option is to place splints on both sides of the injured part to keep the forearm from twisting or rotating **FIGURE 16-3**.

Keep the person's thumb in an upright position so that the two bones in the forearm (the radius and the ulna) do not touch each other. Secure the splint with a roller bandage or several cravats. A pillow or a rolled, folded blanket also can be secured to the arm. Put the arm in a sling and secure it with a swathe (binder) around the body **FIGURE 16-4**. To splint the forearm, follow the steps in **SKILL SHEET 16-6** and **SKILL SHEET 16-7**.

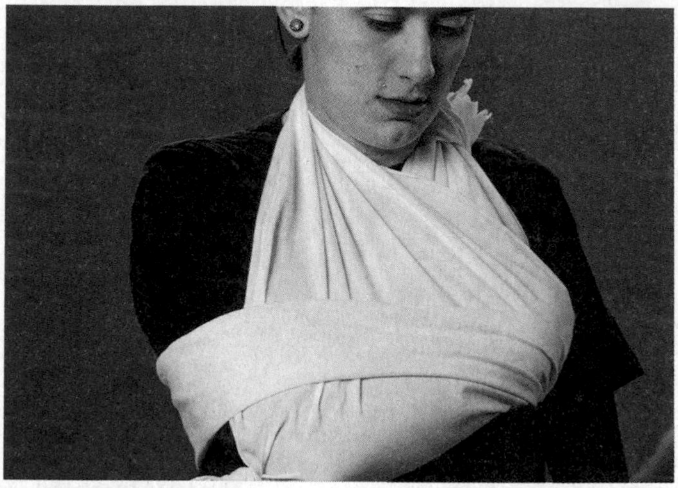

FIGURE 16-4 An arm sling with a swathe (binder) helps stabilize upper extremity injuries.

SKILL SHEET 16-6 Applying a Rigid Splint on a Forearm

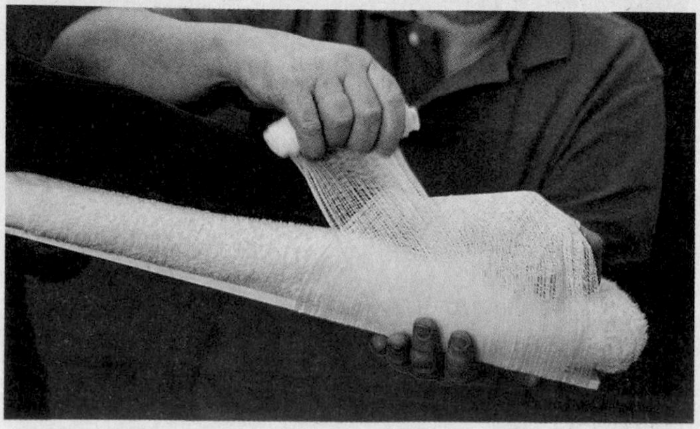

1 Assess CSM before splinting. Place a rigid object (eg, cardboard, wood board, folded newspaper or magazine) under the forearm. Place padding (eg, towel, T-shirt) between the rigid object and the skin, and place padding in the palm (eg, roller bandage, wad of cloth).

SKILL SHEET 16-6 Applying a Rigid Splint on a Forearm (*Continued*)

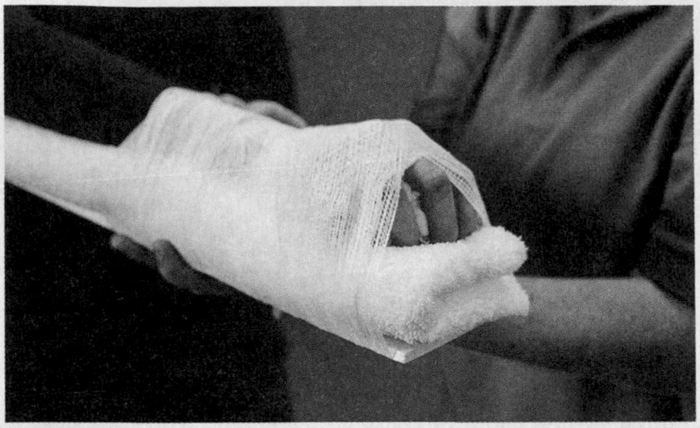

2 Secure the splint onto the arm by using either a roller bandage or folded triangular bandages (known as cravat bandages).

3 Place the arm in a sling with a binder. Assess CSM after splinting.

SKILL SHEET 16-7 Applying a Soft Splint on a Forearm

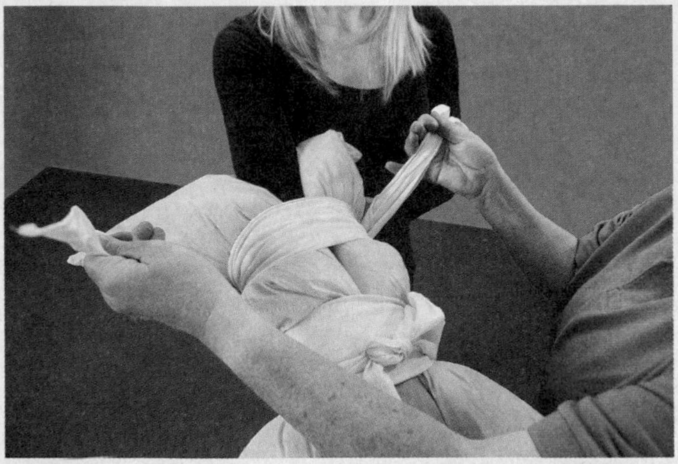

1 Assess CSM before splinting. Wrap a pillow or folded blanket around the forearm.

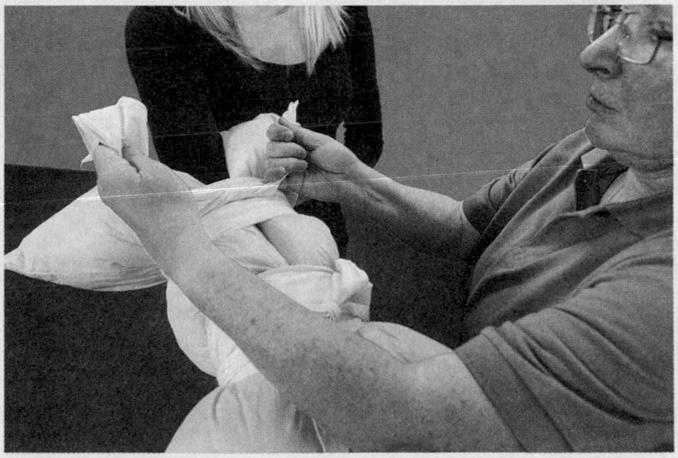

2 Secure the soft splint (eg, pillow) by using folded triangular bandages (known as cravat bandages) or cloth bands.

3 Place the arm in a sling with a binder. Assess CSM after splinting.

Wrist, Hand, and Fingers

To stabilize the wrist, hand, and fingers, use one of the following three methods:

- Place the injured hand in the position of function (hand looks like it is holding a baseball) by placing a rolled pair of socks or a roller bandage in the palm. Then attach a rigid splint that extends past the tips of the fingers along the forearm **FIGURE 16-5**.
- Place the hand in the position of function, mold a pillow around the hand and forearm, and tie the pillow in place with cravats or a roller bandage. Then place the arm in a sling and a swathe (binder), with the thumb in an upright position.
- Splint fingers by taping them together (buddy taping), with gauze separating the fingers.

Pelvis and Hip

If you suspect a pelvis or hip fracture, stabilize the person as you found them. **DO NOT** lift the legs, and wait for EMS to arrive.

Femur (Thigh)

A fractured femur is best splinted with a traction splint, which requires special training to use. Traction splints are seldom available except on ambulances.

Call 9-1-1 immediately. Tell the person not to move. Keep them lying down. **DO NOT** move or attempt to straighten the leg. Apply an ice pack while waiting for EMS. Treat for shock, but **DO NOT** raise the injured leg.

Knee

Always stabilize an injured knee in the position in which you find it. If the knee is straight, splint it straight; if it is bent, splint it bent **FIGURE 16-6**.

For a straight knee, there are three options: (1) tie one long, padded board that extends from the hip to the ankle underneath the leg; (2) tie two boards along the sides of the leg, one between the person's legs that extends from the groin to the foot and the other on the outer side that extends from the hip to the foot; or (3) tie the injured leg to the uninjured one.

For a bent knee, tie a long board extending from just below the hip to just above the ankle to prevent motion of the knee. Or place a pillow or a rolled blanket beneath the knee and tie the injured leg to the uninjured leg.

To splint a knee in the straight position, follow the steps in **SKILL SHEET 16-8**. To splint a knee in the bent position, follow the steps in **SKILL SHEET 16-9**.

Lower Leg

Stabilize the lower leg with two boards that extend from the upper thigh to the bottom of the foot. Or, place a folded blanket or pillow between the person's legs for padding, and then tie the injured leg to the uninjured leg with several swathes, cravats, or bandages.

To splint the lower leg using the self-splint method, follow the steps in **SKILL SHEET 16-10**. To splint the leg using rigid splints, follow the steps in **SKILL SHEET 16-11**.

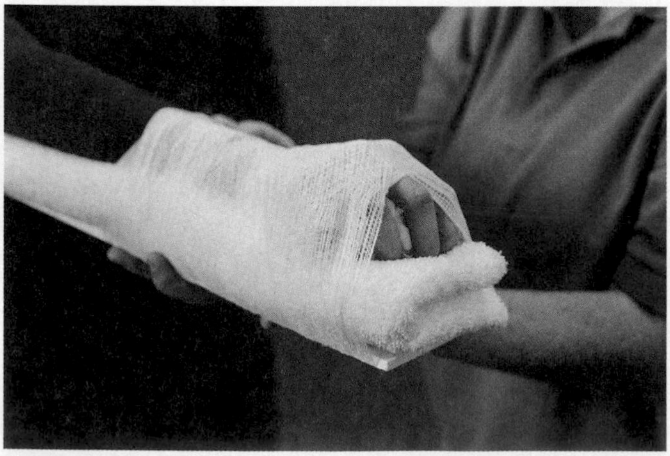

FIGURE 16-5 Splinting a wrist, hand, or finger fracture.

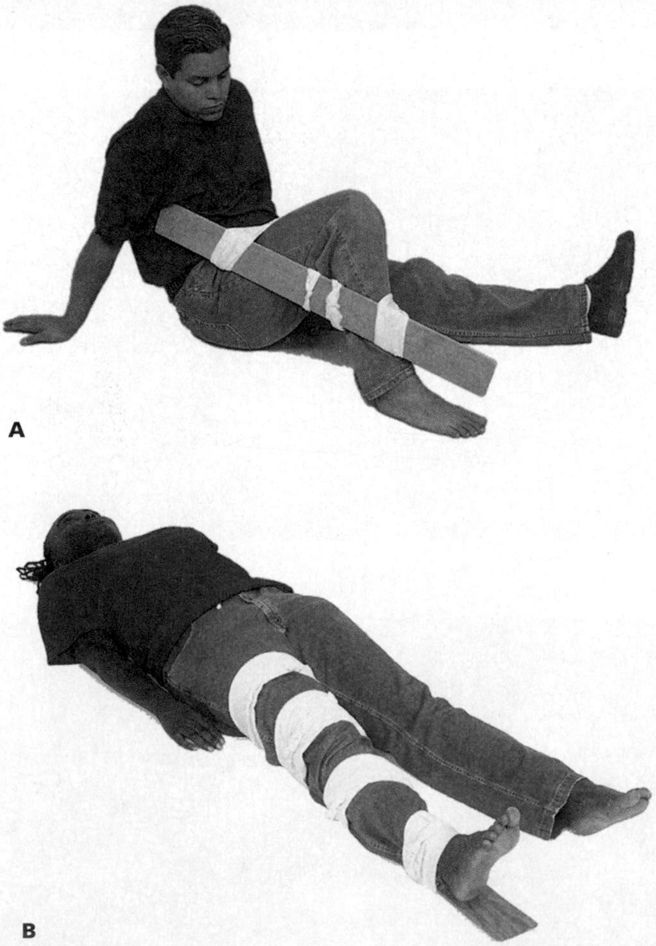

FIGURE 16-6 Splint knee in position found. **A**. If the knee is bent, splint it bent. **B**. If the knee is straight, splint it straight.

SKILL SHEET 16-8 Splinting a Knee in the Straight Position

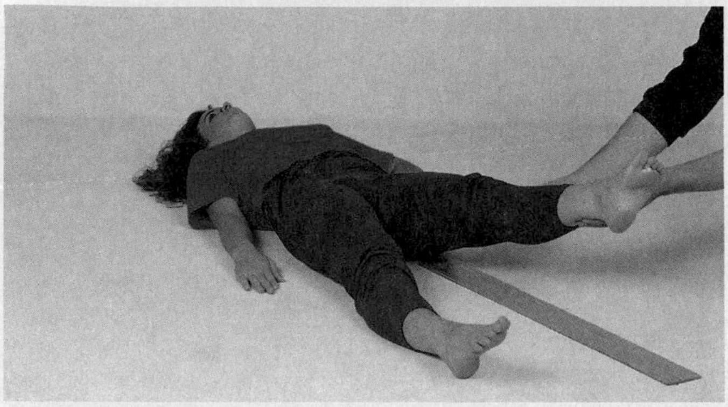

1 Assess CSM before splinting. Lift the injured leg and place a rigid splint (long board) under the leg. The splint should extend from the buttocks to beyond the foot.

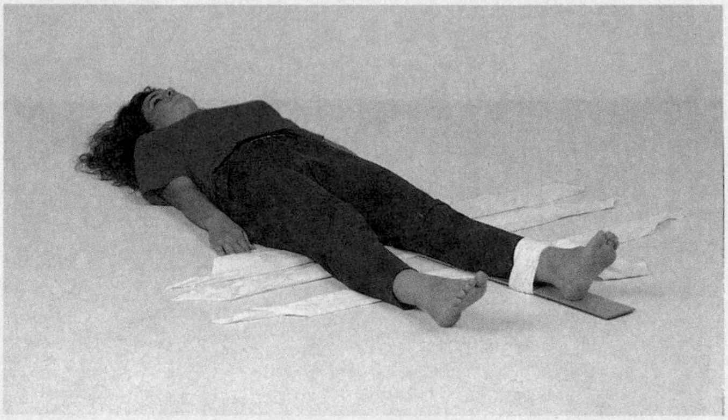

2 Place cravat bandages under the rigid splint and place soft padding under the knee and ankle.

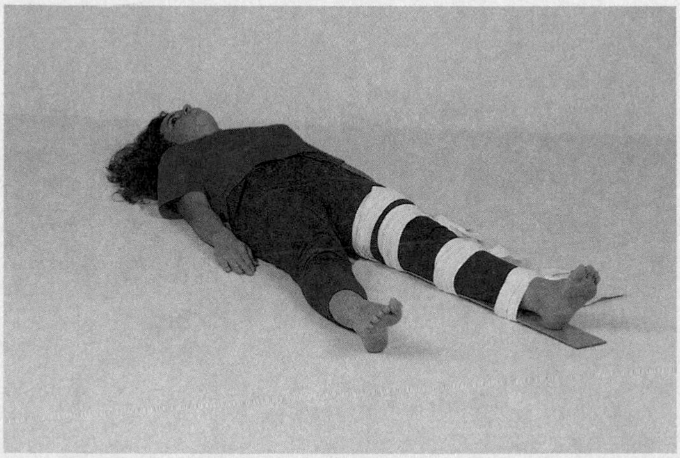

3 Tie the cravat bandages. **DO NOT** tie the knots over the injured area. **DO NOT** tie the knot over skin. All knots should be tied against the splinting material. Assess CSM after splinting.

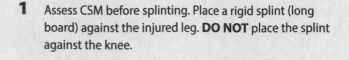

SKILL SHEET 16-9 Splinting a Knee in the Bent Position

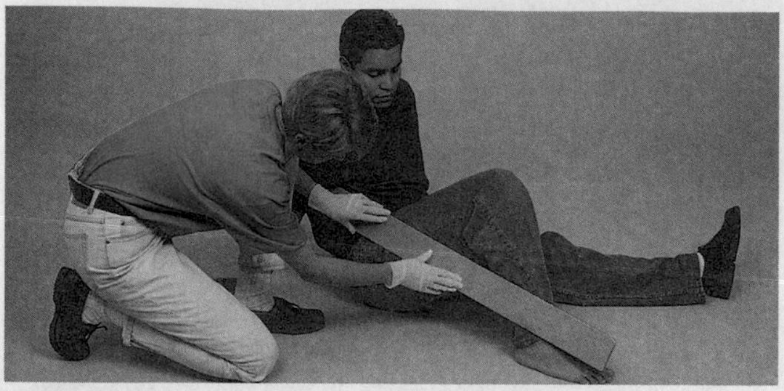

© Jones & Bartlett Learning. Courtesy of MIEMSS.

1 Assess CSM before splinting. Place a rigid splint (long board) against the injured leg. **DO NOT** place the splint against the knee.

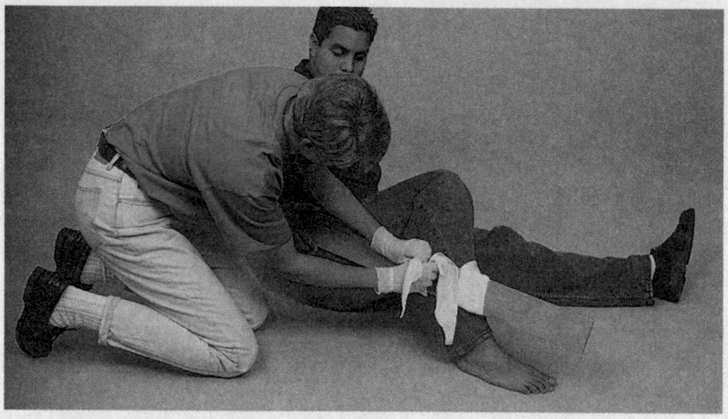

© Jones & Bartlett Learning. Courtesy of MIEMSS.

2 Tie a cravat bandage around the splint and lower leg.

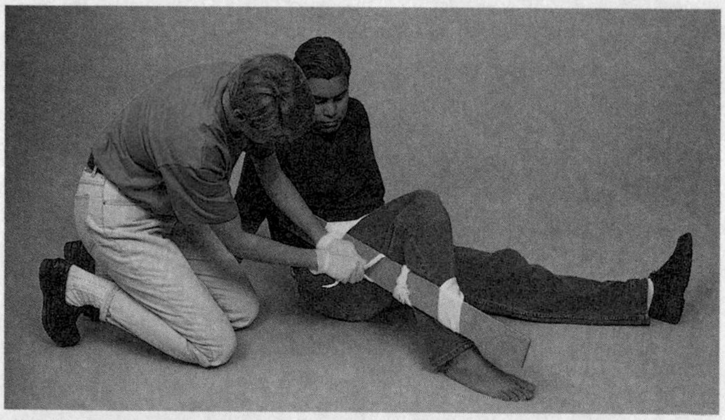

© Jones & Bartlett Learning. Courtesy of MIEMSS.

3 Tie a cravat bandage around the splint and thigh.

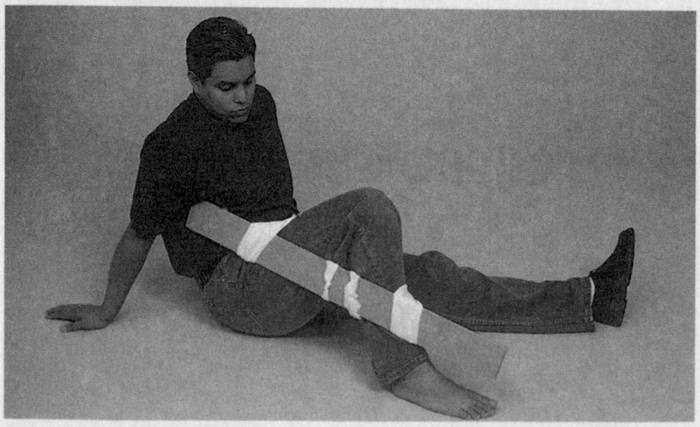

© Jones & Bartlett Learning. Courtesy of MIEMSS.

4 Tie knots over the splint, not over the leg. Assess CSM after splinting.

SKILL SHEET 16-10 Splinting Lower Leg (Self-Splint)

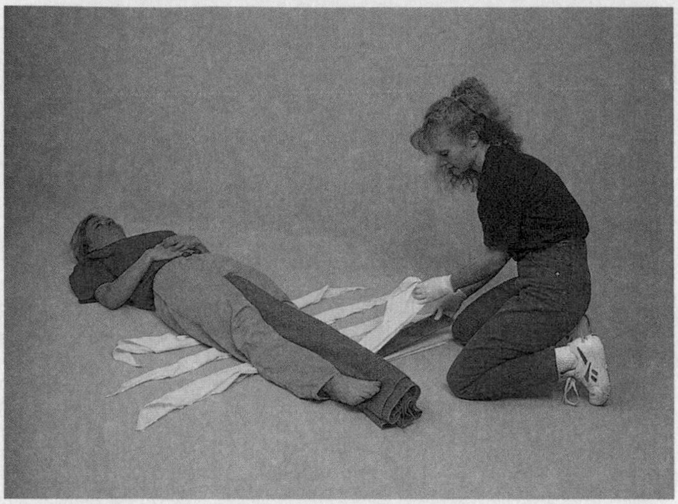

1 Assess CSM before splinting. Place padding (folded blanket) between the legs. Push the cravat bandages under the leg with a thin board.

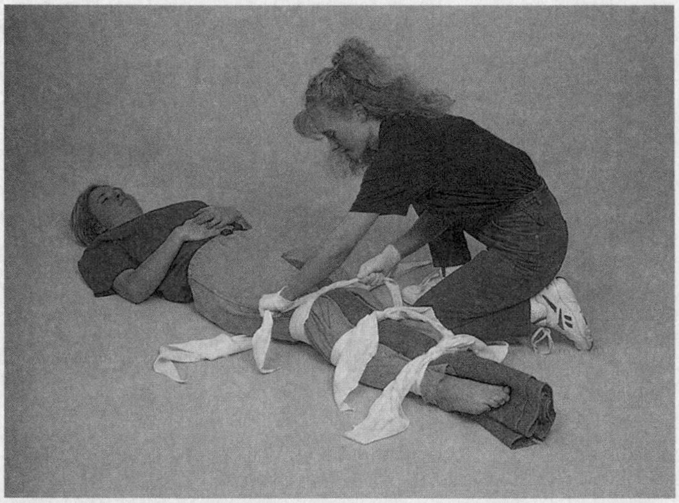

2 Tie the legs together.

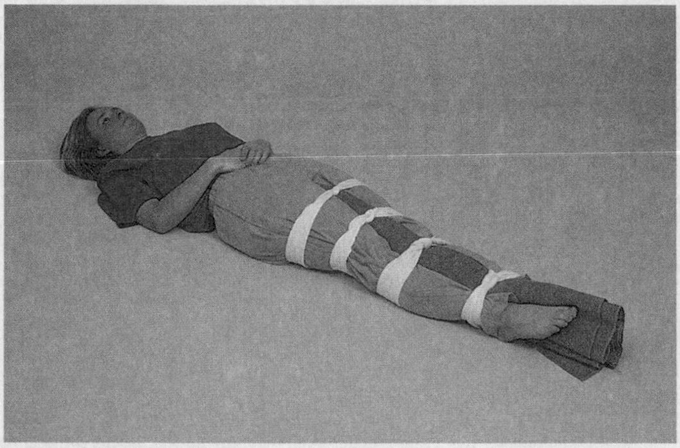

3 Tie knots between the legs, over the padding (folded blanket). Assess CSM after splinting.

SKILL SHEET 16-11 Splinting Leg (Rigid Splint)

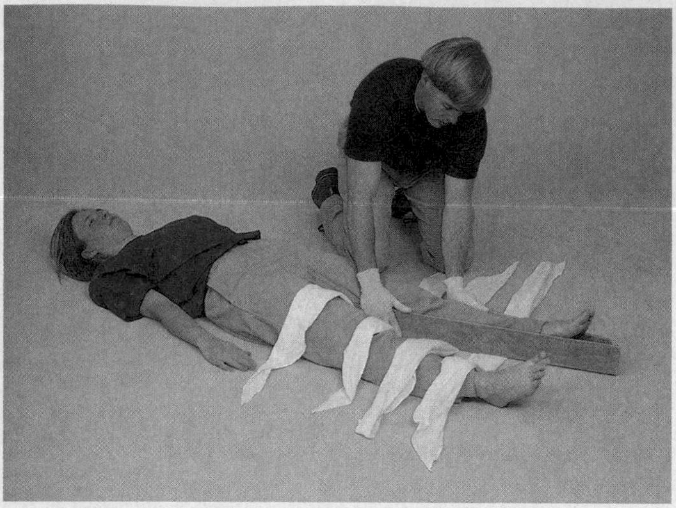

1 Assess CSM before splinting. Place one rigid splint (board) on the outside (lateral) and another inside (medial). Push the cravat bandages under the leg with a thin board.

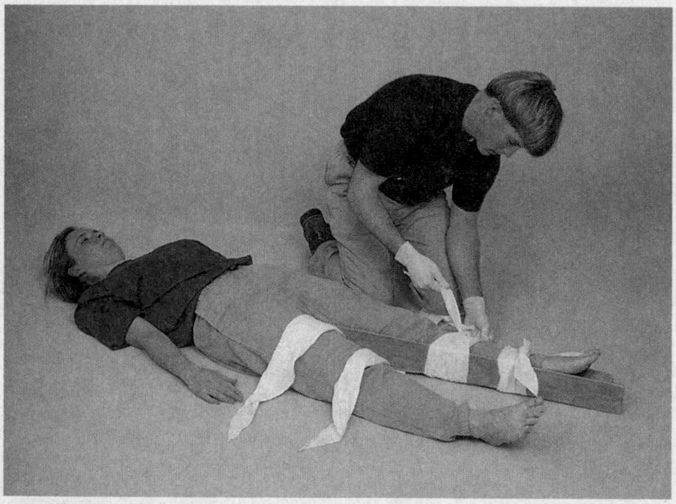

2 Tie both splints and leg together with cravat bandages.

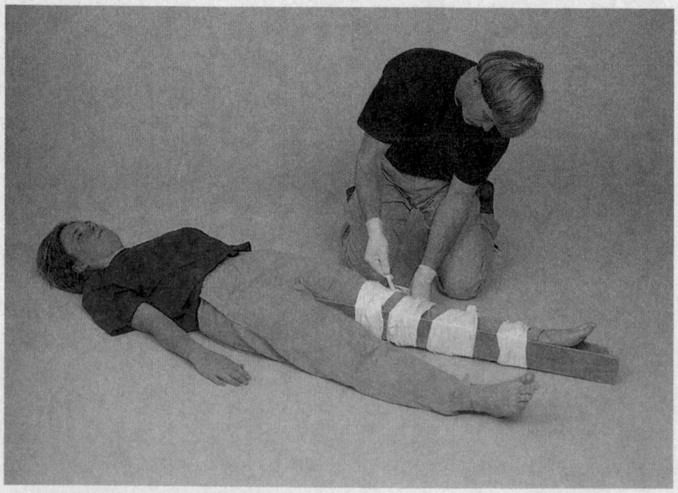

3 Tie knots on top of the splint (board). Assess CSM after splinting.

Ankle and Foot

Treat ankle and foot injuries with the RICE procedure. To further stabilize an ankle, wrap a pillow or folded blanket around the ankle and foot and tie with cravats **FIGURE 16-7** and **FIGURE 16-8**.

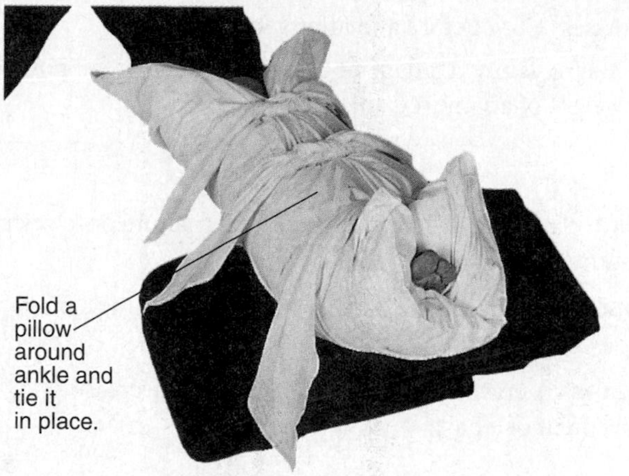
Fold a
pillow
around
ankle and
tie it
in place.

FIGURE 16-7 Splinting an ankle and foot.

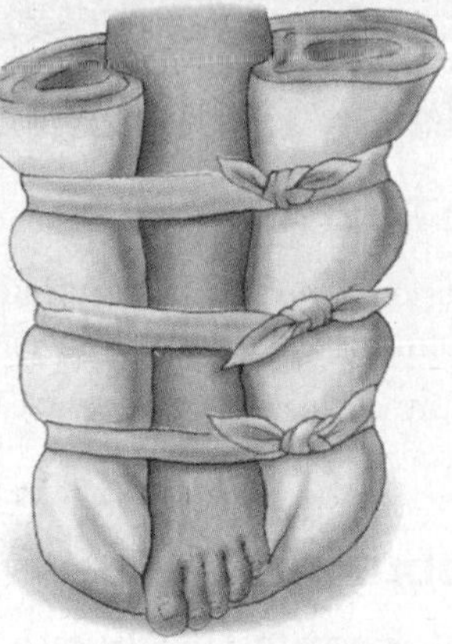

FIGURE 16-8 Splinting an ankle and foot with a rolled or folded blanket in a U shape.

PREP KIT

Ready for Review

- Until professional medical care is available, stabilize the injury by splinting the extremity in the position found.
- A splint is any device used to stabilize a fracture or dislocation.
- When in doubt, apply a splint.
- Assess CSM before and after splinting.
- A sling is any bandage or material that helps support the weight of an injured area.

Vital Vocabulary

rule of thirds A system that divides each long bone into thirds to determine which section or sections of an injured bone should be splinted.

sling A triangular bandage applied around the neck to support an injured upper extremity; any material long enough to suspend an upper extremity by passing the material around the neck; used to support and protect an injury of the arm, shoulder, or clavicle.

splint Any support used to stabilize a fracture or to restrict movement of a part.

stabilize To minimize further injury by holding a body part to prevent movement.

swathe A cravat tied around the body to decrease movement of a part.

Assessment in Action

You are out with your best friend at a dog park, walking her Irish wolfhound. Your friend is animated and engrossed in your conversation. Suddenly, a rabbit leaps out of the hedges and the dog lurches forward, pulling your friend and causing her to trip and let go of the leash. After you regain control of the dog, your friend complains about pain in one of her fingers, which appears to be deformed.

Directions: Circle Yes if you agree with the statement; circle No if you disagree.

1. You should stabilize the finger until professional medical care becomes available.

   YES NO

2. You should splint the finger to prevent a possible closed fracture from becoming an open fracture.

   YES NO

3. Splinting increases blood flow to the fracture, thus speeding up the healing process.

   YES NO

4. If you do not have a commercial splint, you could improvise one.

   YES NO

Check Your Knowledge

Directions: Circle Yes if you agree with the statement; circle No if you disagree.

1. All fractures are complicated to some degree by damage to the soft tissue and structures surrounding the bone.

   YES NO

2. A rigid splint should never be used on an extremity.

   YES NO

3. All fractures and dislocations should be stabilized before the person is moved.

   YES NO

4. Always check the CSM in the extremity.

   YES NO

5. Shoulder injuries can involve the clavicle, the scapula, and the tibia.

   YES NO

6. An elbow must be stabilized in the position in which it is found.

   YES NO

7. Always straighten an injured knee before splinting it.

   YES NO

8. First aid providers should always use traction splints on leg fractures.

   YES NO

9. Buddy taping is when you tape two fingers together with gauze separating the fingers.

   YES NO

10. You can make a temporary sling by pinning a shirt or coat sleeve to the front of the coat or shirt.

    YES NO

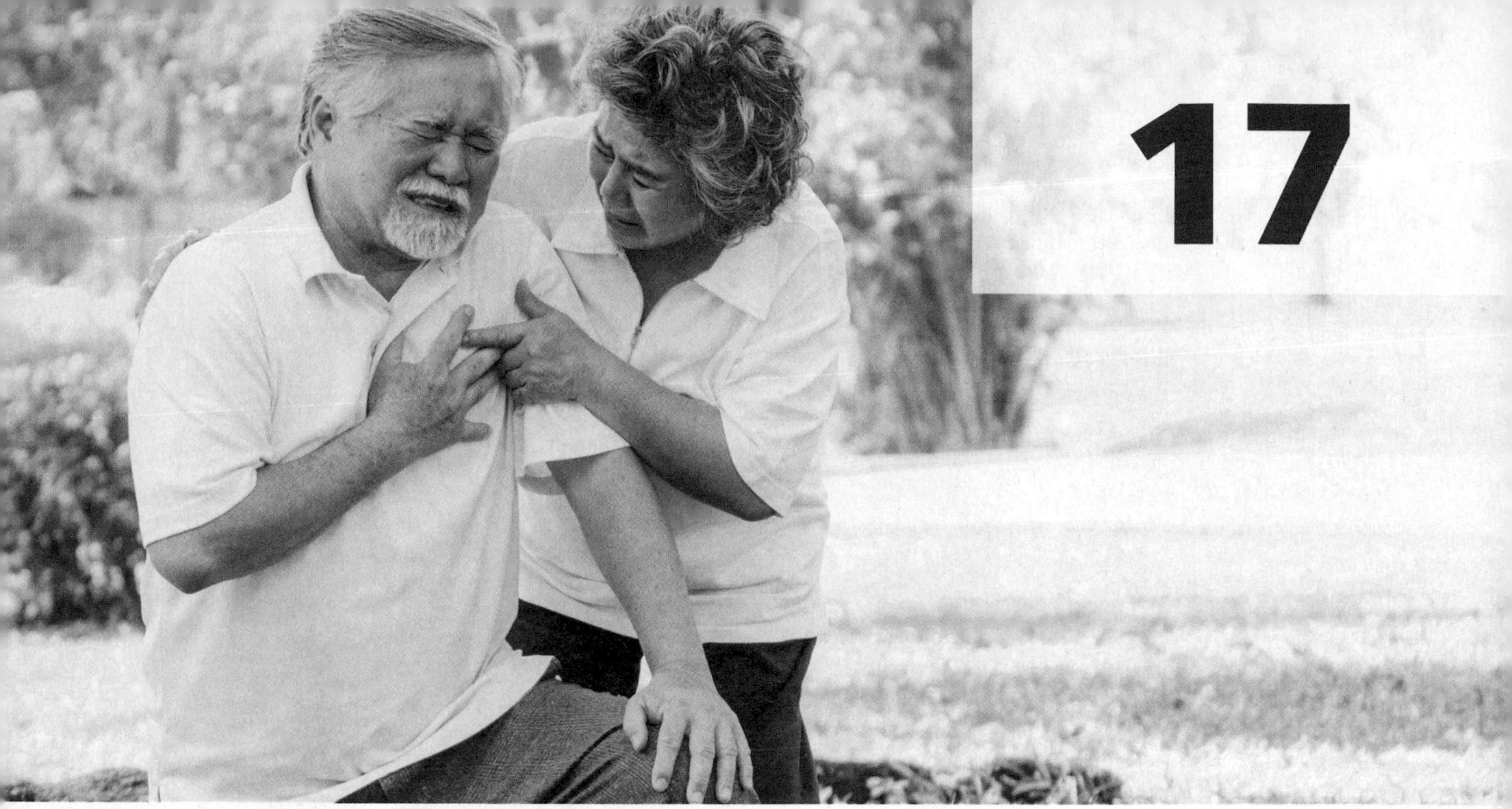

17

Sudden Illness

CHAPTER AT A GLANCE

Unexplained Change in Responsiveness

People can be fully alert (oriented to person, place, and day), can be completely unresponsive (not responding to painful stimuli), or can range anywhere between these two. Not all responsive people are fully alert, and they may respond to different levels of stimulation; for example, a person who does not respond to your voice may react when you squeeze their shoulder muscle. The mental status indicates the level of responsiveness and how well the brain is functioning. The AVPU scale can be used to measure a person's mental status:

A = *Alert.* The person is awake, aware, and can respond to their surrounding environment.

V = *Verbally responsive.* The person's eyes do not open spontaneously, but open in response to verbal stimulus.

P = *Painfully responsive.* The person's eyes do not open spontaneously, but the person responds by moving, moaning, or making noise in response to painful stimulus.

U = *Unresponsive.* The person's eyes do not open spontaneously, and the person does not respond to verbal or painful stimuli.

The main causes for a decrease in a person's alertness and responsiveness are brain injury and lack of either oxygen or glucose reaching the brain. The mnemonic STOP offers clues to the cause(s) of changes in mental status **TABLE 17-1**.

TABLE 17-1 Causes of Changes in Responsiveness: STOP Mnemonic

S	Sugar Seizures Stroke Shock	Blood glucose too low (insulin reaction) or too high (diabetic coma)
T	Temperature	Too high (heatstroke) or too low (hypothermia)
O	Oxygen	Inadequate oxygen or ventilation
P	Poisoning Pressure on brain	Drug/alcohol overdose; carbon monoxide poisoning Head injury

Heart Attack

Heart muscle needs oxygen to survive. The coronary arteries are the vessels that supply blood and oxygen to the heart muscle, the myocardium. When the blood supply is cut off, a **heart attack**, or acute myocardial infarction (AMI), results. Blockage of blood flow occurs as the vessel walls slowly become thicker and harder due to the buildup of plaque (mainly cholesterol). This slow process is known as atherosclerosis **FIGURE 17-1**. If part of the plaque breaks open, a clot can form over it, causing a sudden, complete blockage of the artery, which results in a heart attack.

FYI

Risk Factors for Heart Disease

Several factors contribute to an increased risk of heart attack and stroke. The more risk factors present, the greater the possibility that a person will develop heart disease.

Risk Factors You Cannot Change

- *Heredity.* Tendencies appear in family lines.
- *Sex.* Men have a greater risk, although heart attack is still the leading cause of death among women.
- *Age.* Most people who experience a heart attack are 65 years or older.

Risk Factors You Can Change or Control

- *Cigarette smoking.* Smokers have more than twice the risk of heart attack as nonsmokers.
- *High blood pressure.* This condition adds to the heart's workload.
- *High blood cholesterol level.* Too much cholesterol in the blood can cause a buildup on the walls of the arteries.
- *Diabetes.* This condition affects the blood's cholesterol and triglyceride levels.
- *Obesity.* Being overweight influences blood pressure and blood cholesterol, can result in diabetes, and can place added strain on the heart.
- *Physical inactivity.* Inactive people have twice the risk of heart attack as active people.
- *Stress.* All people feel stress but react in different ways. Excessive, long-term stress can lead to physical conditions in some people.

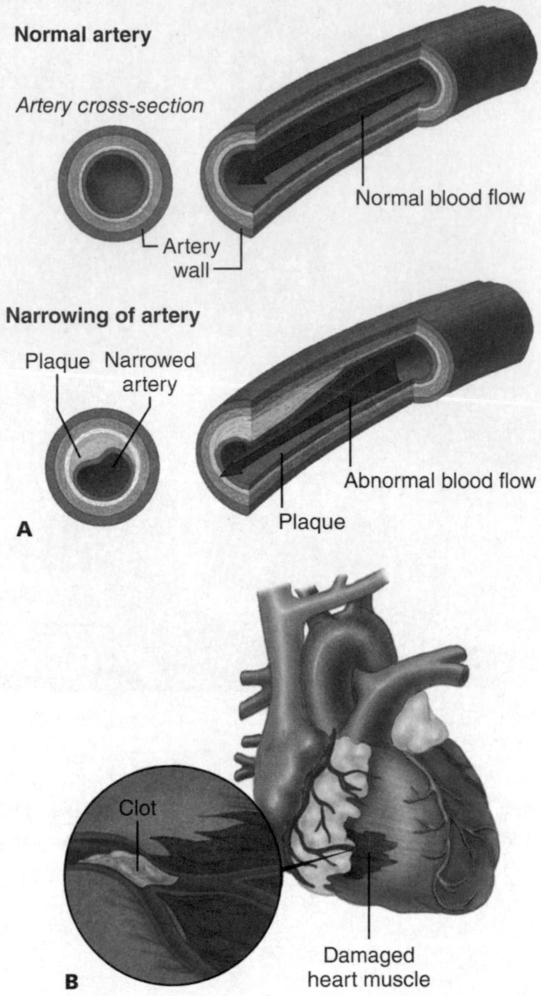

FIGURE 17-1 A. A normal artery with normal blood flow and an artery with plaque buildup. **B**. A heart attack occurs when a clot prevents blood from flowing to a part of the heart.

Heart and blood vessel (cardiovascular) disease is America's number one killer. About one-half of the deaths from heart and blood vessel disease are from impairment of blood flow to the heart, known as coronary heart disease, which includes heart attack.

Difference Between Heart Attack and Cardiac Arrest

The conditions *heart attack* and *cardiac arrest* confuse many people. The two are very different, and so is the first aid and emergency care for them.

- *Heart attack.* When one or more of the arteries delivering blood to the heart becomes blocked, a heart attack results. Oxygen-rich blood cannot reach a portion of the heart muscle, and therefore that portion becomes damaged. This damage to the heart muscle can lead to disturbances of the heart's ability to pump as well as its electrical system. It can also lead to cardiac arrest.
- *Cardiac arrest.* Cardiac arrest occurs either when the heart stops beating (asystole) or when the heart's lower

chambers (ventricles) suddenly develop a rapid irregular rhythm (ventricular fibrillation), causing the ventricles to quiver rather than contract. The quivering motion of the ventricles renders the heart an ineffective pump that can no longer supply the body and brain with oxygen-rich blood. Within seconds, the person becomes unresponsive and has no pulse. Only immediate action such as cardiopulmonary resuscitation (CPR) and external defibrillation can offer hope of survival.

Refer to **FLOWCHART 17-1** for additional information regarding the care of a person with a heart attack.

FYI

No Chest Pain in One-Third of Heart Attacks

A study of hundreds of thousands of people who had experienced heart attacks found that as many as one-third had no chest pain and that these people were less likely to seek help and twice as likely to die.

The study found that women, people of color, people older than 75 years, and people with previous heart failure, stroke, or diabetes were most likely to have painless heart attacks. Although physicians have long known about painless heart attacks, many said they did not realize the number was so high.

Patients with chest pain were more than twice as likely to be diagnosed at admission and to receive clot-busting drugs or undergo angioplasty to open clogged arteries.

Data from Canto JG, Shlipak MG, Rogers WJ, et al. Prevalence, clinical characteristics, and mortality among patients with myocardial infarction presenting without chest pain. *JAMA*. 2000;283:3223–3229.

FYI

Why Don't They Call?

A study asked people who experienced a heart attack and waited for more than 20 minutes before getting help why they delayed. Their answers included the following:

- They thought the symptoms would go away.
- The symptoms were not severe enough.
- They thought it was a different illness.
- They were worried about medical costs.
- They were afraid of hospitals.
- They feared being embarrassed.
- They wanted to wait for a better time.
- They did not want to find out what was wrong.

The average time that elapsed between symptom onset and hospital arrival was 2 hours; 28% waited at least 1 hour, 33% waited 1 to 3 hours, 15% waited 3 to 6 hours, and 23% waited more than 6 hours. Most people reported they were not sure their symptoms were severe enough to merit action as drastic as calling 9-1-1.

The same study concluded that one way to shorten out-of-hospital delay is to encourage people with heart-related symptoms to use emergency medical services (EMS) rather than slower transportation methods.

Reproduced from Meischke H, Eisenberg MS, Schaeffer SM, Larsen MP. Reasons patients with chest pain delay or do not call 911. *Ann Emerg Med*. 1995;25(2):193–197.

What to Look For

Although sometimes difficult to determine, symptoms of a heart attack can include:

- Chest discomfort that feels like pressure, squeezing, or fullness, usually in the center of the chest. It may also be felt in the jaw, shoulder, arms, or back.
- Sweating
- Light-headedness or dizziness
- Nausea or vomiting
- Numbness, aching, or tingling in an arm (most often the left arm)
- Shortness of breath
- Weakness or fatigue, especially in older adults

Women and older adults experience the typical signs and symptoms of a heart attack. However, women and older adults are more likely than men to have milder signs and symptoms of a heart attack that can extend over many hours, days, or weeks leading up to the heart attack, such as:

- Shortness of breath
- Nausea or vomiting
- An ache in the chest
- Sore jaw
- Strange feeling in arm
- Upper back pain
- Flulike symptoms
- Dizziness

What to Do

1. Have the person sit, with knees bent, and lean against a stable but comfortable support (eg, wall, tree trunk, fence post). Try to keep the person calm. **DO NOT** allow the person to walk **FIGURE 17-2**. Doing so can put more stress on the heart.
2. Call 9-1-1 immediately. **DO NOT** drive the person to a medical facility; wait for EMS to arrive.
3. While waiting for EMS to arrive:
   - Loosen any tight clothing.
   - Ask if the person takes any chest pain medication (eg, nitroglycerin) for a known heart condition, and if so, help them take it.
   - If the person is alert, able to swallow, not allergic to aspirin, and has no signs of a stroke (see page 248), help the person take one adult aspirin (325 mg) or two to four low-dose aspirins (81 mg each). Pulverize or have the person chew before swallowing for faster results.
   - Monitor breathing. If the person becomes unresponsive and stops breathing, begin CPR (see Chapter 5, *CPR*). If they are unresponsive and are breathing, place them on their side (recovery position; see pages 70–71.)

Flowchart 17-1 Heart Attack

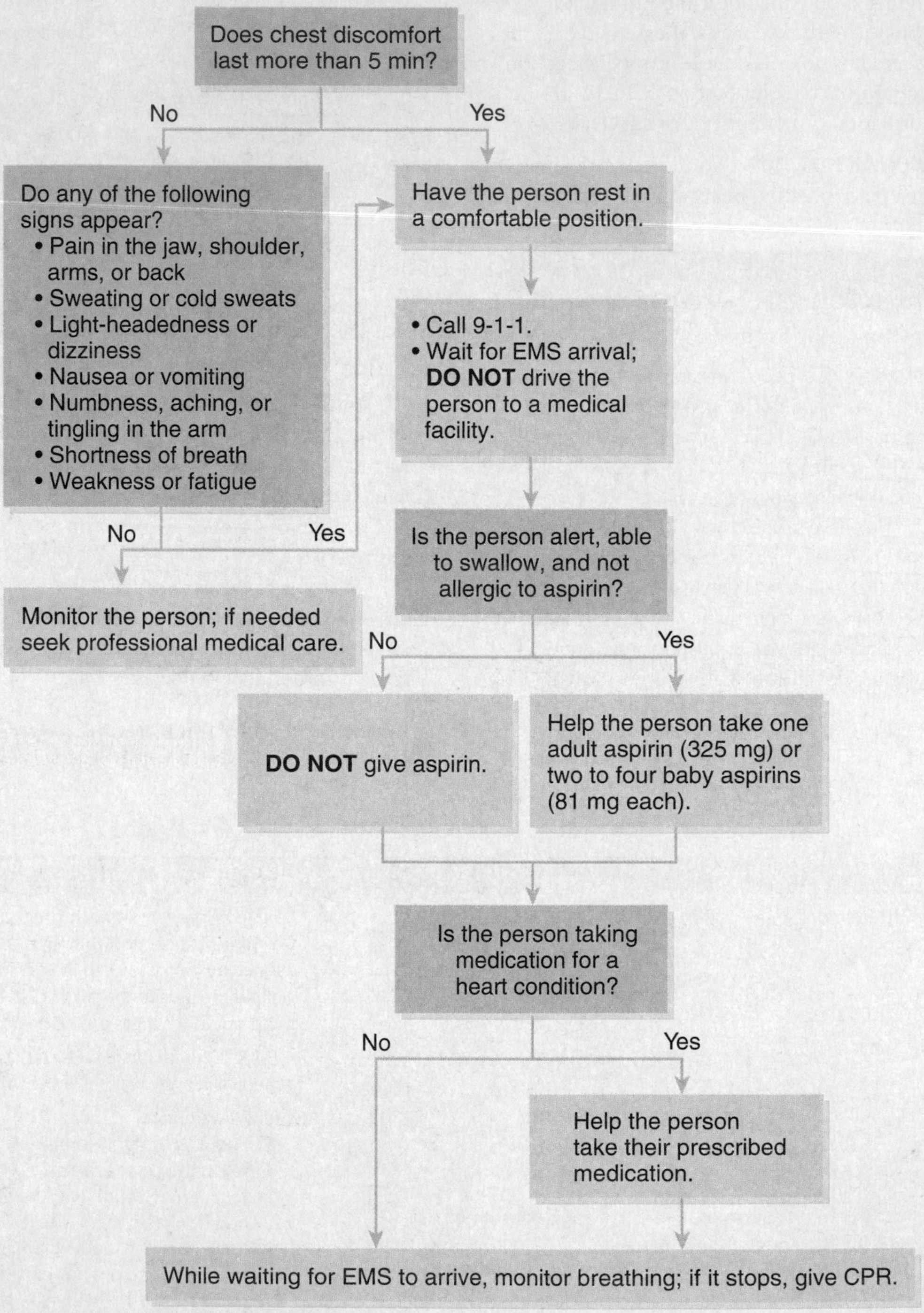
Does chest discomfort last more than 5 min?
No
Yes
Do any of the following signs appear?
• Pain in the jaw, shoulder, arms, or back
• Sweating or cold sweats
• Light-headedness or dizziness
• Nausea or vomiting
• Numbness, aching, or tingling in the arm
• Shortness of breath
• Weakness or fatigue
No
Yes
Monitor the person; if needed seek professional medical care.
Have the person rest in a comfortable position.
• Call 9-1-1.
• Wait for EMS arrival; DO NOT drive the person to a medical facility.
Is the person alert, able to swallow, and not allergic to aspirin?
No
Yes
DO NOT give aspirin.
Help the person take one adult aspirin (325 mg) or two to four baby aspirins (81 mg each).
Is the person taking medication for a heart condition?
No
Yes
Help the person take their prescribed medication.
While waiting for EMS to arrive, monitor breathing; if it stops, give CPR.

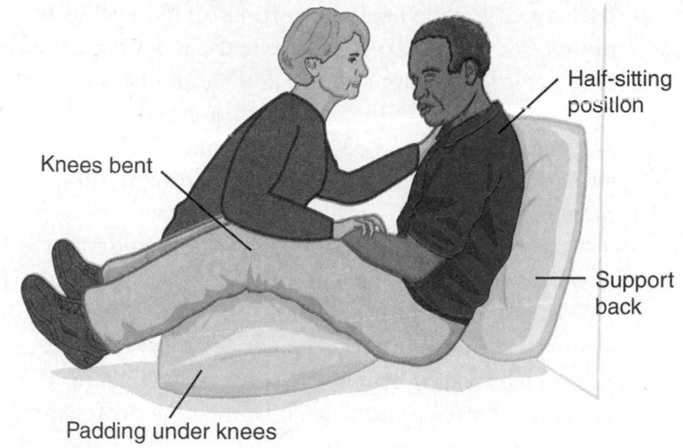

FIGURE 17-2 Help the person into a relaxed position to ease strain on the heart.

Angina

Chest pain called **angina pectoris** results when blood flow to the heart muscle is restricted, but not completely blocked **TABLE 17-2**. Angina occurs when coronary arteries supplying the heart muscle with oxygen-rich blood become narrow and cannot carry sufficient blood to meet the demands during the following situations:

- Physical exertion
- Excitement
- Emotional upset
- Eating of a heavy meal
- Extreme hot or cold temperature exposure
- Cigarette smoking

Angina can be treated with drugs that affect the blood supply to the heart muscle, the heart's demand for oxygen, or both. Drugs that affect the blood supply are coronary vasodilators; they cause blood vessels to relax. When this happens, the opening inside the vessels (the lumen) gets bigger. The blood flow then improves, allowing more oxygen and nutrients to reach the heart muscle.

Nitroglycerin mainly relaxes the veins, but it also relaxes the coronary arteries a little. By relaxing the veins, it reduces the amount of blood that returns to the heart and eases the heart's workload. By relaxing the coronary arteries, it increases the heart's blood supply. Physicians often prescribe nitroglycerin for those with angina. Nitroglycerin should be taken when the person experiences chest pain as long as they are not dizzy, which would indicate hypotension.

TABLE 17-2 Chest Pain

Cause of Pain	Characteristics	Care
Muscle or rib pain from exercise or injury	Reproduced by movement Tender spot when pressed	Rest Aspirin or ibuprofen
Respiratory infection (eg, pneumonia, bronchitis, pleuritis)	Cough Fever Sore throat Production of sputum (mucus)	Antibiotics
Indigestion	Belching Heartburn Nausea Sour taste	Antacids
Angina pectoris	Lasts less than 10 min (but pain is similar to that of a heart attack)	Rest Prescribed medication
Heart attack (myocardial infarction)	Lasts more than 10 min Pressure, squeezing, or pain near center of the chest Pain spreads to shoulders, neck, or arms Light-headedness, fainting, sweating, nausea, shortness of breath	Call 9-1-1 Check breathing Resting position Prescribed medication

What to Look For	What to Do
It can be difficult to differentiate a heart attack from angina, even for physicians. This is why the recommendation for first aid providers is to treat for heart attack even if angina is suspected. The following symptoms can point toward angina rather than heart attack: ▪ Chest pain is described as crushing, squeezing, or like somebody standing on the person's chest. ▪ Pain can spread to the jaw, the arms (frequently the left arm), and the midback. ▪ Pain usually lasts from 3 to 10 minutes, but rarely longer than 10 minutes. ▪ The pain is almost always relieved by the person's prescribed nitroglycerin. ▪ Pain can be associated with shortness of breath, nausea, or sweating. ▪ The person feels anxious.	**1.** Have the person stop what they are doing and sit down. Keep bystanders away. Provide calm reassurance to help reduce the person's anxiety. **2.** If the person has medically prescribed nitroglycerin, either tablets or a spray, let the person use it. Follow the prescription label's directions. If necessary, help them use it. **DO NOT** use nitroglycerin if the person is feeling dizzy, an indication of hypotension. **3.** If the chest pain or discomfort does not improve within 5 minutes after taking one dose of nitroglycerin, call 9-1-1 and administer a second dose. If there is still no relief after another 5 minutes and EMS has not yet arrived, administer a third dose.

Stroke (Cerebral Vascular Accident)

A **stroke**, also known as a cerebral vascular accident (CVA), occurs when there is a sudden interruption of blood flow to the brain. When arteries in the brain rupture **FIGURE 17-3** or become blocked **FIGURE 17-4**, part of the brain does not receive the blood flow it needs. Deprived of oxygen-rich blood, nerve cells in the affected area of the brain cannot function and die within minutes. Because dead brain cells are not replaced, the devastating effects of strokes often are permanent. When nerve cells do not function, the part of the body they control cannot function either. Stroke occurs mostly in older people; however, it is not limited to older people.

Strokes are classified as ischemic or hemorrhagic:

- *Ischemic stroke.* This type of stroke occurs when blood vessels to the brain become narrowed or clogged with fatty deposits called plaque, cutting off blood flow to brain cells. High blood pressure is the most important risk factor for ischemic stroke and should be managed. Ischemic strokes are the most common type of stroke and account for about 85% of all strokes. Ischemic strokes usually occur at night or first thing in the morning.

  Tissue plasminogen activators (tPA) and other clot-busting drugs must be given as soon as possible after stroke onset (within 3 hours). Therefore, it is important to recognize and record the last time the person was seen normal ("last known well") and to recognize a stroke and to seek immediate professional medical care in a stroke center.
- *Hemorrhagic stroke.* About 15% of all strokes happen when a blood vessel ruptures in or near the brain. This kind of stroke is often associated with a very severe headache, nausea, and vomiting. Usually the symptoms appear suddenly.

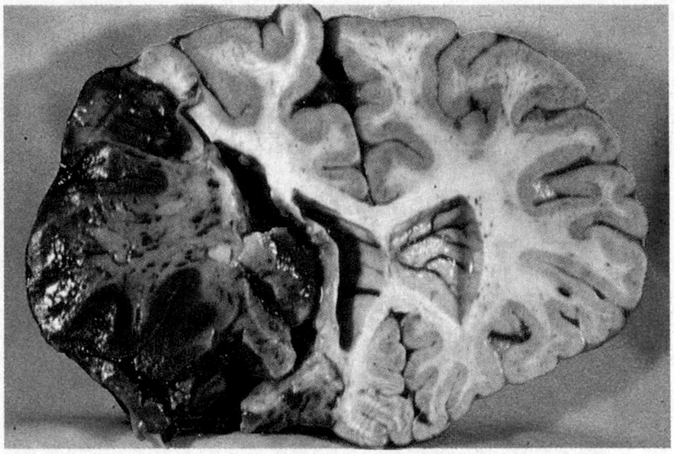

FIGURE 17-3 Severe brain hemorrhage causing a stroke.

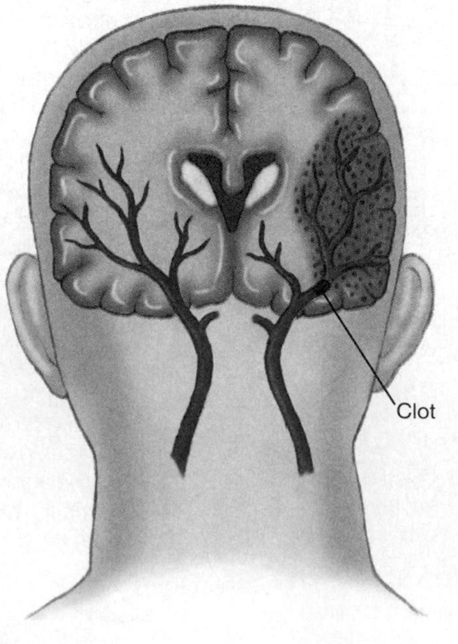

FIGURE 17-4 A blood clot can block the brain's blood supply.

A **transient ischemic attack (TIA)** (also commonly known as a "little stroke" or "mini stroke") is a form of stroke that occurs when a part of the brain is deprived of oxygen-rich blood long enough to cause symptoms but not long enough to cause permanent damage. The person may have similar signs and symptoms of a CVA, but the episode resolves completely within 24 hours. TIAs may be foreshadowing of a serious stroke and should be evaluated in the emergency department.

Immediately seek professional medical care if there is a possibility of stroke. Any or all of the following procedures might be needed:

- Medication to control high blood pressure
- Medication to reduce brain swelling
- Surgery to repair an aneurysm or remove a blood clot

See **TABLE 17-3** for help determining whether a person may be experiencing a stroke. Refer to **FLOWCHART 17-2** for additional information regarding the care of a person who is having a stroke.

TABLE 17-3 Cincinnati Prehospital Stroke Scale

Test	Normal	Abnormal
Facial droop. **FIGURE 17-5.** Ask the person to show their teeth or to smile.	Both sides of face move equally well.	One side of the face does not move as well as the other.
Arm droop. **FIGURE 17-6.** Ask the person to close their eyes and hold out both arms with palms up.	Both arms move the same, or both arms do not move.	One arm does not move, or one arm drifts down compared with the other side.
Speech. Ask the person to say, "The sky Is blue in Cincinnati."	The person uses correct words with no slurring.	The person slurs words, uses inappropriate words, or is unable to speak.

Note: The presence of one of these signs is associated with a high risk of stroke (72%); if all three are present, the risk is as high as 85%.

Flowchart 17-2 Stroke

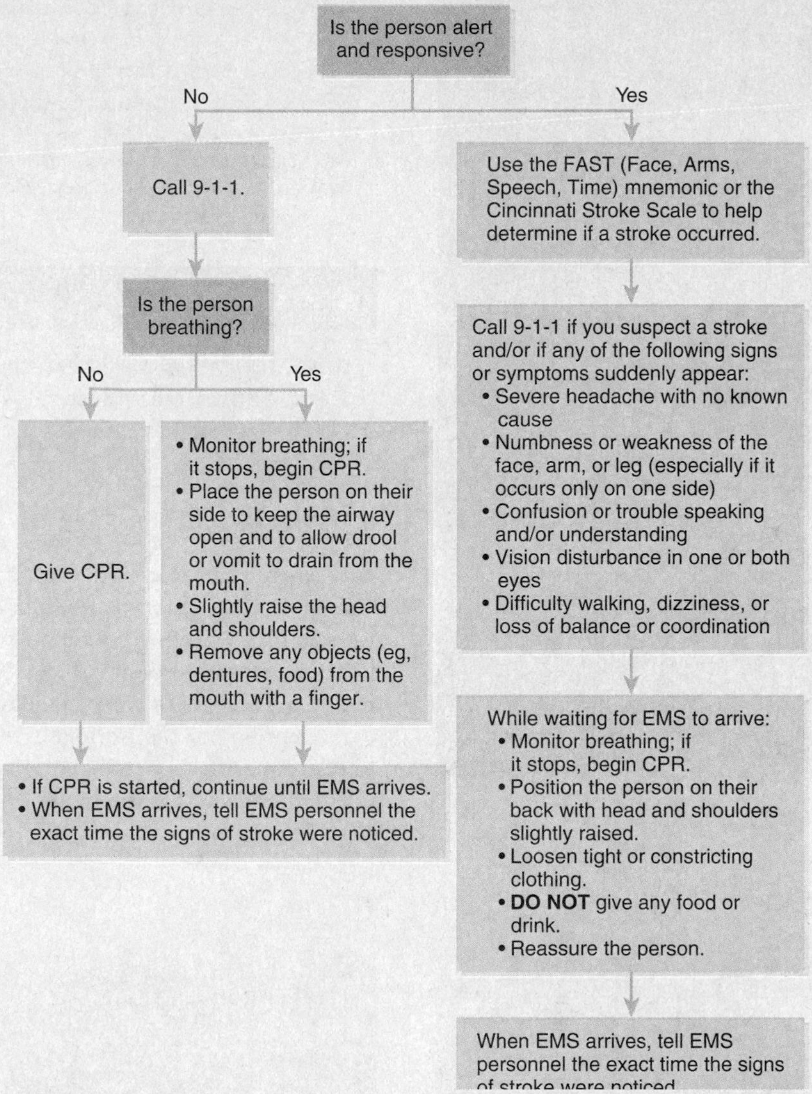
Is the person alert and responsive?
No
Yes
Call 9-1-1.
Is the person breathing?
No
Yes
Give CPR.
• Monitor breathing; if it stops, begin CPR.
• Place the person on their side to keep the airway open and to allow drool or vomit to drain from the mouth.
• Slightly raise the head and shoulders.
• Remove any objects (eg, dentures, food) from the mouth with a finger.
• If CPR is started, continue until EMS arrives.
• When EMS arrives, tell EMS personnel the exact time the signs of stroke were noticed.
Use the FAST (Face, Arms, Speech, Time) mnemonic or the Cincinnati Stroke Scale to help determine if a stroke occurred.
Call 9-1-1 if you suspect a stroke and/or if any of the following signs or symptoms suddenly appear:
• Severe headache with no known cause
• Numbness or weakness of the face, arm, or leg (especially if it occurs only on one side)
• Confusion or trouble speaking and/or understanding
• Vision disturbance in one or both eyes
• Difficulty walking, dizziness, or loss of balance or coordination
While waiting for EMS to arrive:
• Monitor breathing; if it stops, begin CPR.
• Position the person on their back with head and shoulders slightly raised.
• Loosen tight or constricting clothing.
• DO NOT give any food or drink.
• Reassure the person.
When EMS arrives, tell EMS personnel the exact time the signs of stroke were noticed.

What to Look For

Use either the Cincinnati Prehospital Stroke Scale (Table 17-3) or the acronym **F-A-S-T** as an assessment tool to help determine if a stroke may have occurred:

F = Face droops—ask the person to smile. It is abnormal for one side of the face not to move well compared with the other side.

A = Arm weakness—Ask the person to close their eyes and raise both arms with the palms up for a count of 10 seconds. It is abnormal if one arm drifts downward when held extended.

S = Speech difficulty—Ask the person to repeat a simple phrase (eg, "The sky is blue."). It is abnormal if the person slurs words, uses the wrong words, or cannot speak at all.

T = Time to call 9-1-1 if any of the preceding signs occur. The presence of one of these signs is associated with a high risk of stroke (72%); if all three are present, the risk is as high as 85%.

What to Do

1. Call 9-1-1 immediately.
2. Monitor responsiveness and breathing.
   - If the person is unresponsive and not breathing, begin CPR (see Chapter 5, *CPR*).
   - If they are unresponsive and breathing or have fluid or vomit in their mouth, place them on their side (recovery position; see pages 70–71). This will allow any fluids to drain out of their mouth.
   - If they are alert, allow them to find a comfortable position with the head and shoulders above the body.
3. **DO NOT** give the person anything to eat or drink—the throat can be paralyzed, which restricts swallowing and causes choking.
4. Loosen tight clothing (eg, shirt collars, ties).
5. Record the time that the stroke may have occurred and give it to the EMS personnel.

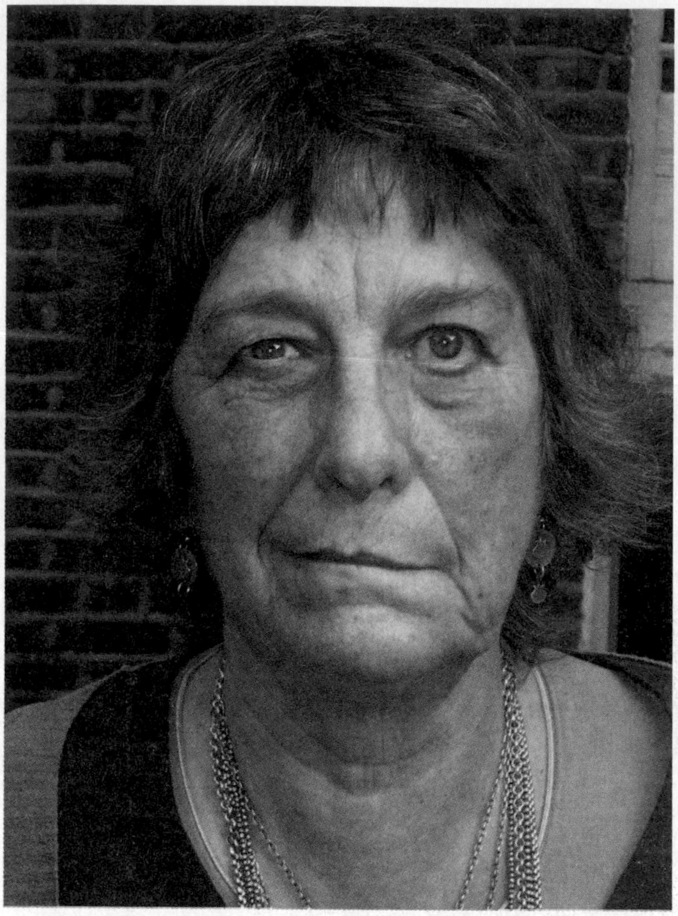

FIGURE 17-5 Facial droop.

FYI

Women and Stroke

Women especially need to know the warning signs of stroke, because they account for over 60% of the deaths from stroke. The most effective treatments for stroke are only available if the stroke is recognized within 3 hours of symptom onset.

Data from Women and stroke. National Stroke Association website. http://www.stroke.org/understand-stroke/impact-stroke/women-and-stroke

CAUTION

DO NOT give a person experiencing a stroke anything to drink or eat. The throat can be paralyzed, which restricts swallowing.

Asthma

Asthma is a chronic (long-term) lung disease that inflames and narrows the airways. Asthma causes recurring periods of wheezing (a whistling sound when a person breathes), chest tightness, shortness of breath, and coughing. The coughing often occurs at night or early in the morning.

According to the National Heart, Lung, and Blood Institute, asthma affects people of all ages, but it most often starts in childhood and has the highest prevalence rate in those ages 5 to 17 years.

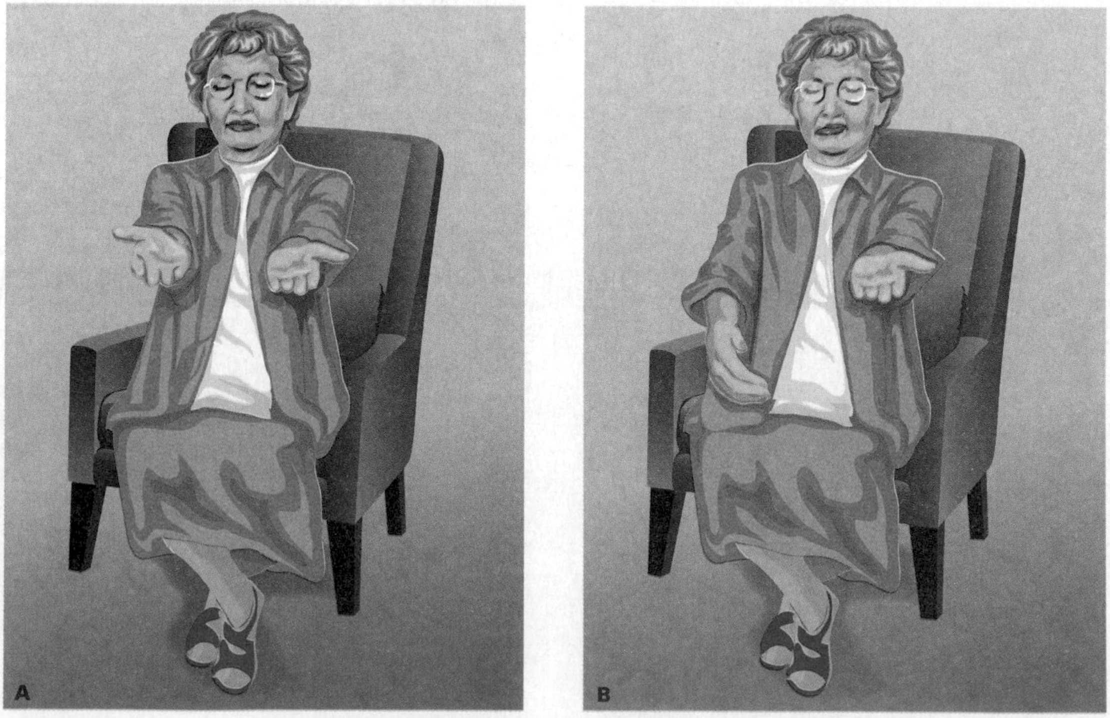

FIGURE 17-6 A. Normal arm position. **B**. Arm droop.

The airways are tubes that carry air into and out of the lungs. Normally, the airways to the lungs are fully open when we breathe, so air moves in and out freely. People with asthma have highly sensitive airways that become inflamed and swollen easily. Asthma episodes or attacks occur when something bothers their airways. When the airways react, the muscles around them tighten. This causes the airways to narrow, allowing less air to flow to the lungs. Swelling makes the airways even narrower. Cells in the airways may make more mucus than normal **FIGURE 17-7**. Mucus is a sticky, thick liquid that can further narrow a person's airways.

During an episode, a person with asthma may cough and wheeze. They may also have difficulty breathing and be gasping for air or become short of breath. Sometimes, an episode is so severe that they need emergency professional medical care to breathe normally again.

For many people with asthma, the same substances (called allergens) that cause allergy symptoms can trigger an asthma attack. These allergens may be inhaled, such as pollen, animal dander, tobacco smoke, mold, dust, or air pollution, or eaten, such as shellfish. Avoiding or limiting exposure to known allergens and secondhand smoke can help prevent asthma attacks.

For some people, an asthma attack can be caused by strenuous physical exercise, certain medications, excitement, stress, and even bad weather such as thunderstorms. No two cases of asthma are exactly alike. Some of the known triggers of asthma are listed in **TABLE 17-4**.

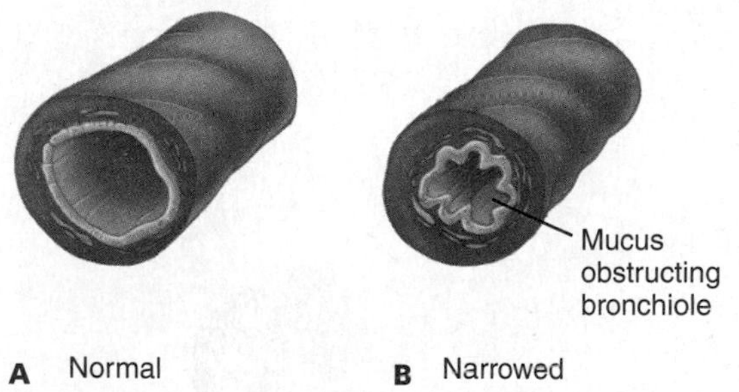

FIGURE 17-7 A. A cross-section of a normal airway. **B**. A cross-section of an airway during asthma symptoms, with the airway narrowed and inflamed, a thickened airway wall, and mucus.

TABLE 17-4 Common Asthma Triggers

Environmental	Drugs or Chemicals	Conditions or Events
▪ Cold air ▪ House dust mites ▪ Cockroaches ▪ Animals (eg, cats, dogs, rodents) ▪ Indoor irritants (eg, wood-burning stoves) ▪ Outdoor air pollution (eg, vehicle emissions) ▪ Indoor or outdoor molds and fungi ▪ Tobacco smoke ▪ Pollen (eg, grass, trees) ▪ Seafood, shellfish	▪ Aspirin ▪ Beta blocker medicine ▪ Food or drug preservatives ▪ Occupational exposure to chemicals ▪ Household cleaning agents ▪ Perfumes	▪ Gastroesophageal reflux ▪ Allergic rhinitis ▪ Panic attacks ▪ Menstruation, pregnancy ▪ Viral respiratory infections ▪ Emotional stress, excitement ▪ Exercise

Not everyone with asthma takes the same medicine. Some medicines are inhaled, or breathed in, and others are taken as a pill. Asthma medicines come in two types: quick-relief (rescue) and long-term. Quick-relief medicines (rescue inhalers) control the symptoms of an asthma attack. Long-term medicines help a person to have fewer and milder attacks, but they are not intended to help treat a person having an asthma attack. Refer to **FLOWCHART 17-3** for additional information regarding the care of a person with asthma.

What to Look For	What to Do
▪ Frequent coughing ▪ Wheezing ▪ Breathing difficulty ▪ Unable to speak in complete sentences without stopping to breathe ▪ Sitting in the tripod position (leaning forward with hands on knees or other support, trying to breathe)	1. Have the person sit in an upright position, leaning slightly forward, and loosen tight clothing. 2. Encourage the person to sit quietly and to breathe slowly and deeply in through the nose and out through the mouth. 3. Ask the person about any asthma medication they use. Most people with asthma have a physician-prescribed quick-relief inhaler often accompanied with a spacer or holding chamber **FIGURE 17-8**. 4. If the person has a quick-relief (rescue) inhaler, help them use it. **DO NOT** borrow or use someone else's inhaler. Quick-relief inhalers may or may not have a spacer (spacers help administer more medicine into the lungs by holding the medicine inside itself for a few seconds so that the user does not have to breathe in and spray at the same time). For an inhaler without a spacer, follow the steps in **SKILL SHEET 17-1**. For an inhaler with a spacer, follow the steps in **SKILL SHEET 17-2**. 5. Improved breathing should occur within 5 to 15 minutes. Additional doses may be needed to stop an asthma attack. **DO NOT** exceed the dose prescribed by the person's doctor. If breathing difficulty still persists, get immediate professional medical help. 6. Call 9-1-1 immediately if: ▪ The person is struggling to breathe, talk, or stay awake. ▪ They are unable to speak one to two words in one breath. ▪ Their lips or fingernails turn blue. ▪ The person asks for professional medical care. ▪ There is no improvement after using their quick-relief inhaler or they do not have a rescue inhaler. ▪ Repeated attacks occur. ▪ A severe and prolonged attack occurs. 7. **DO NOT** assume the person's condition is improving if wheezing is no longer heard.

Flowchart 17-3 Asthma

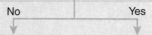

- Place the person in an upright sitting position, leaning slightly forward.
- Encourage the person to breathe slowly and deeply in through the nose and out through the mouth.

↓

Help the person use their physician-prescribed quick-relief (rescue) inhaler, if available.

↓

Does the person:
- Struggle to breath, talk, or stay awake?
- Have blue lips or fingernails?
- Have no medicine?
- Ask for an ambulance?

No → Monitor breathing.

Yes →
- Call 9-1-1.
- While waiting for EMS to arrive, encourage the person to continue using their inhaler, if available.
- Monitor breathing; if it stops, give CPR.

Q&A

Who gets asthma?

Asthma is very common, affecting about 23 million people in the United States, including more than 6 million children. No one knows for sure why some people have asthma and others do not. People who have family members with allergies or asthma are more likely to have asthma.

In young children, boys are nearly twice as likely as girls to develop asthma, but this sex difference tends to disappear in older age groups. Obesity is a newly identified risk factor for asthma.

What causes asthma?

People generally think of asthma in terms of episodes or attacks. Actually, the asthmatic condition is always present, but symptoms may be dormant until triggered by an allergen, respiratory infection, or bad or cold weather. Other triggers may include some medicines, environmental irritants, physical exertion, and some foods and food additives.

Data from Asthma. Centers for Disease Control and Prevention website. http://www.cdc.gov/asthma. Last reviewed December 7, 2020. Accessed January 18, 2021.

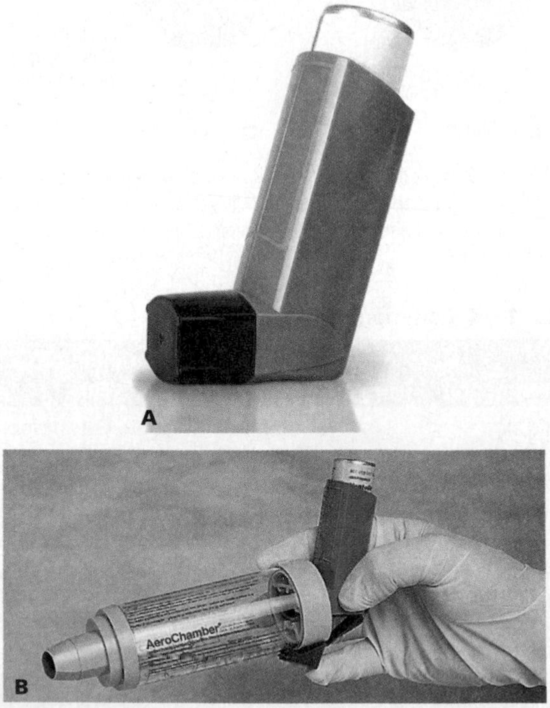

FIGURE 17-8 A. Inhaler without a spacer. **B**. Inhaler with a spacer.

SKILL SHEET 17-1 Using an Inhaler Without a Spacer

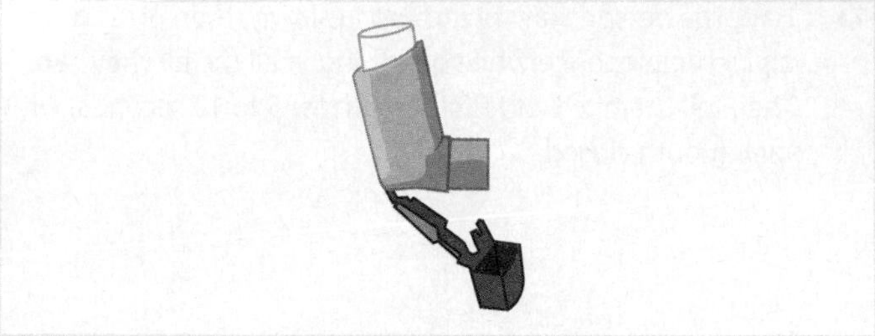

1 Take the cap off the inhaler and make sure the mouthpiece and spray hole are clean.

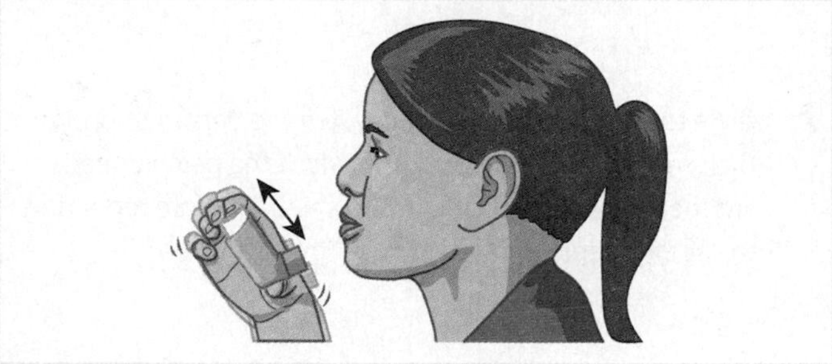

2 Shake the inhaler 10 to 15 times.

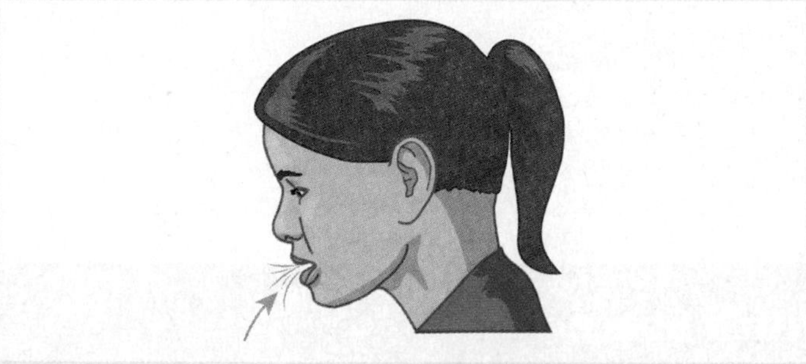

3 Without the inhaler, ask the person to take a deep breath in and then breathe out all the way.

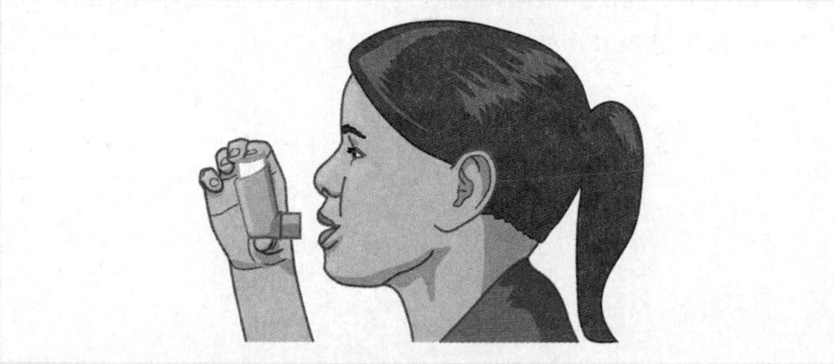

4 Have the person hold the inhaler upright and between their index finger and thumb.

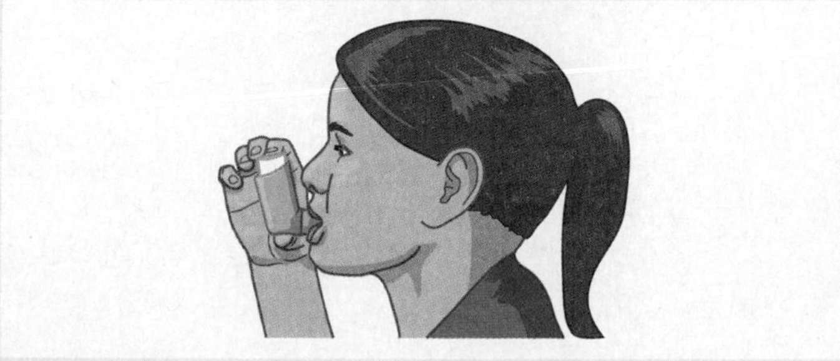

5 Have the person put the mouthpiece of the inhaler in their mouth, above their tongue and between their teeth, and then close their lips around the inhaler.

Continues

SKILL SHEET 17-1 Using an Inhaler Without a Spacer (*Continued*)

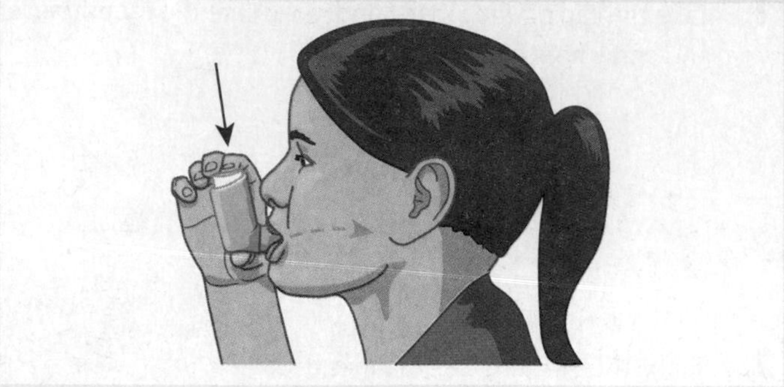

© Jones & Bartlett Learning.

6 Have the person start breathing in slowly, then press down on the inhaler once while breathing in all the air they can. Then tell them to hold their breath for 5 to 10 seconds, with their mouth closed.

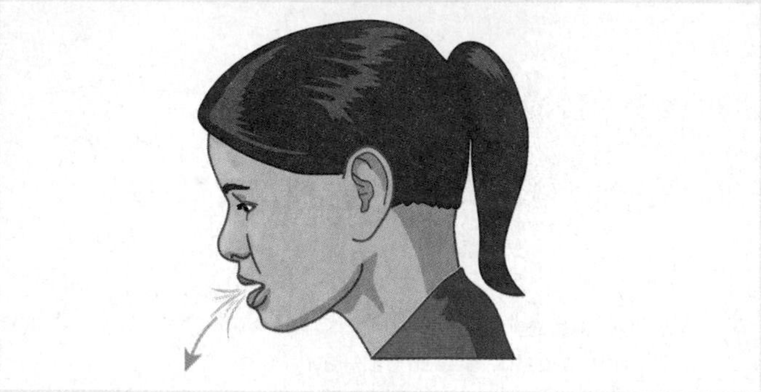

© Jones & Bartlett Learning.

7 Once the 5 to 10 seconds are up, tell the person to open their mouth and breathe out slowly. If the person needs another dose of medicine, wait 1 minute before repeating the above steps.

SKILL SHEET 17-2 Using an Inhaler With a Spacer

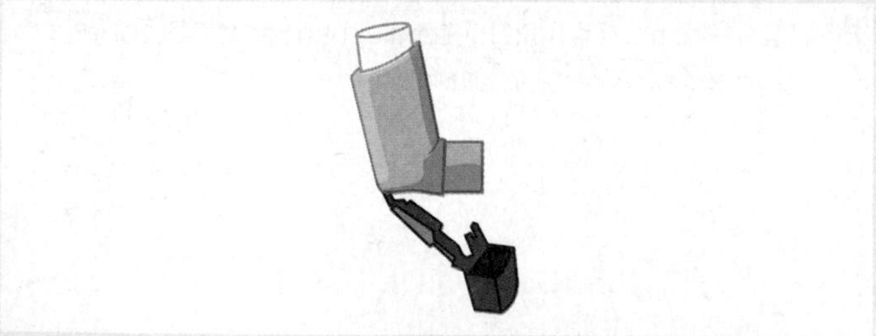

© Jones & Bartlett Learning.

1 Take the cap off the inhaler, and inspect the mouthpiece to ensure that it is clean.

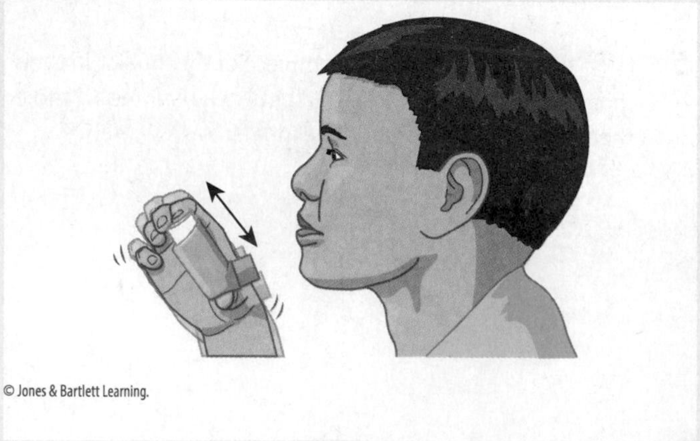

© Jones & Bartlett Learning.

2 Shake the inhaler 10 to 15 times.

SKILL SHEET 17-2 Using an Inhaler With a Spacer (*Continued*)

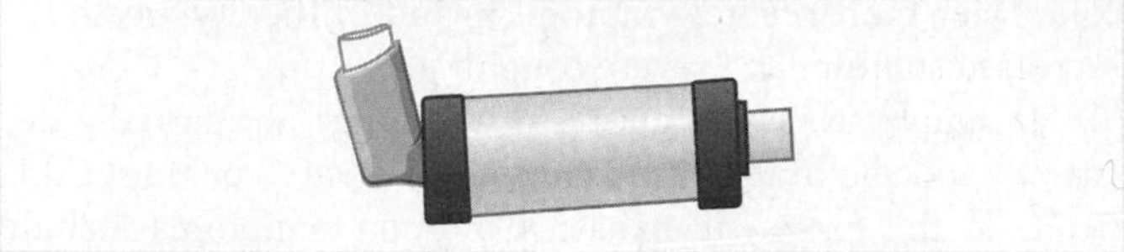

3 Insert the inhaler mouthpiece into the end of the spacer.

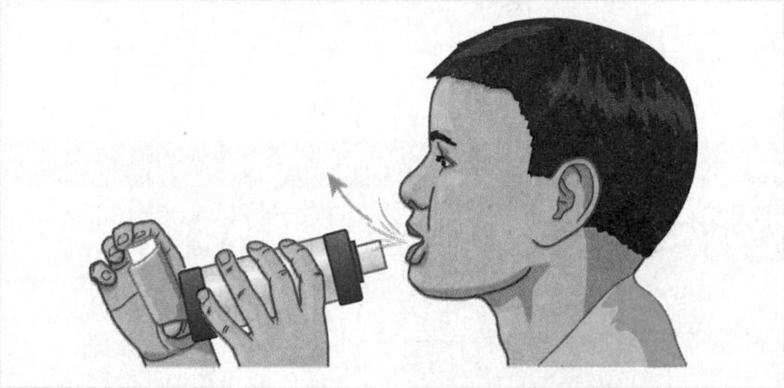

4 Have the person hold the inhaler and spacer between their index finger and thumb. Then, without the inhaler, ask the person to take a deep breath in and breathe out all the way.

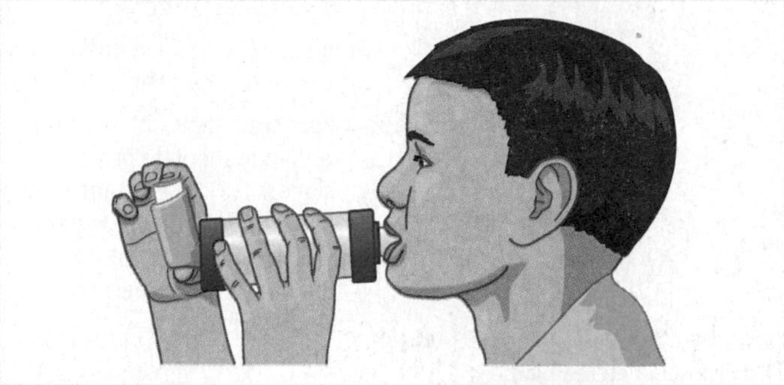

5 Have the person put the mouthpiece of the spacer in their mouth, above their tongue, and then close their lips around the spacer.

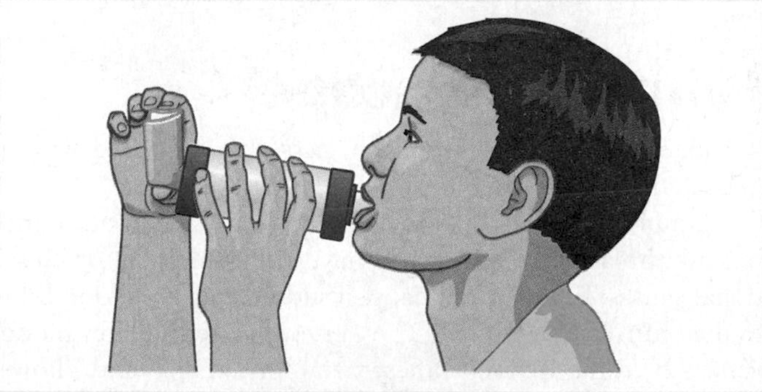

6 Have the person tip their head back slightly toward the ceiling, and press the top of the inhaler to spray one dose of medicine. Tell the person to slowly breathe in all the air they can and hold for 5 to 10 seconds, with their mouth closed.

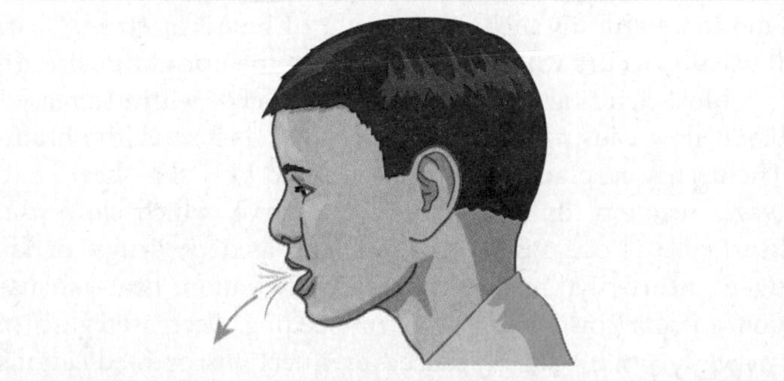

7 Once the 5 to 10 seconds are up, tell the person to open their mouth, move the inhaler away from their mouth, and breathe out slowly. If the person needs another dose of medicine, wait 1 minute before repeating these steps.

Hyperventilation

Excessively fast breathing that occurs during emotional distress is called **hyperventilation**. The result is an abnormal decrease in the blood carbon dioxide level, which causes the symptoms of tingling in the fingers and toes and light-headedness. It is important to rule out other causes of rapid breathing, such as untreated diabetes, severe shock, certain poisons, and brain swelling due to injury or high altitude.

What to Look For	What to Do
■ Shortness of breath ■ Fast breathing (more than 40 breaths per minute) ■ Tingling or numbness of the hands, feet, and around the mouth ■ Dizziness or light-headedness	1. Calm and reassure the person. 2. Take the person to a quiet place or ask bystanders to leave. Have the person sit down. 3. Encourage the person to breathe slowly, using the abdominal muscles: inhale through the nose, hold the full inhalation for 1 to 2 seconds, then exhale slowly through pursed lips.

FYI

Breathing Into a Paper Bag

A popular remedy for anxiety-related hyperventilation was to breathe into a paper bag. **DO NOT** do this. Bag rebreathing may alleviate anxiety, but increase the risk of hypoxemia (below normal levels of oxygen in the blood).

Data from Callaham M. Hypoxic hazards of traditional paper bag rebreathing in hyperventilating patients. *Ann Emerg Med.* 1989;18(6):622–628.

Chronic Obstructive Pulmonary Disease

Chronic obstructive pulmonary disease (COPD) is a broad term applied to emphysema, chronic bronchitis, and related lung diseases (ie, asbestosis, coal miner disease or black lung, World Trade Center disease). COPD describes a disease that makes it hard for a person to breathe because the normal flow of air into and out of the person's lungs is partially obstructed.

The incidence of COPD is very high in North America, and the most common causative factor is cigarette smoking. Because COPD takes many years to develop before a person notices difficulty breathing, it is usually considered a disease of older adults and is most commonly diagnosed in people older than 60 years.

Chronic bronchitis is caused by chronic infection, which can be brought on by irritations such as tobacco smoke. The bronchi become thick, unable to stretch, and partially blocked. Early symptoms include a smoker's cough or a cough due to a cold. Later, more severe symptoms include difficulty breathing, increased sputum, and severe coughing.

In emphysema, the alveoli of the lungs are partially destroyed and the lungs have lost their elasticity, making it difficult for the person to exhale. Common symptoms include coughing, wheezing, and shortness of breath. Breathing is extremely difficult for people with emphysema.

What to Look For	What to Do
The signs and symptoms of COPD are similar to those of asthma: ■ Wheezing ■ Prominent coughing and shortness of breath ■ Person may depend on a constant low level of artificially supplied oxygen to maintain breathing	1. People with COPD usually will have their own physician-prescribed medications. Assist the person to take any prescribed medications. 2. Place the person in the sitting position that provides the greatest comfort. 3. Encourage the person to cough up any secretions. 4. For acute breathing distress, obtain immediate professional medical assistance. The person might need oxygen, which is available from EMS and at hospital emergency departments.

Fainting (Syncope)

A sudden, brief loss of responsiveness not associated with a head injury is known as **syncope** (fainting).

Simple fainting, or **vasovagal syncope**, is common and not life threatening, and it can have either physical or emotional causes. Fainting can happen suddenly when blood flow to the brain is interrupted. The nervous system dilates blood vessels to three to four times their normal size and allows blood to pool in the legs and lower body.

Vasovagal syncope can be precipitated by unpleasant emotional stimuli such as the sight of blood or strong fear. It usually occurs when the person is in the upright position.

Most fainting episodes are associated with decreased blood flow causing deficient oxygen or glucose in the brain. The decreased blood flow can be caused by a slow heart rate (vagal reaction, in which the vagus nerve, which slows the heart rate, is overstimulated by fright, anxiety, drugs, or fatigue), heart-rhythm disturbances, dehydration, heat exhaustion, anemia (low hemoglobin), or bleeding. Decreased glucose (**hypoglycemia**) can be caused by infections or medications used to treat diabetes.

What to Look For	What to Do

▪ Pale skin or lips
▪ Clammy, sweaty skin
▪ Shivering
▪ Shaky and unsteady while standing
▪ Feels warm/hot or cold
▪ Person reports:
  ▪ Ringing in ears
  ▪ Dizziness
  ▪ Abdominal pain
  ▪ Visual disturbance (eg, black spots, blurred vision, narrowing vision)
	1. Assist the person into a sitting or lying position to reduce the risk of falling.
	2. Once in a safe position, the person can use physical counterpressure maneuvers (PCMs) to avoid fainting (syncope).
	PCMs are muscle contractions (squeezing) to elevate blood pressure. Depending upon the situation, lower-body PCMs are more effective than those for the upper body. Examples of PCMs include the following:
	  ▪ Leg crossing with muscle squeezing—while lying down, squeeze the legs together or, if necessary, while standing
	  ▪ Squatting—lower body into a squatting position
	  ▪ Arm tensing—gripping opposing hands with fingers and pulling arms in opposite directions
	  ▪ Isometric handgrip—squeezing fist with or without an item in the hand
	  ▪ Neck flexion—touching chin to chest and tightening the neck muscles
	3. **DO NOT** use PCMs when suspecting a heart attack or stroke.
	4. If no improvement occurs within 2 minutes or if the condition worsens or reoccurs, call 9-1-1.
	5. Monitor breathing.

Sitting or standing for a long time without moving, especially in a hot environment, can cause blood to pool in dilated vessels, which results in a loss of effective circulating blood volume, causing the blood pressure to drop. As the blood flow to the brain decreases, the person has a loss of consciousness and collapses.

Be aware that although syncope is not life threatening, in older adults and those with underlying medical conditions, it can be an indication of a disturbance in the heart rhythm, a stroke, or other serious medical conditions.

Presyncope

If a person says that they feel that they are about to faint or looks as though they are about to faint, this is a condition known as presyncope. Some first aid providers and bystanders may experience fainting when seeing blood or experiencing the stress of an emergency scene. Others may experience the condition when they rapidly move from lying down or sitting to a standing position or have stood for long periods of time, especially in hot weather.

Person Has Fainted

Sometimes you will be able to intervene before the fainting has occurred, other times you may need to provide aid to someone who has already fainted.

Refer to **FLOWCHART 17-4** for additional information regarding the care of a person who has fainted.

Flowchart 17-4 Fainting

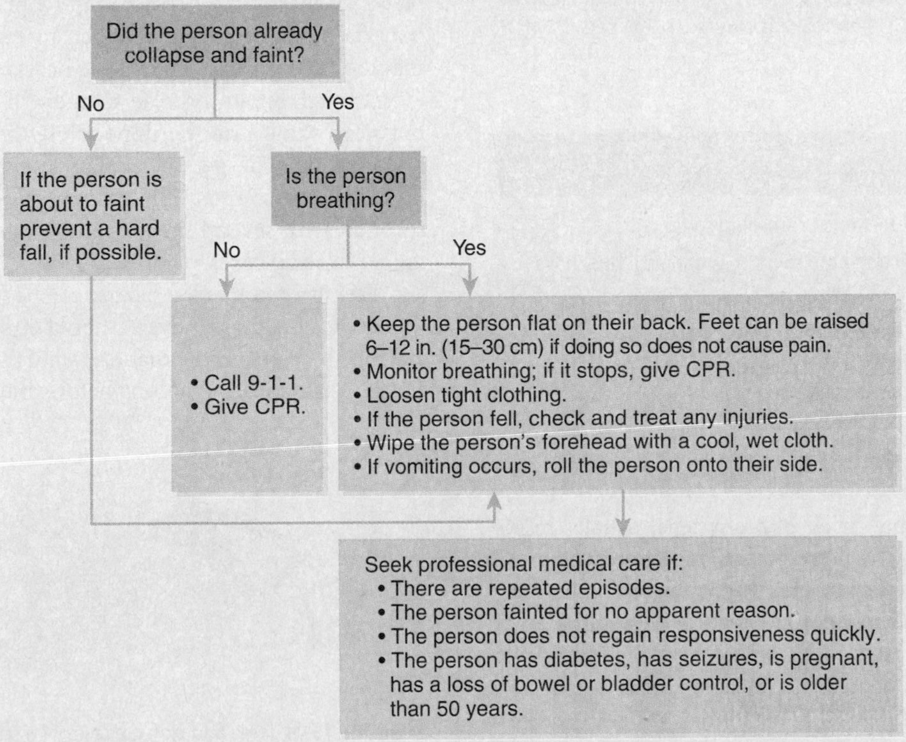

Did the person already collapse and faint?
No
Yes
If the person is about to faint prevent a hard fall, if possible.
Is the person breathing?
No
Yes
• Call 9-1-1.
• Give CPR.
• Keep the person flat on their back. Feet can be raised 6–12 in. (15–30 cm) if doing so does not cause pain.
• Monitor breathing; if it stops, give CPR.
• Loosen tight clothing.
• If the person fell, check and treat any injuries.
• Wipe the person's forehead with a cool, wet cloth.
• If vomiting occurs, roll the person onto their side.
Seek professional medical care if:
• There are repeated episodes.
• The person fainted for no apparent reason.
• The person does not regain responsiveness quickly.
• The person has diabetes, has seizures, is pregnant, has a loss of bowel or bladder control, or is older than 50 years.

What to Look For	What to Do
▪ A person collapsing to the ground ▪ Motionlessness	1. Check breathing. 2. If the person is breathing: ▪ Keep them flat on their back. Feet can be raised 6 to 12 inches (15 to 30 cm) if doing so does not cause pain. ▪ Monitor breathing. ▪ Loosen tight clothing. ▪ If they fell, check for and treat any injuries. ▪ Wipe the person's forehead with a cool, wet cloth. ▪ If vomiting occurs, roll the person onto their side (recovery position). 3. If the person is not breathing: ▪ Place them on their back on a flat and firm surface. ▪ Begin CPR (see Chapter 5, *CPR*). ▪ Call 9-1-1. 4. **DO NOT** use ammonia inhalants or smelling salts. 5. **DO NOT** give the person anything to drink or eat until they have fully recovered and can swallow. 6. **DO NOT** splash or pour water on the person's face. 7. **DO NOT** slap the person's face in an attempt to revive them. 8. Call 9-1-1 if: ▪ The person does not awaken or does not return to normal upon awakening. ▪ There are repeated episodes. ▪ The person fainted for no apparent reason. ▪ The person appears to have a serious health condition (eg, heart attack, diabetes, stroke). ▪ The person has diabetes, has seizures, is pregnant, has a loss of bowel or bladder control, or is older than 50 years.

CAUTION

DO NOT use ammonia inhalants or smelling salts.

DO NOT give the person anything to drink or eat until they have fully recovered and can swallow.

DO NOT splash or pour water on the person's face.

DO NOT slap the person's face in an attempt to revive them.

Seizure

A **seizure** is an abnormal firing of brain cells, usually resulting in jerking movements followed by an unresponsive period. Many different types of seizures exist. People may experience just one type or more than one. The type of seizure a person has depends on which part and how much of the brain is affected by the electrical disturbance that produces seizures. If you witness the seizure, the EMS personnel will want to hear your description of the event.

FYI

Seizures in Medical TV Dramas

About half the time, the physicians and nurses on popular fictional TV medical shows give improper seizure first aid that, in reality, could lead to broken teeth, bruises, or dislocations, according to a study presented at the American Academy of Neurology's annual meeting.

In the study, around 280 hours of recent medical dramas were watched, and when a clip showing a seizure was found, it was reviewed and compared with the Epilepsy Foundation's first aid guidelines for seizures. Fifty-nine seizures were found, and 46% of the actions by the physician and nurse actors were considered inappropriate. They noted such poor medical actions as holding a patient down, attempting to stop involuntary movement, and putting something in a patient's mouth while a seizure was in progress. In about 29% of the cases, the action was medically correct. The remaining seizure incidents were on the screen too briefly to judge.

Data from Moeller A, Moeller JJ, Rahey SR, Sadler RM. Depiction of seizure first aid management in medical television dramas. *Can J Neurol Sci.* 2011;38(5):723–727.

The type of seizure that most first aid providers encounter is a generalized, tonic-clonic seizure (formerly and still commonly called grand mal) **FIGURE 17-9**. The person suddenly becomes completely stiff or tense (sometimes emitting a vocal cry), with arms and legs extended (tonic phase). The person then begins to jerk rigorously, with arms and legs contracting and then relaxing in unison (clonic phase). These two phases make up the convulsion phase.

In a generalized seizure, the person always has a loss of responsiveness. The person may foam at the mouth (sputum may be pink- or red-tinged due to tongue biting), and they may be incontinent. The heart beats during the convulsion, even though breathing may temporarily stop. CPR chest compressions should not be done while the person is still jerking or twitching. The person having a seizure often makes a series of gasping sounds. The gasping generally lasts for 20 to 30 seconds, with several seconds in between gasps, but it can last longer in some cases.

Seeing a generalized seizure can be frightening. Fortunately, the convulsion phase is over in about 60 seconds, usually before a call to 9-1-1 can even be made. Even if the person turns blue, the seizure will typically end long before brain damage would begin.

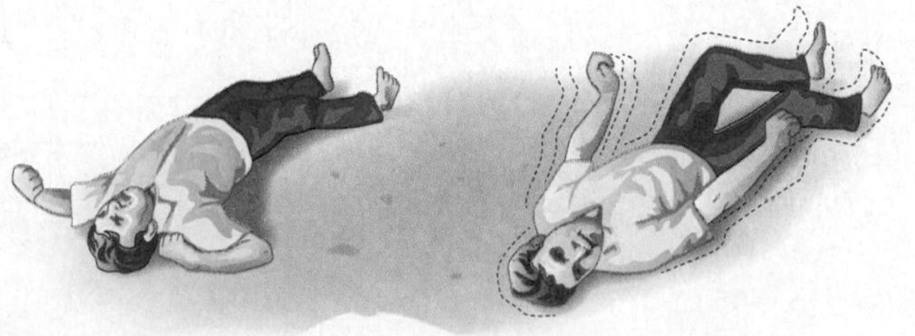

FIGURE 17-9 Tonic and clonic phases of a seizure.

Check for breathing after any convulsive episode has stopped. After the convulsion phase, the person becomes postictal (a state of confusion, sleepiness, and occasionally combativeness). They may have lost control of their bladder and be embarrassed.

There are other types of seizures. In an absence, or staring, seizure (formerly known as a petit mal seizure), the person momentarily becomes mentally absent and appears to be daydreaming.

Several medical conditions increase the instability or irritability of the brain and can lead to seizures, including the following:

- Lack of oxygen
- Heatstroke
- Poisoning
- Electric shock
- Hypoglycemia
- High fever in children
- Brain injury, tumor, or stroke
- Alcohol withdrawal, drug abuse, or overdose

Nearly all seizures resulting from fever occur in children between the ages of 6 months and 5 years (at 23 months, on average). They affect 3% to 5% of all children by the age of 5 years. Febrile seizures may occur in the same child on more than one occasion, but this does not constitute epilepsy. Febrile seizures are very frightening to the child's parents. Although these seizures are not life threatening, they may be a symptom of meningitis, a life-threatening brain infection that requires professional medical care.

Another cause of seizure is cardiac arrest. The brain is quickly affected when it runs out of blood glucose and oxygen. A person may incur irreversible brain damage or even die if the condition is not immediately recognized and the person is not rapidly resuscitated.

Additional causes of seizures include trauma, brain tumors, meningitis, alcohol withdrawal, and drug abuse (especially cocaine and amphetamines). People with diabetes may be prone to seizures when their blood glucose falls below normal levels and they become hypoglycemic due to too much insulin. Severe head injuries can cause rapid swelling of or bleeding into the brain, causing a seizure. Rapid action by surgeons can relieve the condition and be lifesaving.

Epilepsy, in contrast to the aforementioned causes of seizures, is an underlying condition (or permanent brain injury) that affects the delicate systems that govern how electrical energy behaves in the brain, making it susceptible to recurring seizures. Most people with epilepsy have seizures due to an unknown cause. Epilepsy is not a mental illness, nor it is not a sign of low intelligence. It also is not contagious. Between seizures, a person with epilepsy can function as normally as a person who does not have epilepsy. Medication can often help control seizure frequency in people with epilepsy. A frequent cause of a seizure is medication noncompliance—missed dosages of anticonvulsants.

Refer to **FLOWCHART 17-5** for additional information regarding the care of a person with a seizure.

FYI

Knowledge of Epilepsy

A survey found that about one-half of all people have witnessed an epileptic seizure either in person or on television, and about one-third of all people know someone with epilepsy. Even so, relatively few people are familiar with epilepsy, how to respond to a seizure, or the Epilepsy Foundation (www.epilepsy.com).

Reproduced from Kobau R, Price P. Knowledge of epilepsy and familiarity with this disorder in the US population. *Epilepsia.* 2003;44(11):1449–1454.

What to Look For	What to Do
Convulsive seizures (eg, tonic-clonic seizures) typically last for 1 to 2 minutes (but may last longer), and the person may experience the following signs and symptoms: ▪ Sudden falling to the floor or ground ▪ Stiffening of arm and leg muscles followed by jerky movement with arching of the back ▪ Foaming at the mouth ▪ Grinding of teeth ▪ Blue-gray face and lips ▪ Eyes rolling upward ▪ Loss of bladder and bowel control Nonconvulsive seizures (eg, absence or staring seizures) last only a few seconds and are so brief that they often escape detection. The person may experience the following signs and symptoms: ▪ Staring, confusion, or inattentiveness ▪ Frequent eye blinking ▪ Involuntary movements (eg, lip smacking, picking at clothes, fumbling)	**1.** Move nearby objects to avoid injury. **2.** Place something soft under the head such as a rolled towel or flat pillow. **DO NOT** use a soft, fluffy pillow, because it could interfere with breathing. **3.** Time the seizure from start to finish. **4.** Most seizures do not require professional medical care and end in 1 to 2 minutes. Stay with the person until the seizure is over. **5.** Keep bystanders away. **6.** Call 9-1-1 for any of the following: ▪ Seizure lasting longer than 5 minutes ▪ Series of seizures following one another ▪ The person has breathing difficulties after the seizure ▪ The person has diabetes or is pregnant ▪ Seizure happened in water ▪ This is the person's first known seizure ▪ The seizure is injury-related ▪ Slow recovery **7.** After the seizure: ▪ Keep the airway open by placing the person on their side and head on a rolled towel. ▪ Monitor breathing and if it stops, give CPR. ▪ Allow the person to sleep. ▪ Stay with the person until they have fully recovered.

Flowchart 17-5 Seizures

- Move nearby objects to avoid injury.
- Place something soft under the head such as a rolled towel or flat pillow. **DO NOT** use a soft, fluffy pillow.
- Time the seizure from start to finish.
- Keep bystanders away.

↓

Did any of the following occur?

- Seizure lasting longer than 5 min
- Series of seizures following one another
- The person has breathing difficulties after the seizure
- The person has diabetes or is pregnant
- Seizure happened in water
- This is the person's first known seizure
- The seizure is injury-related
- Slow recovery

No →

After the seizure:

- Keep the airway open by placing the person on their side and head on a rolled towel.
- Monitor breathing and if it stops, give CPR.
- Allow the person to sleep.
- Stay with the person until they have fully recovered.

Yes →

Call 9-1-1.

Status Epilepticus

Most seizures end after a few seconds or a few minutes. However, in some cases, they are prolonged or occur in a series, a condition called **status epilepticus**. A lengthy seizure over 5 minutes or two back-to-back seizures without a lucid interval is an emergency situation and requires immediate professional medical care. Repeated, uncontrolled seizures can lead to brain damage, fractures, severe dehydration, and aspiration. In adults, the most common cause of status epilepticus is failure to take prescribed medicines for epilepsy.

CAUTION

DO NOT restrain the person.

DO NOT put anything between the person's teeth during the seizure.

DO NOT splash or pour water or any other liquid on the person's face.

DO NOT move the person to another place (unless it is the only way to protect the person from injury).

DO NOT leave a person until they are fully alert and recovered.

Diabetic Emergencies

Insulin is a hormone produced by the pancreas that assists the body in using energy from food **FIGURE 17-10**. Insulin allows the transportation of glucose from the blood into the cells where it serves as a major source of fuel for the body. When excess glucose remains in the blood and is not transferred to the cells, the cells must rely on fat for fuel. When blood glucose cannot be used, it builds up in the blood. The glucose then overflows into the urine, passing through the body unused. When this occurs, a condition called **diabetes** develops **TABLE 17-5**. In diabetes, insulin is either ineffective or lacking in the body. This condition is not contagious, and in most cases special diet and/or medication can control it.

The body is continuously balancing glucose and insulin **FIGURE 17-11**. Too much insulin and not enough glucose leads to low blood glucose and possibly an insulin reaction. An insulin reaction results from a severely low blood glucose level, causing unconsciousness and possibly death. Too much glucose and not enough insulin leads to high blood glucose, the production of ketones, and possibly **diabetic coma**. Ketones cause a sweet or fruity odor on the breath.

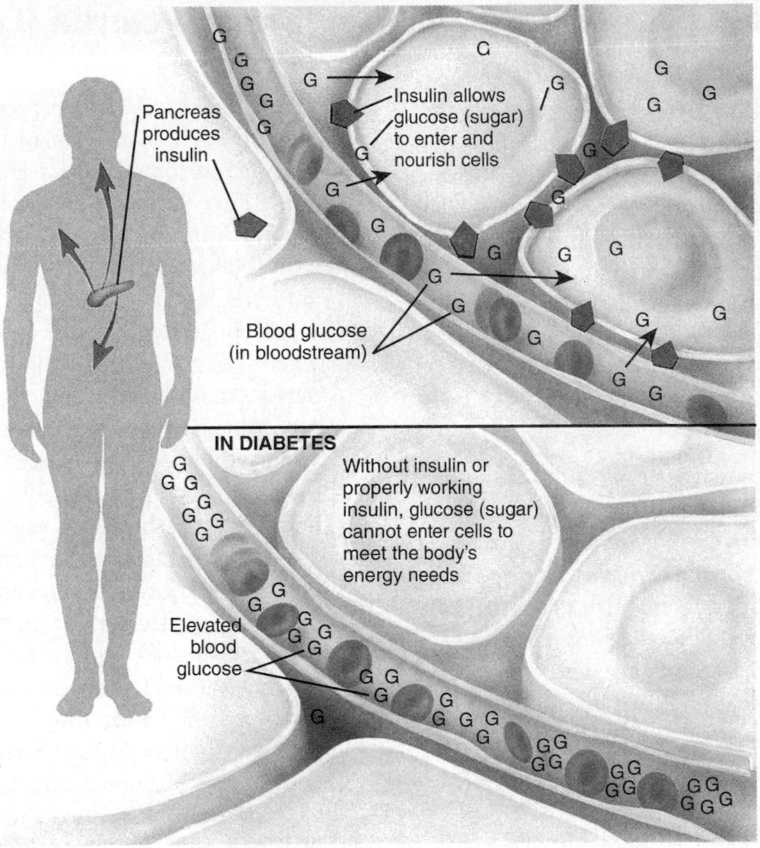

FIGURE 17-10 Normal metabolism (top) and diabetes (bottom).

TABLE 17-5 Diabetic Emergencies

	Hyperglycemia (high blood glucose)	Hypoglycemia (low blood glucose)
Cause	Not enough insulin; too much glucose	Too much insulin; not enough glucose
Insulin level	Insufficient	Excessive
Onset of symptoms	Gradual	Sudden
Skin	Flushed, dry, warm	Pale, clammy
Breath	Fruity odor or an acetone (nail polish remover) smell	Normal
Thirst	Severe	Normal
Urination	Frequent	Normal
Behavior	Normal to disorientation, drowsiness, and change in mood	Appearance of intoxication: combativeness, bad temper, anger, confusion, disorientation
Other symptoms	Drowsiness, vomiting, heavy breathing, eventual stupor or unresponsiveness	Sudden hunger, eventual stupor or unresponsiveness
First aid	If in doubt, give sugar. Give fluids to fight dehydration. Take the person to the hospital.	Give sugar. Seek professional medical care.

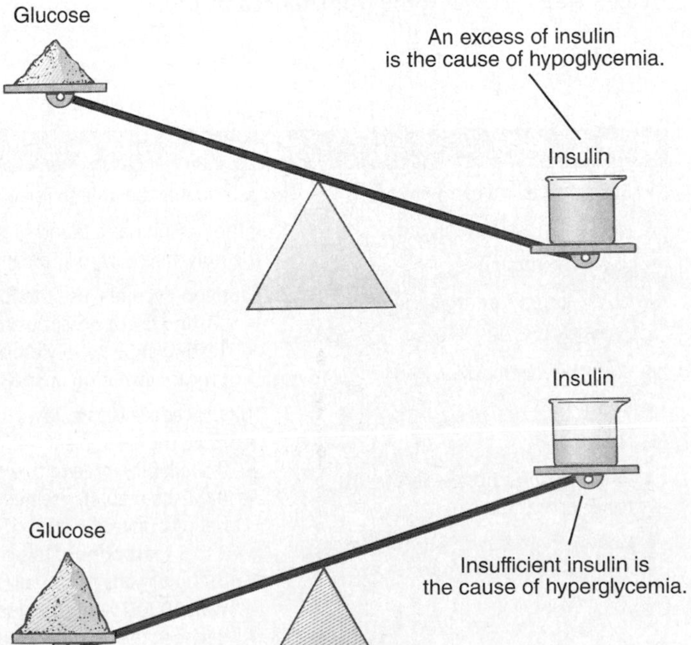

FIGURE 17-11 Diabetic emergencies are caused by either too much or too little insulin.

Types of Diabetes

Type 1 Diabetes

Type 1 diabetes (formerly called juvenile-onset or insulin-dependent diabetes) is most commonly diagnosed in childhood, but it may present at any age in life. This type of diabetes requires external insulin (not made by the body), which enables the glucose to enter the cells. External insulin is necessary because the body is unable to produce the insulin the cells require. When a person with type 1 diabetes is deprived of external insulin, they will become very ill. People with type 1 diabetes will usually be thin or not overweight.

Type 2 Diabetes

Type 2 diabetes used to be known as non–insulin-dependent or adult-onset diabetes. The incidence of type 2 diabetes is reaching epidemic proportions in the United States. Excess body weight and a sedentary lifestyle are widely recognized risk factors. Other risk factors include a family history of type 2 diabetes and age older than 45 years. The age of onset is usually older than 40 years, but it can occur at any age, and type 2 diabetes is being diagnosed in a growing number of children and adolescents. This type of diabetes may require insulin replacement and other medication.

Gestational Diabetes

Gestational diabetes occurs in some pregnancies. It usually ends after a baby is born, but when women who had experienced gestational diabetes get older, type 2 diabetes can develop. Gestational diabetes results from the body's resistance to the action of insulin. This resistance is caused by hormones produced during pregnancy. Gestational diabetes is usually treated with diet, but some women need insulin.

Hypoglycemia (Low Blood Glucose)

Most diabetic-related emergencies are due to low blood sugar (glucose). The condition of low blood glucose, called hypoglycemia, is sometimes referred to as an insulin reaction. This condition occurs in a person with diabetes for several reasons: too much insulin (rapidly depletes sugar), too little or delayed food intake, vomiting, exercising more than usual, alcohol, or any combination of these factors.

Hypoglycemia is not unusual for a person with diabetes who takes glucose-lowering medications, such as insulin. The person must balance injecting the right amount of insulin, eating the right amounts of certain foods, and exercising. The wrong amount of any element can result in too much insulin in the blood, using up available glucose too rapidly. Because the brain's most usable fuel is sugar, it is the first organ at risk.

Hypoglycemia can happen quickly, often within a few minutes. If it is not recognized and treated quickly, the person may die or experience permanent brain injury. Behaviors related to hypoglycemia often mimic those of people who have consumed too much alcohol: the person may stagger, may slur their speech, and may not follow simple commands. Unfortunately, some people with diabetes have been detained for intoxication by law enforcement personnel only to be found dead a few hours later.

Some people with diabetes are not dependent on insulin. Their bodies still make some insulin but not enough; with careful attention to diet and/or oral medication, the condition is more easily controlled. These people rarely become dangerously hypoglycemic.

People experiencing hypoglycemia may drool excessively. Profuse drooling can have the same effect as vomiting. Follow the same instructions as those for managing vomiting: quickly turn the person on their side.

What to Look For	What to Do
▪ Responsive and can swallow ▪ Medical identification tag ▪ Shaky, trembling ▪ Cold, clammy, or moist skin ▪ Confused ▪ Light-headed or dizzy ▪ Sudden hunger ▪ Nauseated ▪ Tingling or numbness in the lips, tongue, or cheeks ▪ Heavy sweating	The person may be able to tell what is wrong and what to do. **1.** If the person has a blood glucose monitor and is capable, have them check their blood glucose level: it is the only sure way to know if a person is experiencing low blood sugar. **FIGURE 17-12**. **2.** For hypoglycemia, use the following procedure, but only when: ▪ Testing is not possible and low blood sugar is suspected. ▪ Testing shows a low blood sugar (glucose) level (below 70 mg/dL). ▪ Profuse sweating or shaking occurs in a person known to have diabetes. **3.** The procedure is as follows (if the person can swallow): ▪ Have the person eat 15 to 20 g of sugar. ▪ If available, three to five glucose tablets is preferred (as directed on the label) **FIGURE 17-13**. ▪ If glucose tablets are not available, give any form of sugar such as glucose gel tube (as directed on label); 4 ounces (½ cup) of fruit juice (eg, orange, apple); 4 ounces (½ cup) of regular soda (not diet); 3 to 5 teaspoons of table sugar or honey; or hard candies, jellybeans, gumdrops (check the food label for how many to consume). ▪ Wait 10 to 15 minutes for the sugar to get into the blood. ▪ Recheck the blood glucose level, or if there is no monitor, look for improvement. ▪ If the blood glucose level is still low or no monitor was used and the person still has symptoms of low blood sugar, give the person an additional 15 g of sugar. **4.** If the person has no gag reflex and cannot swallow, **DO NOT** give anything by mouth. **5.** If there is no improvement or unable to give sugar, call 9-1-1 immediately.

What to Look For	What to Do
	Notes: ▪ Young children usually need less than 15 g of carbohydrates to fix a low blood sugar level (eg, infants, 6 g; toddlers 8 g, small children 10 g). ▪ For a suspected hypoglycemic and uncooperative child who rejects swallowing a form of glucose, glucose placed under the tongue (sublingual) can be attempted. ▪ Many people may want to eat as much as they can until they feel better. This can cause blood sugar levels to shoot way up. Using the procedure described here can help avoid this (high blood sugar levels).
Severe hypoglycemia suspected: ▪ Staggering, slurred speech, and not following simple commands ▪ Unable to swallow ▪ Seizures ▪ Unresponsiveness	1. Call 9-1-1 immediately. 2. If not breathing, begin CPR (see page Chapter 5, *CPR*). 3. If breathing, roll them onto their side (recovery position; see page 70–71) and monitor breathing. 4. **DO NOT** give food or fluids. 5. If unsure which diabetic condition (low blood sugar or high blood sugar) exists, give sugar. **DO NOT** give insulin.

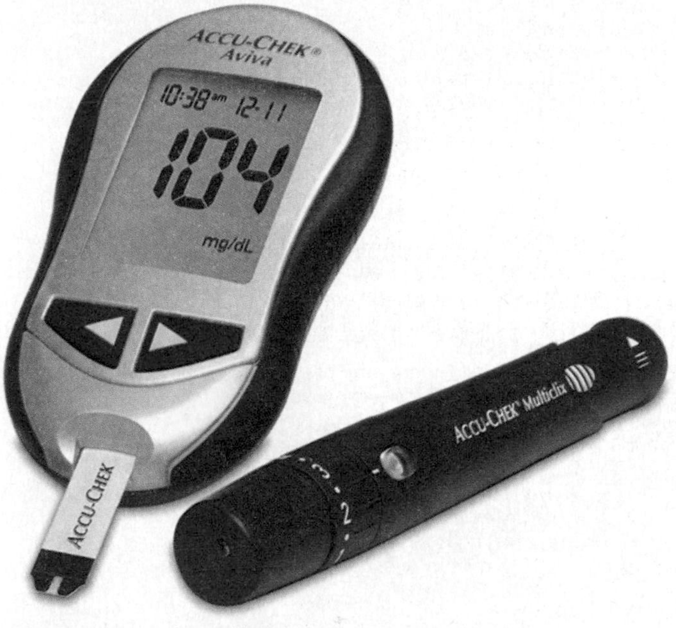

FIGURE 17-12 Blood glucose meter with lancing device.

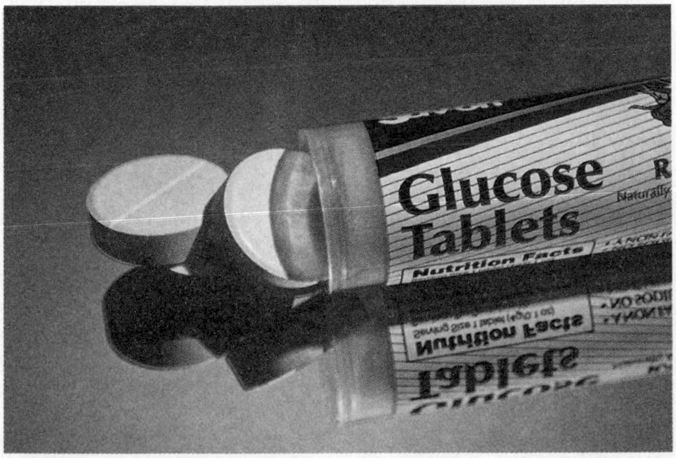

FIGURE 17-13 Glucose tablets.

Hyperglycemia (High Blood Glucose)

The opposite reaction of hypoglycemia is **hyperglycemia**. This condition occurs when a person with diabetes has too much glucose in the blood. Several scenarios can cause this medical condition, including insufficient insulin, overeating, illness, inactivity, stress, or a combination of these factors.

If the lack of insulin goes uncorrected for too long, the person's alertness slowly deteriorates to a state of unresponsiveness from which the person cannot be aroused. This serious condition is called diabetic coma; there is little that first aid providers or even EMS personnel can do to correct it. It requires careful rebalancing of insulin, fluids, and electrolytes in a medical facility, a process that can take days. Because diabetic coma has a generally slow onset and usually occurs in people with previously known diabetes, the person is most often brought to professional medical care long before unresponsiveness occurs.

Refer to **FLOWCHART 17-6** for additional information regarding the care of a diabetic emergency.

What to Look For	What to Do
▪ Medical identification tag ▪ Gradual onset (hours to days) because some sugar is still reaching the brain ▪ Drowsiness ▪ Extreme thirst ▪ Very frequent urination ▪ Warm, red, dry skin ▪ Vomiting ▪ Fruity breath odor (has been described to be like nail polish remover) ▪ Heavy breathing ▪ Eventual unresponsiveness	1. Give frequent, small sips of water if the person with diabetes can swallow. 2. If possible, have a family member check the person's blood sugar level. If uncertain whether the person with diabetes has a high or low blood glucose level, and if they are responsive and able to swallow, use the procedures for giving sugar, as previously described. The extra sugar will not cause significant harm in a person experiencing hyperglycemia. 3. **DO NOT** give insulin unless the person with diabetes can self-administer it. 4. Call 9-1-1 as soon as possible.

Flowchart 17-6 Diabetic Emergencies

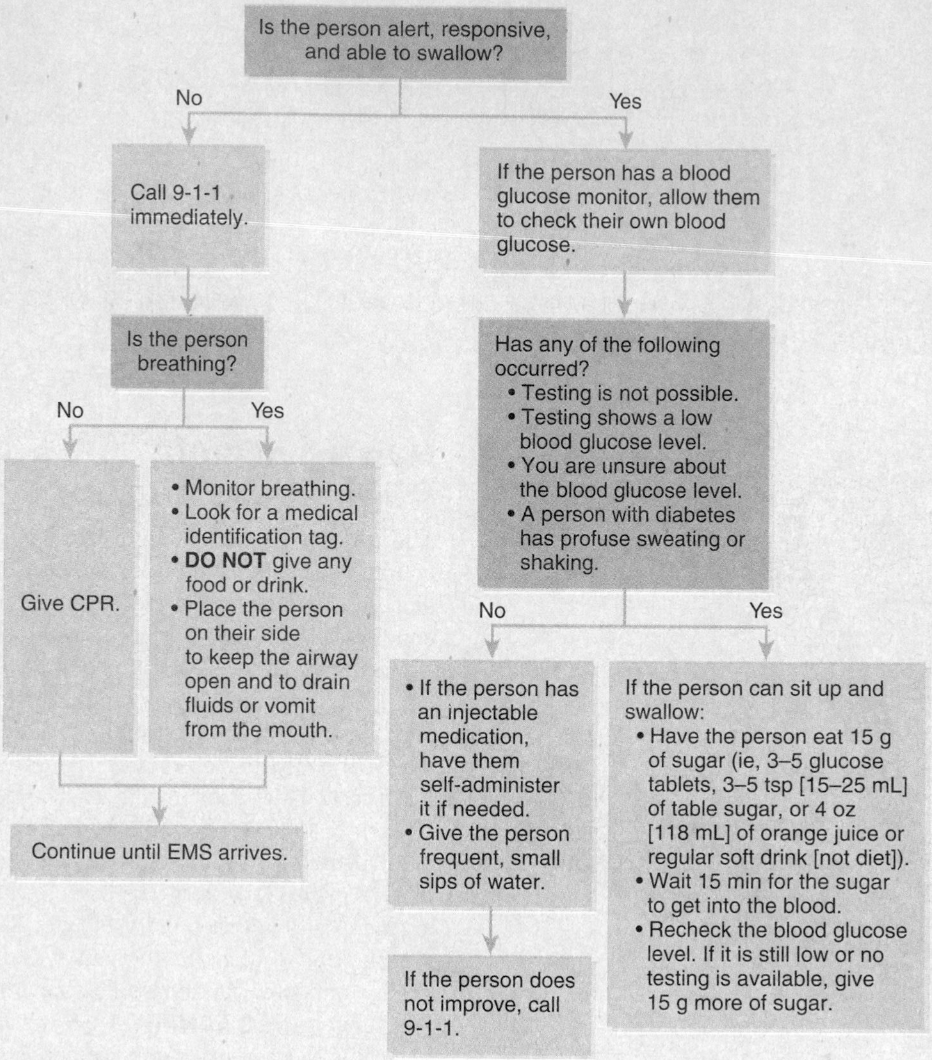

Q&A

How can you tell the difference between hypoglycemia and hyperglycemia?

It is difficult to determine whether a person has hypoglycemia or hyperglycemia. Sugar helps the person with hypoglycemia, but not the person with hyperglycemia. However, do not debate whether to give sugar; sugar will cause no harm in either condition.

Ask the person with diabetes two questions: "Have you eaten today?" and "Have you taken your insulin today?" If the person with diabetes has taken their insulin but has not eaten, suspect hypoglycemia. If the person with diabetes has eaten but has not taken insulin, suspect hyperglycemia. If you are unsure which condition exists, give sugar.

Abdominal Complaints

People with gastrointestinal conditions usually complain about one or more of the following symptoms:

- *Abdominal pain that is aching, cramping, sharp, or dull.* It might be constant, or it can come and go. The pain could indicate a mild condition or an acute condition requiring immediate surgery.
- *Nausea and vomiting.* Vomiting is the ejection of the stomach's contents through the mouth. Nausea is a feeling of the need to vomit.
- *Diarrhea or constipation.* Diarrhea is the frequent passage of loose, watery stools. Constipation is the opposite of diarrhea; stools are infrequent, hard, and difficult to pass.

Abdominal Pain

The abdomen is the area between the diaphragm and the groin. Abdominal organs are either hollow or solid. Hollow organs are tubes, such as the stomach and the intestines, through which material passes, conducting food through the body. Solid organs are solid masses of tissue in which much of the chemical work of the body takes place. The liver, spleen, and pancreas are solid organs. The peritoneum is a thin membrane lining the entire abdominal cavity. Inflammation of the peritoneum is called peritonitis.

There are many possible causes of abdominal pain—some not so serious and some life threatening. They often can be serious enough to require emergency surgery.

Abdominal conditions are so difficult to diagnose that even skilled physicians can have trouble pinpointing an exact cause. It is neither feasible nor useful for a first aid provider to distinguish among the many causes of abdominal pain because first aid usually will be similar regardless of the cause.

What to Look For	What to Do
A first aid provider should ask the following questions: ▪ When did the pain start? Where is it located? ▪ Is the pain constant, or does it come and go? Constant pain can be more serious than a cramping pain. Constant abdominal pain suggests inflammation of an organ; cramping suggests obstruction of a hollow organ. ▪ Does belching or passing gas relieve the pain? If so, the intestine might be affected. ▪ Does the person feel nauseated, or do they have a good appetite? ▪ Is there diarrhea or vomiting? ▪ Does the person feel warm (feverish)? ▪ Does anyone near the person have similar symptoms? ▪ For a woman: Is there any chance of pregnancy? Any pain with pregnancy should be treated as an emergency. ▪ Is the abdomen rigid to the touch? A rigid abdomen can be a sign of an emergency condition.	**1.** Give the person only clear fluids (anything you can see through, except alcohol and caffeinated beverages). Have the person slowly sip the fluids. **2.** Give the person an antacid. **3.** If practical, place a hot-water bottle against the person's abdomen or have the person soak in a warm bath. **4.** Recognize the possibility of vomiting and be prepared for it. Keep the person on their left side to help prevent vomiting. **5.** Keep the person in a comfortable position, usually lying down with knees bent (unless the person is nauseated). **6.** Seek professional medical care if any of the following applies: ▪ Pain is constant and severe. ▪ The person is unable to drink fluids. ▪ The person is or might be pregnant. ▪ The abdomen is rigid and painful. ▪ The abdomen is swollen. ▪ More pain occurs after you press your fingers on the person's abdomen and suddenly release them. ▪ There is bloody, blood-stained, or black stool or vomit. ▪ The person has a fever. ▪ There is light-headedness or fainting. ▪ Pain began around the belly button and later moved to the lower right part of the abdomen. This is a sign of appendicitis.

Nausea and Vomiting

Nausea (upset stomach) and vomiting often occur with conditions such as altitude sickness, motion sickness, brain injury, intestinal viruses, eating or drinking too much, and being emotionally upset. In minor illnesses, nausea and vomiting should clear up in a day. Persistent nausea and vomiting can signal more serious illnesses such as appendicitis, food poisoning, or bowel obstruction. In general, if the condition lasts longer than 1 or 2 days, or if the person vomits multiple times in a short period, the person could become dehydrated (have a loss of too much fluid). Young children and older people can be more seriously affected.

What to Look For	What to Do
Nausea and vomiting. A first aid provider should ask the following questions: ▪ Is there abdominal pain? ▪ Is there blood or brown, grainy material in the vomit? ▪ Is there diarrhea? Vomiting and diarrhea together usually indicate a self-limited viral infection. ▪ Are there signs of dehydration (eg, the person is dizzy when standing; has dry, cracked lips; is very thirsty)? ▪ Does anyone else near the person have similar symptoms? ▪ Has the person had a recent head injury?	**1.** Give the person small amounts of clear fluids (eg, sports drinks; clear soups; flat, decaffeinated soda; apple or cranberry juice), except alcohol and caffeinated beverages. **2.** If the person is able to keep fluids down, offer carbohydrates (eg, bread, cereal, pasta) first; they are easier to digest. Avoid milk products and meats for 48 hours. **3.** Have the person rest and avoid exertion until they are able to eat solid foods easily. **4.** Prevent inhalation of vomit by positioning the person on their side to allow drainage. Inhaled vomit can result in severe pneumonia. **5.** Seek professional medical care if: ▪ Blood or brown, grainy material appears in the vomit. ▪ There is constant abdominal pain. ▪ The person faints when standing. ▪ The person is unable to keep fluids down for more than 24 hours. ▪ The person has severe, projectile vomiting (vomit shoots out in large quantities). ▪ The vomiting follows a recent head injury.
Motion sickness, indicated by: ▪ Nausea ▪ Pale skin ▪ Cold sweats ▪ Vomiting ▪ Dizziness ▪ Headache ▪ Fatigue	**1.** If the person is prone to motion sickness, they should sit near the midsection of a plane, boat, bus, train, or car. People susceptible to motion sickness should look far ahead to the horizon, not to the sides, and they should avoid reading or overeating. **2.** A person prone to motion sickness should try taking dimenhydrinate (Dramamine) or using a physician-prescribed scopolamine patch 1 hour before traveling (follow label directions).

CAUTION

DO NOT give enemas and laxatives, which can worsen the condition or cause complications such as ruptured bowel.

DO NOT give fluids other than clear fluids as long as the pain continues.

DO NOT give solid foods.

DO NOT give milk products.

Diarrhea

Diarrhea is the passage of loose, watery, or unformed stools (usually more than four times a day). Diarrhea can be a symptom of intestinal infection (bacterial, viral, or parasitic), food poisoning, or food sensitivity or allergy, among other ailments. Dehydration can occur if the body loses too much fluid through the stool and the person cannot drink enough fluid to keep up with the fluid losses from the diarrhea. Older people and very young people are especially prone to dehydration, which can result in dangerous chemical imbalances. Replacing fluids and electrolytes such as sodium and potassium is of primary importance for any person with diarrhea. Diarrhea flushes bacteria and parasites out of the body. Letting diarrhea run its course is best because then bacteria or parasites are not trapped in the intestines.

What to Look For	What to Do
Determine the answers to the following questions: ▪ Was the person recently exposed to untreated, possibly contaminated water or food? ▪ Is blood or mucus present in the stool? Their presence can signal more serious conditions. ▪ Are signs of dehydration present (eg, the person is dizzy when standing; has dry, cracked lips; is very thirsty)? ▪ Does the person have cramping abdominal pain? ▪ Has the person been incontinent? ▪ Is the person feverish? ▪ Does anyone else near the person have similar symptoms?	**1.** Have the person drink a lot of clear fluids (8 to 10 eight-oz [240-mL] glasses daily). This is the single most important treatment. **2.** When the person can tolerate clear fluids, give mild foods such as soup and gelatin. Later, the BRAT diet—bananas, rice, applesauce, toast—is recommended. **3.** Bismuth can help in most cases (follow label directions). Be aware that bismuth can turn the stool and the tongue black. People sensitive to aspirin should not use bismuth. **DO NOT** give to children or teenagers. If the person cannot let the diarrhea run its course, over-the-counter medications will calm the bowel, reducing movement through the intestines. **4.** Seek professional medical care if: ▪ The person has bloody stools, which might appear black or tarry. (Keep in mind that bismuth preparations can cause black stools.) ▪ Symptoms do not improve after 24 hours. ▪ The person has a fever. ▪ The person has severe, constant abdominal pain. ▪ The person is severely dehydrated.

CAUTION

DO NOT give milk products and meats for 48 hours after diarrhea stops.

DO NOT give caffeine, which stimulates the intestine and causes urination, furthering dehydration.

DO NOT give soda or fruit juice, because they contain high levels of sugar, which can worsen the condition, and they do not provide electrolytes, which are essential for rehydration. Sports drinks, however, contain the right ratio of sugar and electrolytes to rehydrate without worsening the condition.

Constipation

Constipation is the passage of hard, dry stools. Most physicians define constipation as three or fewer bowel movements per week, where stools are hard, dry, and small, and painful and difficult to pass. Constipation is rarely more than a passing discomfort in otherwise healthy people. Normal bowel movements can occur three times per day or once every 3 days. Minor changes in diet, fluid intake, activity, or emotional state can cause bowel movement changes. Rectifying any of those changes will also relieve constipation in most cases. Bowel stimulants or laxatives are rarely needed.

What to Look For	What to Do
▪ Bloating sensation of abdomen. A very painful or visibly swollen abdomen is a more serious condition than simple constipation. ▪ Hard, dry stools. Small strings of blood are not unusual if the stool was painful to evacuate.	**1.** Have the person eat more fiber (fresh or dried fruits, vegetables, bran). Fiber causes the colon to contract. Over-the-counter fiber products can be used, but the label directions should be followed. **2.** Make sure the person drinks plenty of fluids (8 to 10 eight-oz [240-mL] glasses daily). Excessively hard stools often are the result of dehydration. **3.** Encourage the person to remain active. Activity such as walking stimulates colon contractions. **4.** If symptoms do not improve, try one of the following: ▪ A stool softener (docusate sodium) ▪ Caffeine, which stimulates colon contractions **5.** Seek professional medical care if the person experiences any of the following: ▪ Severe abdominal pain ▪ Visibly swollen or very painful abdomen ▪ Fever ▪ Vomiting

PREP KIT

Ready for Review

- A heart attack occurs when a portion of the heart muscle tissue dies because its blood supply is stopped.
- Angina pectoris results when blood flow to the heart muscle is restricted, but not completely blocked.
- A stroke occurs when part of the blood flow to the brain is suddenly cut off.
- Asthma is a condition marked by recurrent attacks of breathing difficulty, often with wheezing.
- Hyperventilation is fast, deep breathing and is common during emotional stress.
- Chronic obstructive pulmonary disease (COPD) is a broad term applied to emphysema, chronic bronchitis, and related lung diseases.
- Fainting, or syncope, is a sudden brief loss of responsiveness not associated with head injury.
- A seizure results from an abnormal stimulation of the brain's cells, which causes uncontrollable muscle movements.
- Diabetes is a condition in which insulin is lacking or ineffective.
- Hypoglycemia is a very low blood glucose level and can be caused by too much insulin, too little or delayed food intake, exercise, alcohol, or a combination of these factors.
- Hyperglycemia occurs when the body has too much glucose in the blood and can be caused by insufficient insulin, overeating, inactivity, illness, stress, or a combination of these factors.
- People with gastrointestinal conditions usually report pain, nausea, vomiting, diarrhea, or constipation.
- Nausea (upset stomach) and vomiting often occur with conditions such as altitude sickness, motion sickness, brain injury, intestinal viruses, eating or drinking too much, and being emotionally upset. Persistent nausea and vomiting can signal more serious illnesses such as appendicitis, food poisoning, or bowel obstruction.
- Diarrhea is the frequent passage of loose, watery, or unformed stools and can be a symptom of intestinal infection, food poisoning, food allergy, or other ailments.
- Constipation is the passage of hard, dry stools and is rarely more than a passing discomfort in otherwise healthy people.

Vital Vocabulary

angina pectoris A spasmodic pain in the chest, characterized by a sensation of severe constriction or pressure on the anterior chest; associated with insufficient blood supply to the heart, aggravated by exercise or tension, and relieved by rest or medication.

asthma A condition marked by recurrent attacks of breathing difficulty, often with wheezing, due to spasmodic constriction of the air passages, often as a response to allergens or to mucus plugs in the bronchioles.

chronic obstructive pulmonary disease (COPD) A disease that makes it hard for a person to breathe because the normal flow of air into and out of the person's lungs is partially obstructed.

diabetes A condition that develops when glucose builds up in the blood, overflows into the urine, and passes through the body unused.

diabetic coma A state of unresponsiveness caused by a lack of insulin that goes uncorrected for too long.

heart attack A lay term for a condition resulting from blockage of a coronary artery and subsequent death of part of the heart muscle; a myocardial infarction; sometimes called simply "a coronary."

hyperglycemia An abnormally increased concentration of glucose in the blood.

hyperventilation Excessively fast breathing that occurs during emotional distress.

hypoglycemia An abnormally diminished concentration of glucose in the blood.

seizure Generalized, uncoordinated muscular activity associated with a loss of responsiveness; a convulsion; an attack of epilepsy.

status epilepticus The occurrence of two or more seizures without a period of complete consciousness between them or a lengthy seizure lasting more than 5 minutes.

stroke A brain injury due to bleeding in the brain tissue or to a blockage of blood flow, causing permanent damage.

syncope Fainting; a brief period of unresponsiveness.

transient ischemic attack (TIA) A form of stroke that occurs when a part of the brain is deprived of oxygen-rich blood long enough to cause symptoms but not long enough to cause permanent damage; a mini-stroke.

vasovagal syncope A shock-like state due to severe emotional distress; may result in a fainting spell resulting from a transient decrease in blood flow to the brain.

PREP KIT continued

Assessment in Action

You are on a 5-day backpacking trip in the mountains with your friends. On day 3, and after several tough miles of hiking, your friend seems to be disoriented and is stumbling over rocks and tree roots on the trail. He falls to the ground but remains responsive. You know that this friend has type 1 diabetes and did take his insulin that morning.

Directions: Circle Yes if you agree with the statement; circle No if you disagree.

1. This person is very likely suffering from hyperglycemia.
YES **NO**

2. Low blood glucose levels can be caused by too much insulin, too little or delayed food intake, exercise, and alcohol.
YES **NO**

3. To give sugar in this scenario, the person must be known to have diabetes, have an altered mental status, and be awake enough to swallow.
YES **NO**

Check Your Knowledge

Directions: Circle Yes if you agree with the statement; circle No if you disagree.

1. People having a heart attack can experience chest pain.
YES **NO**

2. You can help the person with chest pain take their nitroglycerin.
YES **NO**

3. A responsive person having a stroke should lie down with their head slightly raised.
YES **NO**

4. People with asthma may have a prescribed inhaler.
YES **NO**

5. A person who is breathing fast (hyperventilation) should be encouraged to breathe slowly by holding inhaled air for several seconds and then exhaling slowly.
YES **NO**

6. Immobilize the spine of a person having a seizure.
YES **NO**

7. Some people having a seizure display a rigid arching of the back.
YES **NO**

8. A person having seizures always requires medical attention.
YES **NO**

9. If in doubt about the type of diabetic emergency a person is experiencing, give sugar to a responsive person who can swallow.
YES **NO**

10. Nitroglycerin can relieve chest pain associated with angina.
YES **NO**

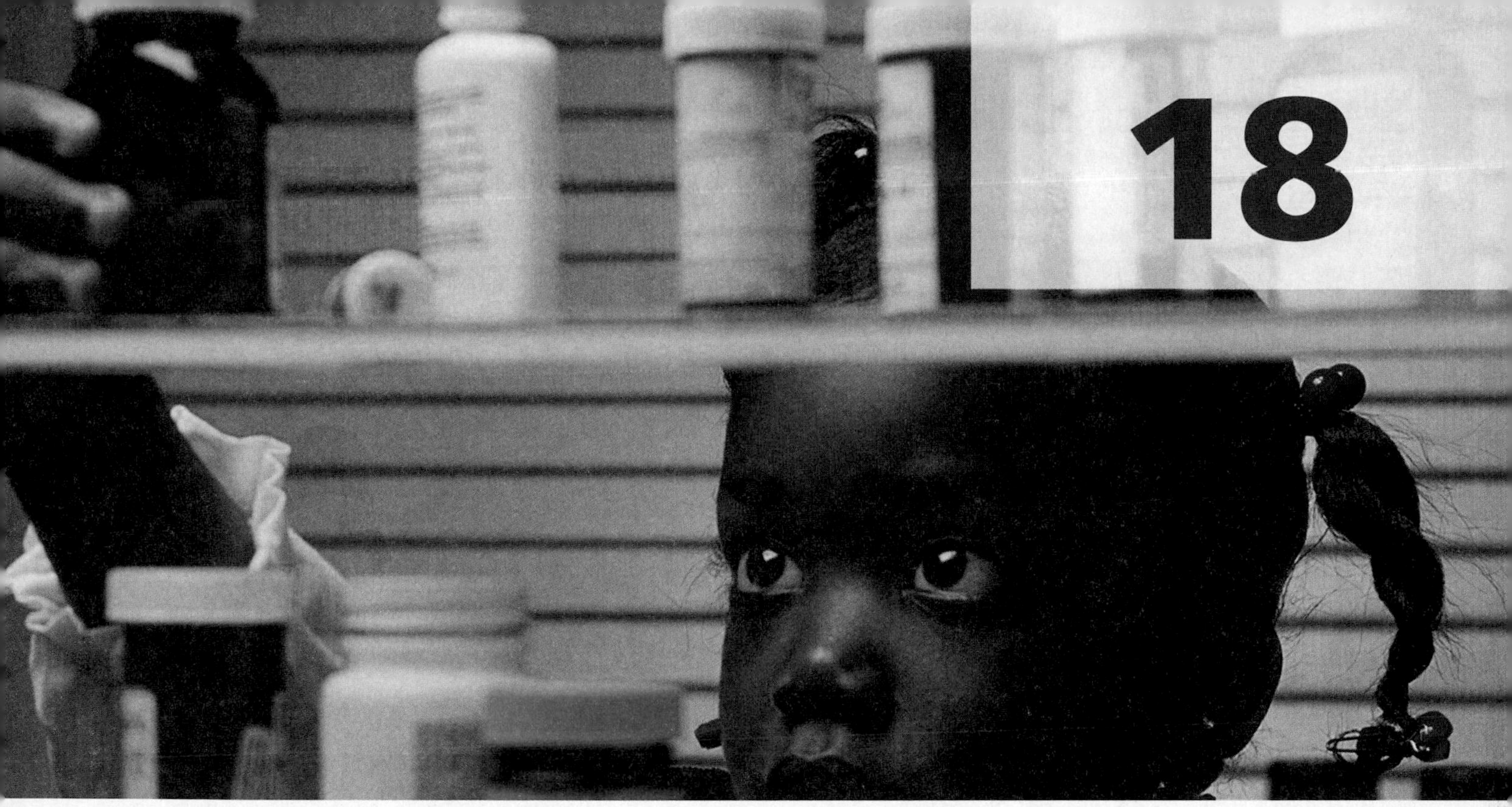

18

Poisoning

CHAPTER AT A GLANCE

- Poison
- Alcohol Emergencies
- Drug Emergencies
- Carbon Monoxide Poisoning
- Plant-Induced Dermatitis

Poison

What Is a Poison?

The American Association of Poison Control Centers (AAPCC) defines a **poison** as anything that can harm someone if it is (1) used in the wrong way, (2) used by the wrong person, or (3) used in the wrong amount. A **toxin** is a poisonous substance produced by bacteria, animals, or plants that acts by changing the normal metabolism of cells or by destroying them.

Poisons can be classified by how they enter the body **FIGURE 18-1**:

- Ingested (swallowed)—through the mouth
- Inhaled (breathed)—through the lungs
- Injected—through a needlelike device (eg, snake's fangs, bee's stinger)
- Absorbed (direct contact)—through the skin or eyes

Poisons come in four forms: solids (eg, medicine pills and tablets, dry powders, batteries, certain plants), liquids (eg, household cleaning products, antifreeze, paint), sprays (eg, spray cleaning products, bug spray), and gases (eg, carbon monoxide, formaldehyde).

Consumer products are typically safe to use as directed by their label; however, if label directions are not followed or are improperly followed, some of these products can be poisonous. The most

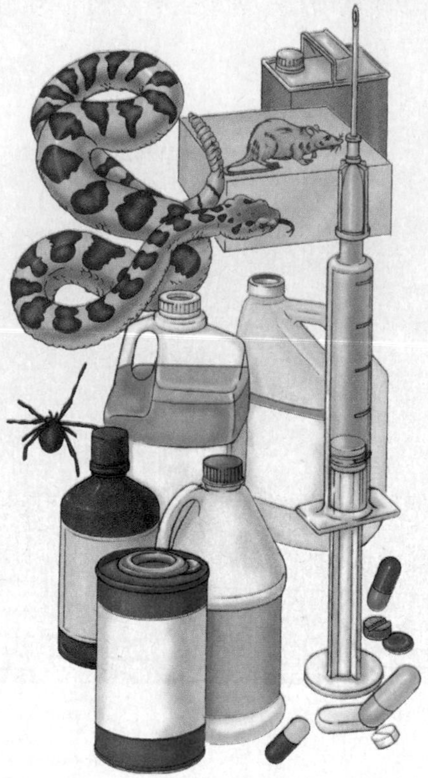

FIGURE 18-1 Sources of poisons.

> **Q&A**
>
> **Are some poisons absorbed through the skin?**
>
> Chemical substances, including some medicines and poisons, are absorbed through the skin. Heavy metals such as mercury and lead pass through the skin and can result in chronic poisoning. Chlordane, malathion, and other pesticides cross the skin barrier and can cause acute and chronic conditions. Cyanide readily absorbs through the skin and can be deadly.

common poisons are not necessarily the most dangerous ones. Some of the more dangerous poisons that could be found in a home include the following:

- Antifreeze and windshield washer products
- Some medicines and medications
- Corrosive cleaners such as drain openers, oven cleaners, toilet bowl cleaners, and rust removers
- Fuels such as kerosene, lamp oil, and gasoline
- Pesticides

Ingested (Swallowed) Poisons

Ingested poisoning occurs when a person swallows a toxic substance. Fortunately, most poisons have little toxic effect or are ingested in such small amounts that severe poisoning rarely occurs. However, the potential for severe or fatal poisoning is always present. According to the AAPCC, more than 80% of all poisonings happen by ingesting a toxic substance.

Swallowing nonfood substances is so common among children that it is unusual for a child to reach the age of 5 years without ingesting a nonfood substance at least once. Although many nonfood substances are not harmful, others present definite health threats. Some have the potential to block the airway. Others are poisonous. Hundreds of thousands of poisonings occur in the United States each year, but only a small percentage progress to severe or life-threatening conditions. The AAPCC reports that approximately 50% of all poisoning cases occur in children younger than 6 years.

People who are prescribed many medications may have difficulty keeping them straight and may inadvertently take an excessive dose if they forget having already taken a medication.

Analgesics (pain medications) account for the largest category of poisoning exposures. Basically, any substance that is accessible to a child is a potential poison. Analgesic products that contain acetaminophen, for example, are involved in poisoning incidents more often than other analgesics are, not because acetaminophen is more toxic but because many products contain acetaminophen and they can be taken concurrently.

It is important not to confuse poisoning frequency with poisoning severity. Most plant and mushroom ingestions are minor, with harmless effects. In contrast, gun-bluing products (agents containing selenious acid that are used to prevent rusting of gun barrels) account for fewer episodes of exposure, but the potential for harm is much greater. Fortunately,

What to Look For	What to Do
▪ Abdominal pain and cramping ▪ Nausea or vomiting ▪ Diarrhea ▪ Burns, odor, or stains around and inside the mouth	**1.** Try to determine: ▪ Person's age and weight ▪ Person's condition ▪ What poison was swallowed ▪ When the poison was taken ▪ How much was taken **2.** For an alert and awake person, call the Poison Control hotline (**Poison Help**) at 1-800-222-1222, even if signs of poisoning are not present **FIGURE 18-2**. Follow their directions. **3.** Place the person lying down on their left side to delay the poison from moving into the intestines and to prevent inhalation of vomit, if vomiting occurs **FIGURE 18-3**. **4.** Monitor breathing, and if absent, begin CPR. See Chapter 5, *CPR*.

What to Look For	What to Do
▪ Drowsiness or unresponsiveness ▪ Difficulty breathing, speaking, or swallowing ▪ Seizure ▪ Poison container nearby	**5.** *Cautions:* ▪ **DO NOT** give mouth-to-mouth breaths. ▪ **DO NOT** come into contact with vomit or body fluids as these may contain the poison and cause injury to the first aider. ▪ **DO NOT** give anything to eat or drink unless advised to do so by Poison Control or a professional health care provider. ▪ **DO NOT** try to cause vomiting by giving syrup of ipecac or by gagging or tickling the back of the person's throat. ▪ **DO NOT** give activated charcoal unless advised to do so by Poison Control or a professional health care provider. ▪ **DO NOT** give water or milk to dilute poisons other than caustic or corrosive substances (acids and alkalis) unless instructed by staff at Poison Control. Fluids can dissolve a dry poison, such as tablets or capsules, more rapidly and fill up the stomach, forcing the stomach contents (the poison) into the small intestine, where it will be absorbed faster. Vomiting and aspiration could occur.

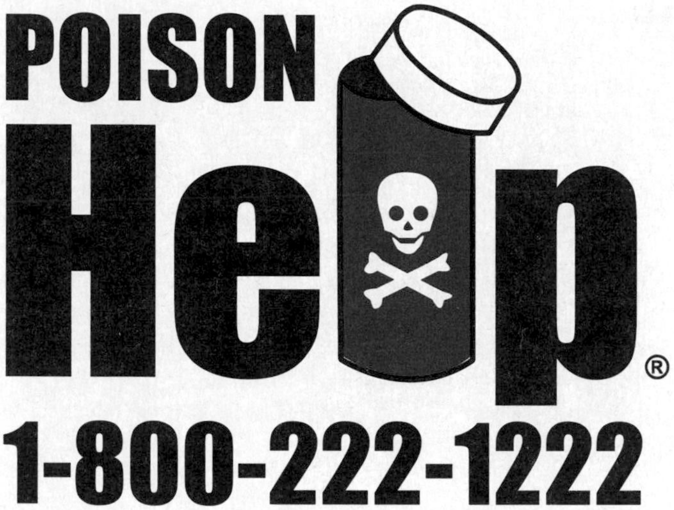

FIGURE 18-2 If you or someone you know may have ingested a dangerous substance, contact poison control immediately at 1-800-222-1222 or go to poisonhelp.org for assistance.

Courtesy of the American Association of Poison Control Centers. To locate your local poison center call 1 (800) 222-1222 or visit aapcc.org.

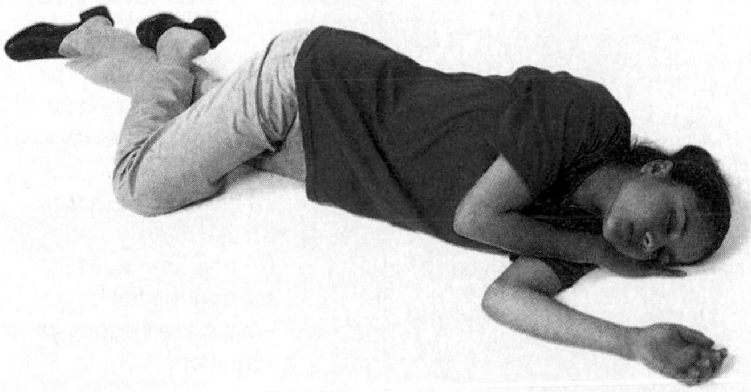

FIGURE 18-3 The left-side position delays the advance of the poison into the small intestine.

most poison ingestions involve products with minor toxic effects or amounts so small that severe poisoning rarely occurs **TABLE 18-1**.

Refer to **FLOWCHART 18-1** for additional information regarding the care of a person who has ingested poison.

TABLE 18-1 Substances Most Frequently Involved in Human Exposures

Substance Category	All Substances	Percentage of Total Exposures*
Analgesics	257,747	10.85
Cleaning substances (household)	185,139	7.28
Cosmetics/personal care products	165,959	6.53
Sedative/hypnotics/antipsychotics	140,692	5.53
Antidepressants	132,807	5.22
Cardiovascular drugs	111,194	4.37
Antihistamines	110,346	4.34
Foreign bodies/toys/miscellaneous	93,197	3.67
Pesticides	83,305	3.28
Alcohols	71,878	2.83
Stimulants and street drugs	71,117	2.80
Anticonvulsants	66,340	2.61
Topical preparations	64,274	2.53
Dietary supplements/herbals/homeopathic	59,259	2.33
Vitamins	58,862	2.32
Hormones and hormone antagonists	56,167	2.21
Cold and cough preparations	54,719	2.15
Antimicrobials	51,767	2.04
Gastrointestinal preparations	47,622	1.87
Chemicals	45,378	1.79
Bites and envenomations	43,337	1.70
Plants	42,495	1.67
Fumes/gases/vapors	34,144	1.34
Other/unknown nondrug substances	31,739	1.25
Electrolytes and minerals	30,046	1.18

*Percentages are based on the total number of substances reported in all exposures ($N = 2{,}577{,}557$).

Reproduced from Mowry JB, Spyker DA, Brooks DE, McMillan N, Schauben JL. 2014 Annual Report of the American Association of Poison Control Centers' National Poison Data System (NPDS): 32nd annual report. *Clin Toxicol* 53(10):962–1147.

Flowchart 18-1 Ingested Poisoning

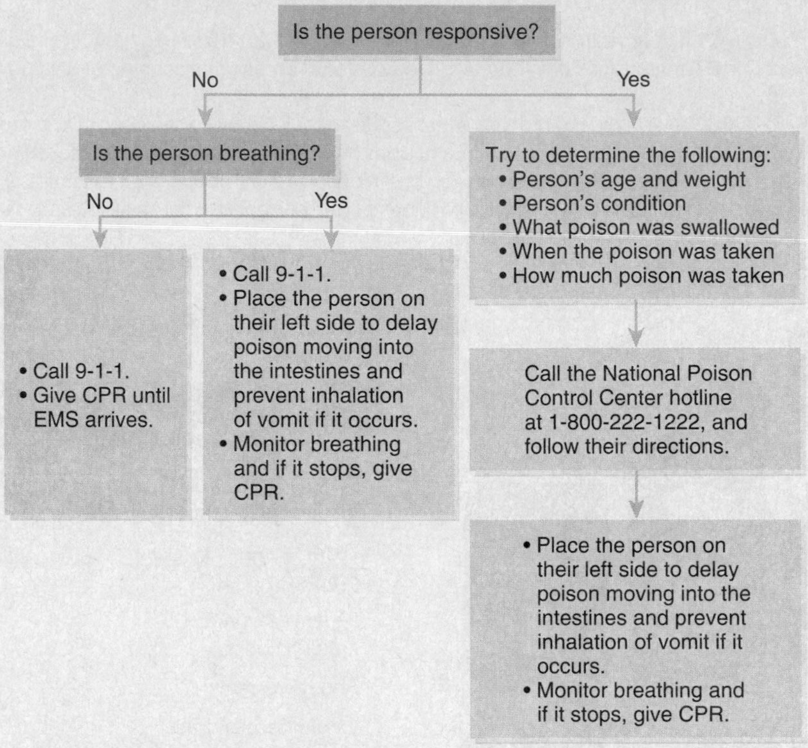

CAUTION

DO NOT give water or milk to dilute poisons other than caustic or corrosive substances (acids and alkalis) unless told to do so by staff at a poison center. Fluids can dissolve a dry poison such as tablets or capsules more rapidly and fill up the stomach, forcing the stomach contents (the poison) into the small intestine, where it will be absorbed faster. Vomiting and aspiration could occur.

DO NOT try to induce vomiting in any way.

DO NOT give dish soap, raw eggs, or mustard powder. They are not effective.

DO NOT use syrup of ipecac.

DO NOT follow the first aid procedures or recommendations on a container label without first getting confirmation from a medical source. Many labels are incorrect or out of date.

DO NOT try to neutralize a poison. Giving weak acids, such as lemon juice or vinegar, is not safe, contrary to the advice given on many drain cleaner and lye product labels. Chemical neutralization releases large quantities of heat that can burn sensitive tissues.

DO NOT think that a specific antidote exists for most poisons. An antidote is a substance that counteracts a poison's effects. Few poisons have specific antidotes that will effectively block their toxic effects.

DO NOT think that there is a universal antidote. No product is effective in treating most or all poisons.

Inhaled Poisoning

If poison has been inhaled, all affected people require professional medical care even if they appear to have recovered. If the scene is not dangerous, immediately move the person into fresh air. **DO NOT** enter the scene unless properly equipped and trained.

What to Look For	What to Do

▪ Headache
▪ Ringing in the ears (tinnitus)
▪ Chest pain (angina)
▪ Muscle weakness
▪ Nausea and vomiting
▪ Dizziness and visual changes (blurred or double vision)
▪ Difficulty breathing, speaking, or swallowing
▪ Unresponsiveness
▪ Respiratory and cardiac arrest
▪ Indications of possible carbon monoxide poisoning:
  ▪ Symptoms that come and go
  ▪ Symptoms that worsen or improve in certain places or at certain times of the day
  ▪ Similar symptoms in people around the person who is ill
  ▪ Pets that seem ill
	1. Call 9-1-1 as soon as possible.
	2. Try to determine the following:
	  ▪ What substance was inhaled?
	  ▪ When did the exposure occur?
	  ▪ For how long was the substance inhaled?
	  ▪ What is the person's condition?
	3. Place the person in a sitting or reclining position, or in whatever position best facilitates breathing and is comfortable. Support the back for easier breathing.
	4. Monitor breathing, and if absent, begin CPR. See Chapter 5, *CPR*.

Poison Control Centers

If someone swallows poison, do not call the hospital emergency department unless the person has become unresponsive or has trouble breathing. Call the poison center. Researchers who made 156 test calls to 52 hospital emergency departments in Illinois found that the advice given was correct only 64% of the time. In addition, calls to the same emergency department on different days for the same condition did not consistently produce the same advice. In contrast, poison centers gave correct advice in 17 of 18 (94%) test calls.

In the United States, there are 55 accredited poison control centers. All of these centers can be reached by calling the same telephone number: 1-800-222-1222. They are staffed by pharmacists, physicians, nurses, and other poison experts who are toxicology specialists, which means that all calls to a center are answered by a trained medical professional. Calling a poison control center will allow a poison expert to decide if the person is in immediate danger. The poison expert will give you the advice you need and may stay on the phone with you while you get help or call you later to follow up. More than 70% of all the calls to a center about a potential poisoning are managed on-site and outside of a hospital or health care facility. This saves costly emergency department visits. If you require a physician or an ambulance, the poison expert will tell you right away.

FYI

Preventing Poisoning

Follow these precautions to reduce the risk of poisoning:

1. Keep household products and medicines out of reach and out of sight of children, preferably in a locked cabinet or closet. When an adult who is using household products or taking medicine leaves the room, even briefly, they should move the containers to a safe place.
2. Store medicines separately from other household products and keep them in their original containers—never in cups or soft drink bottles.
3. Properly label all products and read the label before use.
4. Turn on a light when giving or taking medicine.
5. Because children tend to imitate adults, avoid taking medications in their presence.
6. Refer to medicines and vitamins by their correct names. Do not tell children that medicines are candy; they are not.
7. Use household substances in child-resistant packaging. Prescription medicines should be kept in safety packaging.

To avoid poisonings among older people:

1. Always read the label and follow instructions when taking medicine.
2. Turn on a light at night when taking medicine.
3. Never mix medicines and alcohol, and never take more than the prescribed amount of medicine.
4. Do not borrow a friend's medicine or take old medicines.
5. Inform the physician what other medicines are being taken to avoid the risk of an **adverse drug interaction**.

Data from US Consumer Product Safety Commission.

About 20% of the calls are from a health care facility requesting advice. All calls are kept confidential and can be translated into 161 languages. Calls are free and can be made 24 hours per day, every day of the year. These poison control centers also provide educational outreach poison prevention programs.

Q&A

Why place a person who has ingested poison on their left side?

Placing the person on their left side (recovery position) positions the end of the stomach, where it enters the small intestine, straight up. Gravity will delay (up to 2 hours) the poison from moving into the small intestine, where absorption into the person's circulatory system is faster. This position also helps prevent inhalation into the lungs if vomiting begins.

Alcohol Emergencies

Alcohol is a **depressant**, not a stimulant. It affects a person's judgment, vision, reaction time, and coordination. In very large amounts, it can cause death by paralyzing the respiratory center of the brain.

Alcohol is a commonly used and abused drug. The Centers for Disease Control and Prevention (CDC) cites it as a risk factor for motor vehicle crashes, falls, drownings, burns, and violence, including homicide, suicide, and sexual assault. It directly affects millions of people annually in the United States and causes tens of thousands of deaths, according to the National Institute on Alcohol Abuse and Alcoholism (NIAAA). Alcohol abuse is a major national health problem, ranking with heart disease and cancer **FIGURE 18-4**. Lack of data makes it difficult to assess the actual number of alcohol-related injuries.

Helping an intoxicated person is often difficult because the person could be belligerent and combative. However, it is important that people who abuse alcohol be helped and not labeled as drunks. Their condition can be quite serious, even life threatening.

Occasionally, a person will have consumed so much alcohol that there are signs of central nervous system depression.

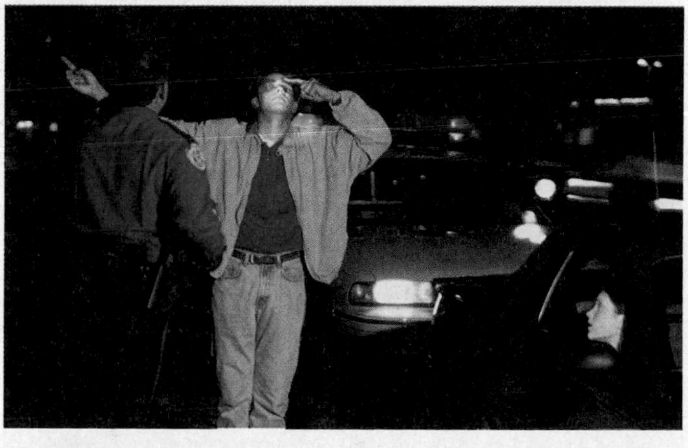

FIGURE 18-4 Field sobriety test.

In such cases, complete respiratory support might be necessary. Death can result from the excessive consumption of alcohol.

The consumption of alcohol is deeply embedded in our society. Because of the widespread use of alcohol, people whose lives are affected directly or indirectly by alcohol abuse should be educated so they can recognize problems and know what to do in an emergency.

What to Look For	What to Do
Although the following signs indicate alcohol intoxication, some might also mean illness or injury other than alcohol abuse, such as diabetes or heat injury: ▪ The odor of alcohol on a person's breath or clothing ▪ Unsteady, staggering walking ▪ Slurred speech and the inability to carry on a conversation ▪ Nausea and vomiting ▪ Flushed face ▪ Seizures (Any seizures related to alcohol require medical evaluation. Hypoglycemia can mimic alcohol intoxication, as can poisoning and neurologic conditions. For additional information, see Chapter 17, *Sudden Illness*.)	1. Look for any injuries. Alcohol can mask pain. 2. Monitor breathing and treat accordingly. 3. If the intoxicated person is lying down, place them in the recovery (left-side) position to reduce the likelihood inhaling vomit if it happens and to delay the absorption of alcohol into the bloodstream. Be sure to check that the person is breathing and does not have a spinal injury before you move them. The recovery position can be used for responsive and unresponsive people. 4. Call the poison center for advice or 9-1-1 for help. It might be best to let emergency medical services (EMS) personnel decide whether the police should be alerted. 5. If the person becomes violent, leave the scene and find a safe place until police arrive. 6. Provide emotional support. 7. Assume that an injured or unresponsive person has a spinal injury and needs to be stabilized against movement. Because of decreased pain perception, a person who is intoxicated cannot be assessed reliably. If you suspect a spinal injury, wait for EMS personnel to arrive. They have the proper equipment and training to stabilize and move a person. 8. Because many intoxicated people have been exposed to the cold, suspect hypothermia (dangerously low body temperature) and move the person to a warm place whenever possible. Remove wet clothing and cover the person with warm blankets. Handle a person with hypothermia gently because rough handling could induce a deadly heart rhythm.

CAUTION

DO NOT let an intoxicated person sleep on their back.

DO NOT leave an intoxicated person alone unless they become violent.

DO NOT try to handle a hostile, intoxicated person by yourself. Find a safe place, and then call the police for help.

Drug Emergencies

Drugs are classified according to their effects on the user as follows:

- *Uppers* are stimulants of the central nervous system. They include amphetamines, cocaine, and caffeine **FIGURE 18-5**.
- *Downers* are depressants of the central nervous system. They include **barbiturates**, **tranquilizers (benzodiazepines)**, marijuana, and **narcotics** **FIGURE 18-6**.
- *Hallucinogens* alter and often enhance the sensory and emotional information in the brain centers. They

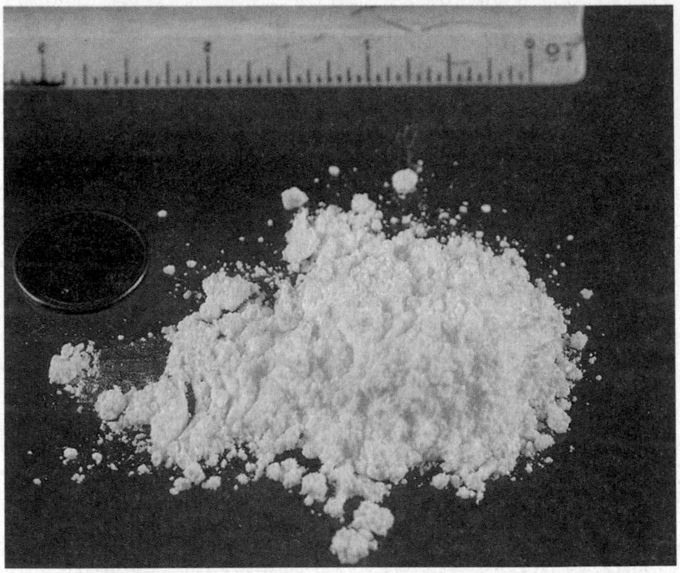

FIGURE 18-5 Cocaine.
Courtesy of DEA.

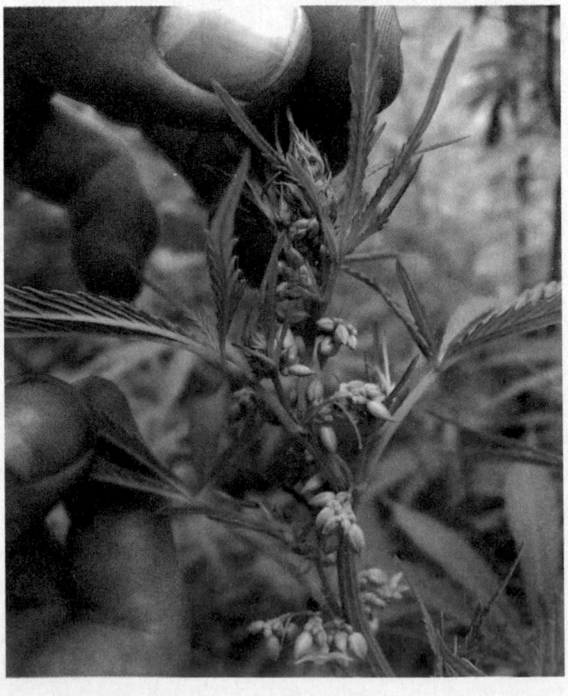

FIGURE 18-6 Marijuana.
© Ben Smith/Shutterstock.

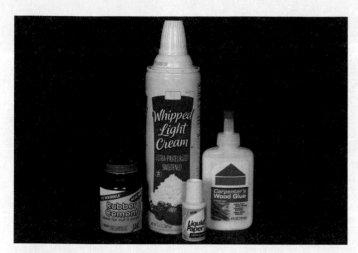

FIGURE 18-7 Inhalants.

include lysergic acid diethylamide (LSD), mescaline, peyote, and phencyclidine hydrochloride (PCP). Marijuana also has some hallucinogenic properties.

- *Inhalants* usually are inhaled and can cause serious damage to many body organs. They include plastic model glue and cement, paint solvent, gasoline, spray paint, and nail polish remover **FIGURE 18-7**.

Sympathomimetics

Sympathomimetics are stimulants. A **stimulant** is any agent that produces an excited state. Amphetamine and methamphetamine are commonly taken by mouth. They are also injected in many cases. They typically are taken to make the user feel good, improve task performance, suppress appetite, or prevent sleepiness. Sympathomimetic drugs are frequently called uppers. Methamphetamine production is dangerous because it is often produced illegally in makeshift labs using hazardous materials and techniques.

Cocaine can be taken in a number of different ways—through the nose, by injection, and by smoking. Crack is a form of cocaine that is smoked. Smoked crack produces the most potent effect. Cocaine is one of the most addictive substances known. It can induce strokes, seizures, and heart attacks. Signs that a person has taken a stimulant include disorganized behavior, hyperactivity, restlessness, and sometimes anxiety or great fear. They may also suffer from paranoia (which can put the user and others in danger) and delusions.

Hallucinogens

Hallucinogens produce changes in mood and sensory awareness; a person using these drugs might "hear" colors and "see" sounds. They can cause hallucinations and bizarre behavior that might make users dangerous to themselves and others. Users of hallucinogens also report visual hallucinations and increased intensity of vision and hearing. Acute intoxication requires medical attention. Users should be protected from hurting themselves. The classic hallucinogen is LSD. Abuse of another hallucinogen, PCP, often called angel dust, is dangerous because it causes severe behavioral changes.

Marijuana

The flowering hemp plant called marijuana is used throughout the world. Signs of marijuana use can include euphoria, relaxation, and drowsiness; impaired short-term memory and capacity to do complex thinking and work; altered perception of time; and anxiety and panic. In very high doses, users can also experience hallucinations.

Abused Inhalants

Inhaling nitrous oxide from spray cans such as whipped cream, inhaling certain glues, or inhaling other solvents (gasoline, lighter fluid, nail polish remover) produces effects similar to those from ingesting alcohol. These effects can include mild drowsiness to unresponsiveness, slurred speech and clumsiness, seizures, and slow breathing rate. A sign that someone might have abused inhalants is the smell of solvents. People who sniff these substances can die of suffocation. In addition, some inhalants can cause death by changing the rhythm of the heartbeat and can cause permanent brain damage.

Depressants

Depressants are often prescribed as a part of legitimate medical treatment. They are easy to obtain, and people intent on misusing them sometimes solicit prescriptions from several physicians. This class of drug includes **opiates** (narcotics) and sedatives (barbiturates and tranquilizers).

Sedatives

Sedatives are prescribed as anesthetics, sleep aids, and anti-anxiety treatments. The effects of sedative drug overdose are similar to those of alcohol. These effects can include drowsiness and sleepiness, slurred speech, and slow breathing rate.

Opioids

Opioids are a classification of drugs that relieve pain. They also trigger the release of endorphins, natural chemicals that boost happiness, and are highly addictive. Like all medications, people can have adverse reactions to opioids. Because opioids slow or even stop breathing, drug overdoses can be fatal.

In recent years as fatalities have soared to tens of thousands per year, there have been numerous efforts to identify and manage opioid users by all levels of law enforcement and first responders.

Most opioids are narcotic pain relievers; they include morphine, heroin, methadone, fentanyl, and oxycodone.

A drug overdose can happen when a person does any of the following:

- Misunderstands the directions for use, unintentionally takes an extra dose, or deliberately misuses a prescription opioid or an illicit drug (eg, heroin)
- Takes an opioid medication prescribed for someone else
- Mixes opioids with other medications, alcohol, or over-the-counter (OTC) drugs

What to Look For	What to Do
▪ Extreme sleepiness or drowsiness ▪ Unresponsiveness ▪ Breathing problems ranging from slow and shallow breathing to no breathing ▪ Lips and nails turning blue ▪ Skin that feels cold and clammy ▪ Extremely small pupils	**1.** When an *unresponsive* person is known or suspected to have taken an opioid drug, check for breathing. ▪ If the person is not breathing or is only gasping and there is someone to help, have the other person call 9-1-1 and get an AED and naloxone too, while you begin CPR. ▪ If the person is not breathing and only gasping for air and you are alone, complete five cycles of CPR (see Chapter 5, *CPR*) before leaving to call 9-1-1 and getting an AED and naloxone. **2.** Give naloxone if available **FIGURE 18-8**. ▪ **Naloxone** is a safe medicine that rapidly reverses a drug overdose. It is easy to use. It only reverses the effects of opioids. It has no effect on other drugs (eg, alcohol, stimulants). **DO NOT** delay giving CPR or compression-only CPR to an unresponsive person who is not breathing while waiting for naloxone to work. ▪ Naloxone is available in different forms: • To administer a prefilled, single-dose *nasal spray* that cannot be reused (Narcan), first place the person flat on their back, with the head tilted back. Then administer the spray into one nostril. If there is no recovery within 2 to 3 minutes and another nasal spray device is available, repeat the dose in the other nostril. • To administer a prefilled, single-dose *auto-injector* that cannot be reused (Evzio), pull the device out of the case. Once activated, the device provides voice directions (similar to automated defibrillators). Inject into the person's outer thigh (similar to an epinephrine auto-injector). It can be given through clothing (eg, pants, jeans) if necessary. If the electronic voice directions do not work, the device can still deliver the naloxone dose. If there is no recovery within 2 to 3 minutes and there is another auto-injector available, repeat the dose. **3.** If naloxone has been given and the person becomes responsive and is breathing, monitor breathing and if breathing stops, begin CPR. Be sure to stay with the person until EMS arrives. The person should receive professional medical care, even if they have recovered. **4.** If naloxone is not available, stay with the person until EMS arrives. Place the person on their side (recovery position; see pages 70–71) to keep the airway open. Monitor breathing and if breathing stops, begin CPR. **5.** If possible to do quickly and safely, try to identify the drug. Look for medicine bottles or ask bystanders. **Important:** ▪ The effects of the opioid often outlast the effect of naloxone and a second dose may be required. ▪ Some opioids are strong and might require multiple doses of naloxone. ▪ Anyone who is taking opioids or is at risk of an overdose should carry naloxone in case of emergencies. ▪ All 50 states allow the purchase of naloxone with a physician's prescription. Most states allow behind-the-counter (without a prescription) purchasing of naloxone.

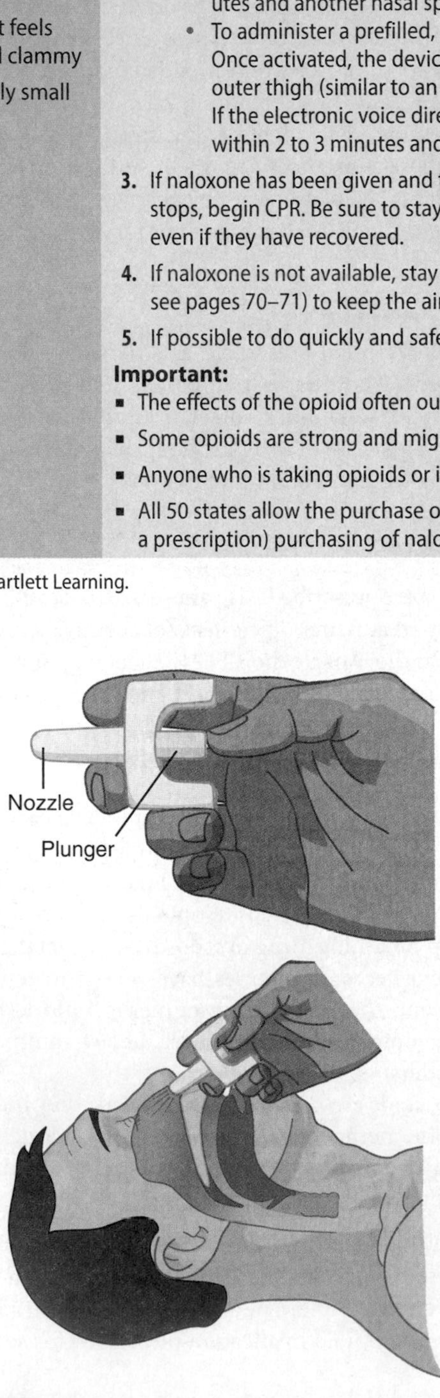

FIGURE 18-8 Nasal spray naloxone administration.

Non-Opioids

For all other non-opioid drug emergencies—sympathomimetics, hallucinogens, depressants, and abused inhalants—follow these instructions:

If person is ...	What to Do
Alert and responsive	**1.** Call the Poison Control hotline at 1-800-222-1222.
Unresponsive and breathing	**1.** Call 9-1-1, monitor breathing and if it stops, begin CPR.
Unresponsive and not breathing	**1.** Call 9-1-1 and begin CPR.
For all drug-overdosed persons	**1.** Provide reassurance and emotional support. **2.** Place the person on their left side (recovery position) to delay poison moving into the intestines and to prevent inhalation of vomit if it occurs. **3.** Check for injuries. **4.** If the person becomes violent, seek safety until law enforcement arrives. Let them handle any dangerous situation.

Carbon Monoxide Poisoning

Carbon monoxide, because of its common presence in our environment, along with its insidious nature, is a leading cause of poisoning death in the United States each year. Carbon monoxide is produced by the incomplete combustion of carbon-based fuels. According to a report from the CDC, each year hundreds of Americans die of unintentional carbon monoxide poisoning. Carbon monoxide poisoning sends tens of thousands to the hospital annually.

What to Look For	What to Do
It is difficult to determine if a person is poisoned by carbon monoxide. Sometimes, a complaint of having flulike symptoms is actually a sign of carbon monoxide poisoning: ▪ Dull headache ▪ Ringing in the ears (tinnitus) ▪ Chest pain (angina) ▪ Muscle weakness ▪ Nausea or vomiting ▪ Dizziness and visual changes (blurred or double vision) ▪ Loss of responsiveness ▪ Respiratory and cardiac arrest The traditionally cited sign of carbon monoxide poisoning is cherry-red skin and lips. This sign is uncommon, however, and occurs only at death; therefore, it is a poor initial indicator of carbon monoxide poisoning. The following are earmarks of possible carbon monoxide poisoning: ▪ The symptoms come and go. ▪ The symptoms worsen or improve in certain places or at certain times of the day. ▪ People around the person have similar symptoms. ▪ Pets seem ill.	1. Get the person exhibiting symptoms and all others out of the toxic environment and into fresh air *immediately*. 2. Call 9-1-1, who will send EMS personnel who will be able to give the person 100% oxygen, improving oxygenation and disassociating the linkage between the carbon monoxide and the hemoglobin. For a responsive person, it takes 4 to 5 hours with ordinary air (21% oxygen) or 30 to 40 minutes with 100% oxygen to reverse the effects of carbon monoxide poisoning. 3. Monitor breathing, and if it stops, give CPR. 4. Place an unresponsive breathing person in the recovery position. 5. Seek professional medical care. All people with suspected carbon monoxide poisoning should obtain a blood test to determine the level of carbon monoxide.

People who ride long distances in older, poorly maintained cars are at increased risk of carbon monoxide poisoning. Rust can damage an automobile's exhaust system and create holes in the car's body, through which carbon monoxide can enter. A common source of carbon monoxide poisoning is motor vehicle exhaust. Some people will attempt suicide by running the engine inside a closed garage and inhaling the fumes. Many unintentional deaths involve people sleeping inside a running car, often after consuming alcohol.

People in a closed room where there is cigarette smoking experience mild increases in the level of carbon monoxide in their blood. Less familiar and, therefore, more dangerous sources of carbon monoxide are faulty furnaces, water heaters, and portable generators. Recreational fires, whether open-flame or charcoal grills, also give off carbon monoxide.

People with carbon monoxide poisoning are often unaware of its presence. The gas is invisible, tasteless, odorless, and nonirritating. It is produced by the incomplete burning of organic material such as gasoline, wood, paper, charcoal, coal, and natural gas.

Carbon monoxide causes hypoxia, or lack of oxygen, in two ways. First, the hemoglobin in red blood cells is about 200 times more likely to bind to carbon monoxide than to oxygen if both are present in the blood; thus, even a small amount of carbon monoxide can greatly reduce the amount of oxygen carried in the bloodstream. Second, carbon monoxide does not allow the cells to use what little oxygen is delivered. In short, carbon monoxide restricts oxygen to the body parts that need oxygen the most—the heart and the brain.

Refer to **FLOWCHART 18-2** for additional information regarding the care of an inhaled poison emergency.

Plant-Induced Dermatitis

Poison Ivy, Poison Oak, and Poison Sumac

According to the American Skin Association, about 85% of the population is sensitive to poison ivy, poison oak, and poison sumac. With more people venturing into the outdoors, episodes of dermatitis caused by exposure to poison ivy **FIGURE 18-9**, poison oak **FIGURE 18-10**, and poison sumac **FIGURE 18-11** are increasing. (Actually, more than 60 plants can cause allergic reactions, but these three are by far the most common offenders.) Of those who do react, 10% to 15% will have incapacitating swelling and blistering eruptions that require professional medical care **FIGURE 18-12**, according to the American Skin Association. There is no routine test to determine a person's degree of sensitivity; a history of dermatitis is the most reliable indicator.

The resin (urushiol) of these plants is a colorless or slightly yellow oil. It runs in resin canals just under the surface, from the roots through the stems, into the leaves and flowers, and just under the surface of the fruit. It is not present in the nectar. The leaves of the plants are fragile and easily ruptured by strong winds or by humans or animals brushing against them. The oil immediately oozes onto the surface.

The light-colored oil generally is not visible on human skin. If present on the sole of a shoe, on the palm of a hand or glove, or on the surface of an animal's fur, it can be spread by direct contact. On some objects, the oil can stay in an active form for months or years. Urushiol can be on the handle of a rake for years and still bond to human skin within 5 or 10 minutes. Poison ivy leaves have been kept for up to 5 years with no loss of potency. Contaminated clothing has caused rashes even after more than 1 year. Smoke from burning plants can produce severe dermatitis. People downwind from these burning leaves can be affected by airborne oil, which can be inhaled and cause airway irritation.

Flowchart 18-2 Inhaled Poisoning

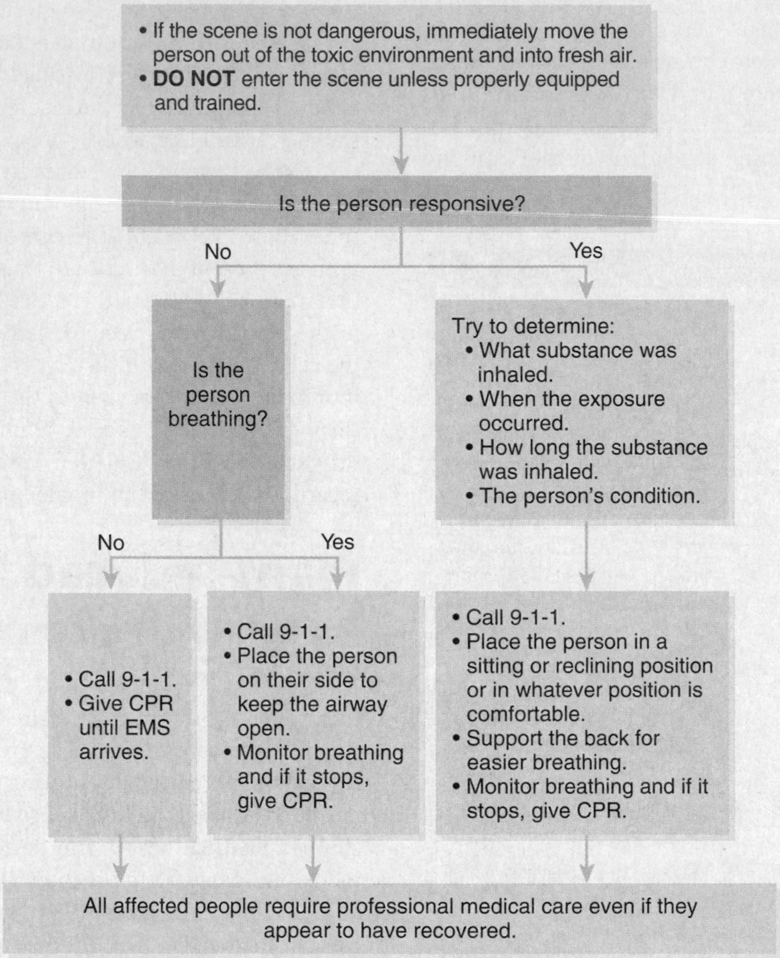
• If the scene is not dangerous, immediately move the person out of the toxic environment and into fresh air.
• DO NOT enter the scene unless properly equipped and trained.
Is the person responsive?
No
Yes
Is the person breathing?
Try to determine:
• What substance was inhaled.
• When the exposure occurred.
• How long the substance was inhaled.
• The person's condition.
No
Yes
• Call 9-1-1.
• Give CPR until EMS arrives.
• Call 9-1-1.
• Place the person on their side to keep the airway open.
• Monitor breathing and if it stops, give CPR.
• Call 9-1-1.
• Place the person in a sitting or reclining position or in whatever position is comfortable.
• Support the back for easier breathing.
• Monitor breathing and if it stops, give CPR.
All affected people require professional medical care even if they appear to have recovered.

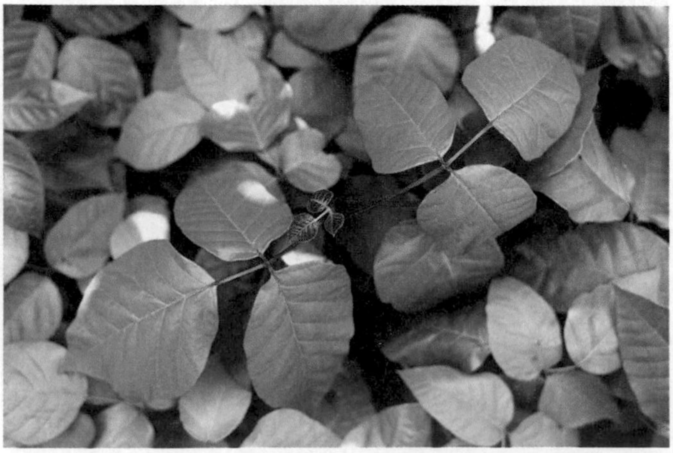

FIGURE 18-9 Poison ivy, found in all 48 contiguous states in the United States.

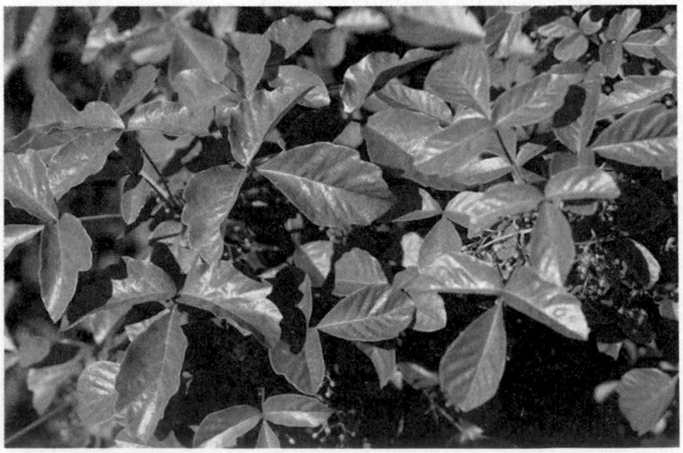

FIGURE 18-10 Poison oak.

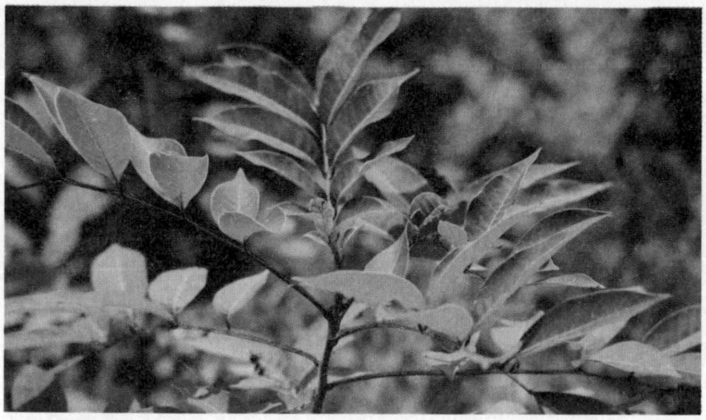

FIGURE 18-11 Poison sumac.
Courtesy of US Fish & Wildlife Service.

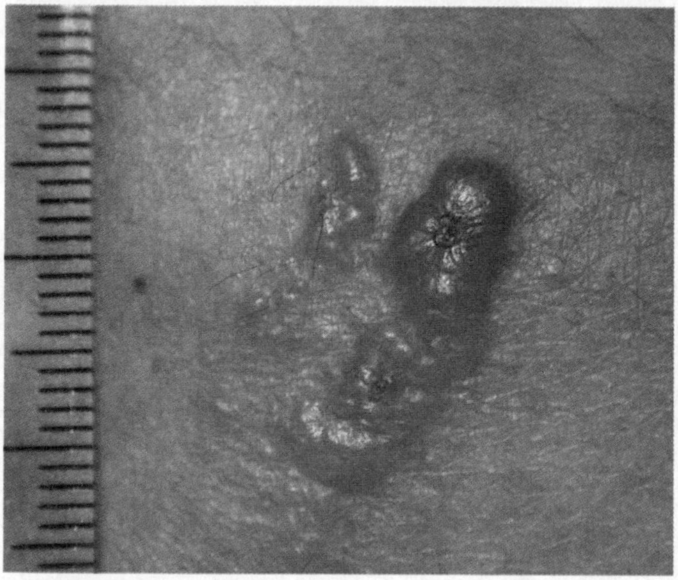

FIGURE 18-12 Poison ivy dermatitis.
© Pinkannjoh/Blickwinkel/Age Fotostock.

Most people cannot identify these irritating plants. Poison ivy and poison oak are low bushes or climbing vines with waxy, broad, green leaves in the summer that change to brown to red in the fall. The leaflets of poison ivy and poison oak grow in groups of three (three leaves radiating from a single attachment point), giving rise to the warning, "leaves of three, let them be." Poison ivy flourishes throughout most of the United States, except in Alaska and Hawaii; poison oak is found on the West and East Coasts and some South Central areas of the United States. Poison sumac is found chiefly in damp, swampy areas in the eastern United States. These plants tend not to grow at elevations higher than 5,000 feet (1,500 m) or in hot, dry deserts. A helpful method of identifying these plants is the black spot test. When the sap is exposed to the air, it turns brown in a matter of minutes and black by the next day.

People can come in contact with the urushiol of these plants from their clothes or shoes, pet fur, or the smoke from burning plants. Contrary to popular belief, no one can develop a rash by touching the fluid from the blisters (their own or others') because the fluid in the blister does not contain the oily resin. Any apparent spreading is actually a delayed reaction to contact with the resin.

Refer to **FLOWCHART 18-3** for additional information regarding the care of plant-induced dermatitis from poison ivy, poison oak, and poison sumac.

FYI

Conducting a Black Spot Test

Most people with poison ivy dermatitis do not recognize the plant. Poison ivy and poison oak leaves have three leaflets; poison sumac has 7 to 13 leaflets per leaf. The mature fruit is an off-white berry. These botanical characteristics explain the axioms, "leaves of three, let them be" and "berries white, poisonous sight!"

The black spot test is another means of identifying these plants. To check a suspicious plant, grasp a leaf and its stem where it attaches to the branch with a folded sheet of white paper (do not touch the leaf). Crush the end of the leaf stalk in the folded sheet of white paper with a rock. The paper needs to be wet with the sap of the leaf stem. The clear sap of poison ivy, poison oak, and poison sumac on the paper will turn dark brown within 10 minutes and black within 24 hours. This test is not conclusive but can strongly suggest that the plant is one of the three plants.

Data from Schram SE, Willey A, Lee PK, Bohjanen KA, Warshaw EM. Black-spot poison ivy. *Dermatitis.* 2008;19(1):48–51.

FYI

Preventing Poisonous-Plant Dermatitis

To reduce the likelihood of poisonous-plant dermatitis developing, follow these suggestions:

- Avoid the plants.
- Wear protective clothing and use appropriate commercial barrier preparations.
- Replenish the barrier protection every 4 to 6 hours, if practical.
- Decontaminate after known exposure with liberal amounts of soap and water, and then reapply the barrier preparation.
- Decontaminate at the end of the day with isopropyl alcohol and a water rinse.
- Dispose of all contaminated clothing and equipment.

CAUTION

DO NOT use OTC anti-itch lotions that also have antihistamines because they can cause further skin irritation. Oral antihistamines often are used in conjunction with prescription creams to help decrease itching.

DO NOT let the person rub or scratch the rash or itching skin.

Flowchart 18-3 Plant-Induced Dermatitis

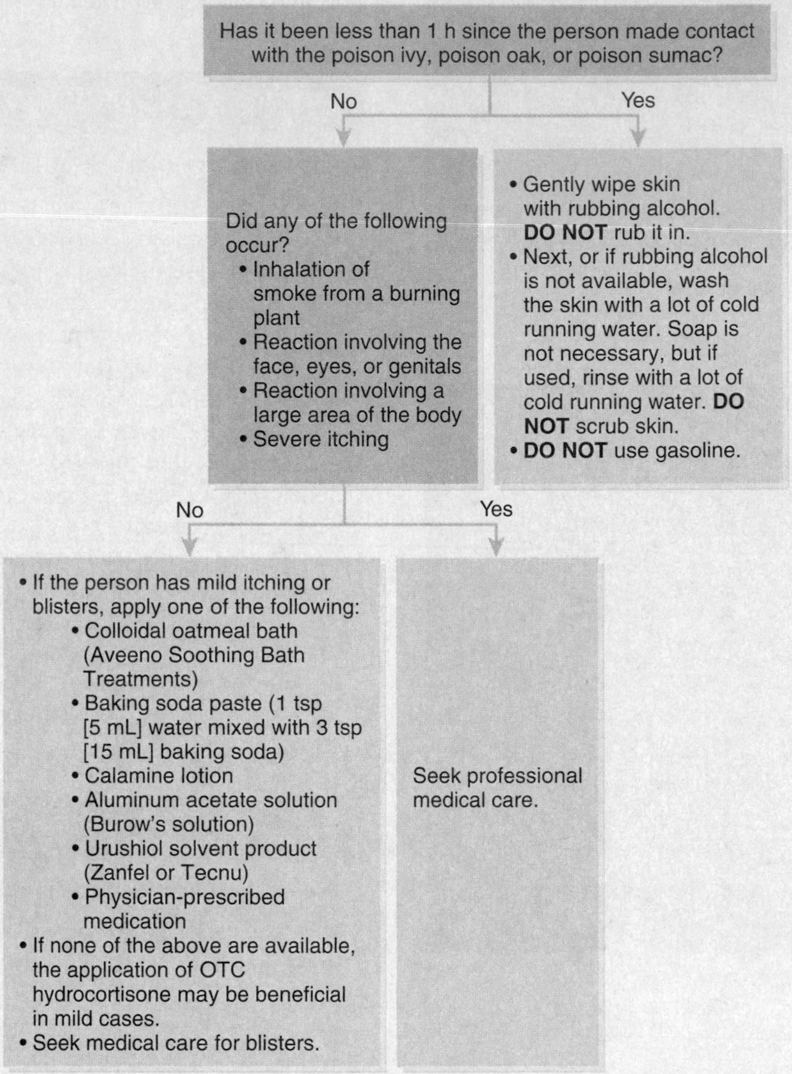
Has it been less than 1 h since the person made contact with the poison ivy, poison oak, or poison sumac?
No
Yes
Did any of the following occur?
• Inhalation of smoke from a burning plant
• Reaction involving the face, eyes, or genitals
• Reaction involving a large area of the body
• Severe itching
• Gently wipe skin with rubbing alcohol. DO NOT rub it in.
• Next, or if rubbing alcohol is not available, wash the skin with a lot of cold running water. Soap is not necessary, but if used, rinse with a lot of cold running water. DO NOT scrub skin.
• DO NOT use gasoline.
No
Yes
• If the person has mild itching or blisters, apply one of the following:
• Colloidal oatmeal bath (Aveeno Soothing Bath Treatments)
• Baking soda paste (1 tsp [5 mL] water mixed with 3 tsp [15 mL] baking soda)
• Calamine lotion
• Aluminum acetate solution (Burow's solution)
• Urushiol solvent product (Zanfel or Tecnu)
• Physician-prescribed medication
• If none of the above are available, the application of OTC hydrocortisone may be beneficial in mild cases.
• Seek medical care for blisters.
Seek professional medical care.

What to Look For	What to Do
Known contact within 5 minutes for people with sensitive skin and up to 1 hour for people with moderately sensitive skin	1. Gently wipe skin with rubbing alcohol. **DO NOT** rub it in. 2. Next, or if rubbing alcohol is not available, wash the skin with lots of cold running water. Soap is not necessary, but if used, rinse with lots of cold running water. **DO NOT** scrub skin. 3. **DO NOT** use gasoline.
Mild dermatitis: itching	1. Apply any of the following: ▪ Colloidal oatmeal bath (Aveeno Soothing Bath Treatments) ▪ Baking soda paste (1 teaspoon [5 mL] water mixed with 3 teaspoons [15 mL] baking soda) ▪ Calamine lotion ▪ Aluminum acetate solution (Burow's solution) ▪ Urushiol solvent product (Zanfel or Tecnu) ▪ Physician-prescribed medication 2. If none of these is available, the application of OTC hydrocortisone may be beneficial in mild cases.
Moderate dermatitis: itching and swelling	1. Treat the same as for mild signs and symptoms. 2. Apply a physician-prescribed steroid ointment.

What to Look For	What to Do
Severe dermatitis: itching, swelling, and blisters	1. Treat the same as for mild and moderate symptoms. 2. Apply a physician-prescribed topical or oral steroid. 3. Seek professional medical care if the person inhales smoke from a burning plant or if the reaction involves the face, eyes, genitals, or large areas of the body.

Stinging Nettle

The stinging nettle plant has stinging hairs on its stem and leaves. The stinging hair is a fine, hollow tube with a bladder at its base that contains a chemical irritant. When the stinging hair is touched, a fine needlepoint that penetrates the skin and injects an irritating chemical is formed.

Stinging nettle affects almost all people. Its effects are not an allergic response, as with poison ivy, but rather result from the direct irritant effect of the plant's sap.

What to Look For	What to Do
▪ Immediate, intense redness, burning, and itching to the exposed area, lasting for an hour or more, depending on the area of the body exposed to the plant. ▪ The thicker skin on the soles and the palms retards the stinging hairs better than areas of thinner skin, such as the backs of the hands and the arms. ▪ Usually, no systemic (whole-body) effects are noted.	1. Wash the exposed area with soap and water to remove irritant chemicals. 2. Apply a cold, wet pack to help soothe the painful itching. Other treatments might include a paste of colloidal oatmeal, an OTC hydrocortisone cream (1%), or calamine lotion. 3. Take an OTC antihistamine, if desired. Be sure to follow package directions, and be aware that antihistamines cause drowsiness. 4. The duration of the stinging nettle reaction is measured in hours, rather than days, so little therapy is needed.

PREP KIT

Ready for Review

- A poison is any substance that impairs health or causes death by its chemical action when it enters the body or comes in contact with the skin.
- Poisons are classified by how they enter the body. They can be ingested, inhaled, absorbed, and injected.
- Ingested poisoning occurs when the person swallows a toxic substance.
- Alcohol is a depressant that affects a person's judgment, vision, reaction time, and coordination.
- Drugs are classified according to their effects on the user as follows:
  - Uppers (stimulants)
  - Downers (depressants)
  - Hallucinogens
  - Inhalants
- Opioids are highly addictive drugs that are used for pain relief. Overdoses can be treated with naloxone.
- Carbon monoxide is a leading cause of poisoning death in the United States each year.
- About 85% of the population is sensitive to poison ivy, poison oak, and poison sumac.

Vital Vocabulary

adverse drug interaction An unintended or harmful response to two or more drugs being taken concurrently.

barbiturates A group of drugs in the class of drugs known as sedatives.

carbon monoxide A colorless, odorless, poisonous gas formed by incomplete combustion, such as in fire.

depressant An agent that produces a depressed or reduced level of stimulation.

hallucinogens An agent that produces false perceptions in any one of the five senses.

ingested poisoning Poisoning caused by swallowing a toxic substance.

naloxone A medication used to counter the effects of opioids.

narcotics A drug that produces sleep or altered mental status.

opiates A drug containing or derived from opium.

opioids A synthetically produced narcotic not derived from opium.

poison Any substance that impairs health or causes death by its chemical action when it enters the body or comes in contact with the skin.

Poison Help A medical facility operated by the National Poison Control Center that provides immediate, free, expert advice any time; can be reached by calling 1-800-222-1222.

sedatives A class of drugs that act as a central nervous system depressant.

stimulant An agent that produces an excited state.

toxin A poisonous substance produced by bacteria, animals, or plants that acts by changing the normal metabolism of cells or by destroying them.

tranquilizers (benzodiazepines) A group of drugs in the class of drugs known as sedatives.

Assessment in Action

You have been helping your sister paint three rooms in her home. While taking a break, your 2-year-old niece enters the room with a small cup of paint used for touch up. There is paint around and inside her mouth.

Directions: Circle Yes if you agree with the statement; circle No if you disagree.

1. Immediately give your niece water or milk to dilute the ingested paint.

   YES **NO**

2. Use syrup of ipecac to induce vomiting.

   YES **NO**

3. Determine how much of the paint was swallowed, when it was swallowed, and the age and size of your niece.

   YES **NO**

4. Call the National Poison Control Center for advice (1-800-222-1222).

   YES **NO**

PREP KIT continued

Check Your Knowledge

Directions: Circle Yes if you agree with the statement; circle No if you disagree.

1. Swallowing a poison can produce nausea.
   YES **NO**
2. Milk should be given to all people who ingest poison.
   YES **NO**
3. A person with alcohol intoxication does not require professional medical care.
   YES **NO**
4. Carbon monoxide has a unique smell.
   YES **NO**
5. Everyone who touches a poison ivy, poison oak, or poison sumac plant will have some type of skin reaction.
   YES **NO**
6. Causing a person who is poisoned to vomit is a recommended first aid practice.
   YES **NO**
7. Some cases of poison ivy, poison oak, or poison sumac require professional medical care.
   YES **NO**
8. Calamine lotion can help relieve itching caused by poison ivy, poison oak, or poison sumac.
   YES **NO**
9. If a person who is intoxicated or drugged becomes violent, leave the area.
   YES **NO**
10. All opioid overdoses require professional medical care.
    YES **NO**

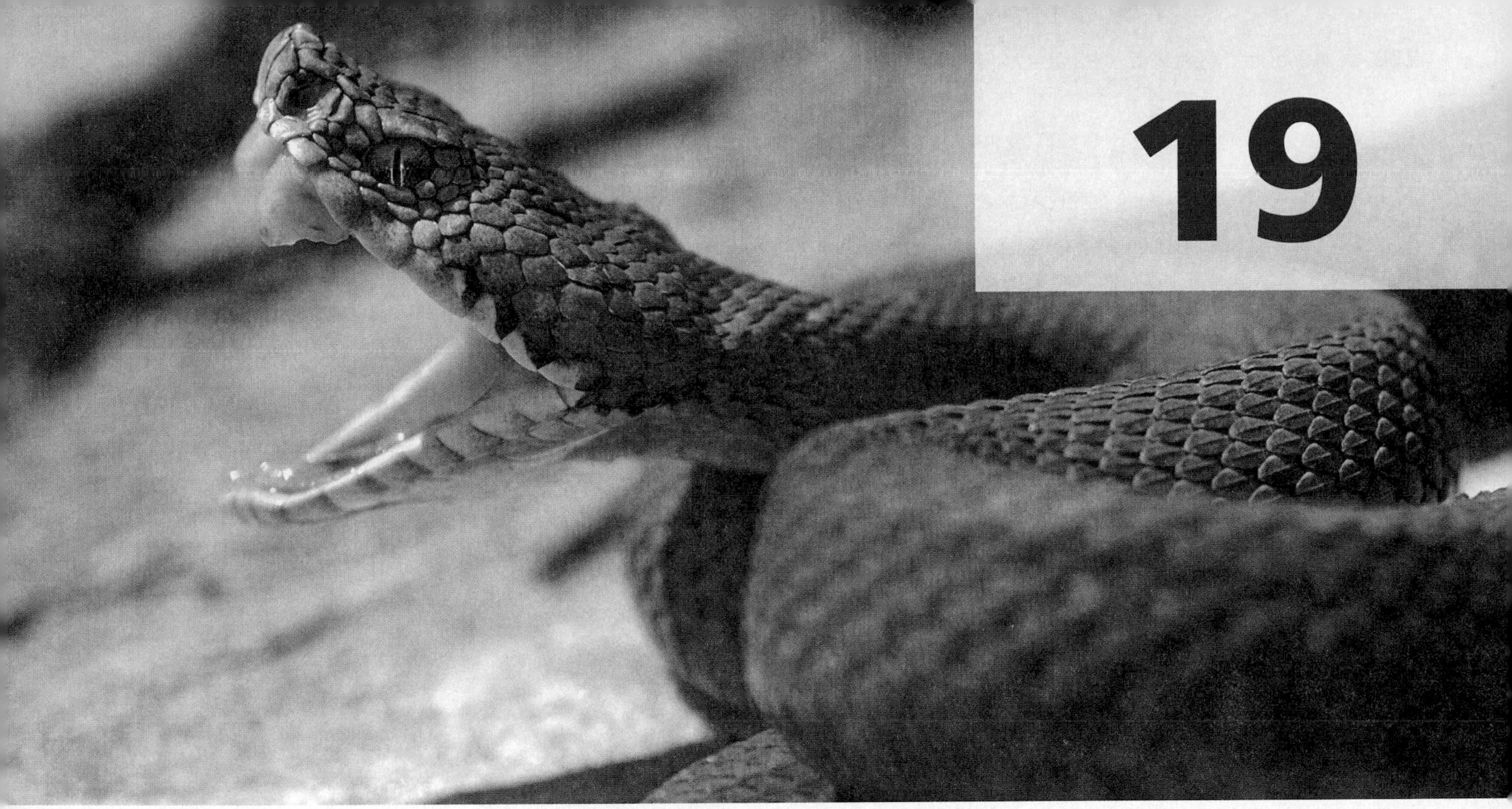

19

Bites and Stings

CHAPTER AT A GLANCE

- Animal Bites
- Snake Bites
- Insect Stings
- Spider and Insect Bites
- Marine Animal Injuries

Animal Bites

Animal bites represent a major, largely unrecognized public health issue. Two concerns result from an animal bite: immediate tissue damage and later infection from microorganisms.

Dogs are responsible for the majority of all animal bite injuries **FIGURE 19-1**. According to the American Veterinary Medical Association (AVMA), about 30 to 40 bite-related deaths occur in the United States each year **TABLE 19-1**. However, 80% of the nearly 5 million dog bites that occur yearly are trivial or minor, and professional medical care is not required or sought, which demonstrates the importance of knowing first aid.

A dog's mouth can carry more than 60 species of bacteria, some of which are dangerous to humans **TABLE 19-2**. Two examples of infection—tetanus and rabies—have been almost eradicated by medical advances, but they still pose a potential issue.

Although cat bites are less mutilating than dog bites, cat bites have a much higher rate of infection than dog bites. Cats have very sharp teeth, which can create deep puncture wounds and involve muscle, tendon, and bone.

Another pet especially likely to bite children is the ferret. These animals are often unpredictable. Ferrets can attack unprovoked, rapidly and repeatedly biting and slashing their target; they can cause severe facial injury to infants.

Besides children, older adults and people unable to help themselves are especially prone to animal bites because they are sometimes

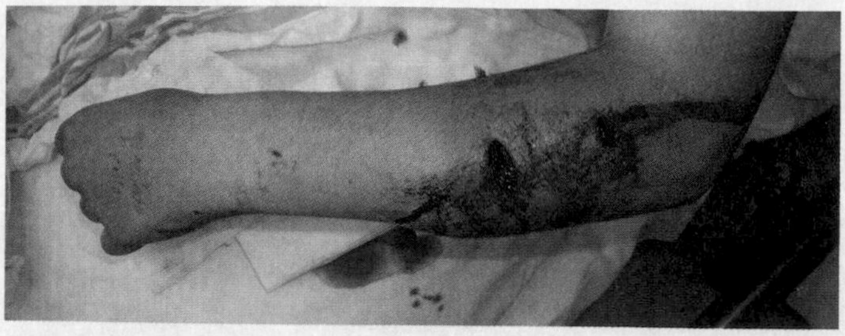

FIGURE 19-1 Dog bite.

TABLE 19-1 Animal-Related Human Deaths in the United States (2008–2015)

	Number of Deaths	Percentage of Deaths (from total)	Average Number of Fatalities per Year
Venomous Animals	686	43	86
Hornets, wasps, and bees	478	30	60
Other venomous arthropods	84	5	11
Venomous spiders	49	3	6
Venomous snakes and lizards	48	3	6
Unspecified venomous animal or plants	22	1	3
Centipedes and venomous millipedes	3	0	<1
Scorpions	2	0	<1
Venomous marine animals and plants	0	0	0
Nonvenomous Animals	924	57	115
Other mammals	576	36	72
Dogs	272	17	34
Other nonvenomous insects or other nonvertebrates	61	4	8
Marine animals	13	1	2
Other reptiles	1	0	<1
Crocodiles or alligators	1	0	<1
Rats	0	0	0
Total	1,610		201

Reproduced from: Forrester JA, et al. Fatalities from venomous and nonvenomous animals in the United States. *Wilderness and Environm Med.* 2018;23(2):146–152. Copyright (2018), with permission from Elsevier.

unable to detect or prevent a dangerous situation. Many animal-related deaths occur when the person is left alone with the offending pet. Contrary to popular belief, wild or stray dogs are seldom involved in fatal attacks.

Damage mostly occurs on the hands, arms, legs, and face. A damaged face presents several issues because the proximity of blood vessels to the skin surface makes the face susceptible to copious bleeding. Facial disfigurement and scarring can result in emotional trauma. Complete or partial loss of an eye also is possible.

TABLE 19-2 Facts About Dog Bites

Carefully choose your pet dog. Evaluate your environment and lifestyle, and speak with a professional to determine the appropriate type of pet.
Dogs should be neutered to reduce aggressive tendencies.
Never leave infants or young children alone with a dog. Be sensitive to cues that a child is fearful or apprehensive about a dog.
Teach children basic safety around dogs, and review regularly.
Dogs with histories of aggression are inappropriate for families with children.
DO NOT play aggressive games, such as wrestling, with your dog.
Never approach an unfamiliar dog. Immediately report stray dogs or dogs displaying unusual behavior.
Remain motionless when approached by an unfamiliar dog—never run or scream.
DO NOT disturb a dog that is sleeping, eating, or caring for puppies.
If knocked down by a dog, lie still and remain in a ball.
If bitten by a dog, immediately report the bite.

Data from: Centers for Disease Control and Prevention. Nonfatal dog bite-related injuries treated in hospital emergency departments—United States 2001. *MMWR Weekly.* 2003;52(26):605-610. www.cdc.gov/mmwr/preview/mmwrhtml/mm5226a1.htm. Accessed December 23, 2015.

Wild animal attacks occur most often in rural or wilderness locations (see Chapter 24, *Wilderness First Aid*, for more information). Not all injuries are bites. Severe injuries result from people being thrown in the air, gored by an antler, butted, or trampled on the ground.

Rabies

Rabies is one of the most ancient and feared of diseases **FIGURE 19-2**. Although human rabies rarely occurs in the United States or in other industrialized nations, it remains a scourge in developing countries. A rabies vaccine is available to those who are at a high risk, which includes veterinarians as well as people who travel to a country where rabies is more prevalent. A virus found in warm-blooded animals causes rabies, which spreads from one animal to another in the saliva, usually through a bite or by licking. Bites from cold-blooded animals such as reptiles do not carry the danger of rabies.

A bite or a scratch is considered a significant rabies exposure if it penetrates the skin. Unprovoked attacks are more likely to have been inflicted by a rabid animal than are provoked attacks. Nonbite exposure consists of contamination of wounds, including scratches, abrasions, and weeping skin rashes.

Consider an animal as possibly rabid if any of the following applies:

- The animal made an unprovoked attack.
- The animal acted strangely, that is, out of character (eg, a usually friendly dog is aggressive, or a wild fox seems docile and friendly).
- The animal was a high-risk species (eg, skunk, fox, raccoon, or bat).

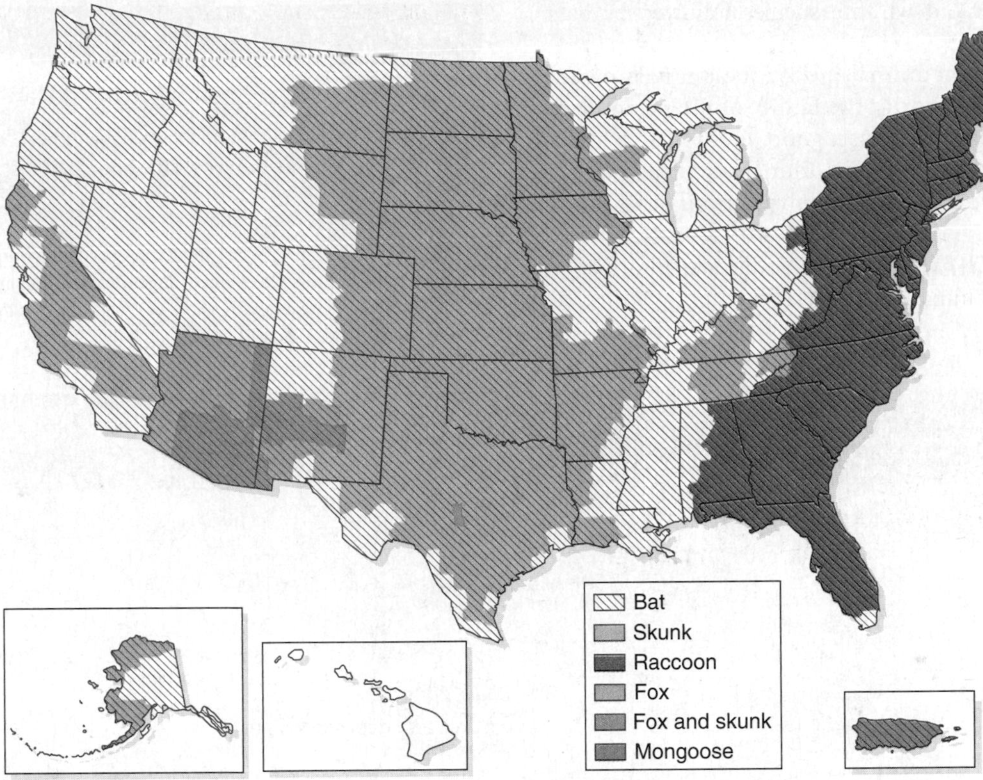

FIGURE 19-2 Distribution of rabies virus among wild animals in the United States, 2013–2017.
Data from Centers for Disease Control and Prevention.

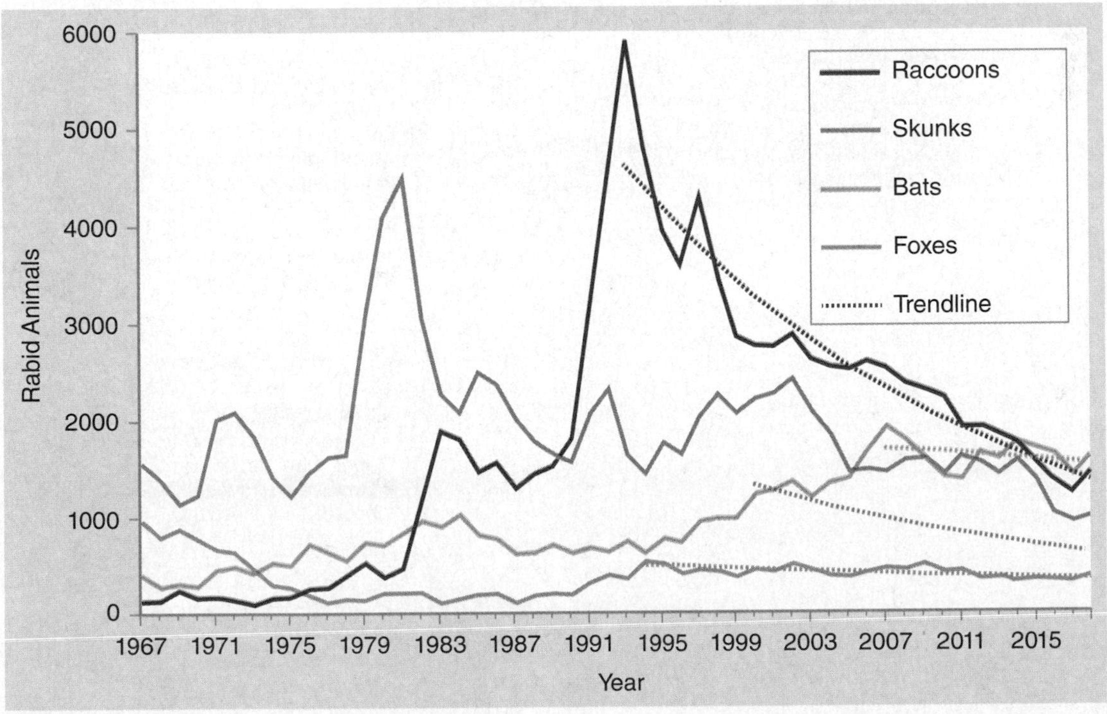

FIGURE 19-3 Rabies in wild animals, 1967–2018.
Data from Centers for Disease Control and Prevention.

Report animal bites to the police or animal control officers; they should be the ones to capture the animal for observation. If a healthy domestic dog or cat that is up to date with its rabies vaccination bit the person, the animal should be confined and observed for 10 days for any illness. If a wild animal bit the person, it should be considered a possible rabies exposure and professional medical care should be sought immediately. According to the Centers for Disease Control and Prevention (CDC), wild animals account for 92% of reported rabies cases in the U.S. **FIGURE 19-3**. Raccoons are the most frequently reported rabid wildlife species followed by bats, skunks, and foxes.

For bites from a pet animal, notify the animal's owner, or, if you are the owner, notify the family of the person who was bitten. When doing so, use good judgment, because encounters may become very emotional and lead to violence. If the bite came from a wild animal, notify the proper authorities.

Refer to **FLOWCHART 19-1** for additional information regarding the care of animal bites.

FYI

Dog Bites: Which Breeds Are Most Dangerous?

The AVMA notes that breed is a poor sole predictor of dog bites. More predictive factors include the dog's past history, training, sex, and neutering status.

Data from American Veterinary Medical Association. Dog bite risk and prevention: The role of breed. https://www.avma.org/KB/Resources/LiteratureReviews/Pages/The-Role-of-Breed-in-Dog-Bite-Risk-and-Prevention.aspx. March 12, 2015.

Flowchart 19-1 Animal Bites

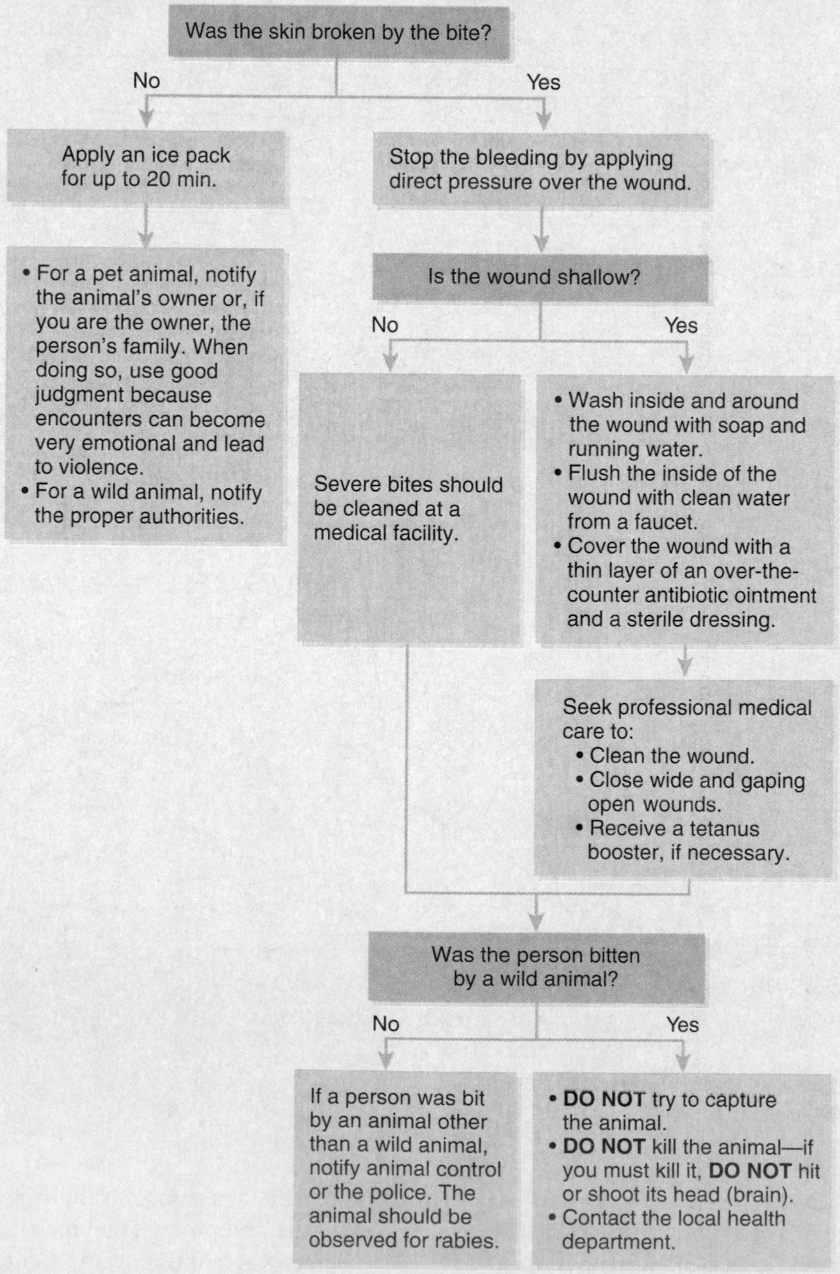

What to Look For	What to Do
Bite that has broken the skin: ▪ Puncture wound from the animal's sharp, pointed teeth ▪ Crushed tissue and skin ▪ Open wound on fingers, knuckles, and/or hand	1. Stop the bleeding by applying direct pressure over the wound. 2. For a shallow wound: ▪ Wash inside and around it with soap and running water. ▪ Flush the inside of the wound with clean running water. ▪ Cover the wound with a thin layer of an over-the-counter (OTC) antibiotic ointment and a sterile dressing. 3. Severe bites should be cleaned at a medical facility. For all bites that break the skin, seek professional medical care to: ▪ Clean the wound. ▪ Close wide and gaping open wounds. ▪ Receive a tetanus booster, if necessary.
Bite that did not break the skin	Apply an ice pack to the skin for up to 20 minutes.
Wild animal bite	1. **DO NOT** try to capture the animal. Instead, try to remember its description and last location so that authorities can manage the animal. 2. **DO NOT** kill the animal. If you must kill it, **DO NOT** hit or shoot its head (brain). Though often impossible, the animal's brain can be tested for the rabies virus. 3. Contact the local health department.

CAUTION

DO NOT try to capture the animal yourself.

DO NOT go near the animal.

DO NOT kill the animal unless absolutely necessary. If it must be killed, protect the head and brain from damage so they can be examined for rabies. Transport a dead animal intact to limit exposure to potentially infected tissues or saliva. The animal's remains should be refrigerated to prevent decomposition.

DO NOT handle the animal without taking appropriate precautions. Infected saliva might be on the animal's fur, so wear heavy gloves or use a shovel if you have to move a dead animal.

FYI

Human Rabies

The number of human deaths in the United States attributed to rabies has declined from 100 or more each year to an average of 1 to 3 each year. Two programs have been responsible for this decline. First, animal control and vaccination programs, which were begun in the 1940s; and second, effective human rabies vaccines and immunoglobulins have been developed.

Data from Centers for Disease Control and Prevention; United States Rabies Surveillance Data.

Human Bites

After dogs and cats, the animal most likely to bite humans is another human. Human bites can cause severe injury, often more so than other animal bites. The human mouth contains a wide range of bacteria and viruses, so the chance of infection is great from a human bite, especially on the hand **FIGURE 19-4**.

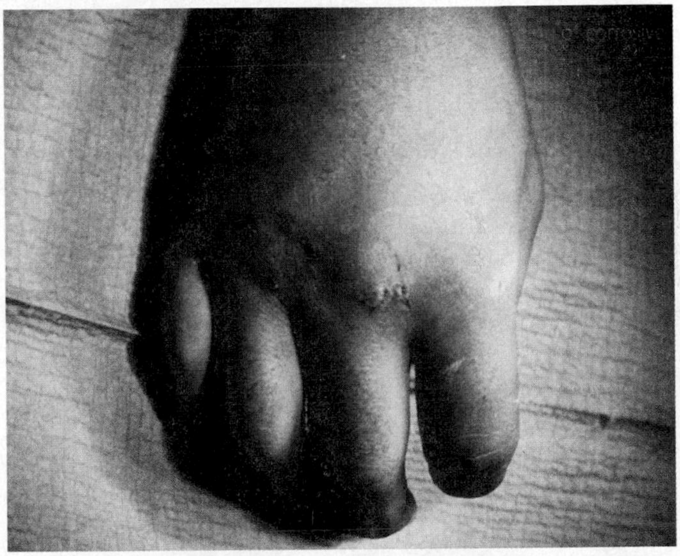

FIGURE 19-4 Human bites can result in serious, spreading infection.

Most human bites are inflicted by fighting youths, by children at play, by people in mental institutions, or during sexual assaults. Embarrassment sometimes causes a person not to seek professional medical care immediately, which greatly increases the risk of infection.

Although most human bites occur during acts of violence, they may also be unintentional or sports-related, sustained by hospital workers trying to restrain children or patients having a seizure, or self-inflicted during nail chewing or thumb sucking. A study published in the *Journal of Emergencies, Trauma, and Shock* reported that men are bitten more often than women, and that bites occur mostly during aggressive altercations, with the peak age being 28 years. The most common injury location is the hand, sustained on a closed fist as the result of a punch.

What to Look For	What to Do

There are two types of human bites:
▪ True bite
  ▪ Part of the body's flesh caught between teeth, usually deliberately
  ▪ Occurs during fights and in cases of abuse (Mandatory reporting laws apply if spousal or child abuse is involved. A schoolyard bite, with one child biting another, generally is not reportable.)
▪ Clenched-fist injury
  ▪ Results from cutting a fist on teeth, usually during a fight (although unintentional injury can happen during sports and play)
  ▪ Associated with a high likelihood of infection
  ▪ Injury usually a laceration over the knuckles
	1. If the wound is not bleeding heavily, wash it with soap and water for 5 to 10 minutes. Avoid scrubbing, which can bruise tissues.
	2. Flush the wound thoroughly with running water under pressure from a faucet.
	3. Control bleeding with direct pressure.
	4. Cover the wound with a sterile dressing. **DO NOT** close the wound with tape or butterfly bandages. Closing the wound traps bacteria in the wound, increasing the chance of infection.
	5. Seek professional medical care for possible further wound cleaning, a possible tetanus shot, and sutures to close the wound, if needed.

Snake Bites

Snake bites are estimated to lead to as many as 9,000 emergency department visits annually in the United States. Venomous snake bites account for about one-third of these visits. Almost all of these bites are from pit vipers **FIGURE 19-5**. Accurate snake bite statistics are difficult to assemble in the United States; however, snake bite deaths are accurate and rarely exceed 10 in any recent year in the United States. People who die of snake bites in the United States usually do so during the first 48 hours after the bite. Only four snake species in the United States are venomous: rattlesnakes **FIGURE 19-6** (which account for about 65% of all venomous snake bites and nearly all the snake bite deaths in the United States), copperheads **FIGURE 19-7**, water moccasins (also known as cottonmouths) **FIGURE 19-8**, and

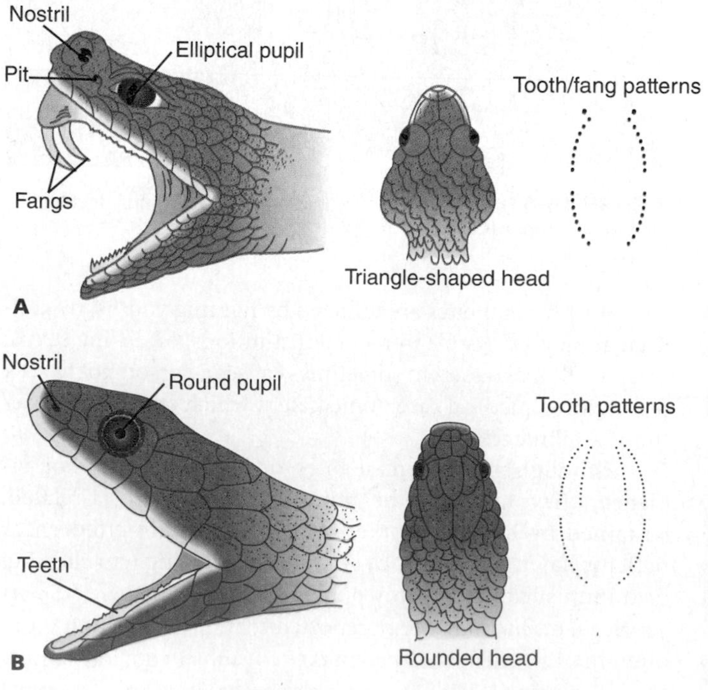

FIGURE 19-5 Characteristic features of venomous snakes (pit vipers) (**A**) and of harmless snakes (**B**).

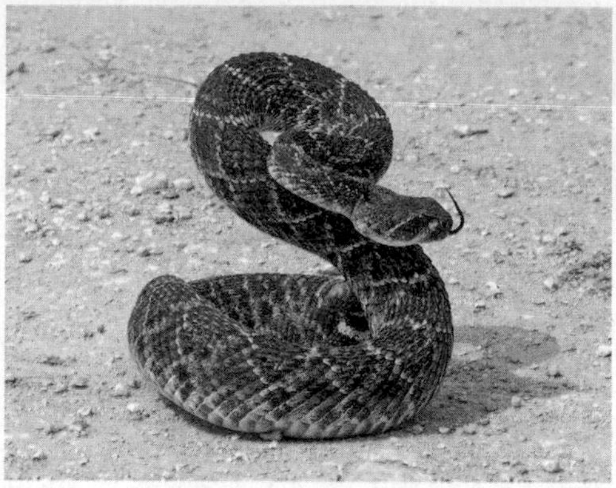

FIGURE 19-6 Rattlesnake.

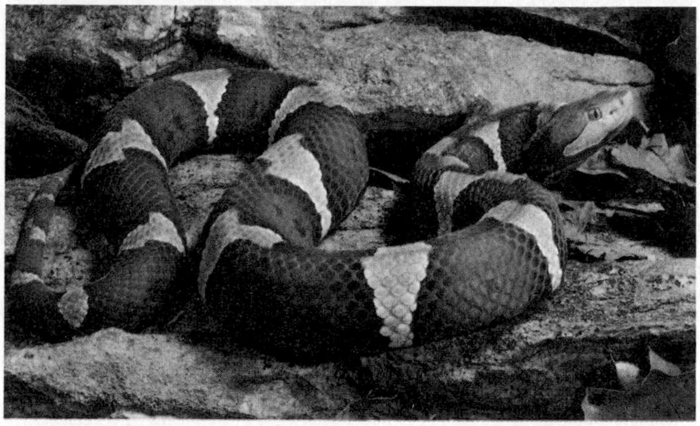

FIGURE 19-7 Copperhead snake.

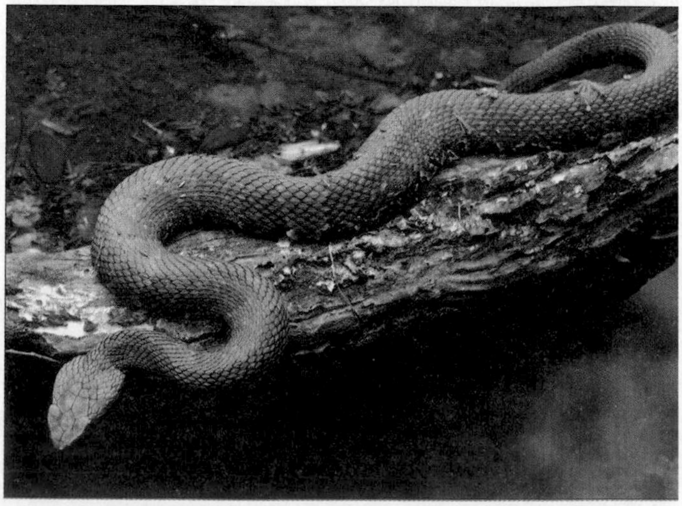

FIGURE 19-8 Water moccasin (cottonmouth).

coral snakes **FIGURE 19-9**. Although uncommon, snake bites can be painful, costly, and potentially deadly. Other than death, disabilities such as partial or complete loss of an extremity or finger or loss of movement in a joint can occur. Most people fully recover.

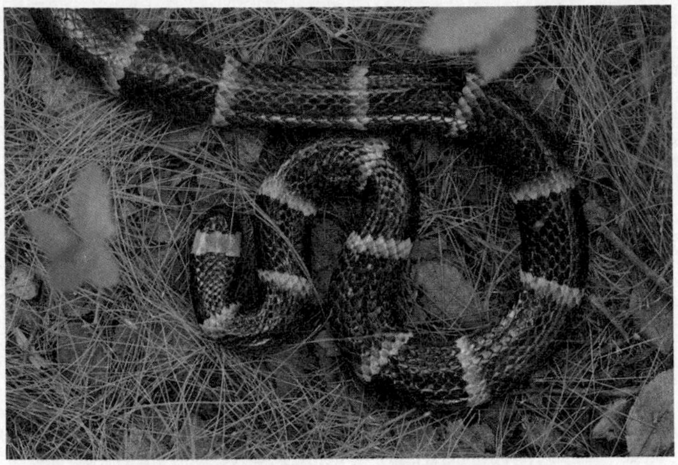

FIGURE 19-9 Coral snake; the United States' most venomous snake.

The first three species of venomous snakes are pit vipers, which have three characteristics in common:

- Triangular, flat heads wider than their necks
- Elliptical pupils (catlike eyes)
- A heat-sensitive pit between the eye and the nostril on each side of the head

The coral snake is small and colorful, with a series of bright red, yellow, and black bands around its body (every other band is yellow). Coral snakes are found in Arizona, the southeastern United States, and Texas.

At least one species of venomous snake is found in every state except Alaska, Hawaii, and Maine **FIGURE 19-10**. Exotic snakes, whether imported legally or smuggled into the United States, can be found in zoos, schools, snake farms, and amateur and professional collections, and account for at least 15 bites per year. Some exotic snakes are venomous.

An accidental snake bite is one in which the person was bitten before the encounter with a snake was recognized or while trying to move away from the snake. They most often involve the lower extremities **TABLE 19-3**.

A provoked snake bite is one in which, before being bitten, the person recognized the encounter with a snake but

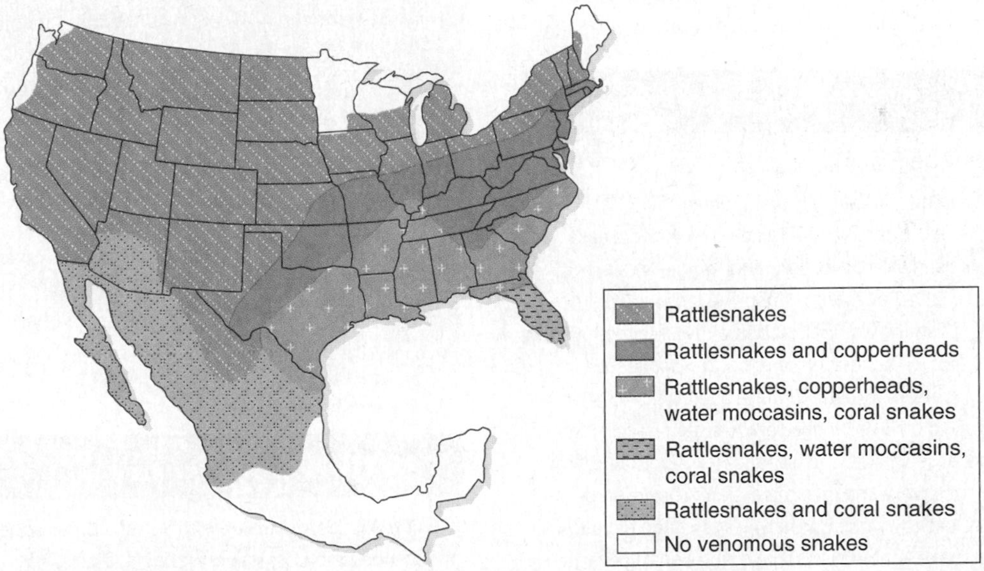

FIGURE 19-10 Location of venomous snakes.

TABLE 19-3 How to Avoid a Snake Bite

■ **DO NOT** handle venomous snakes—keep away. They usually do not have to be killed for identification purposes.
■ Avoid hiking and camping in snake-infested areas; avoid caves, rock crevices, dens, stone walls, and wood piles.
■ Watch where you sit and step; **DO NOT** sit on or step over logs until closely checked. **DO NOT** reach into holes or hidden ledges.
■ Wear protective gear such as boots, gloves, long pants, and long-sleeved shirts when in snake habitats.
■ **DO NOT** handle a dead venomous snake. The reflex action of the jaws can still inflict a bite up to 90 minutes after the snake has been killed, even if decapitated.
■ **DO NOT** surprise or corner a snake. Use a walking stick to prod in front of you while walking, and make noise so that a snake can sense you coming.
■ **DO NOT** keep venomous snakes as pets.
■ When unintentionally encountering a snake, remain silent and motionless. If the snake has not fled, step away slowly and cautiously.

did not attempt to move away from the snake. Most provoked bites occur on the upper extremities. Most bites of this type occur when the person tries to kill, capture, play with, or move a snake. Adult snakes deliver more serious bites because they inject more venom than do young snakes, even though a young snake's venom is two to three times more toxic than an adult's.

Pit Vipers

Pit vipers are found in every state but Alaska, Maine, and Hawaii. Rattlesnakes are the most widespread of the pit vipers. Copperheads are found in the central southeastern United States and westward into the Big Bend of Texas. Water moccasins (cottonmouths) are found in the southeast from Virginia to Florida and into Texas. Snakes benefit us by keeping the rodent population from exploding out of control. They consume hundreds of thousands of mice and rats every year. Few snakes act aggressively toward a human unless provoked. The vast majority of bites are not deadly and can be effectively treated.

According to the Wilderness Medical Society, most people are bitten on the extremities. Alcohol intoxication of the person is a factor in many bites. The majority of bites in the United States occur in the southwestern part of the country, partly due to the near-extinction of pit vipers in the eastern United States. Deaths occur most often in children, in older people, and in people to whom **antivenom** is not given or is inappropriately given.

FYI

Blue Jeans and Snake Bites

Researchers studied whether ordinary clothing (denim material from blue jeans) reduces the amount of venom injected by a rattlesnake.

The investigators used saline solution–filled gloves to simulate human limbs and elicited bites from small and large southern Pacific rattlesnakes. Each snake was videotaped biting a bare glove and a denim-covered glove. The results were that the snakes injected significantly less venom into the denim-covered gloves than into the bare gloves: up to 60% reduction for the small snakes and 66% reduction for the large snakes. The investigators felt that denim interfered with venom delivery and induced a high proportion of dry bites (no venom released), as well as harmless spillage of venom from the fangs of the snakes onto the surface of the denim cover. It was interesting to note that larger rattlesnakes struck more readily, maintained longer fang contact during their bites, and delivered 26 to 41 times more venom into the gloves than did the small snakes. This adds to the body of evidence that indicates large venomous snakes are much more dangerous to humans than small ones.

Wearing long denim pants can be an inexpensive and effective way to reduce the severity of snake bites. Other forms of clothing (eg, high leather boots or other types of long pants) may be equally or more effective at deflecting a bite and preventing a snake bite.

Data from Herbert SS, Hayes WK. Denim clothing reduces venom expenditure by rattlesnakes striking defensively at model human limbs. *Ann Emerg Med.* 2009;54(6):830–836.

In about 25% of venomous snake bites, venom is not injected—only fang and tooth wounds (known as a dry bite) occur. Never assume, however, that the bite is a dry bite.

What to Look For	What to Do
Snake characteristics: ▪ Triangular, flat head that is wider than the neck ▪ Vertical, elliptical pupils (cat's eye) ▪ Heat-sensitive pit located between the eye and nostril Following a bite, the following signs and symptoms may be present: ▪ Severe, burning pain at the bite site ▪ Two small puncture wounds (the person may have only one) **FIGURE 19-11** ▪ Swelling within 10 to 15 minutes; can involve entire extremity ▪ Discoloration and blood-filled blisters possible in 6 to 10 hours ▪ Nausea, vomiting, sweating, and weakness (in severe cases)	1. Get the person and bystanders away from the snake because of the risk of a second bite. A dead snake can still bite even if decapitated. 2. Encourage the person to rest, stay calm, and be still. 3. **DO NOT** try to capture or kill the snake. These actions could lead to a second person being bitten. Try to remember the snake's color and the shape of its head. Taking a good photograph from a safe distance (more than the length of the snake) can help with identifying the snake. 4. Remove any rings, jewelry, or tight clothing from the bitten body part to avoid constriction from swelling. 5. Gently wash the bite with soap and running water and apply a sterile dressing over the fang marks. 6. Call 9-1-1 or transport the person to a medical facility as soon as possible. 7. When possible, carry the person. If alone and capable, walk slowly. 8. **DO NOT** apply a pressure bandage for a pit viper snake bite; this action has not been proven to be beneficial. According to a number of toxicology associations and the Wilderness Medical Society's Practice Guidelines, the application of pressure bandages for pit viper snake bites is not recommended.

CAUTION

DO NOT apply cold or ice to a snake bite. It does not inactivate the venom and poses a danger of frostbite.

DO NOT use the cut-and-suck procedure—you could damage underlying structures (eg, blood vessels, nerves, or tendons). Cutting the skin may cause infection and poor wound healing.

DO NOT apply mouth suction. Your mouth is filled with bacteria, increasing the likelihood of wound infection.

DO NOT use any form of suction.

DO NOT apply electric shock. No medical studies support this method.

DO NOT apply a constriction band—their use remains controversial. They may increase tissue damage. If applied too tightly or if swelling occurs, they can act as a tourniquet.

DO NOT apply a pressure bandage. A number of toxicology associations and the Wilderness Medical Society's Practice Guidelines do not recommend pressure bandages for pit viper snake bites.

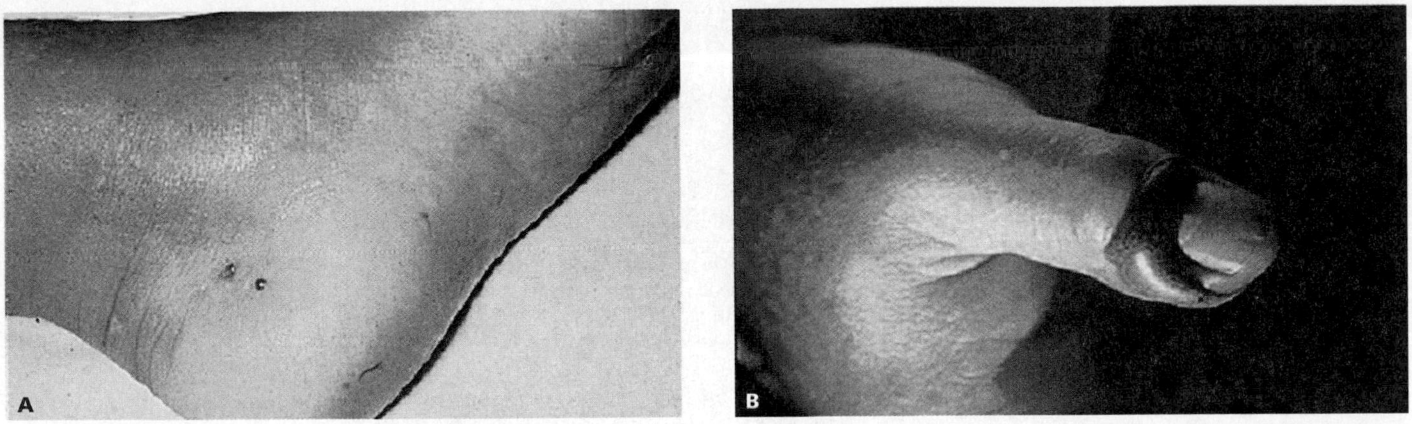

FIGURE 19-11 Rattlesnake bite on the foot (**A**) and thumb (**B**).

Coral Snake Bites

The coral snake is America's most venomous snake, but it rarely bites people. The coral snake has short fangs and tends to hang on and chew its venom into the person rather than to strike and release, like a pit viper. Coral snake venom is a neurotoxin, and symptoms can begin 1 to 5 hours after the bite.

What to Look For	What to Do

Snake characteristics:
▪ Small and colorful, with a series of bright red, yellow, and black bands going all the way around its body
▪ Every alternate band yellow
▪ Black snout
Following a bite, the following signs and symptoms may be present:
▪ Few immediate signs (Absence of immediate symptoms is not evidence of a harmless bite.)
▪ Several hours may pass before the onset of:
  ▪ Nausea
  ▪ Vomiting
  ▪ Sweating
  ▪ Tremors
  ▪ Drowsiness
  ▪ Slurred speech
  ▪ Blurred vision
  ▪ Swallowing difficulty
  ▪ Breathing difficulty
	1. Call 9-1-1. You do not need to capture or kill the snake.
	2. Apply a wide elastic bandage using overlapping turns.
	3. Start wrapping at the end of the bitten arm or leg and wrap upward, covering its entire length.
	4. Use similar tightness as when wrapping a sprained ankle. You should be able to slip a finger under the wrapping.
	5. Stabilize the bitten arm or leg as you would for a broken bone and keep it below heart level.
	6. **DO NOT** cut the skin or use suction.

FYI

Dead Snakes Can Still Bite

Data collected at the Good Samaritan Regional Medical Center in Phoenix show that fatal injuries do not prevent rattlesnakes from biting humans. Of the 34 patients admitted to the Phoenix Center for Rattlesnake Bites in an 11-month period, 5 were bitten by snakes that had been fatally injured and were presumed dead. One patient was bitten on the index finger after picking up a snake he had bludgeoned in the head and assumed was dead. Another was bitten after picking up a snake he had shot, then decapitated.

Data from Suchard JR, LoVecchio F. Envenomations by rattlesnakes thought to be dead. *N Engl J Med.* 1999;340(24):1930.

Nonvenomous Snake Bites

Nonvenomous snakes inflict the most snake bites. If you are not positive about a snake, assume it was venomous. Some so-called nonvenomous North American snakes such as the hognose and garter snakes have venom that can cause painful local reactions but no systemic (whole-body) symptoms.

Refer to **FLOWCHART 19-2** for additional information regarding the care of snake bites.

What to Look For	What to Do
▪ Horseshoe shape of tooth marks on skin ▪ Bleeding ▪ Possible swelling, mild itching, and tenderness	1. Gently clean the bite site with soap and water. 2. Treat the bite the same as you would a shallow wound. (Refer to Chapter 8, *Bleeding*, and Chapter 9, *Wounds*.) 3. Consult with a physician.

Flowchart 19-2 Snake Bites

- Get the person and bystanders away from the snake.
- **DO NOT** try to capture or kill the snake. Try to remember the snake's color and the shape of its head.
- Remove any rings, jewelry, or tight clothing from the bitten body part.
- Gently wash the bitten area with soap and running water and apply a sterile dressing over the fang marks.
- Call 9-1-1 or transport the person to a medical facility as soon as possible.

↓

Does the snake have bright red, yellow, and black bands around its body?

No → Suspect a pit viper.

- Seeking medical care is the most important thing to do.
- Stabilize the bitten arm or leg as you would for a broken bone and keep it below heart level.

Yes → Suspect a coral snake.

- Apply a wide elastic bandage using overlapping turns.
- Wrap the entire length of the bitten arm or leg. Use similar tightness as when wrapping a sprained ankle.
- Stabilize the bitten arm or leg as you would for a broken bone and keep it below heart level.

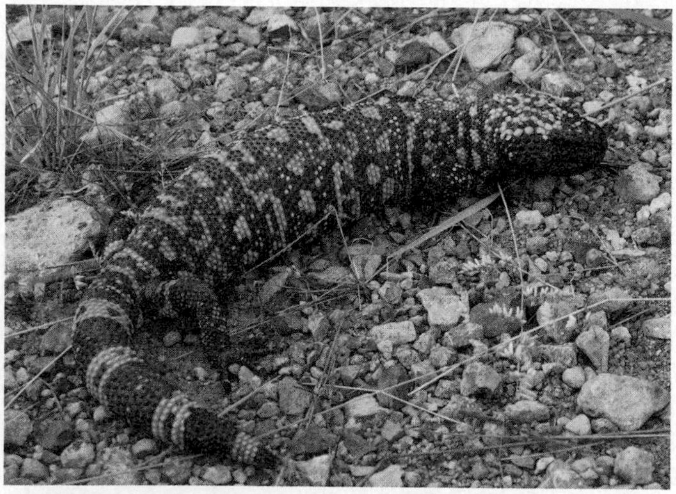

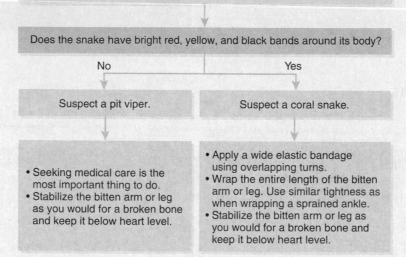

FIGURE 19-12 Gila monster.

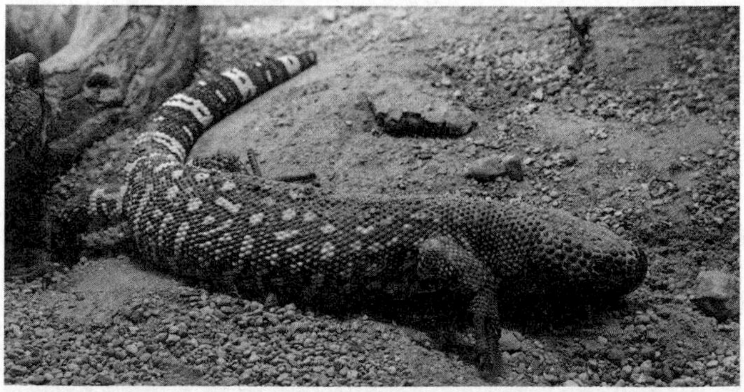

FIGURE 19-13 Mexican beaded lizard.

Other Reptile Bites

Venomous lizards include the Gila monster (United States and Mexico) **FIGURE 19-12** and the Mexican beaded lizard **FIGURE 19-13**. Venomous lizards may firmly hang on during the bite and chew venom into the person's skin.

What to Look For	What to Do
▪ Puncture wounds—teeth may break off ▪ Swelling and pain, often severe and burning ▪ Sweating ▪ Vomiting ▪ Increased heart rate ▪ Shortness of breath	**1.** Give OTC pain medication according to package directions. **2.** Call 9-1-1. **3.** Treat the bite the same as you would for a pit viper bite.

Insect Stings

The stinging insects belonging to the order Hymenoptera include honeybees, bumblebees, yellow jackets, hornets, wasps, and fire ants **FIGURE 19-14**. According to a review published in the *Journal of Allergy and Clinical Immunology*, about 0.4% to 0.8% of children and 3% of adults have life-threatening allergic reactions to Hymenoptera venom. Fortunately, localized pain, itching, and swelling—the most common consequences of an insect bite—can be treated with first aid.

Generally, venomous flying insects are aggressive only when threatened or when their hives or nests are disrupted. Under such conditions, they sting, sometimes in swarms. Honeybees have barbed stingers that become embedded in the person's skin during the sting. After injecting its venom, the bee flies away, tearing and leaving behind the embedded stinger and venom sac, which causes it to die. Honeybees and bumblebees do not release all their venom during the initial injection; some remains in the stinger embedded in the person's skin. If the stinger and venom sac are not removed properly, additional venom can be released and worsen the person's reaction.

In contrast, the stingers of wasps, hornets, and fire ants are not barbed and do not become embedded in the person. Thus, these insects can sting multiple times, and do not die as a result of the stinging. There are two types of yellow jackets: one is a wasp and can sting multiple times; the other is a ground-nesting bee that stings once and then dies, sometimes leaving an embedded stinger like other bees. These bees are smaller than yellow jacket wasps.

Most stings cause only self-limited, local inflammatory reactions consisting of pain, itching, redness, and swelling. These reactions are usually more a nuisance than a medical emergency. However, local reactions can be extensive; for example, involving the person's entire arm. In an extensive reaction, the swelling and redness might peak 2 to 3 days after the sting and last a week or longer. Signs and symptoms of life-threatening reactions include nausea, vomiting, wheezing, fever, and drippy nose. A person might go into **anaphylaxis** almost immediately or after experiencing a variety of symptoms. Most people who have anaphylactic reactions have no history of them. In a study of 400 fatal bee stings published in the *Journal of Allergy and Clinical Immunology*, only 15% of the people had a known history of anaphylaxis. Those with known allergies should carry an epinephrine auto-injector with them.

Reactions generally occur within a few minutes to 1 hour after the sting. People with bee stings who have anaphylactic reactions develop throat swelling and bronchospasm, which are manifested by difficulty speaking, tightness in the throat or chest, wheezing, shortness of breath, and chest pain. Respiratory tract obstruction accounts for the majority of deaths among people with flying insect stings.

For the severely allergic person, a single sting could be fatal within minutes. Although there are accounts of people who have survived some 2,000 stings at one time, 500 stings will usually kill even people who are not allergic to stinging insects.

Massive numbers of stings are rare. They might occur if a person stumbled into a hive or if a truck carrying a load

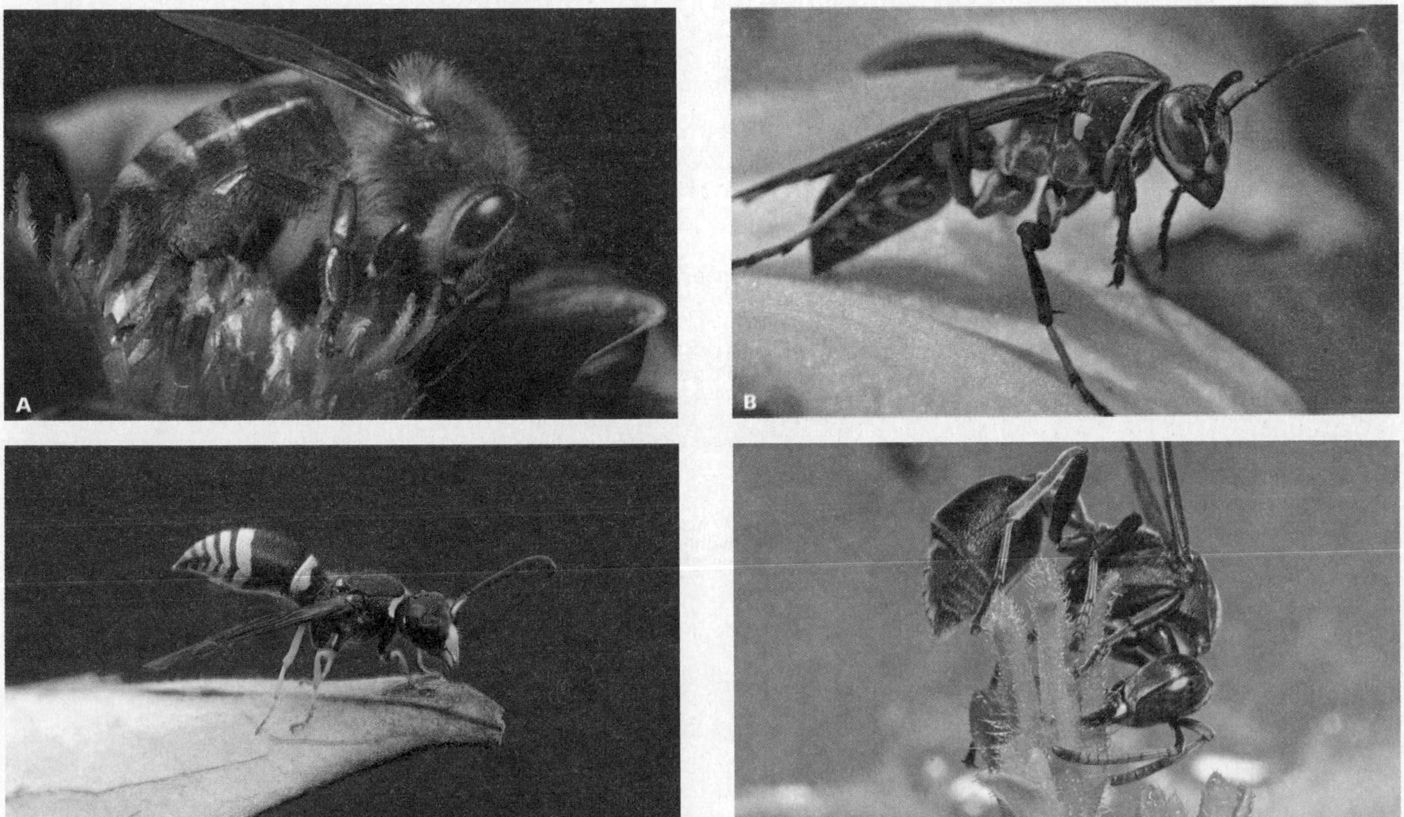

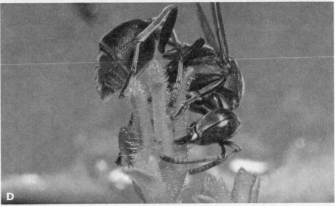

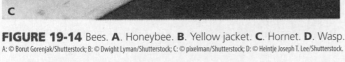

FIGURE 19-14 Bees. **A**. Honeybee. **B**. Yellow jacket. **C**. Hornet. **D**. Wasp.

of honeybee hives crashed. With the slow migration of Africanized bees (so-called killer bees) from South and Central America into the United States, the number of cases involving multiple stings is likely to increase. The venom of the Africanized bee is no more potent than that of the European type; it is just that the African type is extremely aggressive and, thus, more likely to be involved in multiple stings. A number of child deaths have resulted from the multiple stings of fire ants, which are common in the southeastern United States.

A rule of thumb is that the sooner symptoms develop after a sting, the more serious the reaction will be. The seriousness of reactions to stings can be categorized as follows:

- Usual reactions are instant pain, redness around the sting site, and itching.
- Worrisome reactions include hives, swelling of lips or tongue, a tickle in the throat, and wheezing.
- Life-threatening reactions are blue or gray skin color, seizures, unresponsiveness, and an inability to breathe because of swelling and spasm of the airway.

About 60% to 80% of anaphylactic deaths are caused by the person being unable to breathe because swollen airway passages obstruct airflow to the lungs. The second most common cause of death is shock, caused by collapse of blood circulation through the body.

One of the difficulties in dealing with stings is the lack of uniformity in people's responses. One sting is not necessarily equivalent to another, even within the same species, because the amount of venom injected varies from sting to sting. A person who experiences anaphylactic shock after being stung by a hornet might respond to a bee sting with only a small amount of swelling. One person might have a local reaction involving an entire limb, although the more typical response is a small circle of redness and swelling that disappears without incident in a few days. In beekeepers, for whom stings are an accepted occupational hazard, the response is likely to be even less than in most other people, because they have become tolerant to the toxins in the venom from having been stung many times on different occasions. There seems to be no easy way to predict how a person will react. Most people who are stung, however, have local reactions: redness, swelling, and pain.

Stings to the mouth or eye tend to be more dangerous than stings to other body areas. Also, people tend to react more severely to multiple stings, especially 10 or more. The most dangerous single stings in nonallergic individuals are those inside the throat, which can result from swallowing an insect that has dropped into a soft drink can or from inhaling one that flies into the person's open mouth. A sting in the mouth or throat can cause swelling that obstructs the airway even in a person who is not allergic to insect stings. If the sting is not life threatening, have the person suck on ice or flush their mouth with cold water. For a bee sting, dissolve a teaspoon (5 mL) of baking soda in a glass of water. Have the person rinse their mouth and then hold the water in the mouth for several minutes.

Refer to **FLOWCHART 19-3** for additional information regarding the care of insect stings.

Flowchart 19-3 Insect Stings

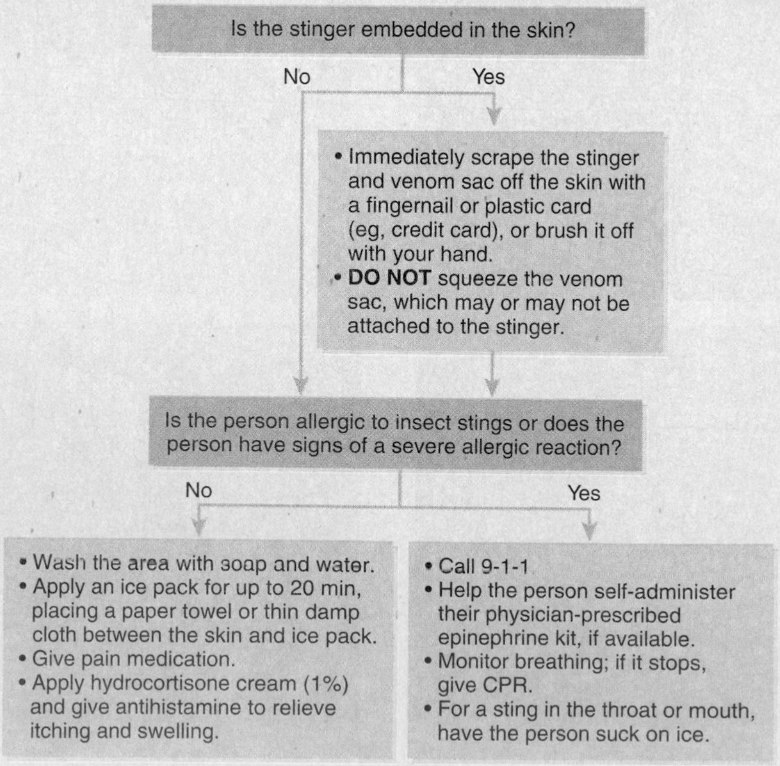

Is the stinger embedded in the skin?
No
Yes
• Immediately scrape the stinger and venom sac off the skin with a fingernail or plastic card (eg, credit card), or brush it off with your hand.
• DO NOT squeeze the venom sac, which may or may not be attached to the stinger.
Is the person allergic to insect stings or does the person have signs of a severe allergic reaction?
No
Yes
• Wash the area with soap and water.
• Apply an ice pack for up to 20 min, placing a paper towel or thin damp cloth between the skin and ice pack.
• Give pain medication.
• Apply hydrocortisone cream (1%) and give antihistamine to relieve itching and swelling.
• Call 9-1-1
• Help the person self-administer their physician-prescribed epinephrine kit, if available.
• Monitor breathing; if it stops, give CPR.
• For a sting in the throat or mouth, have the person suck on ice.

FYI

Fire Ants

Fire ants are aggressive, will defensively attack anything that disturbs them, and can sting repeatedly **FIGURE 19-15**. The fire ant bites by securing itself to the skin of a person with its mandibles, causing pain; then, using its head as a pivot, the ant swings its abdomen in an arc, repeatedly stinging the person with an abdominal stinger. According to a study published in the *Journal of Allergy and Clinical Immunology*, up to 60% of people who live in infested urban areas are stung each year, and more than 80 deaths have been attributed to these insect bites.

The fire ant sting usually produces immediate pain and a red, swollen area, which disappears within 45 minutes **FIGURE 19-16**. A blister then forms, rupturing in 30 to 70 hours, and the area often becomes infected. In some cases, a red, swollen, itchy patch develops instead of a blister. Although the stings are not usually life threatening, they are easily infected and can leave permanent scars.

Some people become sensitive to fire ant stings and should seek the advice of an allergist. Anaphylaxis (a life-threatening allergic reaction) occurs in about 1% to 2% of people stung by fire ants. Therefore, if a sting leads to shortness of breath, tightness and swelling in the throat, tightness in the chest, increased pulse rate, swelling of the tongue and mouth, dizziness, or nausea, the person should be taken to a hospital emergency department immediately. Some people lapse into a coma from even one sting.

First aid for fire ant stings includes placing an ice cube over the sting to reduce the pain and to slow absorption of the venom. A topical corticosteroid cream can help combat local swelling and itching. An antihistamine can prevent some local symptoms if given early, but it works too slowly to counteract a life-threatening allergic reaction. People who are allergic to stings should always carry a kit with antihistamine tablets and a preloaded syringe of epinephrine.

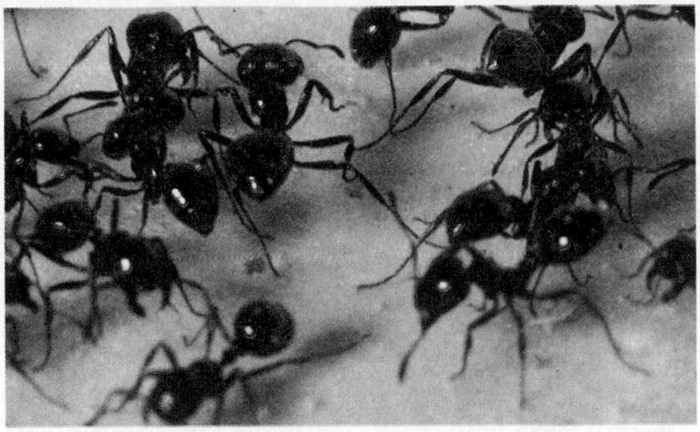

FIGURE 19-15 Fire ants.
Courtesy of Scott Bauer/USDA.

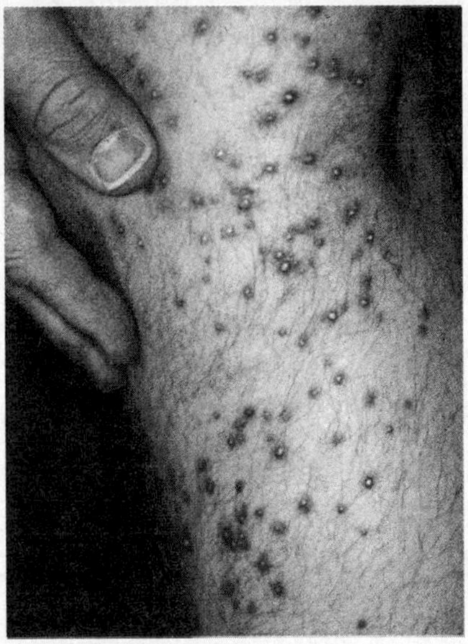

FIGURE 19-16 Fire ant stings.
Courtesy of Daniel Wojcik/USDA.

What to Look For	What to Do

▪ Usual reactions:
  ▪ Instant pain, redness, itching
▪ Worrisome reactions:
  ▪ Hives
  ▪ Swollen lips/tongue
  ▪ Tickle in throat
  ▪ Wheezing
▪ Life-threatening reactions:
  ▪ Blue/gray skin color
  ▪ Seizures
  ▪ Unresponsiveness
  ▪ Inability to breathe because of swollen vocal cords (cause of about 60% to 80% of anaphylactic deaths)
  ▪ Difficulty speaking
	1. Look for a stinger; if found, immediately scrape the stinger and venom sac off the skin with a fingernail or plastic card (eg, credit card), or brush it off with your hand. Only bees leave their stinger embedded. **DO NOT** use tweezers. **DO NOT** squeeze the venom sac, which may or may not be attached to the stinger.
	2. Wash the area with soap and water.
	3. Apply an ice pack to the area for up to 20 minutes, placing a paper towel or thin damp cloth between the skin and ice pack. Baking soda paste may also help, except for wasp stings.
	4. Give OTC pain medication according to package directions.
	5. Apply hydrocortisone cream (1%) and give antihistamine (Benadryl) to relieve itching and swelling.
	6. For a severe allergic reaction, help the person self-administer epinephrine. (See Chapter 7, *Shock*.) A person with a known allergy to insect stings should have a physician-prescribed epinephrine auto-injector to take wherever stinging insects are known to exist. When a person with anaphylaxis does not respond to the first dose, and arrival of EMS will exceed 5 to 10 minutes, consider administering a second dose.
	7. Monitor breathing; if it stops, give cardiopulmonary resuscitation (CPR).
	8. A sting in the throat or mouth can cause swelling even in a person without an allergy; have the person suck on ice or flush their mouth with cold water.

FYI

Preventing Insect Stings

People who know they are allergic to insect stings need to exercise extra care to avoid being stung. They should carry a bee sting kit and follow these guidelines:

- Wear long pants and long-sleeved shirts.
- Because insects are attracted to bright colors and floral patterns, wear white, green, tan, and khaki—the colors least attractive to insects.
- Wear shoes outdoors.
- Avoid yard work and other activities in which insect contact is frequent.
- Keep garbage cans away from the house.
- Remove insect-attracting plants from inside as well as the immediate proximity of the house.
- **DO NOT** use scented soaps, lotions, or perfumes.
- Keep car windows closed.
- If an insect confronts you, avoid quick movements and **DO NOT** provoke it. Turn away, lower your face, and walk away slowly. **DO NOT** run about wildly or move erratically when bees are nearby.
- **DO NOT** eat when bees are nearby.
- Have insect nests around the house removed by professional exterminators.

Spider and Insect Bites

Most spiders are venomous, which is how they paralyze and kill their prey. However, most spiders lack an effective delivery system—long fangs and strong jaws—to bite a human. About 60 species of spiders in North America are capable of biting humans, although only a few species have produced significant poisonings **FIGURE 19-17**.

Most bites are by female spiders. Male spiders are almost always smaller than females and have fangs that are too short and fragile to bite humans. Death rarely occurs and only from bites by brown recluse and black widow spiders.

The number of deaths from spider bites is not accurately known. A spider bite is difficult to diagnose, because most people never see the spider and the bites typically cause little immediate pain. An article in *American Family Physician* cites a study of 600 suspected spider bites, of which 80% were caused by other arthropods (eg, kissing bugs, ticks, fleas, mites, and bedbugs) and disease states (eg, poison ivy, diabetic ulcer, bedsore, Lyme disease, and gonococcus). Spiders rarely bite more than once, and they do not always release venom.

Black Widow Spiders

Black widow spiders are also commonly known as brown widow spiders and red-legged spiders, depending on the species **FIGURE 19-18**. The term *black* widow is actually inaccurate, because only three of the five species of widow spider are actually black; the others are brown and gray. Newly hatched spiders are almost entirely red. Males have white stripes along the outside of the abdomen.

The female black widow spider is one of the largest spiders, with a body that ranges up to 0.5 inch (1 cm) in length and a leg span of up to 2 inches (5 cm). It is her large size that allows the female black widow's fangs to be large and strong enough to penetrate human skin. The female black widow can live as long as 3 years. Black widow spiders have round abdomens that vary from gray to brown to black, depending on the species. In the female black widow, the abdomen is shiny black with a red or yellow spot (often in the shape of an hourglass) or white spots or bands.

The male is only one-third of the size of the female. Contrary to popular myth, the male usually mates safely with the female.

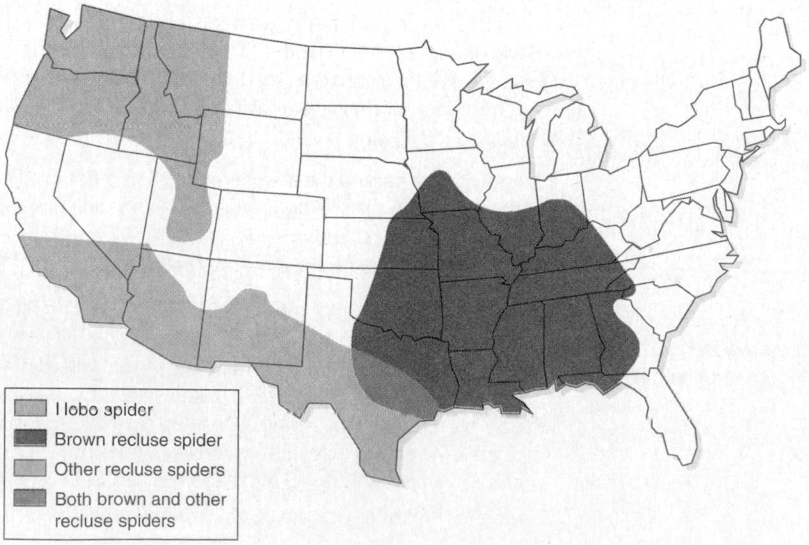

FIGURE 19-17 Map of spider range. Note that, with the exception of Alaska, black widow spiders are present across the U.S.

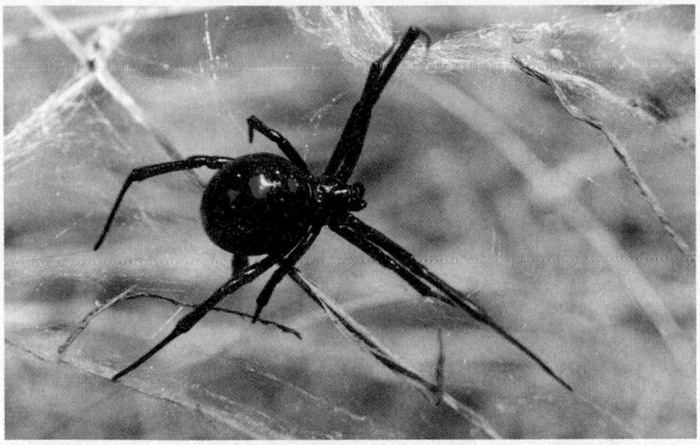

FIGURE 19-18 Black widow spider.
© Sari Oneal/Shutterstock.

Because he is small, his fangs are incapable of penetrating human skin, so bites are from the female. Black widow spiders produce one of the most potent venoms known in terms of volume. The venom is chiefly a neurotoxin in humans, with symptoms most often manifested as severe muscle pain and cramping.

Black widow spiders are found throughout the world. In the Western Hemisphere, they are found from southern Canada, throughout every state in the continental United States and in Hawaii, to the tip of South America.

The web of the black widow spider is an extensive, irregular, shaggy trap for the insects she normally eats. The black widow rarely leaves the web and stays close to her egg mass. She aggressively defends the egg mass and bites if it is disturbed. When she is not guarding eggs, the spider often attempts to escape rather than bite.

Frequent cleaning to remove spiders and their webs from buildings, outbuildings, and outdoor living areas decreases the chance of accidental contact with black widow spiders. Insecticides could decrease the population of the food for the black widows, but they do not usually affect the spiders themselves.

What to Look For	What to Do
▪ Sharp pinprick sensation followed by dull, numbing pain ▪ Two small fang marks seen as tiny red spots ▪ Severe abdominal pain (bites on an arm can produce severe chest pain, thus mimicking a heart attack) ▪ Headache, chills, fever, heavy sweating, nausea, and vomiting	1. Clean with soap and water. 2. Apply an ice pack to the area for up to 20 minutes, placing a paper towel or thin damp cloth between the skin and the ice pack. 3. Give OTC pain medication according to package directions. 4. Seek professional medical care as soon as possible. 5. If facial swelling or anaphylaxis occurs, call 9-1-1 and treat appropriately.

© Jones & Bartlett Learning.

Brown Recluse Spiders

Brown recluse spiders are also known in North America as fiddle-back or violin spiders **FIGURE 19-19**. They have a violin-shaped figure on their backs (several other spider species

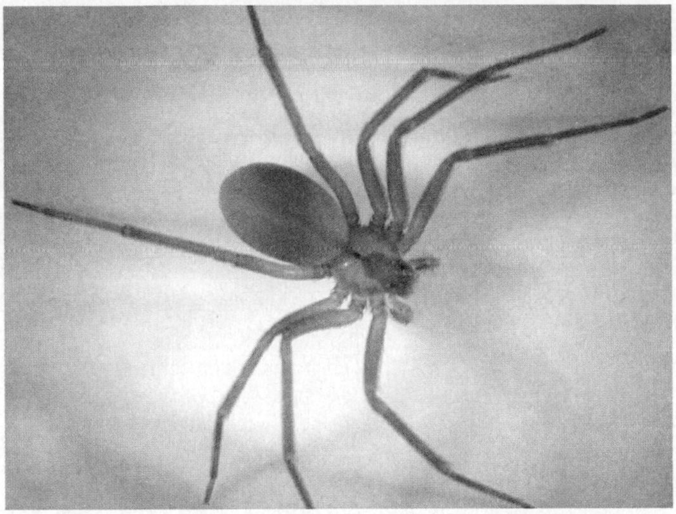

FIGURE 19-19 Brown recluse spider.
Courtesy of Kenneth Cramer, Monmouth College.

have a similar configuration on their backs). Color varies from fawn to dark brown, with darker legs. Male and female spiders are venomous. Brown recluse spiders are found primarily in the southern and midwestern states, with other less toxic but related spiders found throughout the rest of the country. They are absent from the Pacific Northwest.

If you suspect a brown recluse spider bite, remember the following:

- The brown recluse spider bites only when it is trapped against the skin.
- A local reaction usually occurs within 2 to 8 hours with mild to severe pain at the bite site and the development of redness, swelling, and local itching.
- In 48 to 72 hours, a blister develops at the bite site, becomes red, and bursts. During the early stages, the affected area often takes on a bull's-eye appearance, with a central white area surrounded by a reddened area, ringed by a whitish or blue border. A small, red crater remains, over which a scab forms. When the scab falls away in a few days, a larger crater remains. That too scabs over and falls off, leaving a larger crater. The craters are known as volcano lesions. This process of slow tissue destruction can continue for weeks or months. The ulcer sometimes requires skin grafting.
- Fever, weakness, vomiting, joint pain, and a rash could occur.
- Stomach cramps, nausea, and vomiting might occur. Death is rare.

What to Look For	What to Do
▪ Mild to severe pain that occurs within 2 to 8 hours ▪ Blister that develops within 48 to 72 hours; becomes red and bursts; takes on a bull's-eye appearance ▪ Nausea, vomiting, headache, and fever	1. Treat the bite the same as you would a black widow spider bite. 2. If the wound becomes infected, apply antibiotic ointment under a sterile dressing. 3. Seek professional medical care.

© Jones & Bartlett Learning.

Tarantulas

Tarantulas bite only when vigorously provoked or roughly handled **FIGURE 19-20**. The bite varies from almost painless to a deep throbbing pain lasting up to 1 hour. The tarantula, when upset, will roughly scratch the lower surface of its abdomen with its legs and flick hairs onto a person's skin.

What to Look For	What to Do
Varies from mild to severe throbbing pain that lasts up to 1 hour	1. Treat the bite the same as you would a black widow spider bite. 2. For hairs in the skin, remove with sticky tape, wash with soap and water, and apply hydrocortisone cream (1%). 3. Give an antihistamine and OTC pain medication according to package directions.

Common Aggressive House Spider (Hobo Spider)

Another biter is the common aggressive house spider, or hobo spider. It arrived in the Pacific Northwest in 1936 and slowly made its way across Washington State and into surrounding states. In those areas, the hobo spider is the most common large spider. For a common aggressive house spider, look for the same signs as a brown recluse spider and treat the same as you would for a brown recluse bite.

Refer to **FLOWCHART 19-4** for additional information regarding the care of spider bites.

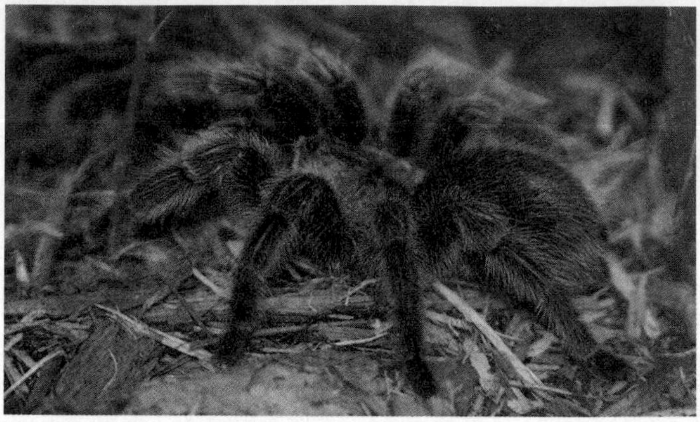

FIGURE 19-20 Tarantula.

Flowchart 19-4 Spider Bites

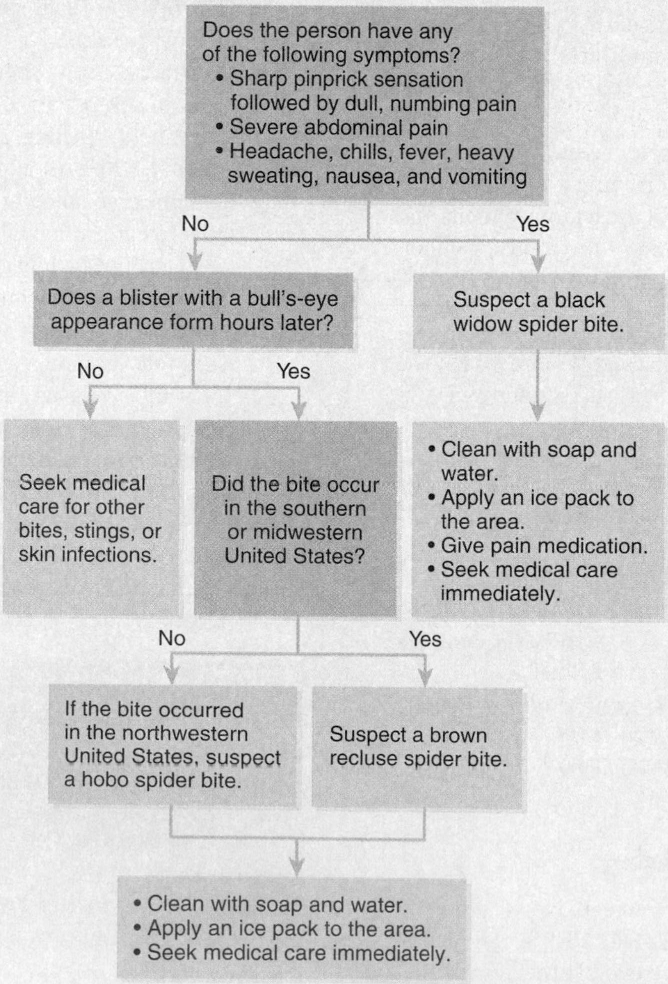
Does the person have any of the following symptoms?
• Sharp pinprick sensation followed by dull, numbing pain
• Severe abdominal pain
• Headache, chills, fever, heavy sweating, nausea, and vomiting
No
Yes
Does a blister with a bull's-eye appearance form hours later?
Suspect a black widow spider bite.
No
Yes
Seek medical care for other bites, stings, or skin infections.
Did the bite occur in the southern or midwestern United States?
• Clean with soap and water. • Apply an ice pack to the area. • Give pain medication. • Seek medical care immediately.
No
Yes
If the bite occurred in the northwestern United States, suspect a hobo spider bite.
Suspect a brown recluse spider bite.
• Clean with soap and water. • Apply an ice pack to the area. • Seek medical care immediately.

Scorpions

Scorpions look like miniature lobsters, with lobsterlike pincers and a long, up-curved taillike appendage with a venomous stinger **FIGURE 19-21**. Several species of scorpions inhabit the southwestern United States, but only the bark scorpion poses a threat to humans. Severe reactions, which usually appear only in children, could include paralysis, spasms, or breathing difficulties. Death due to scorpion stings in the United States is rare.

The bark scorpion is found primarily in Arizona. Rare stings have been reported in other parts of the United States, after the scorpions traveled from Arizona as stowaways in luggage or in car trunks. The bark scorpion is pale tan and is 0.75 to 1.25 inches (2 to 3 cm) long, not including the so-called tail.

Stings to adults usually are not life threatening. Stings to small children, however, are often dangerous. When a child is stung, every effort should be made to get the child to professional medical care as quickly as possible. Pay close attention to make sure the person's airway is open and that they are breathing.

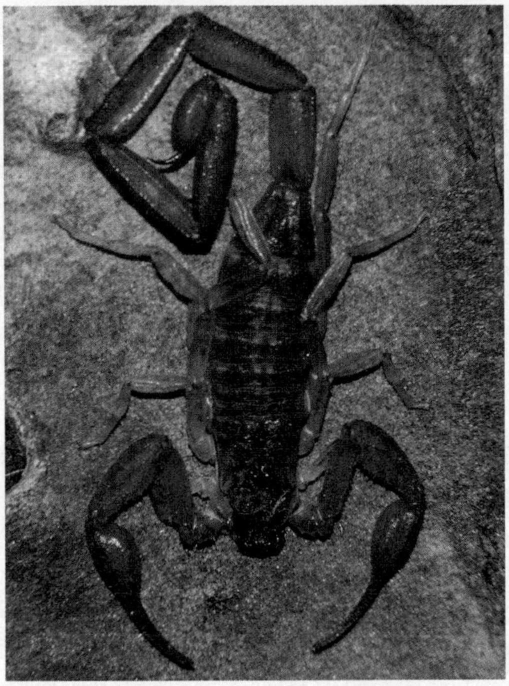

FIGURE 19-21 Bark scorpion.

What to Look For	What to Do
▪ The following symptoms begin from within minutes to one-half hour, reach their height within the first few hours, and usually last from 6 to 24 hours: ▪ Local, immediate pain and burning around the sting site (Tapping a finger over the sting site [the tap test] could serve to indicate a scorpion sting.) ▪ Numbness or tingling that occurs later ▪ Severely affected people will experience: ▪ Pain along the stung arm or leg, even paralysis ▪ Uncontrolled jerking movements of the legs or arms and facial twitching ▪ A fast heart rate ▪ Salivation ▪ Breathing distress	1. Monitor breathing. 2. Gently wash the sting site with soap and water. 3. Apply an ice pack to the sting site to reduce pain and venom absorption. 4. Give OTC pain medication according to package directions. 5. Apply a dressing. 6. Seek professional medical care for severe reactions.

Centipedes

Centipedes come in various sizes and colors and are found all over the United States and throughout the world. The giant desert centipede, which can be up to 8 inches (20 cm) long, is the only centipede in the United States that is dangerous to humans. Do not confuse centipedes with millipedes, which cannot inject venom but can irritate the skin.

Like spiders, any centipede with fangs that can penetrate human skin can inject venom. These arthropods inject toxic substances into the skin from a pair of hollow jaws that act like fangs. Contrary to popular belief, centipedes do not inject venom with their feet. Exaggerated stories about the deadly effects of their bites and reports that the tip of each leg carries a venomous spur have caused many people to have an unreasonable fear of centipedes. Their venom is relatively weak.

What to Look For	What to Do
▪ Burning pain ▪ Local inflammation of the wound ▪ Mild swelling of lymph nodes ▪ The bite of the giant desert centipede causes inflammation, swelling, and redness that last 4 to 12 hours.	1. Clean the wound with soap and water. 2. Apply an ice pack. 3. Give OTC pain medication according to package directions. 4. If symptoms persist, give an antihistamine (Benadryl) or apply hydrocortisone cream (1%) on the bite site. 5. Most bites will get better even without treatment; however, for severe reactions, seek professional medical care.

Mosquitoes

Mosquitoes bite millions of people. Mosquitoes are not only a nuisance, but they also carry many diseases. In developing countries, mosquitoes transmit malaria, yellow fever, and dengue fever; in the United States, they carry West Nile, Zika, and equine encephalitis viruses. There is no evidence that mosquitoes transmit the human immunodeficiency virus (HIV), the virus that causes acquired immunodeficiency syndrome (AIDS).

Female mosquitoes need blood to lay their eggs. Because they breed in water, mosquitoes are most often found in marshes, wetlands, and wooded areas. Mosquitoes usually can be separated into daytime and nighttime biters, but most bite at twilight.

What to Look For	What to Do
▪ Itching ▪ Mild swelling	1. Wash the affected area with soap and water. 2. Apply an ice pack. 3. Apply calamine lotion or hydrocortisone cream (1%) to decrease itching. 4. For a person with numerous stings or a delayed allergic reaction, an antihistamine (Benadryl) every 6 hours or a physician-prescribed cortisone might be helpful.

FYI

Preventing Mosquito Bites

To minimize being bitten by mosquitoes, follow these guidelines:

- Wear protective clothing: pants, long-sleeved shirt, and full-brimmed hat. Mosquito netting draped over a hat will protect the face and neck. Mosquito bed nets should be used when sleeping in unscreened rooms.
- Use insect repellents on exposed skin. DEET (diethyltoluamide)-containing repellents are most effective against mosquitoes and, to a lesser extent, helpful in repelling ticks and black flies.
- DEET is considered to have low toxicity. However, it is absorbed through the skin, and hives, skin rashes, and blisters can result when it is used for prolonged periods or in excessive amounts. The long-acting 35% solution has a polymer that prevents evaporation and skin absorption.
- Products that contain 100% DEET are available but unnecessary, especially for children. Long-acting formulations of 35% DEET seem equally effective in protecting against mosquitoes and have far less potential for toxic effects.
- DEET products can be applied over other creams such as sunscreens and moisturizers. Use DEET only on exposed skin, and avoid the hands of young children because they often put their hands in their mouths. Keep DEET out of the reach of small children because ingestion could be fatal. Children younger than 5 years should not be exposed to concentrations greater than 10%, according to the American Academy of Pediatrics. Children younger than 2 months of age should not have DEET applied to their skin. For children ages 5 or older, the DEET concentration should not exceed 30%.
- Other nontoxic insect repellents seem to be less effective than DEET. They might be only 25% as effective as DEET and might need to be reapplied every half hour. Mixed opinions exist about whether 100 mg of vitamin B_1 (thiamine) taken daily for 1 week before being exposed is an effective preventive agent. Some experts believe that a diet high in garlic will make a person undesirable to a mosquito.
- Permethrin is a pesticide, not a repellent. It should be applied to clothing and not the skin.

FYI

Mosquito Bites

In tropical climates, mosquitoes are carriers of infectious diseases such as malaria and yellow fever. Mosquito bites can also provoke unpleasant skin lesions. In many areas of the world, massive and disturbing mosquito infestations occur. For example, in Alaska it is possible to be bitten by mosquitoes as many as 1,000 times in 1 hour. Under such conditions, complete avoidance of bites is impossible without use of effective repellents and protective clothing. Topical treatment with OTC sticks, creams, and lotions containing antihistamines, hydrocortisone, or other antipruritic agents is common. However, only a few studies have been made regarding the effectiveness of these products.

Data from Reunala T, et al. Treatment of mosquito bites with cetirizine. *Clin Exp Allergy.* 1993;23(1):72–75.

Ticks

Ticks are not insects but are close relatives of mites and spiders. They have eight legs and are classified as hard ticks and soft ticks. Hard ticks are more familiar because of their wide distribution and common occurrence on domestic animals. Soft ticks are found mainly in western states. In the United States, seven kinds of hard ticks and five kinds of soft ticks carry diseases (eg, Lyme disease), are a nuisance (causing itching and swelling), or cause paralysis (toxin injected) **FIGURE 19-22**. Ticks hatch from eggs and grow through three distinct stages: nymph (too small to see), larva (just visible), and adult (ready to lay eggs) **FIGURE 19-23**.

The adult is most likely to be seen. Ticks at any stage of development can use humans for food; at each stage, they need a blood meal before they can grow to the next stage. Ticks are limited in their ability to find their meals. They cannot fly; instead, they crawl very slowly, and, without some help, they cannot travel more than a few yards from where they were hatched. When they are ready for their next meal, they might wait months, years, or even decades for the right host to come along. Bites are nearly painless, so the tick attachment is not noticed until later.

The front part of a tick consists of the head area and the mouthparts. The mouthparts have a central structure, the hypostome, which is shaped like a blunt harpoon. A tick makes a hole in the person's skin with the sharp teeth (barbs) on the front of the hypostome and then inserts it **FIGURE 19-24**. The barbs anchor the tick to the skin and make it difficult to pull the tick out. Some ticks produce a substance that helps cement them to the host. As they feed, some ticks increase in size 20 to 50 times.

Most ticks are harmless, but they can carry diseases (ie, Lyme disease, Rocky Mountain spotted fever, Colorado tick fever, tularemia, etc). The longer the tick stays embedded or the

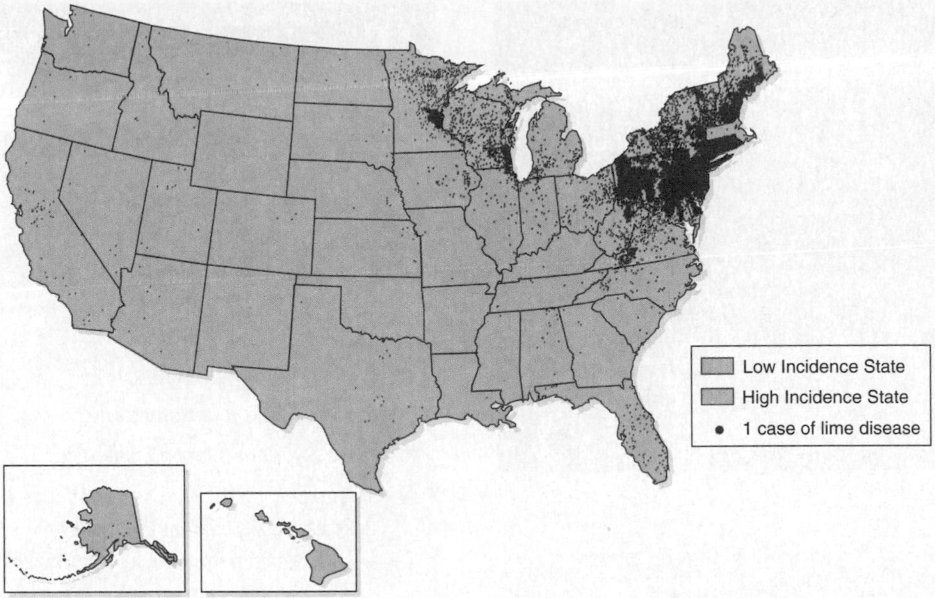

FIGURE 19-22 Reported cases of Lyme disease in the United States, 2018.

Centers for Disease Control and Prevention, Reported Cases of Lyme Disease in the United States, 2018.

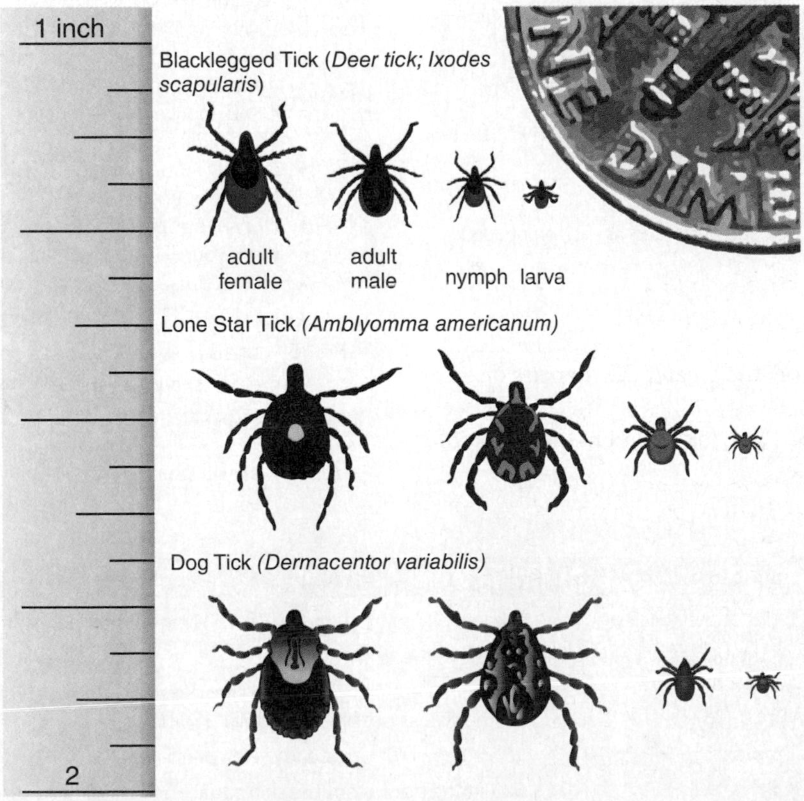

FIGURE 19-23 Life stages of ticks.

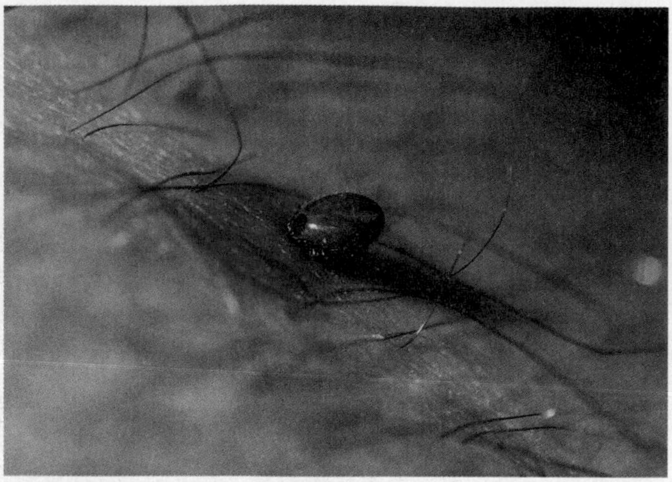

A

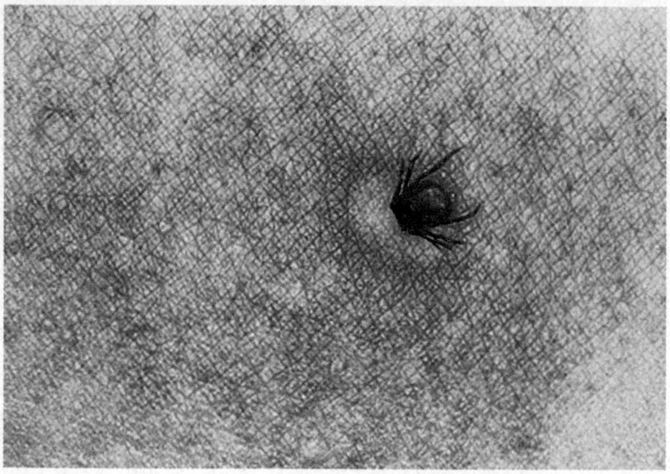

B

FIGURE 19-24 **A**. Tick embedded and engorged. **B**. Tick embedded.

more engorged it is with blood, the greater the chance a disease will be transmitted.

Refer to **FLOWCHART 19-5** for additional information regarding the care of tick bites.

FYI

Preventing Tick Bites

- Wear light-colored clothing so you can see any ticks on your clothes.
- Wear a long-sleeved shirt that fits tightly at the wrists and neck and tuck the shirt into your pants.
- Wear long pants and tuck the pant legs into your boots or socks, or use masking tape to tape the pant legs tightly to your socks, shoes, or boots.
- Check your clothes while you are outdoors and before entering a house. Wash your clothes as soon as possible.
- Inspect your pets for ticks before they come inside.
- After coming indoors, shower or bathe and check your body for ticks, especially in areas that have hair or where clothing was tight. Another person could do the checking.
- Treat your body and clothing with a repellent. The most common, Environmental Protection Agency–approved, and effective tick repellent is DEET.
- You can buy DEET and apply it directly to your skin. Ticks crawling on the treated area are irritated by the repellent and drop off. DEET is most effective against ticks when applied to clothing from a spray can.
- There have been a few reports of adverse toxic reactions to DEET, such as seizures, allergic responses, and skin irritation. To minimize reactions, do the following:
  - Apply DEET sparingly to your skin.
  - Avoid applying high-concentration products (more than 35% DEET) to the skin.
  - **DO NOT** inhale or ingest DEET-containing products or get them in your eyes.
  - **DO NOT** apply DEET to wounds or irritated skin.
  - Wash your skin after coming indoors.
  - **DO NOT** use products with more than 10% DEET on infants and small children (younger than 5 years).
- You can also use 0.5% preparations of permethrin (a pesticide). Permethrin should be applied only to clothing (especially shirt sleeves, pant legs, and collars), never directly on the skin.

What to Look For	What to Do
▪ No initial pain; the tick may go unnoticed for days. ▪ Red area around tick, indicating the tick has punctured the skin and is feeding on the person's blood. ▪ Rash, fever, and chills **FIGURE 19-25** ▪ The bite varies from a small bump to extensive swelling and ulcer.	Ticks are difficult to remove. Partial removal may lead to infection. To remove the tick: **1.** Use tweezers or one of the specialized tick-removal tools to grasp the tick as close to the skin as possible **FIGURE 19-26**. **2.** Pull upward with steady, even pressure. **3.** Lift the tick to tent the skin surface. Hold in this position until the tick lets go (about 1 minute). **4.** Pull the tick away from the skin. Try not to pull hard enough to break the tick apart, which leaves parts of the mouth embedded.

Continues

What to Look For	What to Do
Completely removed tick	1. Wash your hands and the area with soap and water. Apply rubbing alcohol to further disinfect the area. 2. Apply an ice pack to reduce pain. 3. Apply calamine lotion or hydrocortisone cream to relieve itching. 4. Place the tick in a plastic bag and bring it to a physician within 72 hours for identification and possible antibiotic treatment in order to prevent serious illness such as Lyme disease. 5. If a rash, fever, or flulike symptoms (headache, body aches, and/or nausea) occur in 3 to 30 days after the tick's removal, seek professional medical care—with or without the tick.
Tick's mouth parts broke off and remain in the skin	1. If unable to remove the parts, leave them in place and treat with warm soaks and antibiotic ointment. The retained parts will usually expel and the skin will heal. 2. If infection develops, seek professional medical care.

Flowchart 19-5 Tick Bites

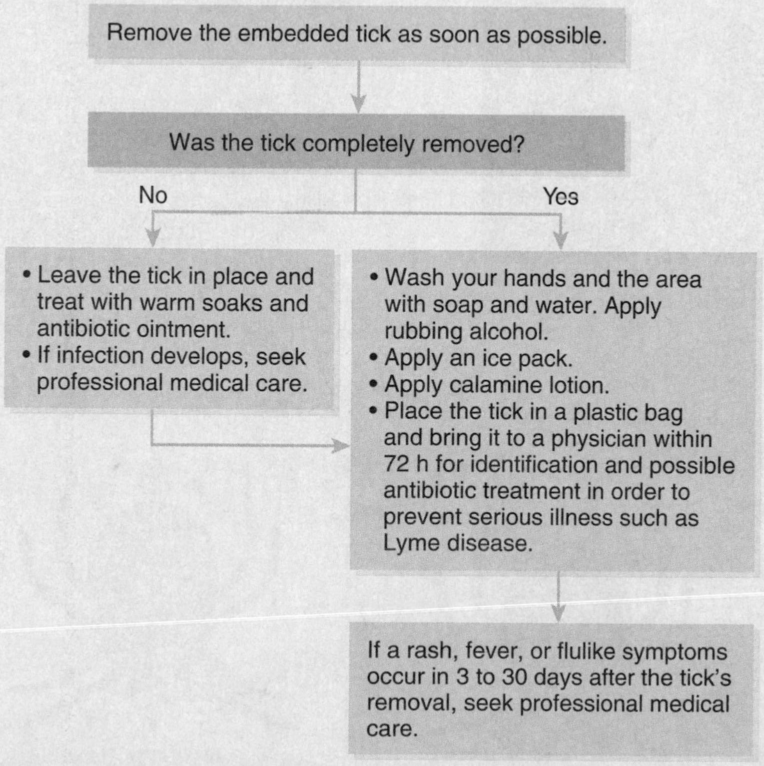

FYI

The Knot Method of Tick Removal

An embedded tick should be removed as soon as possible. The longer an infected tick stays embedded, the more likely it is to transmit a disease. An alternative to using tweezers and special commercial tick removal devices, especially when they are not available, is the knot method. Use cotton thread or dental floss and tie an overhand knot (similar to a shoelace knot without the bows). The open overhand knot is placed over the tick as close as possible to the skin surface and then gently closed to form a loop around the tick. Lift the tick's body over its head in a somersault-type fashion to remove the tick. This method removes the entire tick and is simple and effective.

Data from Celensa A. The knot method of tick removal. *Wilderness Environ Med.* 2002;13(2):181.

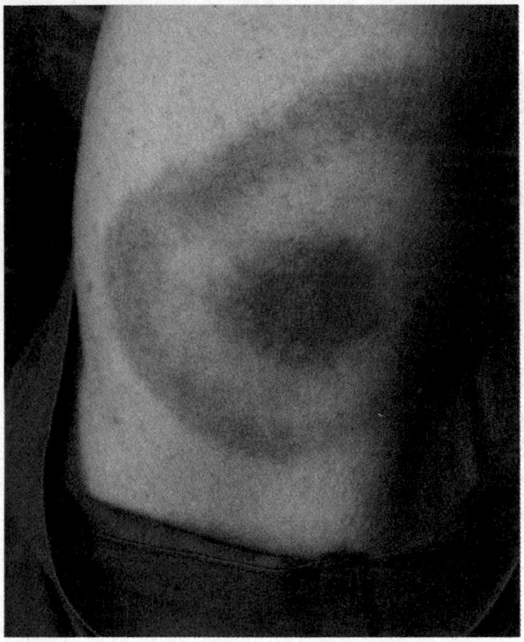

FIGURE 19-25 A bull's-eye rash is a distinctive finding in Lyme disease, but is not always present in people.
Courtesy of James Gathany/CDC.

CAUTION

DO NOT use any of the following ineffective methods to remove a tick:

- Petroleum jelly
- Fingernail polish
- Swabbing tick with a liquid soap-soaked cotton ball
- Rubbing alcohol
- Touching tick with a blown-out hot match, or a heated needle or paper clip
- Gasoline

DO NOT grab a tick at the rear of its body. The tick's internal organs could rupture, resulting in their contents being squeezed into the person, causing infection.

DO NOT twist or jerk the tick, which could result in incomplete removal.

FYI

Lyme Disease

Lyme disease has been reported in every state in the United States, with the Northeast, upper Midwest, and mid-Atlantic regions accounting for a vast majority of cases. It is caused by a bacterium, *Borrelia burgdorferi*, transmitted by the bite of the deer tick. Nearly 30,000 confirmed cases were reported in 2008, easily making Lyme disease the most common insect-borne infection in the United States.

The disease has two distinct phases—early and late. The best-known early symptom, a bull's-eye rash, affects up to 80% of affected people. Other early symptoms include headache, chills and fever, acute arthritis, and heart and spinal nerve root conditions. Lyme disease can include chronic arthritis, peripheral nerve injury, and brain and spinal cord symptoms.

Data from Lipman MM. Lyme disease: beyond the rash. *Consumer Rep Health.* 2010;22(8):11.

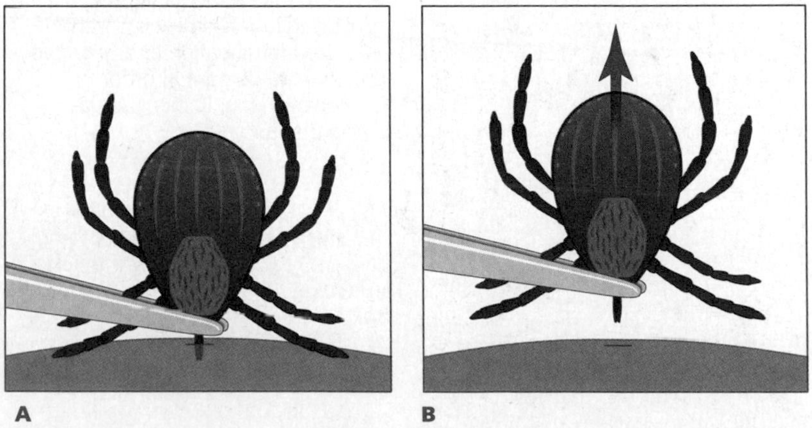

FIGURE 19-26 Removing a tick with tweezers. **A**. Grasp the tick as close to the skin as possible. **B**. Pull upward with steady, even pressure.

Marine Animal Injuries

Most marine animals bite or sting in self-defense, rather than attack. Marine venoms are similar to many venoms found in reptiles and arthropods and can cause anaphylaxis or other types of reactions. The general first aid guidelines are similar to those for any disorder involving trauma, allergy, or cardiopulmonary failure. Serious allergic reactions require primary attention to keeping the airway open.

Sharks

Sharks are the most feared of all marine animals, but, according to the International Shark Attack File, the chance of being attacked by a shark along the North American coastline is rare **TABLE 19-4**. Although exact figures are unavailable, it is estimated that, worldwide, around 50 attacks and fewer than a dozen deaths occur each year. The number of unprovoked shark attacks has grown at a steady rate over the past century.

Most attacks occur within 100 feet (30 m) of shore, and most people are attacked by a single shark without warning. In the majority of attacks, the person does not see the shark before the attack **FIGURE 19-27**. The leg is the most frequently bitten part. Sharks are clearly more attracted to people on the surface than to underwater scuba divers. The greatest attraction for sharks seems to be chemicals found in fish blood sharks can detect them in quantities as small as one part per million parts of water. Shark bite wounds, among the most devastating of all animal bites, are similar to injuries caused by boat propellers and chainsaws. Immediate control of bleeding and treatment for shock are essential.

TABLE 19-4 Preventing Shark Attacks

■ Avoid swimming in areas frequented by sharks or where shark attacks have occurred. (In the United States, the greatest concentration of great white shark attacks is off the northern California coast.)
■ **DO NOT** swim or dive alone.
■ **DO NOT** swim far offshore, in murky water, or along deep drop-offs.
■ People with open wounds should avoid swimming in areas where there is risk of a shark attack.
■ Avoid swimming in the vicinity of seal or sea lion colonies or turtle habitats.
■ **DO NOT** spear fish for an extended period in the same fishing area.
■ Avoid swimming at dawn, dusk, or night in potentially dangerous waters.

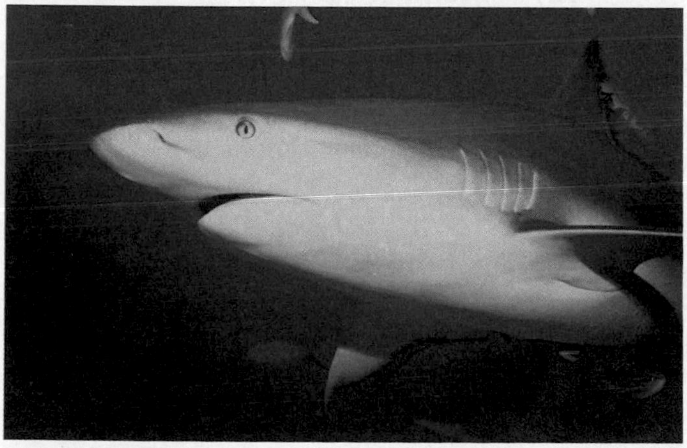

FIGURE 19-27 Shark.

Barracudas and Moray Eels

Barracudas have a fearsome appearance, but they have an undeserved reputation as attackers of humans. The risk of a barracuda bite is exceedingly small. First aid for a barracuda bite is identical to that for a shark bite.

Moray eels also have a fierce appearance. They are frequent biters of divers who handle or tease them, usually in competition for food or in pursuit of lobsters. The multiple puncture wounds created by moray eel bites have a high infection risk. Treat these wounds as you would shark bites.

Marine Animals That Sting

Stings from marine animals lead the list of adverse marine animal encounters. It is important to identify the offending animal, because in many cases, first aid is quite specific. Reactions to being stung vary from mild dermatitis to severe reactions. Most people recover without medical attention.

Jellyfish and Portuguese man-of-wars have long tentacles equipped with stinging devices called **nematocysts**. When cast ashore or onto rocks, detached nematocysts retain their ability to sting for a long time, usually until they are completely dried out.

The Portuguese man-of-war sting is usually in the form of well-defined linear welts or scattered patches of welts with redness, which usually disappear within 24 hours **FIGURE 19-28**. The jellyfish sting produces severe muscle cramping with multiple, thin lines of welts crossing the skin in a zigzag pattern **FIGURE 19-29**. Pain usually is a burning type that lasts 10 to 30 minutes. The welts on the skin usually disappear within an hour.

Anemones are beautiful but potentially dangerous **FIGURE 19-30**. Anemones have an array of tentacles around their mouth that are triggered by touch. Though most species are nonthreatening to humans, some stings can be harmful. Many anemone stings result from the improper handling of aquarium animals.

CAUTION

DO NOT try to rub the tentacles off of the person's skin—rubbing activates the stinging cells.

DO NOT use fresh water for rinsing because it will cause the nematocysts to fire.

DO NOT apply cold packs—they also will cause the nematocysts to fire.

DO NOT touch the tentacles with your bare hands.

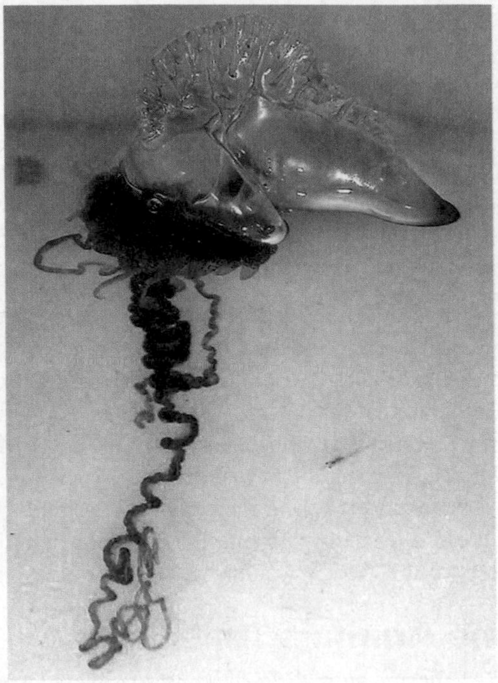

FIGURE 19-28 Portuguese man-of-war.
Courtesy of NOAA.

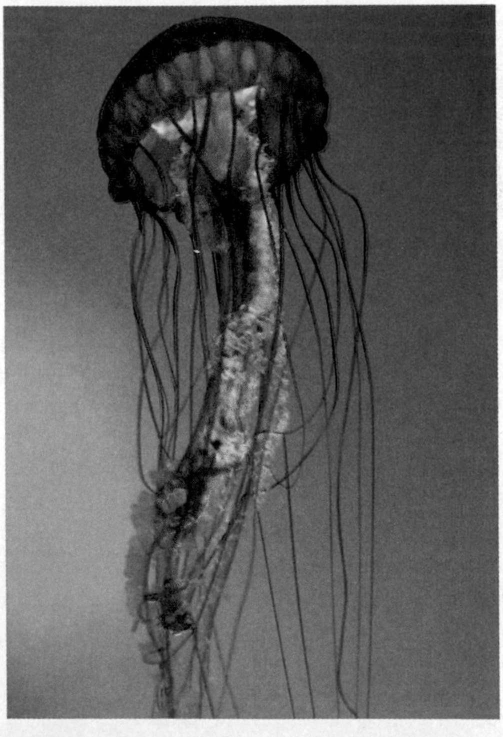

FIGURE 19-29 Jellyfish.
© Real Deal Photo/Shutterstock.

Stingrays

Stingrays, commonly found in tropical and subtropical waters, are peaceful, reclusive bottom feeders that generally lie buried in the sand or mud **FIGURE 19-31**. Most wounds inflicted by stingrays are produced on the ankle or foot when the person steps on a ray. The ray reacts by thrusting its barbed tail upward and forward into the person's leg or foot. According to the American College of Emergency Physicians, approximately 2,000 stingray injuries occur each year in coastal US waters. The stingray's venomous tail barb easily penetrates human skin. The sting usually is more like a laceration because the large tail barb can do significant damage. The venom causes intense burning pain at the site.

Refer to **FLOWCHART 19-6** for additional information regarding the care of marine animal injuries.

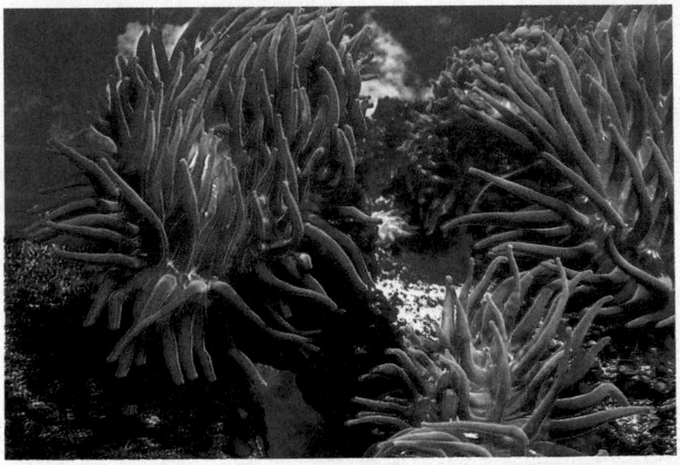

FIGURE 19-30 Anemones.
© fatamorgana-999/Shutterstock.

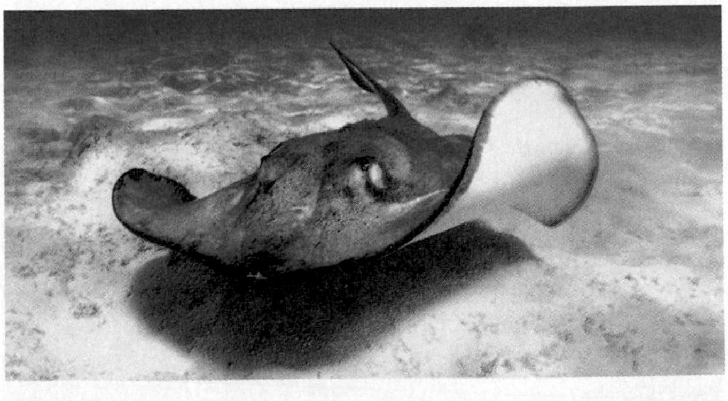

FIGURE 19-31 Stingray.
© AbleStock.

Flowchart 19-6 Marine Animal Injuries

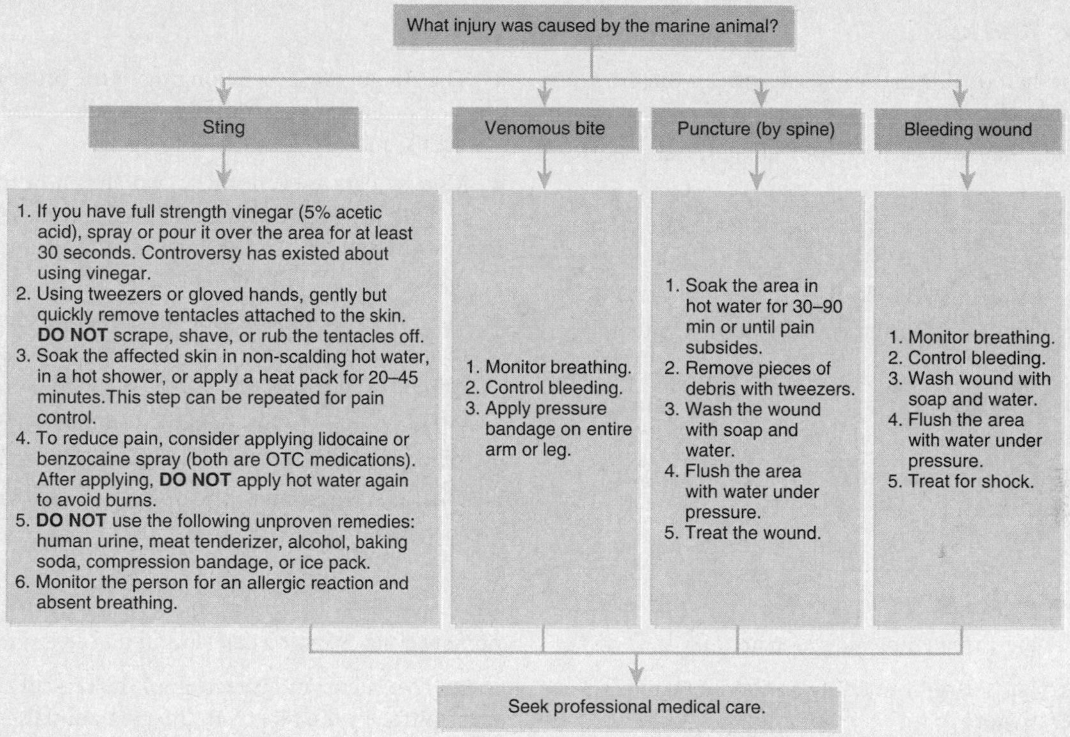

What to Look For	What to Do
Bite, rip, or puncture: ▪ Sharks ▪ Barracudas ▪ Eels ▪ Seals	**1.** Monitor breathing. **2.** Control bleeding. **3.** Wash wound with soap and water. **4.** Flush the area with water under pressure. **5.** Treat for shock.
Sting: ▪ Jellyfish ▪ Portuguese man-of-war ▪ Sea anemone ▪ Fire coral	**1.** If you have full strength vinegar (5% acetic acid), spray or pour it over the area for at least 30 seconds. Controversy has existed about using vinegar. **2.** Using tweezers or gloved hands, gently but quickly remove tentacles attached to the skin. **DO NOT** scrape, shave, or rub the tentacles off. **3.** Soak the affected skin in non-scalding hot water, in a hot shower, or apply a heat pack for 20–45 minutes. This step can be repeated for pain control. **4.** To reduce pain, consider applying lidocaine or benzocaine spray (both are OTC medications). After applying, **DO NOT** apply hot water again to avoid burns. **5.** **DO NOT** use the following unproven remedies: human urine, meat tenderizer, alcohol, baking soda, compression bandage, or ice pack. **6.** Monitor the person for an allergic reaction and absent breathing.
Venomous bite: ▪ Sea snake ▪ Octopus ▪ Cone snail	**1.** Monitor breathing. **2.** Control bleeding. **3.** Apply pressure bandage on entire arm or leg.
Puncture (by spine): ▪ Stingray ▪ Scorpion fish ▪ Stonefish ▪ Starfish ▪ Catfish	**1.** Soak the area in hot water for 30 to 90 minutes or until pain subsides. **DO NOT** use water that is hot enough to burn. **2.** Remove pieces of debris with tweezers. **3.** Wash the area with soap and water. **4.** Flush the area with water under pressure. **5.** Treat the wound.

PREP KIT

Ready for Review

- Almost one-half of all Americans will suffer a bite from either an animal or human.
- In the United States, dogs are responsible for the majority of animal bites.
- After dogs and cats, the animal most likely to bite humans is another human.
- Snake bites are estimated to lead to as many as 9,000 emergency department visits annually in the United States.
- Snakes can be identified as venomous (pit vipers) or nonvenomous.
- Venomous snakes include rattlesnakes, copperheads, water moccasins, and coral snakes.
- The stinging insects belonging to the order Hymenoptera include honeybees, bumblebees, yellow jackets, hornets, wasps, and fire ants.
- Most spiders are venomous, which is how they paralyze and kill their prey. However, most spiders lack an effective delivery system—long fangs and strong jaws—to bite a human.
- Venomous spiders include black widow spiders, brown recluse spiders, tarantulas, and common aggressive house spiders (hobo spiders).
- Other stinging or biting land animals include scorpions, centipedes, mosquitoes, and ticks.
- Most marine animals bite or sting in self-defense, rather than attack.

Vital Vocabulary

anaphylaxis A life-threatening allergic reaction.

antivenom An antiserum containing antibodies against reptile or insect venom.

nematocysts Stinging cells found on certain marine animals.

rabies An acute viral infection of the central nervous system transmitted by the bite of an infected animal.

Assessment in Action

You are enjoying an overnight campout with your family in the springtime. As you get ready for bed, you notice a small lump on your belly and are startled to find an embedded tick.

Directions: Circle Yes if you agree with the statement; circle No if you disagree.

1. You should leave the tick alone because ticks cause no harm to humans.

   YES **NO**

2. Covering the tick with petroleum jelly is very effective for removing the embedded tick.

   YES **NO**

3. You should touch a hot, blown-out match to the tick.

   YES **NO**

4. Grabbing the tick as close to the skin as possible with tweezers and pulling upward is usually effective.

   YES **NO**

5. After removing the tick, clean the wound and use an ice pack to reduce pain.

   YES **NO**

Check Your Knowledge

Directions: Circle Yes if you agree with the statement; circle No if you disagree.

1. Severe abdominal pain is a sign of a black widow spider bite.

   YES **NO**

2. Apply an ice or cold pack over a snake bite.

   YES **NO**

3. Use the cut-and-suck method for a snake bite.

   YES **NO**

4. Remove a bee's stinger by using tweezers to pull it out.

   YES **NO**

5. Apply an ice or cold pack over an insect sting or a suspected spider bite.

   YES **NO**

6. A baking soda paste can help reduce the itching and swelling from an insect sting.

   YES **NO**

PREP KIT continued

7. A person's prescribed epinephrine auto-injector might have to be used if the person has a life-threatening reaction to an insect sting.

YES **NO**

8. Care for stings from marine animals (eg, jellyfish) by pouring hydrogen peroxide on the affected area.

YES **NO**

9. Covering an embedded tick with petroleum jelly causes the tick to back out because of the lack of oxygen.

YES **NO**

10. Ticks can transmit disease.

YES **NO**

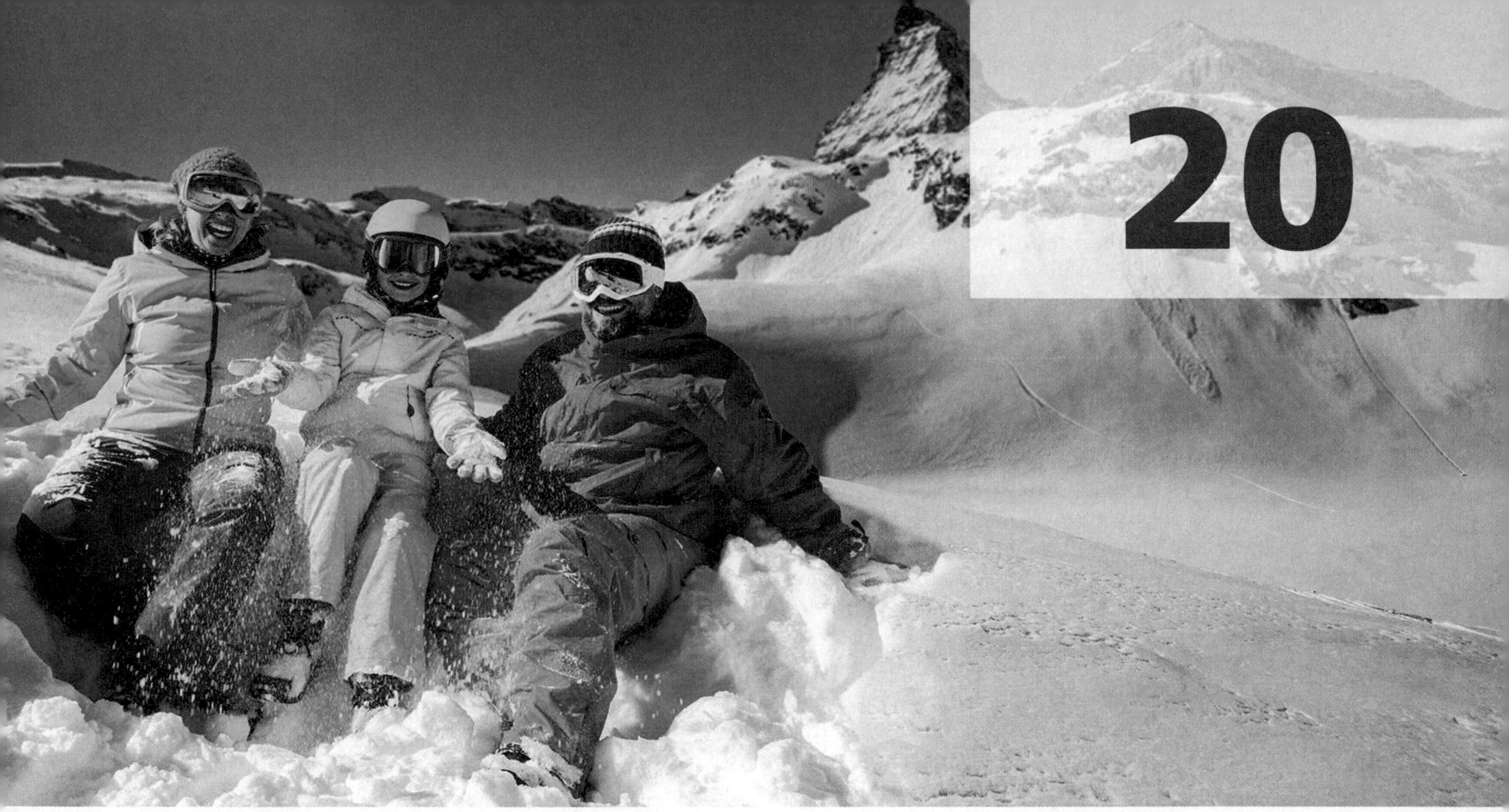

20

Cold-Related Emergencies

CHAPTER AT A GLANCE

Cold-Related Emergencies

Heat flows from an area with a higher temperature to an area with a lower temperature. When a person is surrounded by air or water cooler than body temperature, the body experiences heat loss. If heat escapes faster than the body produces heat, the body's temperature falls. Normal body temperature is 98.6°F (37°C), and if body temperature falls much below that, cold injuries can result. Because the body temperature is so high, you are always losing heat unless you are in a hot tub or living in an extremely hot environment.

How Cold Affects the Body

Humans protect themselves from cold primarily by avoiding or reducing cold exposure through the use of clothing and shelter. When that protection proves inadequate, the body has biologic defense mechanisms to help maintain correct body temperature. The internal mechanisms to maintain body temperature during cold exposure include vasoconstriction and shivering. Triggering of these responses is a signal that clothing and shelter are inadequate.

Vasoconstriction is the tightening of blood vessels. During cold exposure, vasoconstriction occurs in the exposed skin. The reduced blood flow in the skin conserves body heat but can lead to discomfort, numbness, loss of dexterity in the hands and fingers, and, eventually, cold injuries.

Cold triggers shivering, which increases internal heat production and helps offset the heat loss. Shivering is the body's main involuntary defense against the cold. Shivering produces body heat by forcing muscles to contract and relax rapidly. About 80% of the muscle energy used in shivering is turned into body heat. When the core temperature rises, shivering is no longer needed and is shut down by the brain. When the core temperature falls to about 86°F to 90°F (30°C to 32.3°C), the shivering reflex stops. Likewise, when there is no further fuel for the body, shivering stops. This is why people who are malnourished or have hypoglycemia (lower blood sugar) are more susceptible to cold injuries. The body needs both oxygen and glucose to produce energy and heat. Several drugs suppress the shivering response, including barbiturates, narcotics, beta blocking agents, and alcohol.

Internal heat production is also increased by physical activity; the more vigorous the activity, the greater the heat production. In fact, heat production during intense exercise or strenuous work usually is sufficient to compensate completely for heat loss, even when it is extremely cold. However, high-intensity exercise and hard physical work are fatiguing and cannot be sustained indefinitely. Heat is lost from the body 25 times faster when wet compared to dry, so if clothes become wet with sweat, heat loss is markedly increased.

Susceptibility to cold injuries can be minimized by maintaining proper hydration and nutrition; avoiding alcohol, caffeine, and nicotine; limiting periods of inactivity in cold conditions; and wearing appropriate layers of clothing that cover the head and other exposed areas. Humans do not acclimatize to cold weather nearly as well as they acclimatize to hot weather.

The colder the surrounding temperature, the greater the potential for body heat to escape. When the skin is exposed to cold, the brain signals the blood vessels in the skin to constrict, and blood flow to the skin decreases. This is the body's attempt to prevent heat inside the body from being carried to the skin, where heat loss will occur. However, because of reduced blood flow to the skin, the skin temperature falls.

When cold exposure lasts more than an hour (or less if conditions are wet or windy in addition to cold), cooling of the skin and reduced blood flow to the hands will blunt sensation, touch, and pain, and will cause a loss of dexterity and agility. These changes can impair a person's ability to perform manual tasks and, because symptoms could go unnoticed, can lead to more severe cold injuries.

Heat Loss From the Body

Normal body temperature is maintained by a balance of heat production and heat loss. Heat is produced by food metabolism and muscle activity, and shivering can increase heat production up to 500%. Shivering causes a large increase in heat production, but it rapidly consumes calories stored in the liver and muscles as glycogen. Lack of food limits the body's ability to produce heat; when **glycogen** stores are depleted, heat output decreases.

Heat loss occurs primarily through the skin. Blood flow to the skin varies in different parts of the body, and some areas allow more heat loss than others. The constriction of blood vessels caused by cold conserves heat.

Body heat loss can occur via five mechanisms **FIGURE 20-1**:

- **Conduction** , or direct contact with a colder object (eg, lying on the snow or on cold ground), normally accounts for only a small fraction of heat loss. The exception is immersion in cold water, in which heat loss can be 25 to 30 times greater than in air and even more in moving water.
- **Convection** is the loss of heat from the body by air blowing over the skin or through porous clothing. **Windchill** is the combined effect of the ambient temperature and wind speed.
- **Evaporation**, or conversion of liquid on the skin to a vapor, normally accounts for about 20% of heat loss (two-thirds through sweating and one-third through breathing).
- **Radiation** is the primary method of heat loss, accounting for about 65% of the body's heat loss. A warm object gives off (radiates) heat to cooler air.
- **Respiration** is when you inhale cold air, warm it with your body, and lose heat when it is exhaled.

Q&A

How is shivering related to the muscular system?

Shivering is the body's natural way of keeping warm and can actually serve as a lifesaver in extreme cold. Shivering produces heat by forcing skeletal muscles to contract and relax rapidly. About 80% of the muscle energy used in this process is turned into body heat. Studies have shown that applying hot water bottles or hot objects can actually be harmful in some cases of hypothermia because the shivering reflex is shut down.

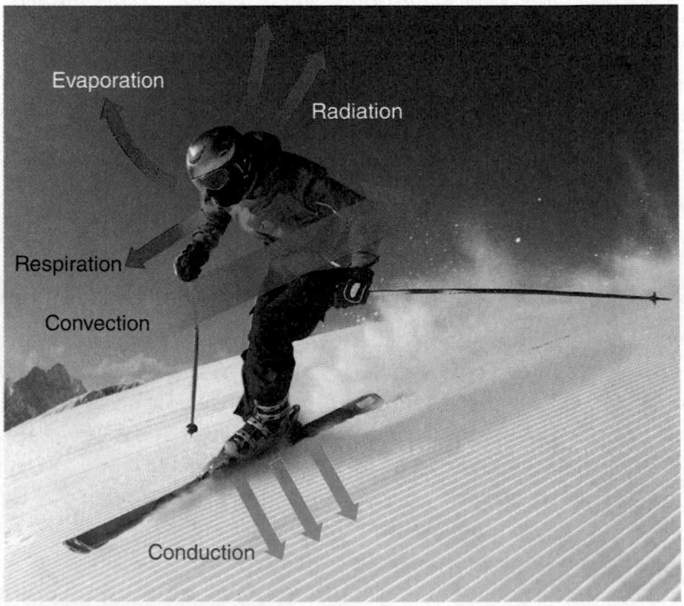

FIGURE 20-1 Sources of heat loss.

FYI

How Cold Is It?

In addition to cold, two other factors account for body heat loss: moisture and wind. Moisture, whether from rain, snow, submersion in water, or perspiration, speeds the conduction of heat away from the body.

Wind causes sizable amounts of body heat loss. If the thermometer reads 20°F (−6.7°C) and the wind speed is 20 mph, the exposure is comparable to 4°F (−15.6°C). This is called the windchill factor. Use the following rough measures of wind speed: if you feel the wind on your face, wind speed is at least 10 mph; if small branches move or if dust or snow is raised, it is 20 mph; if large branches are moving, it is 30 mph; and if a whole tree bends, it is about 40 mph.

Use the following steps to determine the windchill factor:

1. Estimate the wind speed by checking for the aforementioned signs.
2. Look at an outdoor thermometer reading (in degrees Fahrenheit).
3. Match the estimated wind speed with the actual thermometer reading in **FIGURE 20-2**.

Susceptibility to Cold Injury

A person's susceptibility to cold injury is affected by many factors. People who are physically unfit are more susceptible to cold injury. They tire more quickly and are unable to stay active to keep warm for as long as people who are physically fit.

Dehydration reduces blood flow in the skin, which increases susceptibility to cold injury. Fat functions as an insulator against heat loss because it has less blood flow than muscle and loses less heat. Therefore, a very lean person may be more susceptible to the effects of cold if clothing is inadequate or wet or if the person is relatively inactive. Older people are less tolerant of the cold than younger people because of a decline in physical fitness, poor circulation, other illnesses, and medications that affect thermoregulation.

Alcohol and, to a lesser extent, caffeine, cause the blood vessels in the skin to dilate, which can accelerate body heat loss. Also, alcohol and caffeine both increase urine formation, leading to dehydration, which can further degrade the body's defense against cold. Most important, alcohol blunts the senses and impairs judgment, so a person may not feel the signs and symptoms of developing cold injury.

Because nicotine decreases blood flow to the skin, smoking and chewing tobacco can increase susceptibility to frostbite. Inadequate nutrition, illness, and injury compromise the body's responses to cold and a person's ability to recognize and react appropriately to the symptoms of developing cold injury. People with a previous history of cold injury are at greater risk of experiencing another cold injury.

Effects of Altitude

Assessing weather conditions in mountainous regions must include altitude considerations, especially if the assessment is based on weather measurements obtained at lower elevations. Temperatures, windchill, and the risk of cold injury at high altitudes can differ considerably from those at lower elevations.

In general, it can be assumed that air temperature drops 3.6°F every 1,000 feet above the original measurement site. Winds usually are more severe at high altitudes, and there is less cover above the tree line. People are more susceptible to frostbite and other cold injuries at altitudes above 8,000 feet than at sea level because of lower temperatures, higher winds, and less oxygen.

Wind Chill Chart

Effective 11/01/01

Wind (mph) / Calm	40	35	30	25	20	15	10	5	0	-5	-10	-15	-20	-25	-30	-35	-40	-45
5	36	31	25	19	13	7	1	-5	-11	-16	-22	-28	-34	-40	-46	-52	-57	-63
10	34	27	21	15	9	3	-4	-10	-16	-22	-28	-35	-41	-47	-53	-59	-66	-72
15	32	25	19	13	6	0	-7	-13	-19	-26	-32	-39	-45	-51	-58	-64	-71	-77
20	30	24	17	11	4	-2	-9	-15	-22	-29	-35	-42	-48	-55	-61	-68	-74	-81
25	29	23	16	9	3	-4	-11	-17	-24	-31	-37	-44	-51	-58	-64	-71	-78	-84
30	28	22	15	8	1	-5	-12	-19	-26	-33	-39	-46	-53	-60	-67	-73	-80	-87
35	28	21	14	7	0	-7	-14	-21	-27	-34	-41	-48	-55	-62	-69	-76	-82	-89
40	27	20	13	6	-1	-8	-15	-22	-29	-36	-43	-50	-57	-64	-71	-78	-84	-91
45	26	19	12	5	-2	-9	-16	-23	-30	-37	-44	-51	-58	-65	-72	-79	-86	-93
50	26	19	12	4	-3	-10	-17	-24	-31	-38	-45	-52	-60	-67	-74	-81	-88	-95
55	25	18	11	4	-3	-11	-18	-25	-32	-39	-46	-54	-61	-68	-75	-82	-89	-97
60	25	17	10	3	-4	-11	-19	-26	-33	-40	-48	-55	-62	-69	-76	-84	-91	-98

Frostbite Times: 30 minutes; 10 minutes; 5 minutes

Wind Chill (°F) = $35.74 + 0.6215T - 35.75(V^{0.16}) + 0.4275T(V^{0.16})$

Where, T = Air Temperature (°F); V = Wind Speed (mph)

FIGURE 20-2 Windchill chart.

Courtesy of the National Weather Service/NOAA.

Effects of Water

Water can conduct heat away from the body much faster than air of the same temperature. When clothing becomes wet because of snow, rain, splashing water, or accumulated sweat, the body's loss of heat is accelerated up to 25 times. Swimmers and people working or wading in water can experience a great deal of body heat loss, even when the water temperature is only mildly cool. People entering very cold water should be closely watched because sudden plunging into cold water can produce an irregular heartbeat, gasping, and hyperventilation, which can cause inhalation of water, heart failure, and drowning.

Effects of Wind

For any given air temperature, the potential for body heat loss, skin cooling, and decreased internal temperature is increased by wind. Wind increases heat loss from skin exposed to cold air, in effect lowering the temperature. The windchill index integrates wind speed and air temperature to provide an estimate of the cooling power of the environment and the associated risk of cold injury.

Windchill temperatures obtained from weather reports do not take into account artificial wind, which worsens the windchill effect of natural wind. For example, riding in an open vehicle can subject the passengers to dangerous windchill, even when natural winds are low.

Effects of Metals and Liquid Fuels

Metal objects and liquid fuels that have been left outdoors in the cold pose a serious hazard. Both can conduct heat away from the skin rapidly. Fuels and solvents remain liquid at very low temperatures. Skin contact with fuel or metal at below-freezing temperatures can result in nearly instantaneous freezing. Fuel handlers must use great care and not allow exposed skin to come into contact with spilled fuels or metal objects.

Minimizing Effects of Cold on the Body

When adequately protected, humans can tolerate temperatures as low as −72°F (−57.8°C). Adequate clothing maintains the microclimate surrounding the body. Air is an excellent insulator, and the basis for most clothing is to trap a layer of air around the body. Layering, which has been used for centuries, allows the removal or opening of a garment to vent excess heat during times of greater activity or changes in environment, and it accommodates individual needs and preferences. Wearing layered clothing is especially important for people who frequently change environments by going in and out of buildings or who periodically undertake vigorous physical activity **FIGURE 20-3**.

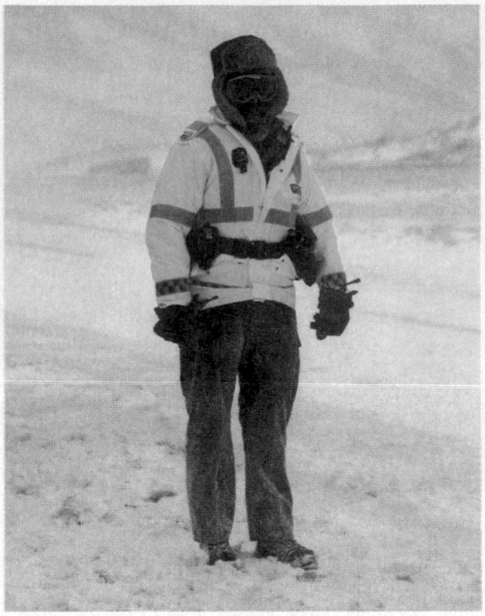

FIGURE 20-3 Wearing layered clothing allows you to retain or release body heat to maintain comfort in changing conditions.

Three important layers are recommended for most outdoor activities. The inner layer (undergarments) removes perspiration from the skin, the middle layer (or layers) insulates, and the outer layer or outer shell protects against wind and water. By understanding this principle, people can vary their clothing for protection and comfort.

For the inner layer, use underwear that wicks away perspiration; that is, it stays dry by drawing moisture away from the skin to the next layer of clothing. Wet clothing transfers heat away from the body. Cotton holds moisture next to the skin, so the person feels cold and clammy. Silk feels warm and soft, but it also retains moisture. Fabrics such as polypropylene or newer types of polyesters such as Capilene or Thermax should be considered.

The middle layer can be a synthetic pile or fleece jacket that is warm and dries quickly or a wool or synthetic sweater. Synthetic insulating materials, unlike down or wool, provide warmth without bulk or heavy weight. Insulation should be effective even when wet. In that respect, synthetics are clearly superior to natural fibers and natural products. Duck or goose down, for example, is virtually useless when wet, and it dries slowly. One exception, however, is the insulating ability of wool, even when wet.

People who are physically active can sweat even in extremely cold weather. Therefore, the best choice for an outside layer is a jacket that is waterproof, wind resistant, and breathable. Materials such as Gore-Tex allow perspiration to evaporate. A zipper is preferable, so the clothing can be opened easily to increase ventilation. Nylon and vinyl are poor choices because they produce a sauna effect by holding in perspiration.

Nonfreezing Cold Injuries

Nonfreezing cold injuries can occur when conditions are cold and wet (air temperatures between 32°F and 55°F [0°C and 12.8°C]) and the hands and feet cannot be kept warm and dry. The most prominent nonfreezing cold injuries are chilblain and trench foot.

Chilblain

Chilblain is a nonfreezing cold injury that, while painful, causes little or no permanent damage. Chilblain can develop in 3 to 6 hours in skin exposed to cold and moisture.

What to Look For	What to Do
▪ Swollen skin ▪ Skin that is tender, hot to the touch, and possibly itchy ▪ Blisters ▪ Condition can worsen to an aching, prickly (pins and needles) sensation and then numbness.	1. Get the person out of the cold.

Trench Foot/Immersion Foot

Trench foot (also called immersion foot) is a serious, nonfreezing cold injury that develops when the skin on the feet is exposed to moisture and cold for prolonged periods (12 hours or longer). Wearing wet boots or shoes and socks causes trench foot; likewise, prolonged immersion of the feet in cold water causes immersion foot. The combination of cold and moisture softens the skin, causing tissue loss and, often, infection. The risk of this potentially crippling injury is high during wet weather. People who wear rubberized or tight-fitting boots in cold weather are at risk for trench foot regardless of weather conditions because sweat accumulates inside the boots and keeps the feet wet.

What to Look For	What to Do
▪ Itching, numbness, or tingling pain ▪ Swollen feet and pale skin that feels cold when touched ▪ Red or blue blotches on the skin, sometimes with open weeping or bleeding	1. Dry the skin. 2. Rewarm the foot gradually. 3. Care for open weeping areas by cleansing with mild soap and water and applying breathable dressings.

Q&A

What is the origin of the term *trench* or *immersion foot*?

The term *immersion foot* was coined during World War I to describe an injury that occurred to people who were shipwrecked and isolated in a lifeboat for a prolonged period of time. Similarly, the term *trench foot* was coined during World War I to describe an injury that occurred to soldiers who were stuck for a prolonged period of time in trenches filled with cold mud and water.

Both conditions occur after prolonged exposure to a wet and cold environment. Temperatures range from just above freezing to about 60°F (10°C). The duration of exposure usually exceeds 10 to 12 hours.

Data from Stewart C. Local cold injuries in children: Diagnosis, management, and prevention. *Pediatr EM Rep* 1991;4:1

Freezing Cold Injuries

Freezing cold injuries can occur whenever the air temperature is below freezing (32°F [0°C]). Freezing limited to the skin surface is **frostnip**. Freezing that extends deeper through the skin and into the flesh is **frostbite**. The key difference between frostbite and frostnip is that, with frostnip, the skin remains pliable when frozen and will not be injured upon warming.

Frostbite is prevalent during military campaigns and is a known hazard for outdoor workers, the homeless, mountain climbers, and explorers. As more people pursue cross-country skiing, snowmobiling, and other outdoor winter sports, the number of frostbite cases probably will increase.

Frostnip

Frostnip is caused when water on the skin surface freezes. Frostnip should be taken seriously because it could be the first sign of impending frostbite. It may be difficult to tell the difference between frostnip and frostbite.

What to Look For	What to Do
▪ Yellow to gray skin color ▪ Frost (ice crystals) on the skin ▪ Initial tingling or numbness that may become painful	1. Get the person out of the cold and to a warm place. 2. Gently warm the affected area by placing it against a warm body part (eg, have the person put bare hands under the armpits) or by applying a warm chemical heat pack covered by a cloth. For the nose, breathe with cupped hands over the nose. 3. **DO NOT** rub the area.

Frostbite

Frostbite happens only in below-freezing temperatures. Tissue is not composed of water alone, so it will not freeze until it has been cooled to about 28°F (−2.2°C). Tissue is damaged in two ways: (1) actual tissue freezing, which results in the formation of ice crystals within the tissue (the ice crystals expand as they freeze, damaging cells), and (2) the obstruction of the blood supply to the tissue, which causes sludged blood clots and further prevents blood from flowing to the tissues. The second type of tissue damage is more extensive than the first. In severely cold temperatures, flesh can freeze in less than a minute **FIGURE 20-4**.

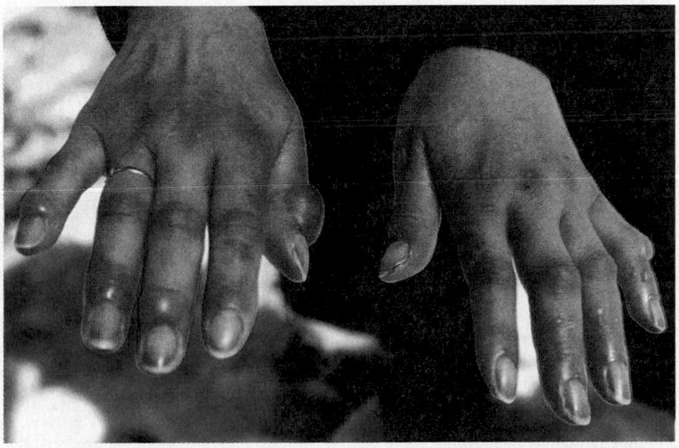

FIGURE 20-4 Frostbitten fingers 6 hours after rewarming in 100°F to 104°F [38°C to 40°C] water.
Courtesy of Neil Malcom Winkelmann.

Frostbite affects mainly the feet, hands, ears, and nose. These areas do not contain large heat-producing muscles and are some distance from the body's heat-generation sources. The severity and extent of frostbite are difficult to judge until hours after thawing. The most severe consequences of frostbite occur when tissue dies (**gangrene**), and the affected part might have to be amputated. The longer the tissue stays frozen, the worse the injury. Check for hypothermia in any person with frostbite.

Refer to **FLOWCHART 20-1** for additional information regarding the care of frostbite.

Flowchart 20-1 Frostbite

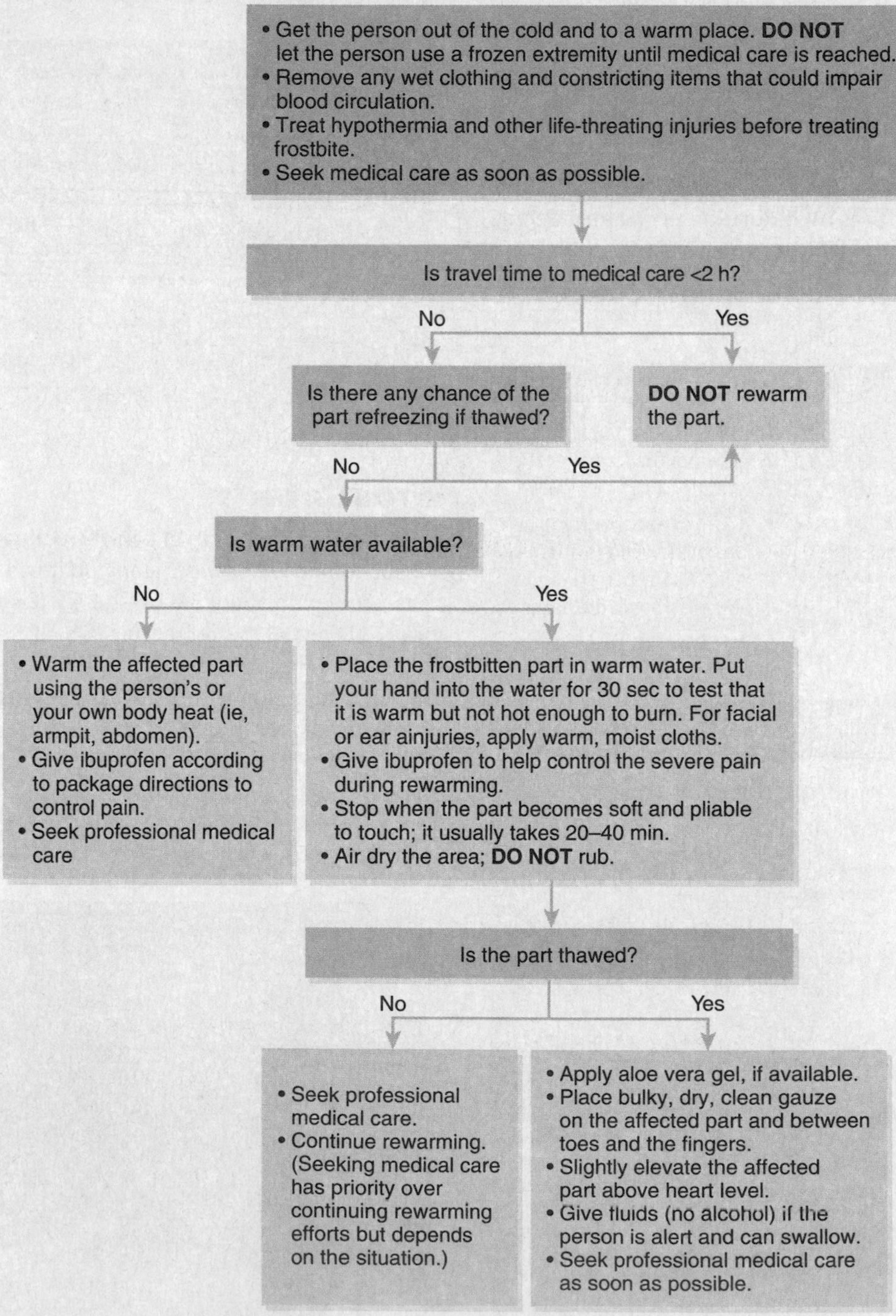

What to Look For	What to Do

Before thawing, frostbite can be classified as superficial or deep:
▪ Superficial frostbite:
  ▪ Skin is white, waxy, or gray-yellow.
  ▪ The affected part feels very cold and numb. There might be tingling, stinging, or an aching sensation.
  ▪ The skin surface feels stiff or crusty and the underlying tissue feels soft when depressed gently and firmly.
▪ Deep frostbite:
  ▪ The affected part feels cold, hard, and solid and cannot be depressed; it feels like a piece of wood or frozen meat.
  ▪ Skin in the affected body part is pale and waxy.
  ▪ A painfully cold part suddenly stops hurting.
	1. Get the person out of the cold and to a warm place. If possible, do not let the person use a frozen extremity until professional medical care is reached.
	2. Remove any wet clothing and constricting items, such as rings, that could impair blood circulation.
	3. **DO NOT** attempt to thaw the part if:
	  ▪ Medical care is less than 2 hours away.
	  ▪ The affected area has thawed.
	  ▪ Shelter, warm water, and a container are not available.
	  ▪ Risk of refreezing exists.
	4. Use the wet, rapid rewarming method if:
	  ▪ Medical care is more than 2 hours away.
	  ▪ There exists no further risk of refreezing of the affected area.
	  ▪ Shelter, warm water, and a container are available.
	Although wet, rapid rewarming is recommended, you may be unable to avoid slow thawing; you should allow slow thawing if it is the only method available.
	5. *Wet, rapid rewarming method:* Place the frostbitten part in warm (100°F to 104°F [38°C to 40°C]) water. **DO NOT** use other heat sources (eg, fire, space heater, oven). If you do not have a thermometer, you can put your hand into the water for 30 seconds to test that it is warm but not hot enough to burn. Maintain water temperature by adding warm water as needed. Rewarming usually takes 20 to 40 minutes or until the part becomes soft and pliable to touch. Air dry the area; **DO NOT** rub. To help control the severe pain during rewarming, give the person ibuprofen as directed on the label. For ear or facial injuries, it is best to apply warm, moist cloths, changing them frequently.
	Cautions:
	  ▪ **DO NOT** rub or massage the affected area.
	  ▪ **DO NOT** apply ice, snow, or cold water to the affected area.
	  ▪ **DO NOT** rewarm the affected area with a stove or vehicle's tailpipe exhaust, or over a fire.
	  ▪ **DO NOT** break blisters.
	  ▪ **DO NOT** allow the person to smoke or drink alcohol.
	  ▪ **DO NOT** rewarm if a possibility of refreezing exists.
	  ▪ **DO NOT** allow the thawed part to refreeze because this will result in greater damage (eg, gangrene).
	  ▪ **DO NOT** place chemical warmers directly on the affected area because this can cause burns.

After thawing, frostbite can be categorized by degrees, similar to the classification of burns:
▪ First-degree frostbite
  ▪ The affected part is warm, swollen, and tender.
▪ Second-degree frostbite
  ▪ Blisters form within minutes to hours after thawing and enlarge over several days **FIGURE 20-5**.
▪ Third-degree frostbite
  ▪ Blisters are small and contain red-blue or purple fluid. The surrounding skin may be red or blue and might not blanch when pressure is applied.
	After thawing:
	1. If the feet are affected, do not allow the person to walk. The feet will be impossible to use after they are rewarmed unless only the toes are affected.
	2. Protect the affected area from contact with clothing and bedding.
	3. Place bulky, dry, clean gauze on the affected part and between the toes and the fingers to absorb moisture and keep them from sticking together.
	4. Slightly elevate the affected part above heart level to reduce pain and swelling.
	5. Apply aloe vera gel to promote skin healing.
	6. Give ibuprofen according to package directions to limit pain and inflammation.
	7. Give fluids if the person is alert and can swallow.
	8. Seek professional medical care as soon as possible.

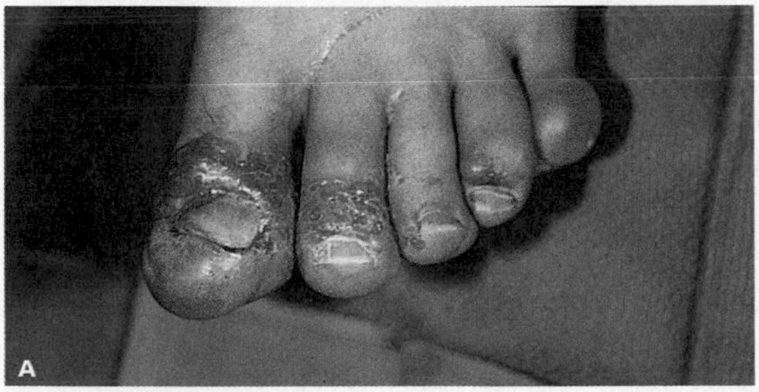

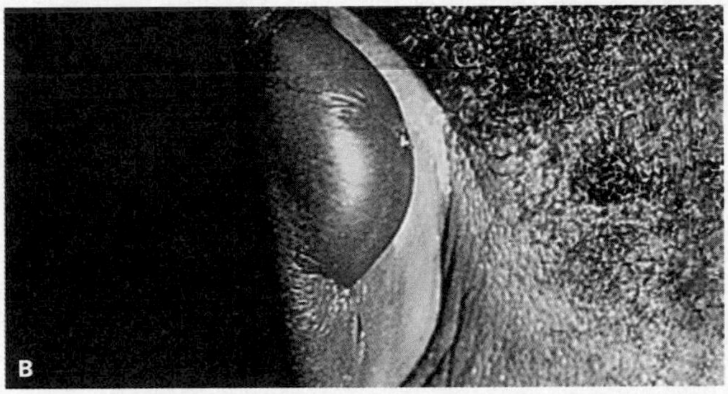

FIGURE 20-5 Second-degree frostbite. **A**. Toes. **B**. Ear.

CAUTION

DO NOT use water hotter than 104°F (40°C)—burns can result.

DO NOT use water cooler than 100°F (37.8°C)—it will not thaw frostbite rapidly enough.

DO NOT break any blisters.

DO NOT rub or massage the affected part—ice crystals can be pushed into body cells, rupturing them.

DO NOT rub the affected part with ice or snow.

DO NOT rewarm the part with a heating pad, hot-water bottle, stove, sunlamp, radiator, exhaust pipe, or over a fire. Excessive temperatures cannot be controlled, and burns can result.

DO NOT allow the person to drink alcoholic beverages. Alcohol dilates blood vessels and causes loss of body heat.

DO NOT allow the person to smoke. Smoking constricts blood vessels, thus impairing circulation.

DO NOT rewarm if there is any possibility of refreezing.

DO NOT allow the thawed part to refreeze because the ice crystals formed will be larger and more damaging. If refreezing is likely or even possible, it is better to leave the affected part frozen.

DO NOT use the dry rewarming technique (putting the person's hands in your armpits) because that takes three to four times longer than the wet, rapid method to thaw frozen tissue. Slow rewarming results in greater tissue damage than rapid rewarming.

DO NOT rewarm if close to a medical facility.

Hypothermia

Cold Stress

Cold stress develops when a person has been exposed to a cold environment. They may be shivering but will be alert and can move and care for themselves. Many people in the outdoors can mistake being cold as being hypothermic. **DO NOT** mistake cold stress for hypothermia. If not paying attention, a cold-stressed person can become hypothermic.

If ...	Then ...
A person has been exposed to a cold environment and has these signs: ▪ Alert and shivering ▪ Can move and care for themselves	Suspect *cold stress*, but *not* hypothermia. 1. Allow the person to remove their own wet clothing and to put on dry clothing. 2. Give high-calorie food or drink. 3. Move around; exercise to warm up. 4. Consider using a warm shower or bath.

Hypothermia

Body temperature falls when the body cannot produce heat as fast as it is lost. **Hypothermia** is a life-threatening condition in which the body's core temperature falls below 95°F (35°C). Generally, the core temperature will not fall until after hours of continuous exposure to cold air if the person is healthy, physically active, and reasonably dressed. However, because wet skin and wind accelerate body heat loss and the body produces less heat during inactive periods, the core body temperature can fall even when the air temperature is above freezing if conditions are windy, clothing is wet, or the person is inactive.

Hypothermia can occur year-round. Most people think of hypothermia as related only to cold outdoor exposure. Nonetheless, hypothermia can happen indoors, in the southern states, and even on a summer day. It does not require subfreezing temperatures.

Hypothermia happens when heat loss occurs faster than heat production. Most people will die if the body temperature falls to 80°F (26.7°C). Hypothermia can occur in indoor or outdoor situations. Hypothermia occurs rapidly during cold-water immersion (1 hour or less when the water temperature is less than 45°F [7.2°C]). Because water has a tremendous capacity to drain heat from the body, prolonged immersion (several hours) in even slightly cool water (less than 70°F [21.1°C]) can cause hypothermia. Hypothermia is a medical emergency. Untreated, it can result in death.

Even though people with severe hypothermia might have no heartbeat, breathing, or response to touch or pain, they may not be dead. Sometimes, the heartbeat and breathing of a person with hypothermia will be so faint or slow that they are not detected. If the person has no signs of life, begin cardiopulmonary resuscitation (CPR) immediately. If hypothermia has resulted from submersion in cold water, CPR should be started without delay. People with hypothermia should be treated as gently as possible because rough handling can cause life-threatening disruptions in heart rhythm, or ventricular fibrillation. All people with hypothermia, even those who do not seem to be alive, must be evaluated by a physician.

In the past, the people believed most vulnerable to hypothermia were hunters, hikers, backpackers, careless drinkers, and people who had been in an accident. However, disadvantaged urban dwellers exposed to the elements and older people with impaired thermoregulatory mechanisms also are susceptible. Lightly clad people almost anywhere can quickly become chilled outdoors when it is raining, even at temperatures that are merely cool, and people immersed for some time in cool or cold water can sustain rapid heat loss. Even well-conditioned athletes such as long-distance runners can experience hypothermia. Hypothermia should be considered whenever the person's behavior and history and the weather conditions indicate abnormal heat loss. Hypothermia is an underreported cause of death in the United States. In most cases, death is attributed to other factors, with hypothermia considered a secondary cause.

The person's history may be sufficient to determine hypothermia has occurred. Hypothermia is likely if a person is reported by companions to be acting strangely and is shivering after exposure to cold or moisture or if they have been immersed in cold water. Hypothermia is not likely if the person is shivering but able to function well and to care for themselves. If there is any doubt, assume that the person has hypothermia.

Predisposing factors are important: drinking alcoholic beverages is commonly associated with hypothermia. A typical scenario involves one or more people in lightweight garments who drink too much, fall asleep outdoors or in a poorly heated shelter, become chilled by cold air or moisture, and remain exposed for many hours. Certain medications predispose people to hypothermia because they interfere with the hypothalamus, which acts as the brain's thermostat in regulating body heat.

Especially vulnerable to hypothermia are very old and very young people. Infants and children have a small muscle mass, so the shivering response is poor in children and nonexistent in infants. They also have less body fat. Younger children need help to protect themselves against the cold because they cannot put on or take off clothes. People who are less fit are also more likely to become hypothermic.

Types of Exposure

There are three classifications of cold exposure:

- Acute exposure (also known as immersion) occurs when body heat loss occurs very rapidly, usually in water. Acute exposure is considered to be 6 hours or less.
- Subacute exposure (also known as mountain or exhaustion exposure) occurs when exposure ranges from 6 to 24 hours; it can be land- or water-based.
- Chronic exposure (also known as urban exposure) involves long-term cooling. It generally occurs on land and exceeds 24 hours.

Recognizing Hypothermia

Consider hypothermia in all people who have been exposed to cold and who have an altered mental status. Suspect hypothermia in any person who has a body temperature of less than 95°F (35°C). (Keep in mind that some thermometers do not measure below 95°F [35°C].) Shivering is a good clue, but it could be suppressed when energy stores (glycogen) are depleted. Suspect hypothermia in people with frostbite and those injured in a cold environment.

Some people die of hypothermia because they or those around them do not recognize the symptoms, which are difficult to recognize in the early stages. Here are some signs to watch for:

- *Altered mental status.* This is one of the first symptoms of developing hypothermia. People may no longer be alert and exhibit signs such as disorientation, apathy, and changes in personality, such as unusual aggressiveness.
- *Shivering.* Shivering is the first, and most important, body defense against a falling body temperature. Shivering starts when the body temperature drops 1°F and can produce more heat than many rewarming methods. As the core temperature continues to fall, shivering decreases and usually stops at about 86°F (30°C). Shivering also stops as body temperature rises. If shivering stops as responsiveness decreases, assume that the core temperature is falling. If, on the other hand, shivering stops while the person is becoming more coordinated and feeling better, assume that the core temperature is rising.
- *Cool abdomen.* Place the back of your hand between the clothing and the person's abdomen to assess the person's temperature. When the person's abdominal skin under clothing is cooler than your hand, consider the person to have hypothermia until proven otherwise.
- *Low core body temperature.* The best indicator of hypothermia is a thermometer reading of the core body temperature. The ability to reliably measure core temperature depends on the availability of an appropriate thermometer and access to the person's rectum. Normal thermometers do not register below 94°F (34.4°C) and so do not indicate whether the hypothermia is mild or severe. Because first aid for mild hypothermia is different from that for severe hypothermia, it is helpful to have a rectal thermometer that registers below 90°F (32.2°C). Oral and axillary (armpit) temperatures are influenced by too many external factors to make them reliable. Measuring rectal temperatures in wilderness or remote locations is seldom done, mainly because low-reading rectal thermometers usually are not readily available. However, taking a rectal temperature can be difficult, inconvenient, and embarrassing to the person and first aid provider. If done outdoors, such a procedure can further expose the already cold person.

Types of Hypothermia

The difference between mild, moderate, and severe hypothermia is based on the core body temperature, but taking a rectal temperature often is not possible for several reasons, including: (1) rectal thermometer not available, (2) embarrassment and/or unwillingness to undress a person, (3) lack of knowledge about the procedure, or (4) not being in a warm environment could worsen the condition if left in the cold. The second most significant difference is that with moderate and severe hypothermia, the person becomes so cold that shivering stops, which means the person's body cannot rewarm itself internally and requires external heat for recovery.

Refer to **FLOWCHART 20-2** for additional information regarding the care of hypothermia.

Q&A

What is the coldest body temperature?

The lowest recorded body temperature with a full recovery was 56.6°F (13.7°C). This was the temperature of Anna Bagenholm, age 29, who was trapped under ice for 80 minutes in May 2000, while skiing with friends near Narvik, Norway.

Data from Martin DS. 2009. From an icy slope, a medical miracle emerges. CNN Health. http://edition.cnn.com/2009/HEALTH/10/12/cheating.death.bagenholm/index.html. Accessed January 20, 2021.

Flowchart 20-2 Hypothermia

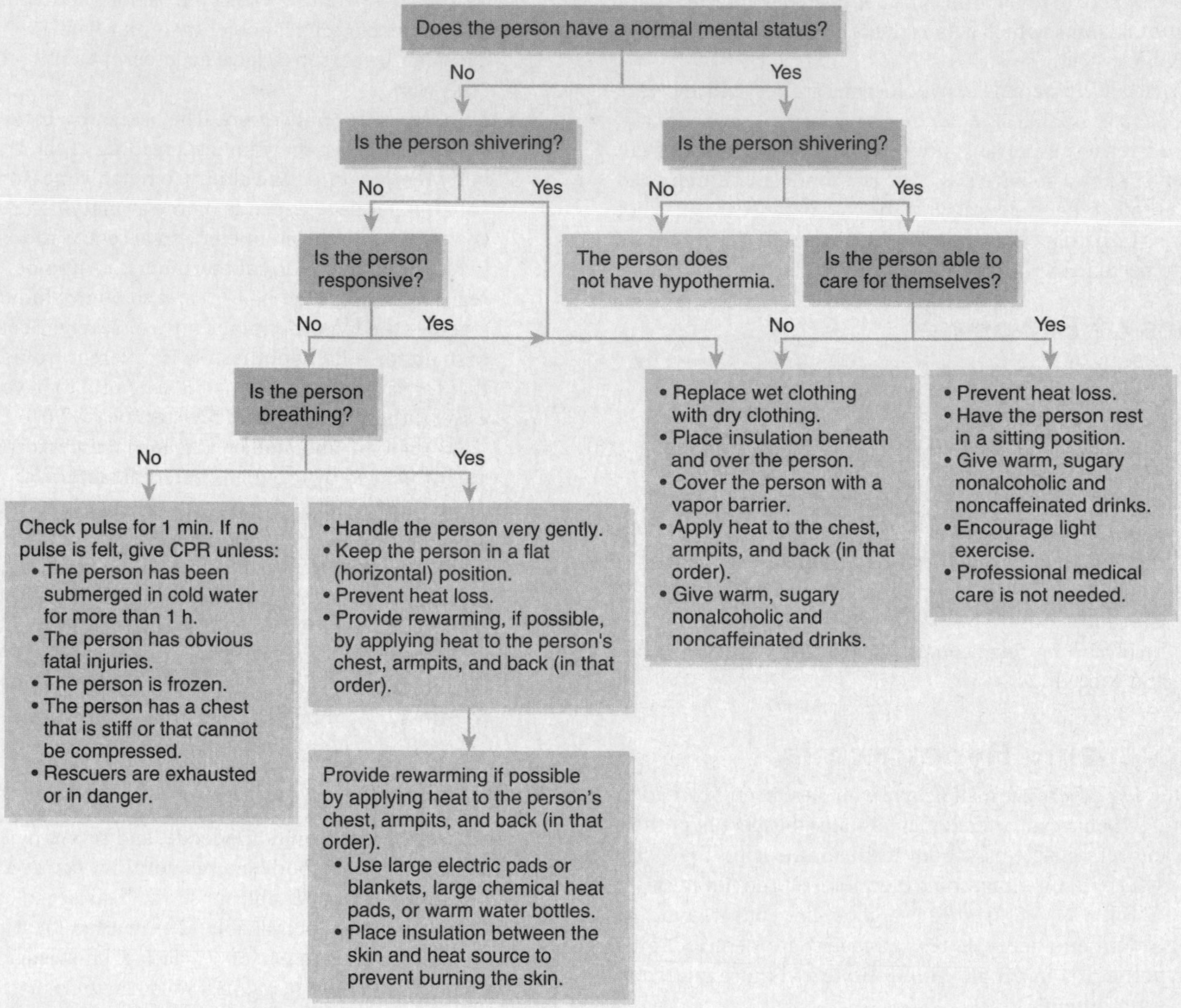
Does the person have a normal mental status?
No
Yes
Is the person shivering?
No
Yes
Is the person shivering?
No
Yes
Is the person responsive?
No
Yes
The person does not have hypothermia.
Is the person able to care for themselves?
No
Yes
Is the person breathing?
No
Yes
• Replace wet clothing with dry clothing.
• Place insulation beneath and over the person.
• Cover the person with a vapor barrier.
• Apply heat to the chest, armpits, and back (in that order).
• Give warm, sugary nonalcoholic and noncaffeinated drinks.
• Prevent heat loss.
• Have the person rest in a sitting position.
• Give warm, sugary nonalcoholic and noncaffeinated drinks.
• Encourage light exercise.
• Professional medical care is not needed.
Check pulse for 1 min. If no pulse is felt, give CPR unless:
• The person has been submerged in cold water for more than 1 h.
• The person has obvious fatal injuries.
• The person is frozen.
• The person has a chest that is stiff or that cannot be compressed.
• Rescuers are exhausted or in danger.
• Handle the person very gently.
• Keep the person in a flat (horizontal) position.
• Prevent heat loss.
• Provide rewarming, if possible, by applying heat to the person's chest, armpits, and back (in that order).
Provide rewarming if possible by applying heat to the person's chest, armpits, and back (in that order).
• Use large electric pads or blankets, large chemical heat pads, or warm water bottles.
• Place insulation between the skin and heat source to prevent burning the skin.

What to Look For	What to Do
Any of the signs of mild, moderate, or severe hypothermia	Take the following actions for all people with suspected hypothermia: **1.** Get the person out of the cold. Treat hypothermia before treating frostbite. **2.** Handle the person gently. **3.** Replace wet clothing with dry clothing only when the person is inside or has other protection from the cold. **4.** Add insulation (eg, extra clothing, blankets, towels, pillows, sleeping bag) beneath and around the person. Cover the person's head (eg, stocking cap, hood). **5.** Cover the person with a vapor barrier (eg, tarp, trash bags with a hole cut out for the face) to prevent heat loss. **DO NOT** cover the mouth or nose. If the person's clothing is dry or damp, leave it on if you know that EMS will arrive in less than 30 minutes. If the clothing is very wet, there is shelter, and EMS is more than 30 minutes away, remove the wet clothing. If unable to remove wet clothing, place the vapor barrier between clothing and insulation. For a dry person, the vapor barrier can be placed outside the insulation. Ideally, using two vapor barriers (one against the person and one outside the insulating layer) offers more protection.

Continues

What to Look For	What to Do

Signs of mild hypothermia:
▪ Vigorous, uncontrollable shivering
▪ Awake and alert
▪ Complains of feeling cold—painful hands and feet
▪ Can answer questions intelligently
▪ The "umbles" beginning to appear:
  ▪ Grumbles
  ▪ Mumbles
  ▪ Fumbles
  ▪ Stumbles
  ▪ Tumbles
	1. If in a warm dry shelter, have the person sit or lie down for at least 30 minutes.
	2. Warm the arms up to the elbows and the lower legs up to the knees in 107°F to 113°F (42°C to 45°C) water.
	3. Give high-calorie (sugary) nonalcoholic and noncaffeinated food or drinks. Shivering rewarms a person who is cold-stressed or mildly hypothermic. They should be well insulated from the cold to retain the generated heat. An alert person who is shivering and can swallow should be given high-calorie nonalcoholic and noncaffeinated liquids and/or food. They provide calories needed to maintain the shivering. Liquids and food may be warmed but should not be hot enough to burn the person's mouth or throat.
	4. Apply heat to the chest, armpits, and back (in this order). Upper torso rewarming is more effective than extremity rewarming. Use large electric pads, electric blankets, or warm water bottles. Place thin insulation between the skin and heat source to prevent burning the skin. Check the skin every 20 to 30 minutes for signs of burning.
	5. **DO NOT** use warm showers or baths for rewarming. This method may be considered for persons who are cold stressed, but not for even a mildly hypothermic person. It causes too many medical complications.
	6. **DO NOT** use small chemical heat packs for rewarming. These packs (eg, used for hand and foot warming) do not provide sufficient heat to affect core body temperature. They can cause burns.
	7. Use the body-to-body method for a mild hypothermic person when there will be a long delay (eg, remote wilderness locations) in getting professional medical care. In such a case, the person must be warmed by any available external heat source.
	8. Monitor for at least 30 minutes.
	9. Call 9-1-1 or transport to a medical facility if no improvement.

Signs of moderate hypothermia: ▪ Shivering stops ▪ The "umbles" worsen ▪ Does not want to move much; may be sleepy ▪ Confused and indifferent to surroundings ▪ Skin is pale or blue and cold when touched	**1.** Call 9-1-1. **2.** Handle gently. **3.** Keep the person flat (horizontal). **DO NOT** raise the legs. **4.** **DO NOT** allow standing or walking. **5.** **DO NOT** massage the person's body. **6.** **DO NOT** give any drink or food. **7.** Insulate and apply a vapor barrier. **8.** Apply heat to the chest, armpits, and back (in that order). Upper torso rewarming is more effective than extremity rewarming. Use large electric pads, electric blankets, or warm water bottles. Place thin insulation between the skin and heat source to prevent burning the skin. Check the skin every 20 to 30 minutes for signs of burning.

Signs of severe hypothermia:
▪ Barely responsive or unresponsive
▪ Rigid and stiff muscles
▪ Skin feels ice cold and appears blue
▪ Slow, shallow, or absent breathing and a weak, slow, or absent pulse (heartbeat)
▪ Appears dead. The signs of life—heartbeat (pulse) and breathing—may be very difficult to detect.
	1. Call 9-1-1.
	2. Treat as moderate hypothermia.
	3. Provide resuscitation if needed. Feel for a pulse at the carotid artery (next to the hard lump [larynx] at the front of the throat) for 1 minute. If no pulse is felt after 1 minute, begin CPR. See Chapter 5, *CPR*. An automated external defibrillator (AED) can be used.
	4. **DO NOT** start CPR if the person:
	  ▪ Has been submerged in cold water for more than 1 hour.
	  ▪ Has obvious fatal injuries.
	  ▪ Is frozen (eg, ice in mouth and throat).
	  ▪ Has a chest that is stiff and cannot be compressed.

Dehydration

Dehydration occurs because of unperceived fluid loss combined with inadequate fluid intake. In very cold weather, the humidity approaches zero, and large quantities of fluid loss occurs through exhaled breath.

People in a cold environment must drink even when they are not thirsty. Inactive people in comfortable climates need 2 quarts (about 2 L) of water per day to prevent dehydration.

A person's hydration status can be monitored by noting the color and the volume of the urine. The lighter the color, the better hydrated; dark yellow urine is a definite indication that fluid consumption should be increased.

Unmelted snow and ice should not be consumed for water. Eating snow and ice irritates the mouth, wastes body heat, and, if enough is consumed, lowers body temperature. When snow and ice are the only available sources of water, they should be melted before being consumed. Melted snow or ice should not be considered drinkable until it has been appropriately disinfected (by boiling, filtering, or using chemicals).

PREP KIT

Ready for Review

- When a person is surrounded by air or water cooler than body temperature, body heat loss occurs.
- Humans protect themselves from cold primarily by avoiding or reducing cold exposure through the use of clothing and shelter.
- Nonfreezing cold injuries can occur when conditions are cold and wet and the hands and feet cannot be kept warm and dry.
- Freezing cold injuries can occur whenever the air temperature is below freezing.
- Hypothermia is a life-threatening condition in which the body's core temperature falls below 95°F (35°C).
- Dehydration occurs because of unperceived fluid loss combined with inadequate fluid intake.

Vital Vocabulary

chilblain A nonfreezing cold injury that, while painful, causes little or no permanent damage.

cold stress An injury that develops when a person has been exposed to a cold environment; can cause shivering, however the person affected will be alert and can move and care for themselves; not to be confused with hypothermia.

conduction The process by which heat is directly transmitted from one object to another.

convection The transfer of heat by the circulation or movement of heated parts of a liquid or gas.

dehydration Loss of water from the tissues of the body.

evaporation Conversion of water or another fluid from a liquid to a gas.

frostbite The damage to tissues as a result of prolonged exposure to extreme cold.

frostnip The reversible freezing of superficial skin layers that is usually marked by numbness and yellow to gray skin.

gangrene Permanent damage or death of tissue.

glycogen Main form in which carbohydrate is stored in the liver and then broken down into glucose (sugar) for energy.

hypothermia Decreased body temperature; severe hypothermia is life threatening.

radiation The transfer of heat to colder objects in the environment by radiant energy.

respiration The inhalation of cold air that is warmed by the body, leading to heat loss when exhaled.

trench foot A serious nonfreezing cold injury that develops when the skin on the feet is exposed to moisture and cold for prolonged periods (12 hours or longer); also called immersion foot.

vasoconstriction The narrowing of the diameter of a blood vessel.

windchill The relationship of wind velocity and temperature in determining the effect of cold on living organisms.

Assessment in Action

You are on a winter hike with five friends high in the mountains. The snowshoeing has been great, but it is very cold. At the trailhead, the temperature was 15°F (–9°C), and it has not warmed up much during your hike. One of your friends wore only tennis shoes but has not been complaining. When you return to the trailhead and begin to warm up in your car, your friend begins to complain of tingling and aching in his toes.

Directions: Circle Yes if you agree with the statement; circle No if you disagree.

1. It is difficult to determine if your friend has frostnip or frostbite.

   YES **NO**

2. Frostbite requires freezing temperatures (below 32°F [0°C]).

   YES **NO**

3. The skin and underlying tissue affected by superficial frostbite feel hard and solid.

   YES **NO**

4. As long as there is no danger of refreezing, you could begin warming his toes in warm water.

   YES **NO**

5. If you do not have warm water, you could rub his toes to increase circulation.

   YES **NO**

PREP KIT continued

Check Your Knowledge

Directions: Circle Yes if you agree with the statement; circle No if you disagree.

1. Shivering is a signal that clothing and shelter are inadequate to protect the body from the cold.
   YES NO
2. Up to 100% of the body's total heat production can be lost by radiation through a person's unprotected head.
   YES NO
3. Physically unfit people are more susceptible to cold injury.
   YES NO
4. Frostnip is caused when water on the skin surface freezes.
   YES NO
5. Shivering produces body heat.
   YES NO
6. Rub a frostbitten part to rewarm it.
   YES NO
7. Rewarm a person with hypothermia quickly in a hot shower or with small chemical heat packs.
   YES NO
8. Replace any wet clothing with dry clothing for a person with hypothermia.
   YES NO
9. Seek professional medical care for a person with severe hypothermia.
   YES NO
10. Below-freezing temperatures are required for hypothermia to occur.
    YES NO

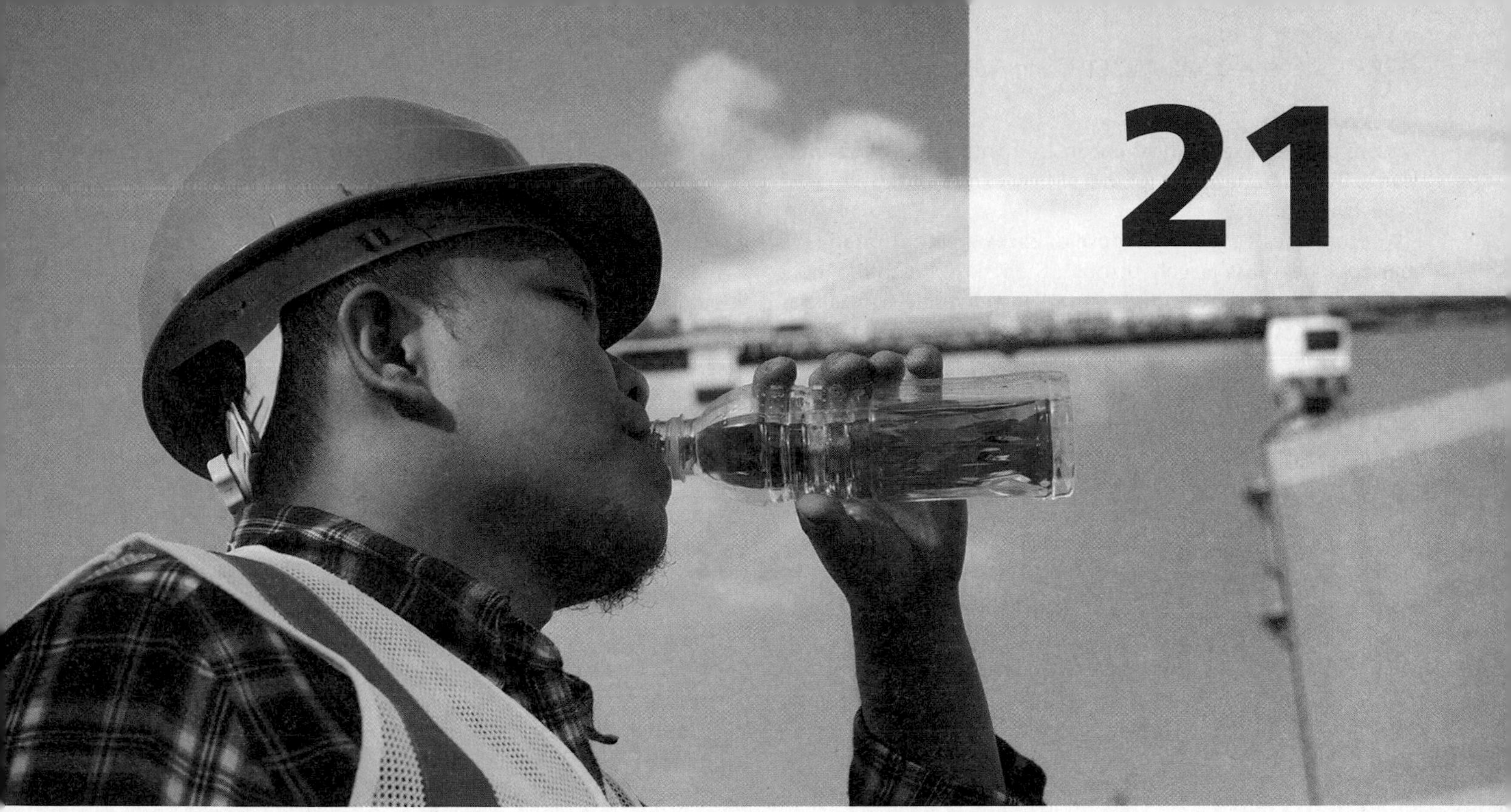

21

Heat-Related Emergencies

CHAPTER AT A GLANCE

Heat-Related Emergencies

When the temperature goes up, a multitude of issues can—and do—arise. Given the right (or wrong) conditions, anyone can develop a heat illness. Some people will develop **heat cramps**, while others may be sickened by **heat exhaustion** or even die from **heatstroke**.

How the Body Stays Cool

The human body is constantly engaged in a life-and-death struggle to disperse the heat that it produces. If allowed to accumulate, the heat would quickly increase your body temperature beyond its comfortable 98.6°F (37°C). That does not normally happen, because your body experiences enough heat loss to maintain a steady temperature. Usually, you are aware of this struggle only during hard labor or exercise in a hot environment, when your body produces heat faster than it can lose it. In certain circumstances, your body can build up too much heat, your temperature might rise to life-threatening levels, and you can become delirious or experience a loss of consciousness. This condition is called heatstroke, and it is a serious medical emergency. If you do not rid your body of excess heat fast enough, damage to the brain and other vital organs will result. Heatstroke is often fatal. Before your temperature reaches heatstroke level, however, you might experience heat exhaustion with its flulike symptoms. By treating the symptoms of heat exhaustion, you avoid heatstroke.

How does the body dispose of excess heat? Humans experience heat loss largely through their skin, much like heat loss occurs in a car through its radiator. Exercising muscles warms the blood, just as the car's hot engine warms its radiator fluid. Warm blood travels through the skin's dilated blood vessels, losing heat by evaporating sweat to the surrounding air, just as the car loses engine heat through the radiator.

When blood delivers heat to the skin, the body loses heat primarily in two ways: radiation and evaporation. When the air temperature is 70°F (21.1°C) or less, the body releases heat into its surroundings by radiation. As the environmental temperature approaches the body's temperature, however, heat loss through radiation is greatly reduced. In fact, people working or exercising on a hot summer day actually gain heat through radiation from the sun, leaving evaporation as the only way to control body temperature effectively.

FYI

World Record: Highest Body Temperature

The person with the highest recorded body temperature who lived to tell about it is Willie Jones. On July 10, 1980, a day when the temperature reached 90°F (32.2°C) with 44% humidity, Mr. Jones was admitted to Grady Memorial Hospital, Atlanta, Georgia, with heatstroke. His temperature was 115.7°F (46.5°C). The record temperature was obtained after he had been immersed for 25 minutes in cold water. The attending physician said that his body temperature may have exceeded 120°F (48.9°C) when he first arrived at the hospital. After 24 days in the hospital, he was discharged. A body temperature of 109°F (42.8°C) can be fatal.

Data from Craig Glenday, *Guinness World Records 2008*, p. 112. New York, 2008, Bantam Books.

Water Loss

Water makes up about 50% to 60% of an adult's body weight. You lose about 2 quarts (about 2 L) every day through breathing, urinating, bowel movements, and sweat. This fluid loss must be replaced. Although the amount of water used each day varies from person to person, an adult requires about 2 quarts (about 2 L) per day from water, other beverages, and food (about 70% of most food is water). A working adult can produce 2 to 3 quarts (about 2 to 3 L) of sweat per hour for short periods and up to 10 to 15 quarts (about 10 to 15 L) per day. When the body's water absorption rate of 1.5 quarts (about 1.5 L) per hour is pitted against a sweat loss of 2 quarts (about 2 L) per hour, dehydration results—drinking water cannot keep up with sweat losses.

An early sign of dehydration is a headache. When you are thirsty, you are already dehydrated. Thirst is not a good guide for when to drink water. In fact, in hot and humid conditions, people could be so dehydrated by the time they become thirsty that they have trouble catching up with their fluid losses. One guideline regarding water intake is to monitor urine output. You are getting enough water if you are producing clear urine at least five times per day. Cloudy or dark urine or urinating fewer than five times per day probably means you should drink more.

If possible while working, especially in hot weather, drink 1 cup (8 ounces) of water every 20 minutes. Usually, 1 pint (16 ounces) is the most a person can comfortably drink at once. It takes time for water to pass from the stomach into the blood, so you cannot catch up by drinking extra water later; about 1 quart (about 1 L) of water per hour can pass out of the stomach.

Cool water (50°F [10°C]) is easier for the stomach to absorb than warm water, and a little flavoring can make the water tastier. The best fluids are those that leave the stomach fast and contain little sodium and less than 8% sugar. Coffee and tea should be avoided because they contain caffeine, a diuretic that increases water loss through urination. Alcoholic beverages also dehydrate by increasing urination. Soda pop contains about 10% sugar and, therefore, is not absorbed as well as water or commercial sports drinks (which contain about 5% to 8% sugar). Fruit juices range from 11% to 18% sugar and have an even longer absorption time. It is important to read the label to decide what the best choice for drinks that help prevent dehydration.

Electrolyte Loss

Sweat and urine contain potassium and sodium, essential electrolytes that control the movement of water into and out of the cells. These electrolytes can be found in many everyday foods. Bananas and nuts are rich in potassium, and most American diets have up to 10 times as much sodium as their bodies need. Acclimatizing to heat (heat exposure 1 to 2 hours per day for 10 to 14 days) can reduce sodium loss tenfold. Getting enough salt (sodium chloride) is rarely an issue in the typical American diet. In fact, most Americans consume an excessive amount of sodium, averaging 5 to 10 grams of sodium per day, although humans probably require only 1 to 3 grams. Sodium loss, therefore, is seldom an issue, unless a person is sweating profusely for long periods and drinking large amounts of water (more than 1 quart [about 1 L] per hour).

For hydration, most people require only water most of the time. Commercial sports drinks can be useful for participants in vigorous physical activity lasting longer than 1 hour. The human body needs water more than it needs salt. Whenever extra sodium is added to a diet, more water should be consumed. Otherwise, excessive sodium can draw water out of the cells, accelerating dehydration.

Drinking large amounts of water (more than 1 quart [about 1 L] per hour) and profuse sweating for long periods can lead to a condition called water intoxication, in which electrolytes (ie, sodium) are flushed from the body. Symptoms of water intoxication include frequent urination, behavior changes (irrationality, combativeness, seizures, and coma), weight gain, and puffiness to the face (edema). These symptoms are the result of inadequate sodium in the body, a condition known as **hyponatremia**.

Effects of Humidity

Sweat can cool the body only if it evaporates. In dry air, you will not notice sweat evaporating. The higher the humidity, the less sweat can evaporate. It drips off the skin without cooling the body. At about 75% humidity, sweating is ineffective in cooling the body.

Because humidity can significantly reduce evaporative cooling, a very humid but mildly warm day can be more stressful than a very hot, dry day. The higher the humidity, the lower the temperature at which heat risk begins, especially for people generating heat with vigorous work.

Who Is at Risk?

Everyone is susceptible to heat illness if environmental conditions overwhelm the body's temperature-regulating mechanisms. Heat waves can set the stage for multiple cases of heatstroke. For example, in the 1995 Chicago heat wave, the death toll reached over 700 people in 5 days. Several groups are at particular risk, including people with obesity, people with a chronic illness, and people with alcoholism.

In addition, older people are at higher risk because of impaired cardiac output and decreased ability to sweat. Infants and young children are also susceptible to heatstroke. Children (and pets) are especially vulnerable when they are left in automobiles. The temperature in a parked car can soar to 150°F (65.6°C), even when a window is open. The fluid loss and dehydration resulting from physical activity put outdoor laborers and athletes at particular risk.

Certain medications predispose people to heatstroke. They include drugs that alter sweat production (eg, antihistamines, antipsychotics, and antidepressants) and those that interfere with **thermoregulation**.

FYI

Heat-Related Deaths of Young Children in Parked Cars

Each year, many young children in the United States die of heatstroke caused by being enclosed in parked motor vehicles. Researchers located and analyzed 171 heat-related deaths in children younger than 5 years:

- 39% involved a child forgotten by a caregiver.
- 27% involved a child playing in an unattended vehicle.
- 20% involved a child intentionally left in a vehicle by an adult.
- 14% involved unclear circumstances.

Data from Guard A, Gallagher SS. Heat-related deaths to young children in parked cars: An analysis of 171 fatalities in the United States. *Inj Prev* 2005;11(1):33–37.

Heat Illnesses

Heat illnesses include a range of disorders. Some of them are common, but only heatstroke is life threatening. People with untreated heatstroke always die.

FYI

Hot Weather Precautions

These simple preventive measures can reduce heat stress:

1. Keep cool indoors.
   - Stay in air conditioned areas, if available.
   - Take cool baths or showers.
   - Use your stove and oven less.
2. Wear lightweight, loose-fitting clothing.
3. If you must go outdoors, put on sunscreen of SPF 15 or higher 30 minutes prior to going out.
4. Limit your outdoor activity to the morning and evening, and make sure to rest often in shady areas.
5. Increase intake of fluids, regardless of your activity level.
   - Thirst is not always a good indicator of adequate fluid intake.
   - People who engage in strenuous activities, such as sports, should drink 2 to 4 glasses of cool fluids each hour in hot weather.
   - People for whom fluid is restricted or who are taking water pills should consult their physicians for instructions on appropriate fluid intake.
   - **DO NOT** drink liquids that contain alcohol or large amounts of sugar.
   - Monitor your urine color. Urine color that is pale yellow or light yellow indicates a person is hydrated; dark yellow urine may be a sign of dehydration
6. Stay in contact with other people and monitor those who are at greater risk of suffering from heat-related illnesses, such as infants, young children, older adults, and people who are overweight, ill, or taking certain medications.
7. Listen or watch local news and weather stations for weather updates and recommended procedures and precautions.
8. **DO NOT** leave infants, children, or pets unattended in a parked car.

Data from Extreme heat prevention guide. Centers for Disease Control and Prevention. http://emergency.cdc.gov/disasters/extremeheat/heat_guide.asp. Published May 31, 2012. Updated September 22, 2015.

Heat Exhaustion

Heat exhaustion is characterized by heavy perspiration with a normal or slightly above-normal body temperature. Heavy sweating causes water and electrolyte losses. Some experts believe that a better term would be *severe dehydration*. Heat exhaustion affects workers and athletes who do not drink enough fluids while working or exercising in hot environments. Symptoms include severe thirst, heavy sweating, fatigue, headache,

Q&A

What is the difference between fever and hyperthermia?

Fever and hyperthermia have different causes. Body temperature is regulated by a natural thermostat in the part of the brain called the hypothalamus. If the "set point" is increased by illness or certain drugs, a fever results. In other words, in a fever, the body is trying to raise the temperature above normal to fight a disease (eg, a virus).

Hyperthermia is related to environmental heat exposure. It occurs when the body absorbs more heat than it can handle. It is caused by an inability to cool the body. Hyperthermia can rapidly progress to heatstroke if not corrected.

What to Look For	What to Do
Painful muscle spasms affecting the muscles in the back of the leg or abdomen that happen suddenly during or after physical exertion	Relief may take several hours. 1. Have the person rest in a cool area. 2. Give lightly salted cool water (dissolve ¼ teaspoon [1.25 mL] of salt in 1 quart [about 1 L] of water) or a commercial sports drink. **DO NOT** give salt tablets. 3. Stretch any cramped muscle.

nausea, vomiting, and sometimes diarrhea. The affected person often mistakenly believes they have the flu.

Heat exhaustion differs from heatstroke because the person has no altered mental status and their skin is clammy, not hot. However, like heatstroke, you should still cool the person, just not as aggressively as for heatstroke. Uncontrolled heat exhaustion can evolve into heatstroke. A person with heat exhaustion will have (1) no altered mental status and (2) skin that is clammy, but not hot **FIGURE 21-1**.

What to Look For	What to Do
▪ Pale or ashen skin ▪ Clammy or sweaty skin, but not hot ▪ Severe thirst ▪ Fatigue ▪ Dizzy ▪ Flulike symptoms (headache, body aches, nausea, and sometimes vomiting) ▪ Shortness of breath ▪ Rapid heart rate	1. Move the person from the hot environment to a cooler, shaded place. 2. Remove excess clothing. 3. Spray or douse cold water on the person's skin and fan vigorously. 4. If the person is able to swallow, give a commercial sports drink, fruit juice, or lightly salted water; if none of these options are available, give cold water. **DO NOT** give salt tablets. 5. Call 9-1-1 if improvement does not occur within 30 minutes.

Heatstroke

Two types of heatstroke exist: classic and exertional **TABLE 21-1**. Classic heatstroke, also known as the "slow cooker," can take days to develop. It is often seen during summer heat waves and typically affects people who are poor, older, chronically ill, and those with alcoholism or obesity. Because older people, who often have medical conditions, are frequently afflicted, this type of heatstroke has a death rate of over 50%, even with professional medical care. It results from a combination of a hot environment and dehydration. Under normal conditions, temperature and humidity are the most

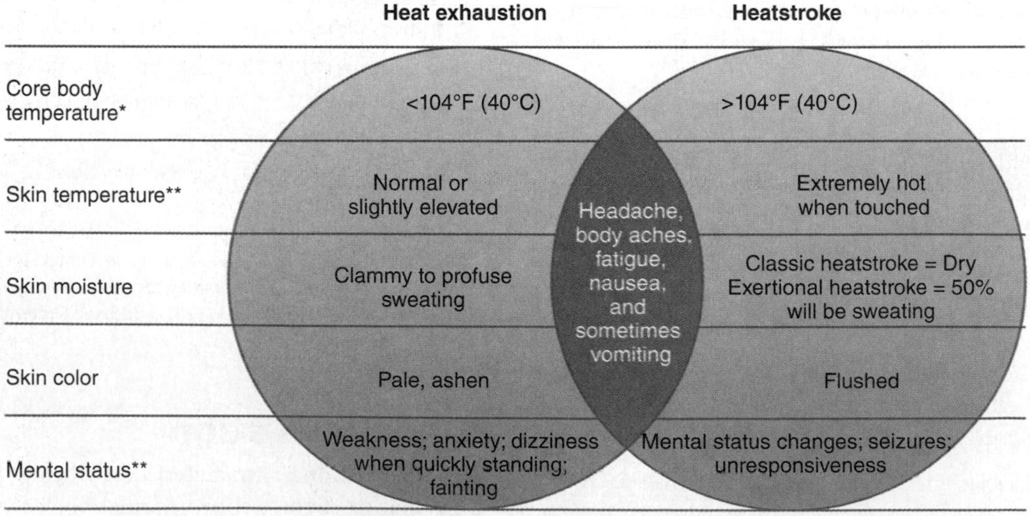

Heat exhaustion
Heatstroke
Core body temperature*
<104°F (40°C)
>104°F (40°C)
Skin temperature**
Normal or slightly elevated
Extremely hot when touched
Skin moisture
Clammy to profuse sweating
Classic heatstroke = Dry
Exertional heatstroke = 50% will be sweating
Skin color
Pale, ashen
Flushed
Mental status**
Weakness; anxiety; dizziness when quickly standing; fainting
Mental status changes; seizures; unresponsiveness
Headache, body aches, fatigue, nausea, and sometimes vomiting

*Measured by using a rectal thermometer.
**Evaluating a person's skin temperature and mental status are the two best ways to determine if a person has heat exhaustion or heatstroke.

FIGURE 21-1 Heat exhaustion versus heatstroke.

important elements influencing body comfort. The heat index compiled by the National Weather Service lists apparent temperatures (how hot it feels) at various combinations of temperature and humidity **FIGURE 21-2**.

Exertional heatstroke is also more common in the summer. It is frequently seen in athletes, laborers, and military personnel, all of whom often sweat profusely. This type of heatstroke is known as the "fast cooker." It affects healthy, active people who are strenuously working or playing in a warm environment. Because its rapid onset does not allow enough time for severe dehydration to occur, 50% of people with exertional heatstroke usually are sweating. (People with classic heatstroke may not be sweating.)

There are several ways to tell the difference between heat exhaustion and heatstroke.

- If the person's body feels extremely hot when touched, suspect heatstroke.
- Altered mental status occurs with heatstroke, ranging from slight confusion and disorientation to coma. Between those extreme conditions, people usually become irrational, agitated, or even aggressive, and they might have seizures.
- In severe heatstroke, a coma can occur in less than 1 hour. The longer a coma lasts, the lower the chance for survival.
- Rectal temperature can also help distinguish heatstroke from heat exhaustion, although obtaining a rectal temperature is usually not practical. A responsive person with heatstroke might not cooperate, taking a rectal temperature can be embarrassing to the person and the first aid provider, and rectal thermometers are seldom available.

TABLE 21-1 Classic or Exertional Heatstroke?

Characteristics	Classic	Exertional
Age group usually affected	Older people	Men, 15–45 years
Claims many people at the same time	During heat waves	During athletic competition
Health status of people	Chronically ill	Healthy and physically fit
Activity at the time of incident	Sedentary	Strenuous exercise
Medication use	Common	Usually none
Sweating	Absent	Often present (50% of people)

FYI

Heat Illness Among High School Athletes

Heat illness during practice or competition is a leading cause of death and disability among high school athletes in the United States. The 100 schools sampled by the CDC reported a total of 118 heat illnesses among high school athletes resulting in at least 1 day of time lost from athletic activity (ie, time-loss heat illness). The highest rate of time-loss heat illness was among football players at a rate 10 times higher than the average rate for the eight other sports surveyed. Time-loss heat illnesses occurred most frequently during August and while practicing or playing football.

Consistent with guidelines from the National Athletic Trainers' Association (NATA), to reduce the risk for heat illness, high school athletic programs should implement heat-acclimatization guidelines (eg, set limits on summer practice duration and intensity). All athletes, coaches, athletic trainers, and parents/guardians should be aware of the risk factors for heat illness, follow recommended strategies, and be prepared to respond quickly to symptoms of illness. Coaches should also continue to stress to their athletes the importance of maintaining proper hydration before, during, and after sports activities.

Data from Centers for Disease Control and Prevention. Heat illness among high school athletes—United States, 2005–2009. *MMWR Morb Mortal Wkly Rep* 2011;59(32):1009–1013.

Temperature (°F)

Relative Humidity (%)	80	82	84	86	88	90	92	94	96	98	100	102	104	106	108	110
40	80	81	83	85	88	91	94	97	101	105	109	114	119	124	130	136
45	80	82	84	87	89	93	96	100	104	109	114	119	124	130	137	
50	81	83	85	88	91	95	99	103	108	113	118	124	131	137		
55	81	84	86	89	93	97	101	106	112	117	124	130	137			
60	82	84	88	91	95	100	105	110	116	123	129	137				
65	82	85	89	93	98	103	108	114	121	128	136					
70	83	86	90	95	100	105	112	119	126	134						
75	84	88	92	97	103	109	116	124	132							
80	84	89	94	100	106	113	121	129								
85	85	90	96	102	110	117	126	135								
90	86	91	98	105	113	122	131									
95	86	93	100	108	117	127										
100	87	95	103	112	121	132										

Likelihood of Heat Disorders with Prolonged Exposure or Strenuous Activity

Caution | Extreme caution | Danger | Extreme danger

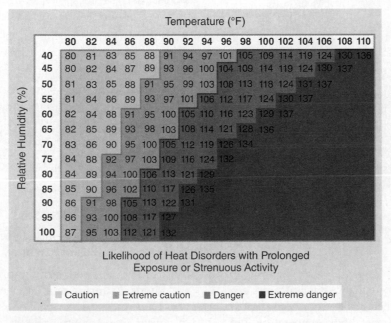

FIGURE 21-2 Heat index.

Courtesy of NOAA.

What to Look For	What to Do
▪ Extremely hot skin ▪ Skin that is usually dry, but may be wet from sweating related to strenuous work or exercise ▪ Altered mental status ranging from slight confusion, agitation, and disorientation to possible seizures or unresponsiveness. ▪ Flushed skin ▪ Flulike symptoms (headache, body aches, nausea, and sometimes vomiting) ▪ Body temperature, usually above 104°F (40°C) causing a feeling of burning up	1. Move the person from the hot environment to a cooler, shaded place. 2. Call 9-1-1 immediately. 3. A person who cannot be taken to a medical facility quickly should be cooled by any means possible. The order of effective cooling is: ▪ **Whole body cold-water immersion.** First, remove clothing down to the person's underwear and then: • Submerge the person's body and extremities up to the neck in a bath of cold water or tub of ice water. The colder the water, the faster the rate of cooling. **OR** • Have the person sit or lay down on a plastic sheet or tarp. Hold the sides up and apply water and crushed ice. Keep the sides upright to keep the mixture in place and move the tarp to keep the water moving around the person. **OR** • Use a natural body of water (eg, stream, pond, river, or lake) to submerge a person and help cool them off. **DO NOT** leave someone suffering from heatstroke in a body of water alone because it is dangerous. ▪ **Spray or douse cold water** repeatedly on the person's skin and fan vigorously. This method is half as fast as immersion cooling **FIGURE 21-3**. ▪ **Ice packs.** Ice packs should cover the entire body. If chemical cold packs are used, they should be applied to the cheeks, palms, and soles rather than the skin covering the neck, armpits, and groin. Note that placing cold packs near the groin or armpits is not harmful, but the other locations previously mentioned cool faster. Ice packs have greater cooling capacity than chemical cold packs. 4. Stop cooling when mental status improves, after 20 minutes, or when emergency medical services (EMS) arrives. 5. **DO NOT** give ibuprofen or aspirin. While helpful in cases of high body temperatures caused by infectious diseases, they are not effective in heat-related illnesses.

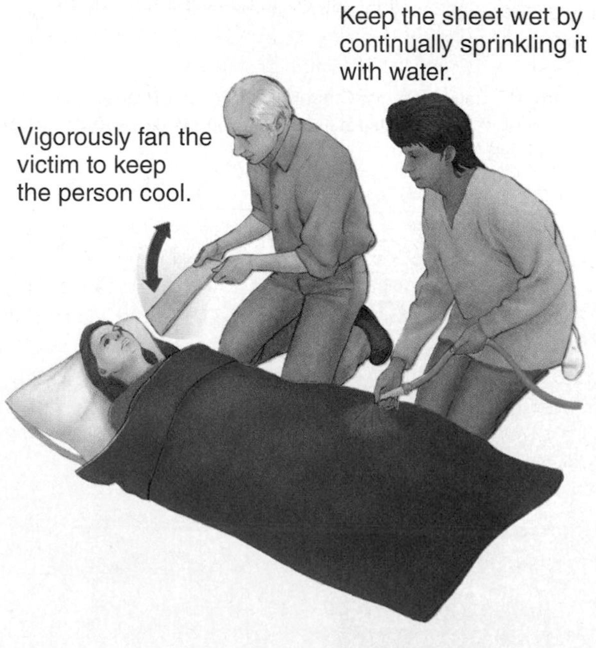

Keep the sheet wet by continually sprinkling it with water.
Vigorously fan the victim to keep the person cool.

FIGURE 21-3 Spraying with water and fanning are effective in low humidity conditions.

However, it is important to note that oral temperature can be inaccurate in distinguishing heatstroke from heat exhaustion and may grossly underestimate body temperature and therefore delay proper treatment.

CAUTION

DO NOT delay initiating cooling while waiting for an ambulance. The longer the delay, the greater the risk of tissue damage and prolonged hospitalization.

DO NOT continue cooling after the person's mental status has improved. Unnecessary cooling could lead to hypothermia.

DO NOT use rubbing alcohol to cool the skin. It can be absorbed into the blood and cause alcohol poisoning. Also, the vapors are a potential fire hazard.

DO NOT give the person aspirin, acetaminophen, or nonsteroidal anti-inflammatory drugs. The brain's temperature control center is not elevated, as it is with fever caused by diseases, so these products are not effective for lowering body temperature.

Other Heat Illnesses

Less-serious heat illnesses include heat cramps, heat syncope, heat edema, heat rash, and exertional hyponatremia.

- Heat cramps are painful muscle spasms that occur suddenly during or after vigorous exercise or activity.
- Heat syncope occurs when someone faints or feels dizzy after strenuous physical activity in a hot environment.

Flowchart 21-1 Heat-Related Emergencies

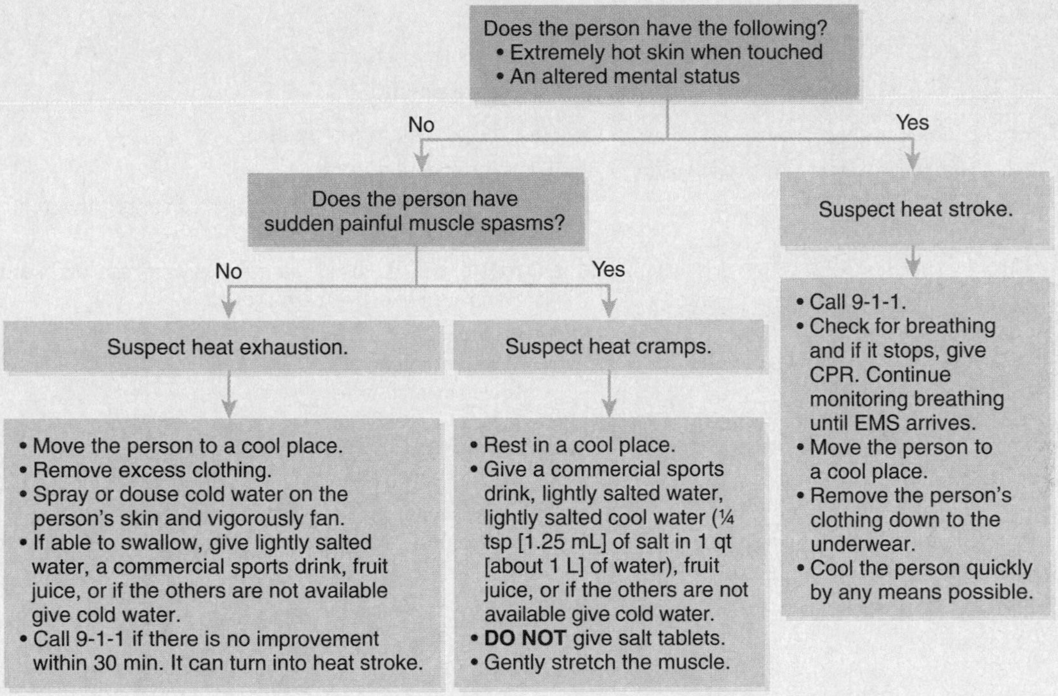
Does the person have the following?
• Extremely hot skin when touched
• An altered mental status
No
Yes
Does the person have sudden painful muscle spasms?
Suspect heat stroke.
No
Yes
Suspect heat exhaustion.
Suspect heat cramps.
• Call 9-1-1.
• Check for breathing and if it stops, give CPR. Continue monitoring breathing until EMS arrives.
• Move the person to a cool place.
• Remove the person's clothing down to the underwear.
• Cool the person quickly by any means possible.
• Move the person to a cool place.
• Remove excess clothing.
• Spray or douse cold water on the person's skin and vigorously fan.
• If able to swallow, give lightly salted water, a commercial sports drink, fruit juice, or if the others are not available give cold water.
• Call 9-1-1 if there is no improvement within 30 min. It can turn into heat stroke.
• Rest in a cool place.
• Give a commercial sports drink, lightly salted water, lightly salted cool water (¼ tsp [1.25 mL] of salt in 1 qt [about 1 L] of water), fruit juice, or if the others are not available give cold water.
• DO NOT give salt tablets.
• Gently stretch the muscle.

- Heat edema occurs when hands or feel are swollen after sitting or standing for a long time in the heat.
- A heat rash, or prickly heat can be caused by hot, humid weather, usually after prolonged sweating.
- Exertional hyponatremia, a decreased concentration of sodium in the blood, results from drinking too much water. It is referred to as water intoxication. It occurs during or up to 24 hours after prolonged and/or extreme physical activity.

Refer to **FLOWCHART 21-1** for additional information regarding care for heat-related emergencies.

What to Look For	What to Do
Signs of heat cramps: ▪ Painful muscle spasms in abdominal muscles or the back of the leg (calf and hamstring muscles) during or after vigorous exercise or physical activity ▪ Heavy sweating *Note*: Some experts believe that heat cramps are caused by water and electrolyte losses during times of excessive sweating. People who experience heat cramps might be drinking fluids without adequate salt content. However, other experts disagree, because the typical American diet is already heavy with salt.	**DO NOT** confuse this condition with a strained muscle. Lightly stretching can relieve a muscle cramp but not a muscle spasm caused by heat cramps. Relief from heat cramps may take several hours. **1.** Have the person rest in a cool place. **2.** Give lightly salted cool water (dissolve ¼ teaspoon [1.25 mL] of salt in 1 quart [about 1 L] of water or a commercial sports drink. **3.** **DO NOT** give salt tablets. **4.** Lightly stretch and massage the cramped muscles. **5.** Apply an ice pack to the cramped muscles.
Signs of heat syncope: ▪ Dizziness ▪ Fainting	**1.** If the person is unresponsive, check their breathing. A person with heat syncope will usually recover quickly. **2.** If the person fell, check for injuries. **3.** Have the person rest and lie down in a cool area. **4.** Wet the skin with a cool, damp cloth or by splashing water on the face. **5.** If the person is not nauseated and is alert and able to swallow, give lightly salted cool water (dissolve ¼ teaspoon [1.25 mL] of salt in 1 quart [about 1 L] of water) or a commercial sports drink. **DO NOT** give salt tablets.

Continues

Continued

What to Look For	What to Do
Signs of heat edema: ▪ Swollen ankles and feet that occur during the first few days in a hot environment	**1.** Have the person wear support stockings. **2.** Elevate the person's legs.
Signs of heat rash: ▪ Itchy rash on skin that is wet from sweating	**1.** Dry and cool the person's skin. **2.** Limit heat exposure.
Signs of exertional hyponatremia: ▪ Person reports drinking too much water (>1 quart [about 1 L] per hour) during the previous several hours ▪ Sweaty skin ▪ Clear urine ▪ Dizziness, weakness, fatigue, headache, nausea, and vomiting ▪ Bloated feeling ▪ Altered mental status ▪ Severe sodium loss may result in seizures or unresponsiveness and can be fatal	**1.** Move the person to a cool location. **2.** Give salty foods and snacks. **3.** **DO NOT** give salt tablets because they can irritate the stomach and cause nausea and vomiting. **4.** **DO NOT** give fluids. Avoid sports drinks which are low in sodium and high in water and are ineffective for this condition. **5.** Call 9-1-1 for: ▪ No improvement ▪ Altered mental status ▪ Seizure ▪ Vomiting ▪ Shortness of breath ▪ Collapse **6.** **DO NOT** confuse exertional hyponatremia with heat exhaustion or heat stroke.

PREP KIT

Ready for Review

- Given the right conditions, anyone can develop a heat illness.
- The human body is constantly dispersing the heat that it produces.
- Heat illnesses include a range of disorders from heat cramps to heatstroke. Heatstroke is life threatening.

Vital Vocabulary

heat cramps A painful muscle cramp resulting from excessive loss of salt and water through sweating.

heat exhaustion A prostration caused by excessive loss of water and salt through sweating; characterized by clammy skin and a weak, rapid pulse.

heatstroke An acute and dangerous reaction to heat exposure characterized by high body temperature and altered mental status.

hyponatremia A condition that occurs when the level of sodium in the body is inadequate.

thermoregulation The body's ability to maintain a normal body temperature despite environmental conditions of heat or cold.

Assessment in Action

You decide to watch your local high school football team practice before its first game in late August. The coach has the defense running sprints for the last 30 minutes without rest breaks. At the end of the sprints, all but one player walk over to the water station. That player falls to the ground and you are the first to respond. The person is responsive and his skin is moist and clammy.

Directions: Circle Yes if you agree with the statement; circle No if you disagree.

1. The person is most likely suffering from heatstroke.

   YES NO

2. The first thing you should do is to help the coach and athletic trainer move the person out of the heat and to a cool place.

   YES NO

3. The person should drink cool water or a sports drink.

   YES NO

4. Giving several salt tablets, if available, should always be considered.

   YES NO

5. Removing the player's jersey, shoulder pads, and helmet and sponging him with cool water is recommended.

   YES NO

6. The coach and/or athletic trainer should seek professional medical care if there is no improvement within 30 minutes.

   YES NO

Check Your Knowledge

Directions: Circle Yes if you agree with the statement; circle No if you disagree.

1. For heat cramps in the legs, stretch the cramped muscle.

   YES NO

2. Commercial sports drinks can be given to people experiencing heat-related emergencies.

   YES NO

3. Move a person with a heat-related illness to a cool place.

   YES NO

PREP KIT continued

4. People with heatstroke need immediate professional medical care—it is a life-threatening condition.

   YES **NO**

5. Rapidly cool a person with heatstroke, including the use of ice packs applied to the neck, armpits, and groin.

   YES **NO**

6. Fruit juices are digested quickly and rehydrate the body most rapidly.

   YES **NO**

7. You can drink too much water and cause water intoxication.

   YES **NO**

8. Humidity cannot significantly reduce evaporative cooling.

   YES **NO**

9. Certain medications may predispose people to heatstroke.

   YES **NO**

10. Heat exhaustion can feel like the flu.

    YES **NO**

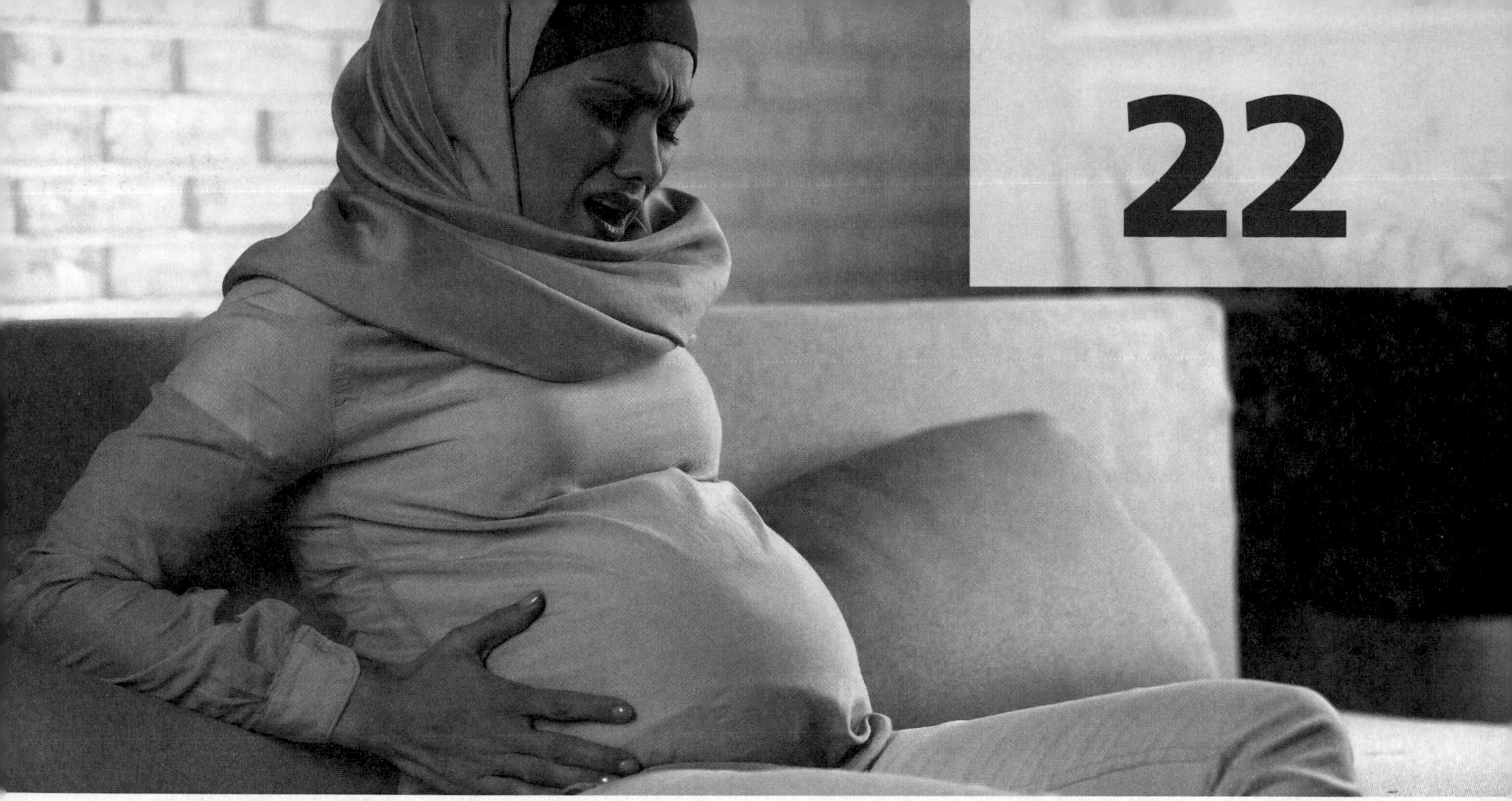

Childbirth and Gynecologic Emergencies

CHAPTER AT A GLANCE

Childbirth and Gynecologic Emergencies

Handling childbirth and gynecologic situations of pregnancy requires that a first aid provider be familiar with the terminology used to describe female reproductive anatomy and physiology.

- The **birth canal** includes the vagina and the lower part of the uterus.
- The **cervix** is the small opening at the lower end of the uterus through which the baby passes.
- The **placenta** (afterbirth) is the organ through which the mother and the fetus exchange nourishment and waste products during pregnancy. It is expelled after the baby's birth.
- The **umbilical cord** is the extension of the placenta through which the **fetus**, the developing offspring, receives nourishment while in the uterus.
- The **amniotic sac** (bag of waters) surrounds the fetus inside the uterus. Amniotic fluid in the sac cushions the fetus and helps protect it from injury.
- **Crowning** occurs when the fetus's head presses against the vaginal opening and begins to bulge out.
- **Bloody show** is the mucus and blood that might be discharged from the vagina as labor begins.

- **Labor** is the process of childbirth (defined in three stages), from the first regular uterine muscle contractions until delivery of the placenta.
- A **miscarriage** (medical term is *spontaneous abortion*) is the delivery of a fetus before it can live independent of the mother.
- **Vena cava syndrome** is a set of symptoms that occur when blood flow to the **inferior vena cava**, the large vein located between the spine and the abdominal organs, is compressed or blocked.
- A **breech** presentation occurs when the baby's buttocks or lower extremities emerge before the head or shoulders.
- **Fontanelles** are the soft spots on the top and back of the infant's head.

Predelivery Emergencies

Ectopic Pregnancy

A fertilized egg that implants in one of the **fallopian tubes** instead of in the uterus is called an **ectopic pregnancy**. The embryo is not viable and must be removed as soon as the condition is identified to avoid serious complications, such as rupture of the fallopian tube.

Pelvic pain and vaginal bleeding or spotting in a woman of childbearing age should be treated as an ectopic pregnancy until the condition is ruled out by a physician. Call 9-1-1 and seek professional medical care for a suspected ectopic pregnancy. Predisposing factors for ectopic pregnancy are previous ectopic pregnancies, surgeries, pelvic infections, and failure of an intrauterine device (IUD). Common signs and symptoms are vaginal bleeding and abdominal tenderness.

Miscarriage

Miscarriages usually occur during the first 3 months (first trimester) of pregnancy. Most occur because the fetus was not developing properly and was unable to survive. The woman will be emotionally upset. She might be hesitant about confiding in a stranger, especially a man; obtaining help from a woman, if possible, might be wise.

What to Look For	What to Do
▪ Cramping pain in lower abdomen resembling menstrual cramps ▪ Aching in the lower back ▪ Vaginal bleeding, which could be sudden and heavy ▪ Passage of tissue from the vagina	1. Be supportive of the woman. 2. Help her into a comfortable position with legs bent. 3. Have the woman place a sanitary pad over the outside of the vagina. **DO NOT** place pads in the vagina. Replace blood-soaked pads or dressings. 4. Any tissue that passes through the vagina should be transported with the woman to the hospital. **DO NOT** try to pull tissue out of the vagina; instead, cover it with a sterile pad. 5. Seek professional medical care. 6. Call 9-1-1 if bleeding is heavy or signs of shock are present.

Vaginal Bleeding

Vaginal Bleeding During Pregnancy

A woman experiencing vaginal bleeding, with or without abdominal pain, late in her pregnancy (third trimester, or last 3 months) constitutes an emergency and will require professional medical care. Find out how long she has been bleeding and how many sanitary pads she has used so that you can report the information to medical personnel. An increase in pulse rate of more than 20 beats per minute, from baseline, when the woman goes from a lying-down to a sitting position suggests blood loss of more than 1 pint (473 mL). The woman might feel embarrassed. She might be hesitant about confiding in a stranger, especially a man; therefore, obtaining help from a woman might be wise.

What to Look For	What to Do
▪ Bleeding may be mild spotting but can indicate a severe condition. ▪ Bleeding may be heavy. ▪ Signs of shock may be present.	To care for someone with vaginal bleeding during late pregnancy, do the following: 1. Place the woman on her left side to relieve pressure from the fetus on the inferior vena cava (large vein between the spine and the abdominal organs). 2. Have the woman place a sanitary pad over the outside of the vagina. 3. Call 9-1-1 immediately. 4. Treat for shock (eg, maintain body temperature, avoid giving fluids).

Vaginal Bleeding Caused by Injury

It is difficult to determine the source of the bleeding. Vaginal bleeding can be difficult to care for because of the woman's modesty and pain.

What to Look For	What to Do
▪ Injuries of the external female genitalia, including all types of soft-tissue injuries (such as wounds or contusions) ▪ Severe pain ▪ Blood in the vaginal area ▪ Massive vaginal bleeding	1. Use direct pressure over a bulky dressing or sanitary pad to control external bleeding from a laceration or other injury. 2. Apply an ice pack to reduce swelling and pain. 3. Never place or pack dressings into the vagina. It is useless and dangerous to introduce packs blindly into the vagina in an attempt to control bleeding. 4. Place the woman on her left side to help prevent aspiration of vomitus, and, if the woman is pregnant, to relieve pressure on the inferior vena cava from the fetus. 5. In the case of a sexual assault, sympathetically explain that evidence needs to be preserved and that the person should not change clothes, wash, urinate, defecate, or douche. 6. Seek professional medical care.

Q&A

Are pregnant women more susceptible to injury?

More injuries are seen in pregnant women because many of them are active and often work and travel throughout all stages of pregnancy. In addition, there is a significant incidence of violence toward pregnant women.

Changes to the female body that occur during pregnancy predispose a woman to injury in early pregnancy from fainting episodes, hyperventilation, and becoming easily fatigued. In the last trimester, an enlarged abdomen changes the woman's center of gravity, making her more susceptible to falls and pelvic pressure can cause leg pain.

Motor vehicle crashes in which the seat belt is not used or is used in an improper position are also a common cause of injury.

Non-Injury-Related Vaginal Bleeding

Bleeding from the vagina in women of childbearing age who are not pregnant is most likely to be menstrual bleeding. However, such bleeding can indicate more serious conditions (eg, miscarriage, childbirth, infection, cervical cancer, uterine fibroids, and vaginitis).

What to Look For	What to Do
▪ Abdominal cramps ▪ Blood in the vaginal area	1. Support the woman. 2. Help her into a comfortable position with legs bent. 3. Have the woman place a sanitary pad over the outside of the vagina. 4. Seek professional medical care.

Emergency Childbirth

Emergency childbirth occurs when a baby is born at an unplanned time or at an unplanned place. Most babies in the United States are delivered in a hospital. Occasionally, the birth process moves along faster than expected. Because emergency childbirth is encountered infrequently, taking care of an anxious mother and her newborn infant is a stressful event for a first aid provider. On the other hand, assisting in the birth of a baby is one of the few situations in which first aid providers have the opportunity to participate in a happy event rather than an unpleasant one.

Imminent Delivery

Consider transporting the woman to a hospital only if she does not have the urge to push or the baby is not crowning and this is her first delivery. Making a hasty decision to transport the woman means that the delivery could take place under the worst possible circumstances. When there is enough time to transport the woman to a hospital, the woman should wear a seat belt. Neither the lap belt nor the shoulder harness should be worn alone: both should be worn at the same time to avoid rupturing the uterus if a crash occurs. If she needs to lie down, place her on her left side. This position prevents a possible drop in blood pressure caused by pressure of the fetus on the inferior vena cava, which reduces venous blood returning to the heart.

If the woman has the urge to push or the baby is crowning, the woman has had previous pregnancies, and there is not enough time to get to the hospital, you must prepare to assist in the delivery. First, call (or have a bystander call) 9-1-1. Then, if the woman is in a crowded or public place, try to find a private, clean area unless the baby is crowning. Never move a woman when the baby is crowning as this could result in injury. The mother might find it reassuring to have a companion, such as her partner, a friend, or a relative, present. Follow these guidelines:

- Wear medical exam gloves. If available, wear a mask, a gown, and eye protection.
- **DO NOT** touch the vaginal area except during delivery and, if possible, with a witness present.
- **DO NOT** let the mother use the toilet.
- **DO NOT** hold the mother's legs together.

If the baby's head is not the presenting part (the first part to come out of the birth canal), the delivery will be complicated. Tell the mother not to push during contractions and attempt to calm and reassure her. Call 9-1-1 if you have not already done so.

Stages of Labor

Labor is a three-stage process that begins with the first regular uterine contractions, includes delivery of the baby, and ends with delivery of the placenta. The first stage usually lasts several hours (possibly 12 hours or more for a first baby), from the first contraction until the cervix is fully open (dilated). The cervix gradually stretches until it is large enough to let the baby pass through. (Outside a hospital setting, first aid providers cannot safely check for dilation of the cervix.) The contractions usually begin as acutely aching sensations in the small of the back; in a short time, they turn into cramplike pains recurring regularly in the lower abdomen. At first, the contractions are 10 to 15 minutes apart, are not very severe, and last less than 1 minute. Gradually, the intervals between contractions grow shorter, and the contractions increase in intensity. A slight, watery, blood-stained discharge (bloody show) from the vagina might accompany contractions or might occur before labor begins.

At the end of the first stage of labor, the amniotic sac breaks, and 1 pint (473 mL) or more of watery fluid, the amniotic fluid, discharges. Sometimes the amniotic sac breaks during the first stage of labor, but this is no cause for concern because it usually does not affect labor. If the amniotic sac breaks prematurely and labor does not begin within 24 hours, the risk of infection to mother and baby is great, and professional medical care should be sought.

The second stage usually lasts from 30 minutes to 2 hours. It begins when the neck of the cervix is fully open and ends with the actual birth of the baby. The baby is normally head down; once the head gets through the pelvis, the rest of the

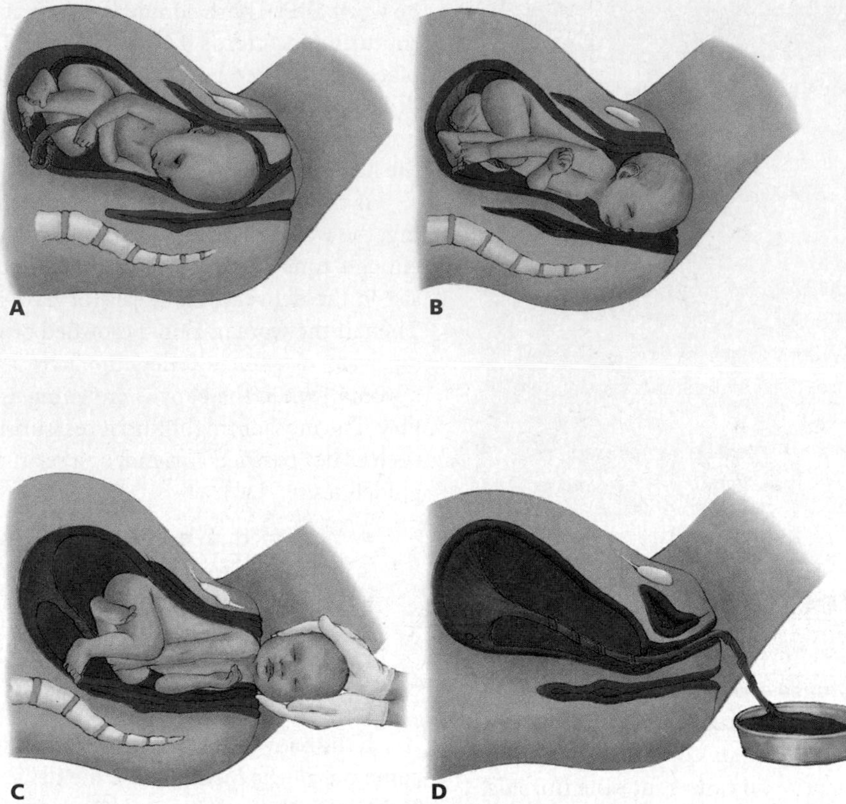

FIGURE 22-1 Normal stages of childbirth. **A**. End of the first stage of labor. **B**. Head delivers facedown. **C**. Support the head. **D**. Placenta is expelled in 5 to 20 minutes.

body should follow easily, one shoulder at a time. During the third stage, which lasts about 15 minutes or more, the afterbirth (placenta) is expelled **FIGURE 22-1**.

Recognizing Signs of Imminent Delivery

At the scene of a woman in labor, you will need to determine whether delivery is imminent or whether there is time to transport the woman to the hospital. To make that decision, answer the questions in the following table. Only if the answers to these questions seem to indicate an imminent birth should you examine the mother for crowning. Look to see if there is bulging at the vaginal opening or if part of the baby is visible. Crowning indicates that the baby is about to be born and that there is no time to get to a hospital before delivery. Because this step might be embarrassing to the mother, other parent, bystanders, or even you, it is important that you explain fully what you are doing and why. Make every effort to protect the woman from embarrassment during such an examination by removing only enough clothing to expose the vaginal area. Use something to shield the woman from prying eyes; for example, a blanket used to make a tent, or even a human shield, with people standing with their backs toward her.

FYI

Supplies for Delivery

Ideally, you should have the following supplies for delivery:

- Clean sheets, towels, and blankets to cover the mother and baby
- Plastic bag or towel to wrap the placenta for delivery to the hospital
- Clean, unused medical exam gloves to reduce the likelihood of infection
- Sanitary pads
- Newspapers, plastic, or a cloth sheet to place under the woman to provide a clean delivery area
- Rubber bulb syringe for suctioning the baby's mouth and nostrils
- Sterile gauze pads for wiping blood and mucus from the baby's mouth and nose
- Strips of gauze, new or clean shoelaces, or similar materials to tie the cord. (**DO NOT** use thread, wire, or string because they might cut through the cord.)

What to Look For	What to Do
To determine whether delivery is imminent or whether there is time to transport the woman to the hospital, answer the following questions: ▪ Has the woman given birth before? Labor during a first delivery is usually longer than in subsequent pregnancies. If this is her first delivery, there might be more time for transport to a hospital. ▪ How frequent are the contractions? Contractions more than 5 minutes apart are a good indication that there will be enough time to get the mother to a nearby hospital. Contractions less than 2 minutes apart that last 45 to 60 seconds, especially in a woman who has had more than one pregnancy, signal imminent delivery. ▪ Has the amniotic sac ruptured? If so, when? Labor usually proceeds more rapidly after rupture. If the sac ruptures more than 24 hours before birth occurs, the likelihood of fetal infection increases, and the hospital staff should be alerted. Delivery might be more difficult when the amniotic sac ruptures prematurely because amniotic fluid serves as a lubricant. ▪ Does the mother feel as though she has to move her bowels? That sensation is caused by the fetal head in the birth canal pressing against the rectum and indicates that delivery is imminent.	If you are faced with an imminent delivery, follow the steps in **SKILL SHEET 22-1**: **1.** Take standard precautions by washing your hands thoroughly and wearing medical exam gloves. If possible, wear a mask, a gown, and eye protection. **2.** Have the mother lie on her back with her head slightly elevated, knees drawn up, and legs spread apart. The mother might want to be in a different position. Other safe positions for childbirth include the following: ▪ Sitting up or squatting, with someone behind supporting her. These two positions place less tension on the vaginal tissues, reducing the likelihood of a tear, and allow the force of gravity to help. ▪ Lying on her left side, which improves blood return to her heart and prevents aspiration should she vomit. Have someone hold the woman's right leg up out of the way. ▪ Kneeling in a knee-chest position, which is used in many countries and in cases of breech presentations. **3.** Remind the woman to take short, quick breaths during each contraction. Between contractions, she should rest and breathe deeply through her mouth. **4.** Place absorbent, clean materials (such as sheets or towels) under the mother's buttocks. **5.** Elevate her buttocks with blankets or a pillow. **6.** When the baby's head appears, place the palm of your hand on top of the head and exert very gentle pressure to prevent an explosive delivery. Have the woman stop pushing. **DO NOT** push on the fontanelles (soft spots on the top and back of the infant's head). **7.** If the amniotic sac does not break or has not broken, tear it with your fingers and push it away from the baby's head and mouth as they appear. The baby could suffocate if the sac is not removed. **8.** As the baby's head emerges from the vagina, determine whether the umbilical cord is wrapped around the baby's neck. If it is, gently slip the cord over the baby's head. If you cannot do that, attempt to alleviate pressure on the cord. **9.** Support the baby's head as it emerges. **10.** Suction the baby's mouth and then the nostrils two or three times with the bulb syringe. Use caution to avoid contact with the back of the baby's mouth. If a bulb syringe is not available, wipe the baby's mouth and then the nose with gauze. **11.** As the torso and full body emerge, support the baby with both hands—the baby will be slippery. **12.** **DO NOT** pull on the baby, which could cause cervical spine damage. **DO NOT** put your fingers in the baby's armpits; pressure on the nerve centers there could cause paralysis. **13.** Keep the baby level with the vagina, slightly head down, to improve drainage from the mouth and nose. **14.** Wipe blood and mucus from the baby's mouth and nose with sterile gauze; suction the mouth, and then suction the nose again. **15.** Dry the infant to reduce heat loss and help stimulate breathing. Rub the baby's back or flick the soles of the feet to stimulate breathing. The baby should breathe within 30 seconds, especially after the cord stops pulsating. (**DO NOT** hold the baby up by the feet and slap its buttocks, which could cause an increase in intracranial pressure.) If breathing does not start within 30 seconds, begin cardiopulmonary resuscitation (CPR). **16.** Wrap the infant in a warm blanket and place on their side, head slightly lower than the trunk. Keep the infant level with the mother's vagina until the cord is cut. Raising the baby above the mother's abdomen (location of the placenta) while the umbilical cord is intact will allow the baby's blood to drain out and might result in shock in the baby. Holding the baby below the mother's abdomen allows her blood to flow into the baby, and the extra blood cells can cause serious conditions such as jaundice. **17.** When the umbilical cord stops pulsating, tie it with gauze (or similar material) or a clean shoelace between the mother and the infant. **18.** If the mother is going to the hospital soon after the birth, and it was a normal delivery, there is no need to cut the cord. Keep the infant warm and wait for EMS personnel, who will have the proper equipment to clamp and cut the cord. If you are in a remote location, you might have to cut the cord yourself. In such a situation and after cord pulsations stop, tie the cord about 7 inches (18 cm) away from the baby and make a second tie 5 inches (13 cm) from the first tie. Cut the cord between the two ties.

What to Look For	What to Do
	19. Watch for delivery of the placenta, which usually takes a few minutes, but could take as long as 30 minutes. **DO NOT** pull on the end of the umbilical cord to speed the delivery of the placenta. **20.** When the placenta is delivered, wrap it in a towel with three quarters of the umbilical cord and place the towel in a plastic bag. Keep the bag at the level of the infant. Take the placenta to the hospital, where it will be examined for completeness. This procedure is necessary because pieces of placenta retained in the uterus can cause persistent bleeding or infection. The cord should be cut by this point. **21.** Place a sterile pad over the vaginal opening, lower the mother's legs, and help her hold them together. **22.** Gently massage the woman's abdomen, just below the navel, to help control bleeding.

SKILL SHEET 22-1 Childbirth

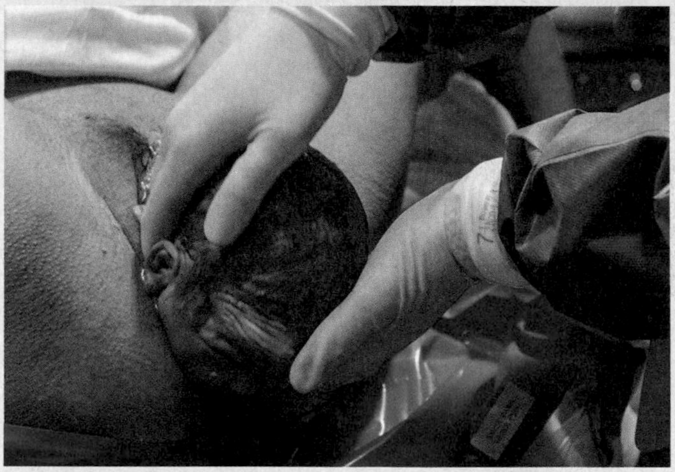

1 Support the baby's head and suction its mouth and nose.

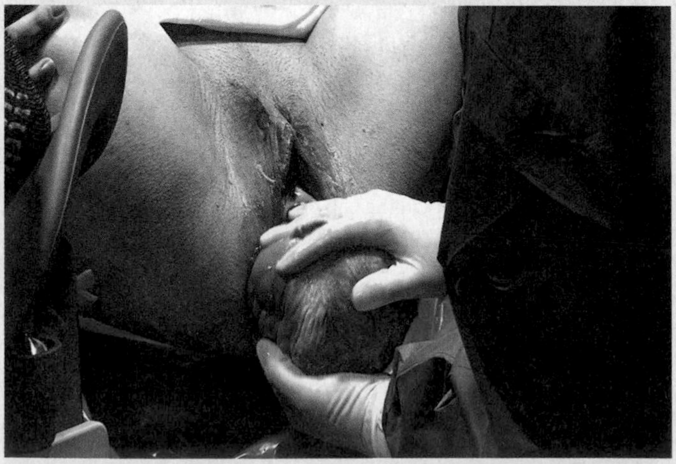

2 Once the head delivers, the baby turns and moves downward to allow the upper shoulder to deliver.

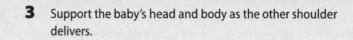

SKILL SHEET 22-1 Childbirth (*Continued*)

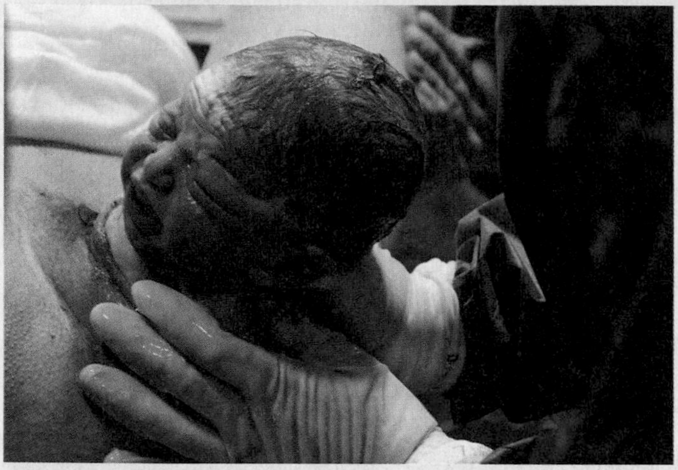
© University of Maryland Shock Trauma Center/MIEMSS.

3 Support the baby's head and body as the other shoulder delivers.

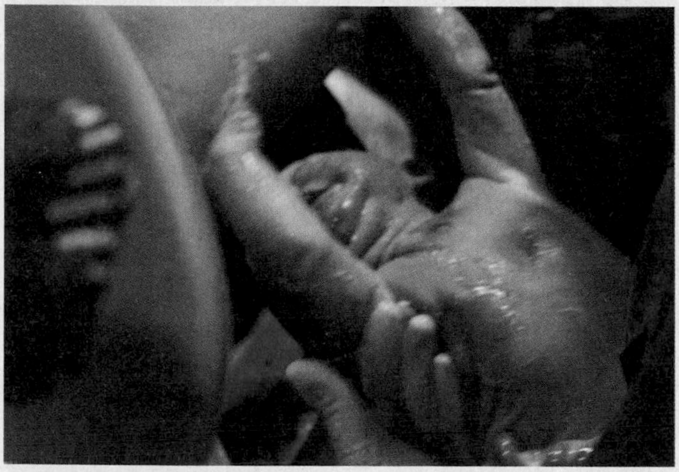
© University of Maryland Shock Trauma Center/MIEMSS.

4 Clean and dry the infant to reduce heat loss and stimulate breathing.

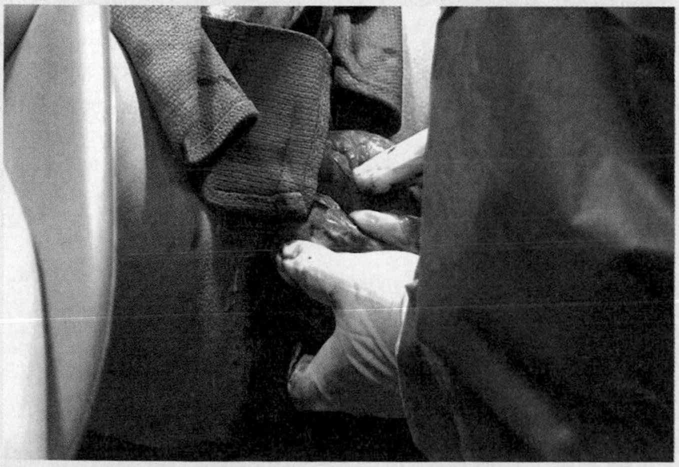
© University of Maryland Shock Trauma Center/MIEMSS.

5 Allow the placenta to deliver. **DO NOT** pull on the umbilical cord.

Delivery Aftercare

After delivery, monitor the mother's breathing and pulse. Replace any blood-soaked sheets and blankets while awaiting transport. A woman can expect from 1 to 2 cups (300 to 500 mL) of blood loss after delivery. You should be aware of this amount of blood loss so it does not cause undue psychological stress to the new mother or to you. If blood loss continues, massage the uterus. Uterine massage stimulates the uterus to contract, thus constricting blood vessels within its walls and decreasing bleeding. You can also let the mother try to nurse the infant as this will also stimulate uterine contraction. To perform uterine massage, do the following:

1. Use your hand with your fingers fully extended.
2. Place the palm of your hand on the lower abdomen, where you should be able to feel a grapefruit-sized mass.
3. Gently massage over the area with a firm, circular motion.
4. If bleeding continues, check your massage technique.
5. The mother can also breastfeed the baby following delivery of the placenta to stimulate uterine contractions and thus help control bleeding.

Initial Care of the Newborn

Normal findings in a newborn are a pulse rate of more than 100 beats per minute (feel the brachial artery, which runs between the shoulder and elbow) and a respiratory rate of more than 40 breaths per minute. The baby often will be crying. The most important care is positioning, drying, keeping warm, and stimulating the newborn to breathe. Wrap the newborn in a blanket, making sure the head is covered. Newborns are at risk for hypothermia; premature and low-weight newborns are at greater risk. Repeat suctioning if necessary, and continue to stimulate the newborn if they are not breathing (flick the soles of the feet and rub the infant's back).

If the newborn is motionless, tap the infant on the bottom of a foot or a shoulder for a response. If the infant does not respond and is not breathing or is only gasping, begin CPR starting with 30 chest compressions followed by two breaths. Initially, give a total of five sets of 30 chest compressions and two breaths before calling 9-1-1 unless a bystander has already called. Continue sets of 30 chest compressions and two breaths until EMS personnel take over. (See Chapter 5, *CPR*.)

Abnormal Deliveries

Most childbirths are normal and natural. Sometimes, however, complications arise. It is essential that you be calm, deliberate, and gentle in a situation that becomes even more stressful because of complications. Call 9-1-1 for all of these situations.

Prolapsed Cord

A **prolapsed cord** is a condition in which the umbilical cord comes through the birth canal before delivery of the head. The cord is squeezed between the baby's head and the mother's body (vaginal wall), and oxygen supply to the baby could be stopped. This puts the baby in danger of suffocation **FIGURE 22-2**. This situation is rare and very dangerous.

FYI

Emergencies During Pregnancy

What Medical Specialties Take Care of Women?

A gynecologist specializes in treating conditions related to the female reproductive tract. An obstetrician specializes in treating pregnant women. A pediatrician specializes in treating newborn babies, toddlers, and teens.

How Is Emergency Care for a Pregnant Woman Different?

Emergency care of a pregnant woman involves both the mother and the fetus. Even minor trauma to the mother's abdomen can result in life-threatening consequences. All pregnant women with trauma to the abdomen need a medical examination in a hospital emergency department and often need fetal monitoring. Fetal viability is determined by maternal viability. Position the mother on her left side to help venous blood return to the heart. Care for the pregnant woman the same way you would treat a nonpregnant woman.

What Are Some Indications of Pregnancy Emergencies?

- The three key warning signs of a serious condition are bleeding, abdominal cramps, and weakness.
- Sickness, swollen ankles, and urinary tract infections are not usually dangerous, but call the physician anyway.
- If a pregnant woman is spotting (small amount of vaginal bleeding), have her lie down immediately. Call for professional medical attention. Spotting can signal the onset of a miscarriage.

What to Look For	What to Do
The umbilical cord can be seen before the baby's head.	1. Position the woman with her head down or buttocks raised to use gravity to lessen pressure in the birth canal. 2. Insert fingers of your gloved hand into the vagina, placing fingers on either side of the cord to hold pressure from the presenting part (most often the head) of the fetus away from the pulsating cord. Continue until EMS arrives. **DO NOT** push the cord back into the vagina. This is one of only two circumstances for putting your fingers into the vagina. 3. Call 9-1-1 immediately.

CAUTION

DO NOT attempt to push the cord back into the vagina.

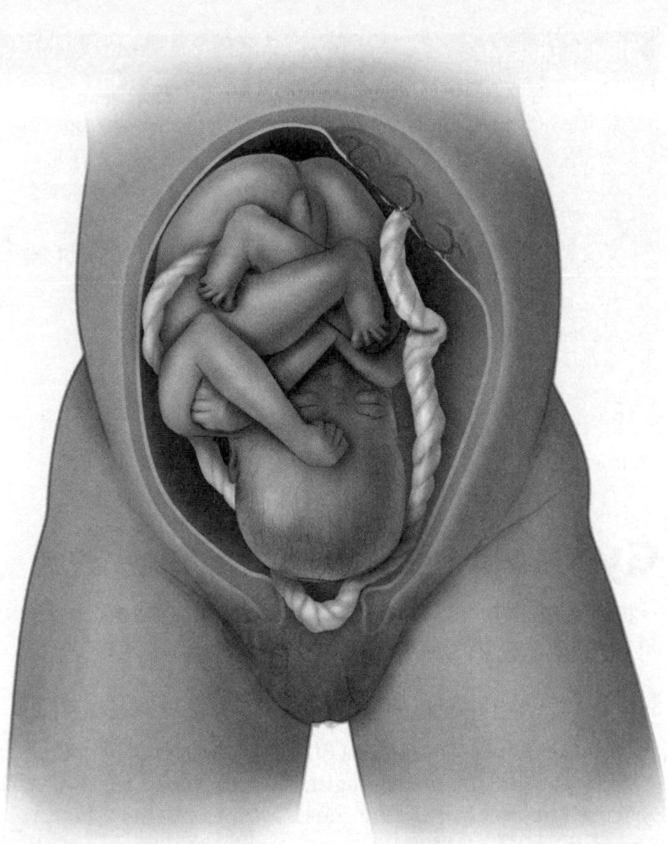

FIGURE 22-2 Prolapsed cord.

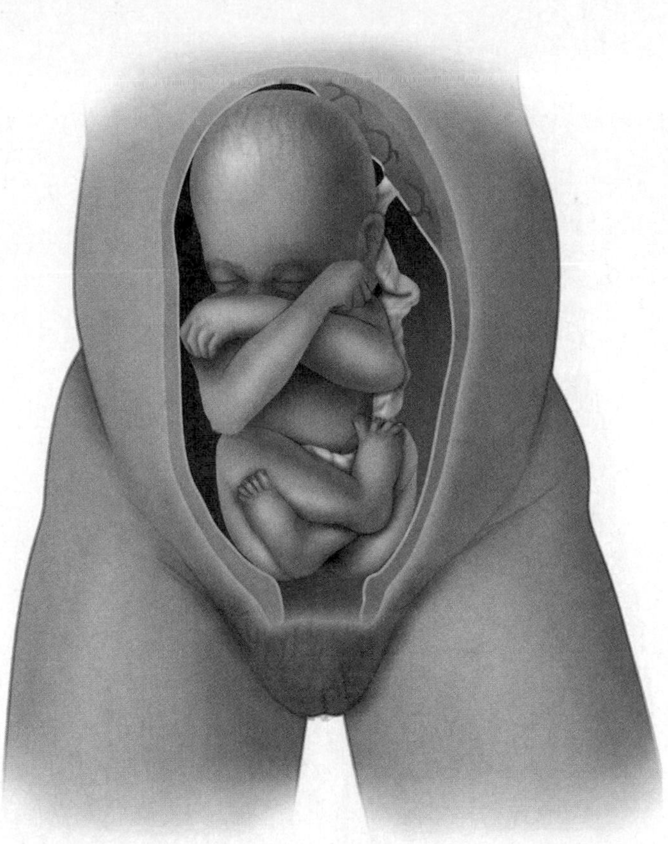

FIGURE 22-3 Breech presentation.

Breech Birth Presentation

A breech presentation occurs when the baby's buttocks or lower extremities emerge before the head or shoulders. Breech presentation is the most common type of abnormal delivery and occurs in 3% to 4% of all deliveries. Place the mother in a kneeling, head-down position, with her pelvis elevated, and seek professional medical care immediately **FIGURE 22-3**.

In a breech presentation, if the baby's head is not delivered within 3 minutes of the body, you must act to prevent suffocation of the baby. Suffocation can occur when the baby's face is pressed against the vaginal wall or when the umbilical cord is compressed by the baby's head in the vagina.

What to Look For	What to Do
The baby's buttocks come out first.	1. Have someone call 9-1-1 immediately. 2. To establish an airway, do the following: ▪ Place one hand in the vagina, positioning the palm toward the baby's face. This is one of only two circumstances for putting your fingers into the vagina. ▪ Form a V with your fingers on either side of the baby's nose. ▪ Push the vaginal wall away from the baby's face until the head is delivered. 3. Have the woman continue to push with contractions and attempt to deliver the baby.

CAUTION

DO NOT pull out the baby's head during a breech delivery.

Limb Presentation

Limb presentation occurs when an arm, leg, or foot of the infant protrudes from the birth canal. A foot more commonly presents when the infant is in a breech presentation **FIGURE 22-4**.

What to Look For	What to Do
An arm, leg, or foot appears first.	1. Place the mother in a head-down position with the pelvis elevated. **DO NOT** pull on the baby or attempt to push the limb back into the vagina. 2. Call 9-1-1 immediately. The baby cannot be delivered in this position by a first aid provider.

Meconium

Meconium is the baby's first feces (bowel movement) and can be present in the amniotic fluid. Its presence is associated with fetal distress during labor and a greater risk for infant death and therefore a need for infant resuscitation. The danger to the baby is the possibility of breathing the meconium into the lungs, where it can cause severe respiratory conditions.

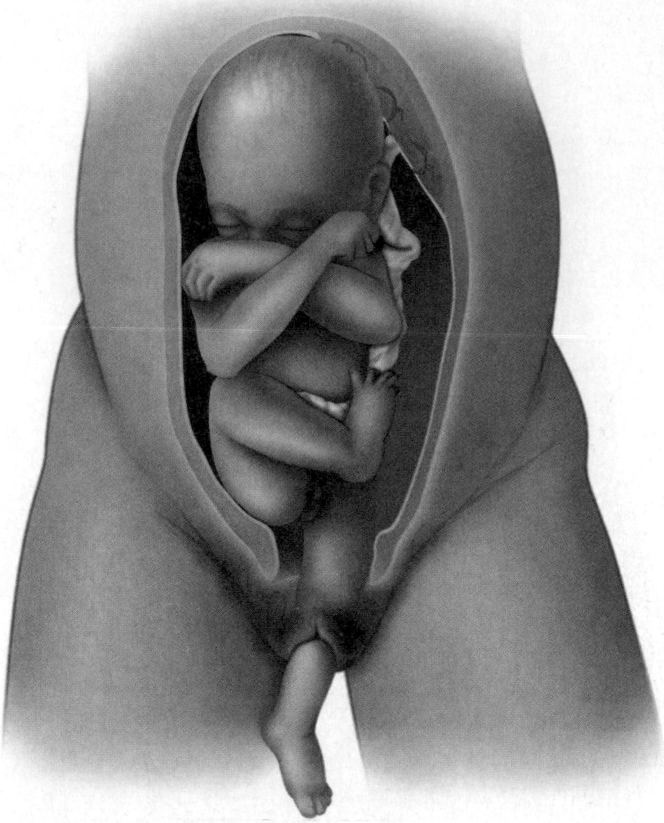

FIGURE 22-4 Limb presentation.

What to Look For	What to Do
Amniotic fluid that is: ▪ Green or brown-yellow ▪ Tarry ▪ Almost odorless	1. Keep the infant in a moderately head-down position to aid with drainage. 2. Suction the mouth and nostrils thoroughly, or the baby will inhale meconium with its first breath into the lungs. Clear amniotic fluid, however, is harmlessly absorbed through the baby's lungs. Try not to stimulate the infant to breathe before suctioning. 3. Maintain the baby's open airway. 4. Call 9-1-1 immediately.

Premature Birth

Any baby born prior to 37 completed weeks of pregnancy is defined as premature and will require special care. Premature babies develop conditions because they are smaller and less developed than full-term infants. For example, their cardiovascular and respiratory systems are often immature.

Refer to **FLOWCHART 22-1** for additional information regarding emergency childbirth.

What to Look For	What to Do
▪ A premature infant will be smaller and thinner than a full-term infant. ▪ A premature infant has a head proportionately larger in comparison with the rest of the body. ▪ The cheesy, white coating on the skin (vernix caseosa) of a full-term infant will be minimal or absent on the premature infant.	1. Keep the baby warm. Premature babies are especially at risk for hypothermia. 2. Keep the mouth and nose clear of mucus. 3. Monitor breathing and perform CPR, if necessary.

Gynecologic Emergencies

Gynecologic emergencies are reproductive system conditions that occur in nonpregnant women.

Pelvic Inflammatory Disease (PID)

Pelvic inflammatory disease (PID) is caused by the spread of microorganisms from the vagina and cervix to reproductive organs. The organisms (the most common being *Chlamydia* and *Neisseria gonorrhoeae*) are typically sexually transmitted. A person with PID can have more than one sexually transmitted disease (STD) at the same time. Other important conditions (eg, ectopic pregnancy, acute appendicitis) may cause confusion about the condition. The inflammatory response can range from mild to severe. No reliable signs or symptoms exist, but may involve vaginal discharge and abdominal tenderness. Because the consequences of unrecognized and untreated PID can be severe, professional medical care should be sought.

Q&A

What should be done about urinary tract infections?

- Women, especially during pregnancy, are very susceptible to urinary tract infections. Often, when one infection clears, another replaces it.
- Seek advice from a physician. Self-care measures to help relieve the burning pain include taking shallow, lukewarm sitz baths sprinkled with baking soda; urinating while standing in the shower; and practicing good personal hygiene. Wiping from front to back after going to the bathroom helps keep bacteria, including *Escherichia coli*, away from the urinary tract. Drinking more fluids helps prevent and treat urinary tract infections. Some experts report that drinking cranberry juice (tablets are also available with fewer calories) might help inhibit urinary tract infections.
- A urinary tract (bladder) infection can lead to the more serious kidney infection. Signs of a kidney infection include pain in the lower back or flank, fever, and nausea or vomiting.

Flowchart 22-1 Emergency Childbirth

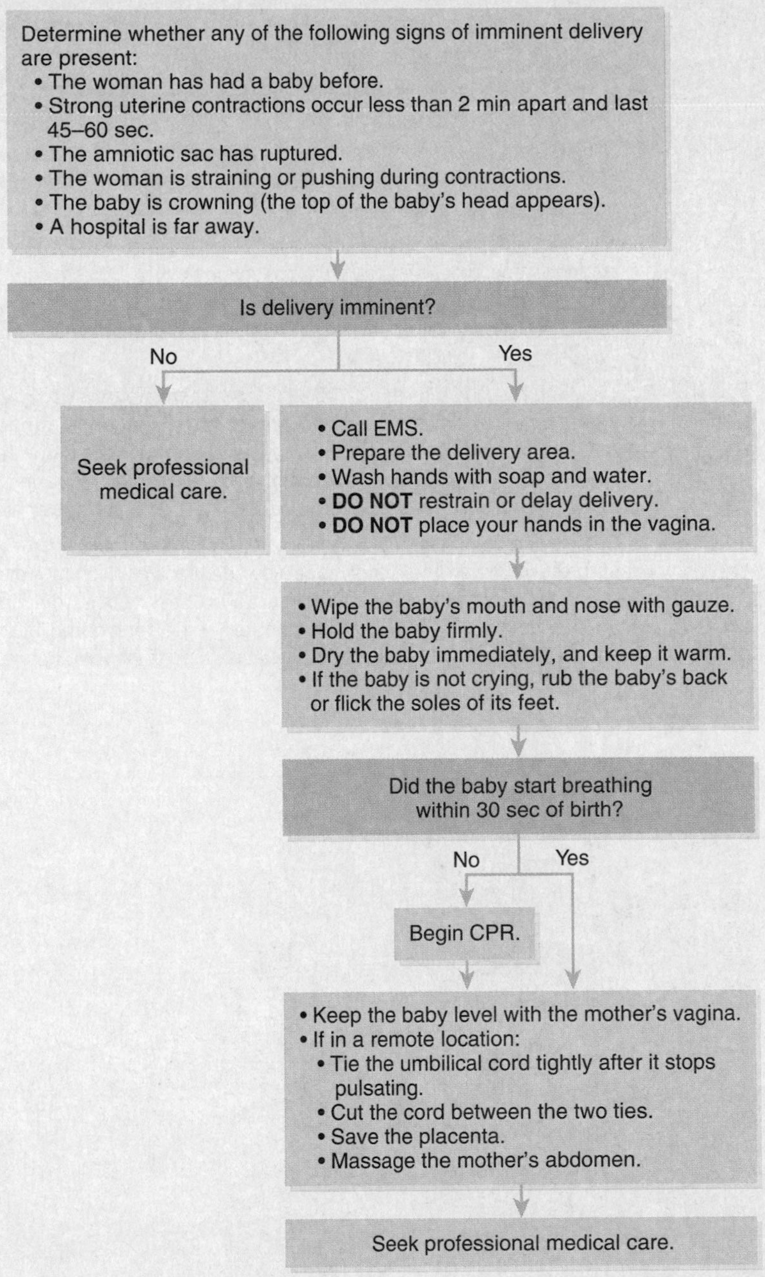
Determine whether any of the following signs of imminent delivery are present:
• The woman has had a baby before.
• Strong uterine contractions occur less than 2 min apart and last 45–60 sec.
• The amniotic sac has ruptured.
• The woman is straining or pushing during contractions.
• The baby is crowning (the top of the baby's head appears).
• A hospital is far away.
Is delivery imminent?
No
Yes
Seek professional medical care.
• Call EMS.
• Prepare the delivery area.
• Wash hands with soap and water.
• **DO NOT** restrain or delay delivery.
• **DO NOT** place your hands in the vagina.
• Wipe the baby's mouth and nose with gauze.
• Hold the baby firmly.
• Dry the baby immediately, and keep it warm.
• If the baby is not crying, rub the baby's back or flick the soles of its feet.
Did the baby start breathing within 30 sec of birth?
No
Yes
Begin CPR.
• Keep the baby level with the mother's vagina.
• If in a remote location:
• Tie the umbilical cord tightly after it stops pulsating.
• Cut the cord between the two ties.
• Save the placenta.
• Massage the mother's abdomen.
Seek professional medical care.

Sexual Assault and Rape

Perhaps one of the most difficult emergency situations that a first aid provider might have to deal with is sexual assault. According to the Rape, Abuse & Incest National Network (RAINN), the majority of sexual assault cases are not reported to authorities. In most cases, the sexual assault survivor is a woman. The Centers for Disease Control and Prevention (CDC) reports that 1 in 5 women in the United States have been raped at some point in their life. It should be noted, however, that men, heterosexual and homosexual, also can be raped.

There are many definitions of rape, but in general, rape involves the criminal act of penetrating another person without their consent. Related physical injury is common, but the psychological trauma may be more damaging. It is essential that you be calm and sympathetic when dealing with a person who has experienced sexual assault. You should also notify the police so appropriate reporting and investigating can occur. (For more information, see Chapter 23, *Emotional Emergencies and Abuse*.)

What to Look For	What to Do
A person who has been sexually assaulted might display: ▪ Headaches ▪ Sleeplessness, nightmares ▪ Nausea and/or muscle spasms ▪ Confusion ▪ Depression ▪ Anxiety, jumpiness	1. **DO NOT** ask a lot of questions. Confine your questions to an assessment of the person's injuries, not a detailed description of the events. Ask questions based on the SAMPLE history (see Chapter 4, *Finding Out What Is Wrong*). 2. **DO NOT** blame the survivor in any way or talk about what might have been done or what you would have done. Be supportive. Remind them that they are safe now. 3. Determine which injuries require immediate care. Whenever it is necessary that a woman disrobe, try to have another woman present. 4. **DO NOT** expose the genitalia unless an injury in that area requires immediate care (eg, severe bleeding). Examining genitalia, except when childbirth is imminent, has serious legal implications, and therefore usually should be avoided. 5. Try, if possible, to preserve evidence but leave the actual investigation to the police. To preserve evidence, encourage the person not to change clothes, wash, urinate, defecate, or douche. Explain to the person in a sympathetic way that it would be best not to clean up. Keep in mind that a person who has been raped, like any other person, has the right to refuse first aid and transport to a hospital. 6. Even if the person refuses aid, **DO NOT** leave them alone. Try to have a trusted friend or relative stay with the person. Protect the privacy of the person. Emotional support is vital. Most large communities have rape crisis centers; furnishing the person with the name and number of the nearest center (check online) is probably as important as treating any physical injuries. Trained volunteers can talk to the person and give you and the person information about what to do next. 7. Get the person professional medical care. The person could be in shock and unaware of the severity of their injuries. Strongly encourage a person who has been raped to receive medical care, even if the person does not show any signs of injury and does not want medical care. However, be aware that the medical exam following a rape is intrusive and, for women, includes a full gynecologic exam. The person will need information about what is going to happen before receiving medical care.

PREP KIT

Ready for Review

- Miscarriages usually occur during the first trimester of pregnancy.
- If a woman experiences vaginal bleeding late in her pregnancy, it usually constitutes an emergency.
- Emergency childbirth occurs when a baby is born at an unplanned time or at an unplanned place.
- In most cases, childbirth is normal and natural. Sometimes complications can arise.
- Perhaps one of the most difficult emergency situations that a first aid provider might have to deal with is sexual assault.

Vital Vocabulary

amniotic sac A thick, transparent sac that holds the fetus suspended in the amniotic fluid.

birth canal The vagina and the lower part of the uterus.

bloody show The bloody mucus plug that is discharged from the vagina when labor begins.

breech Birth presentation where the baby's buttocks or lower extremities emerge before the head or shoulders.

cervix The small opening at the lower end of the uterus through which the baby passes.

crowning The stage of birth when the presenting part of the baby is visible at the vaginal orifice.

ectopic pregnancy A pregnancy that develops outside the uterus, typically in a fallopian tube.

fallopian tubes The tubes that connect each ovary with the uterus.

fetus The developing, unborn offspring inside the uterus.

fontanelles Areas where the infant's skull has not fused together; usually disappear at approximately 18 months of age.

inferior vena cava Large vein located between the spine and the abdominal organs.

labor The process or period of childbirth; especially, the muscular contraction of the uterus designed to expel the fetus from the mother.

meconium A dark green material in the amniotic fluid that can indicate fetal distress; the infant's first bowel movement.

miscarriage Delivery of the fetus before it is mature enough to survive outside the womb (about 20 weeks), from either natural (spontaneous abortion) or induced causes.

placenta The vascular organ attached to the uterine wall that supplies oxygen and nutrients to the fetus; also called afterbirth.

prolapsed cord A condition in which the umbilical cord comes out of the vagina before the infant.

umbilical cord The flexible structure that connects the fetus to the placenta.

vena cava syndrome A set of symptoms that occur when blood flow to the inferior vena cava is compressed or blocked.

Assessment in Action

You are visiting a local museum when you respond to calls for help in the exhibit hall. A young woman has gone into labor. When you arrive on scene, she tells you this is her third child and that her due date is next week. She says she thought she would have time to get to the hospital when the contractions started. However, the contractions intensified and got closer together very quickly. Contractions are now less than 2 minutes apart and last up to 60 seconds. A hospital is 10 minutes away.

Directions: Circle Yes if you agree with the statement; circle No if you disagree.

1. Labor during a third pregnancy is usually longer than in previous pregnancies.

   YES NO

2. Allow the woman to use the toilet.

   YES NO

3. With contractions less than 2 minutes apart, you should have time to get her to the hospital.

   YES NO

4. Call 9-1-1 and immediately prepare a delivery area.

   YES NO

5. If the baby is crowning, you should not restrain or delay delivery.

   YES NO

PREP KIT continued

Check Your Knowledge

Directions: Circle Yes if you agree with the statement; circle No if you disagree.

1. An aching in the lower back is a sign of a miscarriage.
   YES **NO**
2. It is normal for a woman to experience vaginal bleeding in her last trimester.
   YES **NO**
3. Most babies in the United States are delivered at home.
   YES **NO**
4. Place a pregnant woman on her left side when transporting her to the hospital.
   YES **NO**
5. Labor is a four-stage process.
   YES **NO**
6. The second stage of labor lasts from 30 minutes to 2 hours.
   YES **NO**
7. New or clean shoelaces can be used to tie the umbilical cord.
   YES **NO**
8. A prolapsed umbilical cord is a normal occurrence.
   YES **NO**
9. The placenta is also called the afterbirth.
   YES **NO**
10. Whether or not the woman has given birth before will usually affect the length of the labor.
    YES **NO**

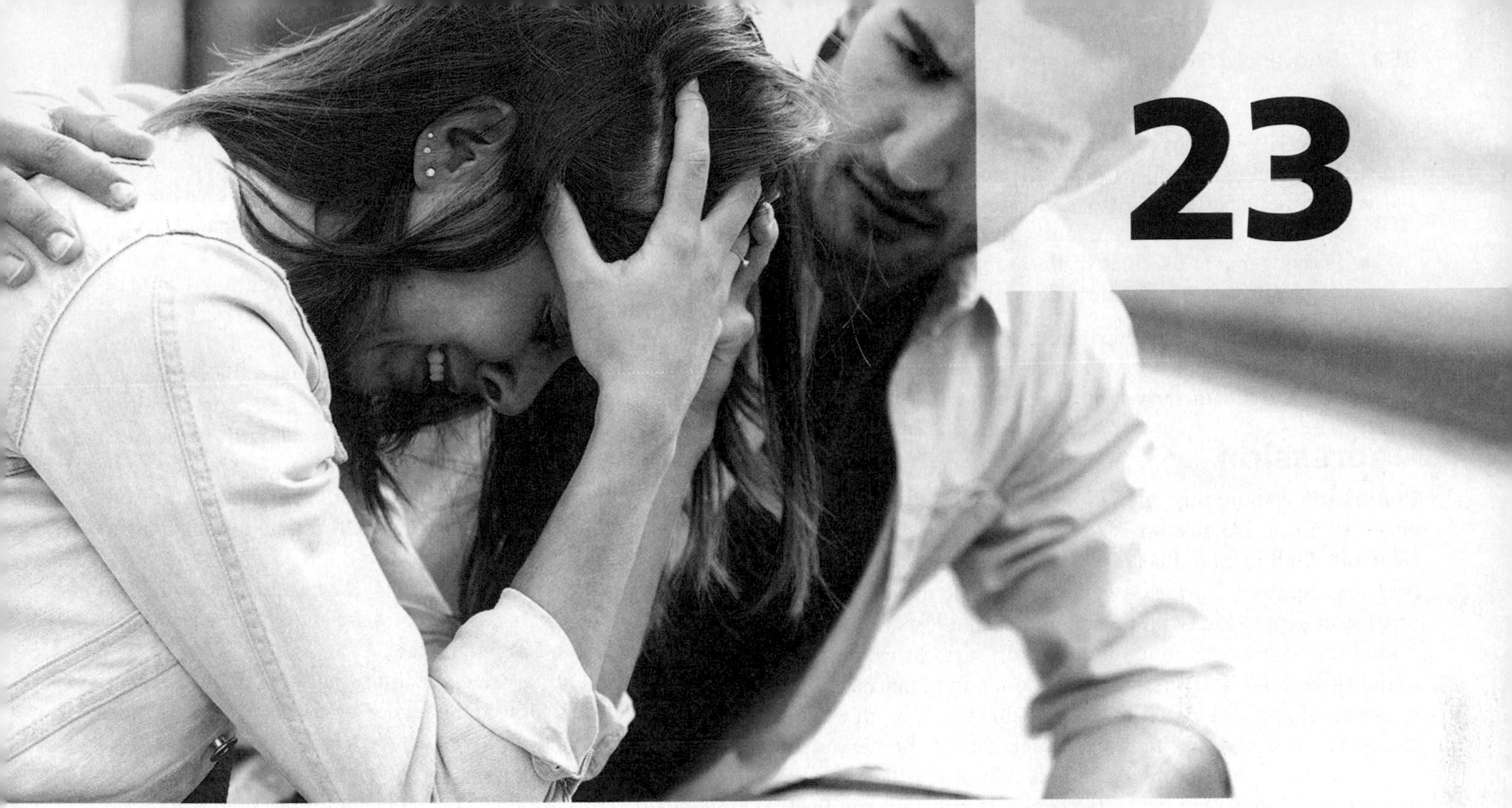

23

Psychological Emergencies and Abuse

CHAPTER AT A GLANCE

- Psychological Emergencies
  - Depression
  - Suicide
  - Emotional Injury
- Abuse
  - Sexual Assault and Rape
  - Child Abuse and Neglect
  - Domestic Violence
  - Elder Abuse

Psychological Emergencies

Behavior is how a person acts. Although each person acts or behaves differently, sometimes a person exhibits unacceptable or intolerable behavior. The abnormal behavior may be due to a psychological condition (such as a mental illness) or a physical condition. For example, a person with diabetes who has an uncorrected low blood glucose level can display aggressiveness, restlessness, or anxiety. Because the brain lacks energy in the form of blood glucose, altered mental status results. Likewise, lack of oxygen and inadequate blood flow to the brain also cause altered mental status, resulting in similar behavior.

Several factors can change a person's behavior, including situational stresses, medical illnesses, psychiatric conditions, alcohol, and drugs. Any situation in which a person is experiencing extreme distress, is unable to cope with everyday life, or is in danger of hurting themselves or others is known as a **psychological emergency**. The following are common reasons for psychological and emotional changes:

- Low blood glucose level in a person with diabetes (hypoglycemia)
- Lack of oxygen (hypoxia)
- Inadequate blood flow to the brain
- Head trauma
- Excessive cold (hypothermia)

- Excessive heat (hyperthermia)
- Infection (eg, bladder infection, pneumonia)
- Mind-altering substances, such as alcohol, depressants, stimulants, hallucinogens, and narcotics
- Psychogenic or psychiatric illness that leads to psychotic thinking, anxiety, depression, or panic

First aid providers should rule out or follow up on the potential medical factors before considering that an alteration in mental status is due to a psychological emergency.

Depression

Depression is more than the sad feeling that everyone experiences at times. Depression is one of the most common and treatable of all mental illnesses. There are several types of depression: reactive depression (following tragic events), major or clinical depression (with no apparent cause, lasts more than 2 weeks, and prevents functioning in top form at work or in social situations), and bipolar depression, a type that includes episodes of euphoria. Depression is believed to be due to a chemical imbalance in the brain, which causes the nerves in the brain to work improperly. This is why it is often treated using medications that act on the brain. Depression can lead to suicide; in fact, untreated depression is the main cause of suicide.

What to Look For	What to Do
Not everyone who is depressed experiences every symptom. Severity of symptoms varies with people and also varies over time. ▪ Persistent sad, anxious, or empty moods ▪ Feelings of hopelessness, pessimism ▪ Feelings of guilt, worthlessness, helplessness ▪ Loss of interest or pleasure in hobbies and activities that were once enjoyed, including sex ▪ Decreased energy, fatigue, feeling slowed down ▪ Difficulty concentrating, remembering, making decisions ▪ Insomnia, early morning awakening, or oversleeping ▪ Appetite and/or weight loss or overeating and weight gain ▪ Thoughts of death or suicide; suicide attempts ▪ Restlessness, irritability ▪ Persistent physical symptoms that do not respond to treatment such as headaches, digestive disorders, and chronic pain	1. Some depressed people do not feel like talking. In such cases, saying, "You look very sad," often allows the person to talk about the depressed feelings. The person might burst into tears. **DO NOT** discourage the crying. Maintain a sympathetic silence and let the person "cry it out." 2. Provide empathetic attention and reassurance. Let the person know you are concerned. 3. Attempt to interview the person in private because the presence of several people may make the person uncomfortable. Ask open-ended questions such as, "Tell me how you feel." 4. Tell the person that many people have periods of unhappiness, but they can be helped to feel better. Mention community resources where such help can be found.

Suicide

Suicide is defined as any willful act that ends one's own life. Suicide in the United States is increasingly an issue for adolescents, college-age students, and older adults.

The Centers for Disease Control and Prevention (CDC) reports the rate for suicide in men is four times that for women. It is most common in men who are single, widowed, or divorced. Slightly more than one-half of all people who die by suicide, both men and women, use firearms. The next most common method is hanging. Poisoning by solids or liquids is the most common method used by people who attempt but do not die by suicide. Jumping from high places, carbon monoxide poisoning by auto exhaust, drowning, and self-inflicted (non-firearm) wounds are less common methods.

The number of suicides peaks during spring months and is lowest in the winter. Suicide rates are lowest in the Northeast and highest in the Mountain States.

Suicide attempts are eight times more common than suicides. In addition, although men die by suicide four times more often than women, women are reported to attempt suicide three times more often, according to the American Foundation for Suicide Prevention (AFSP). It is not known if men are more reluctant to seek help and, thus, less likely to report their attempts. It also is not known if the lower rate of suicide among women results from their choice of less-lethal methods.

Suicide is often attempted by people who are have depression or have alcoholism. The AFSP reports that about 60% of all people who die by suicide have previously attempted suicide, and that about 75% gave clear warning that they intended to kill themselves. Typically, a suicide attempt occurs when a person's close emotional attachments are in danger or when a significant family member or friend dies. People who are contemplating suicide often feel unable to manage their lives. Frequently, they lack self-esteem.

Many people who are planning to die by suicide make last-minute attempts to communicate their intentions. When a person phones to threaten suicide, try to keep the person on the line until EMS reaches the scene.

If you encounter a person who is attempting or threatening suicide, discreetly remove any dangerous articles. Talk quietly with the person and encourage the person to discuss the situation. Ask the following: "Have you attempted suicide before? Have you made any concrete plans for a method of suicide? Has any family member died by suicide?" People who have made a previous suicide attempt, who have detailed suicide plans, or who have a close relative who died by suicide are more likely to try to kill themselves. They must be reassured and taken to professional medical help, usually at a medical facility. **DO NOT** leave them alone under any circumstances.

When a person attempts suicide, first aid care has priority. Drug overdoses must be managed. Bleeding from slashed wrists must be controlled. As you give first aid, try to encourage the person to talk about the situation. If a drug overdose is involved, collect any medication containers, pills, or other drugs found on the scene and take the items to the hospital ED with the person. In all cases, law enforcement authorities should be contacted.

Risk Factors

A combination of individual, relationship, community, and societal factors contribute to the risk of suicide. Risk factors are those characteristics associated with suicide and might not be direct causes. The Centers for Disease Control and Prevention (CDC) identifies the following as suicide risk factors:

- Family history of suicide
- Family history of child maltreatment
- Previous suicide attempt(s)
- History of mental disorders, particularly clinical depression
- History of alcohol and substance abuse
- Feelings of hopelessness
- Impulsive or aggressive tendencies
- Cultural and religious beliefs (e.g., belief that suicide is noble resolution of a personal dilemma)
- Local epidemics of suicide
- Isolation, a feeling of being cut off from other people
- Barriers to accessing mental health treatment
- Loss (relational, social, work, or financial)
- Physical illness
- Easy access to lethal methods
- Unwillingness to seek help because of the stigma attached to mental health, substance abuse, or suicidal thoughts

What to Look For	What to Do
A person who is: ▪ Getting their affairs in order (paying off debts, making or changing a will) ▪ Giving away articles of either personal or monetary value ▪ Exhibiting signs of planning a suicide such as obtaining a weapon or writing a suicide note A person who says: ▪ "Life is not worth living." ▪ "My family would be better off without me." ▪ "Next time I will take enough pills to do the job right." ▪ "Take my (prized collection, valuables); I do not need this stuff anymore." ▪ "I will not be around to deal with that." ▪ "You will be sorry when I am gone." ▪ "I will not be around much longer." ▪ "I just cannot deal with everything—life is too hard." ▪ "Nobody understands me; nobody feels the way I do." ▪ "There is nothing I can do to make it better." ▪ "I would be better off dead." ▪ "I feel like there is no way out."	**1.** If someone tells you they are thinking about suicide, take the distress seriously **TABLE 23-1**. **2.** Ways to be helpful to someone who is threatening suicide include the following: ▪ Be direct. Talk openly and matter-of-factly about suicide. ▪ Be willing to listen. Allow expressions of feelings. Accept the feelings. ▪ Be nonjudgmental. **DO NOT** debate whether suicide is right or wrong. ▪ Get involved. Become available. Show interest and support. ▪ **DO NOT** dare them to do it. ▪ **DO NOT** act shocked. This will put distance between the two of you. ▪ **DO NOT** be sworn to secrecy. Seek support. ▪ Offer hope that alternatives are available but **DO NOT** offer glib reassurance. ▪ Take action. Remove means of suicide, such as guns or stockpiled pills. ▪ Get help from people or agencies specializing in crisis intervention and suicide prevention, such as the National Suicide Prevention Lifeline, at 1-800-273-8255, which is available 24/7 for anyone in suicidal crisis or emotional distress. (By July 2022, 9-8-8 will be the nationwide number).

CAUTION

DO NOT ignore a suicide threat. Every suicidal act or gesture should be taken seriously and the person referred to a mental health professional.

Although most emotional reactions are temporary, lasting only minutes, hours, or, at the most, a few days, they are seriously disabling and may upset others. It is important to know that first aid can be applied to emotional as well as to physical injuries.

Typical Reactions

With few exceptions, all people experience fear in the face of an emergency. Feeling shaky, perspiring profusely, and becoming nauseated are common. Such reactions are normal and no cause for concern. Most people are able to regain their composure reasonably quickly.

Extensive training is not needed to recognize severe, abnormal reactions. To determine whether a person needs help, find out whether they are doing something that makes sense and if are able to take care of themselves. For the most part, emotional first aid measures are simple and easy to understand **TABLE 23-2**.

Emotional Injury

First aid for an emotional injury means being supportive of people with emotional injuries, whether the injuries are from physical injury or excessive or unbearable strain on the person's emotions.

Emotional first aid often goes hand in hand with physical first aid because a physical injury and the circumstances surrounding it may actually cause emotional injury. On the other hand, emotional injury may occur when there is no physical injury. Emotional injuries usually are not as obvious as physical injuries, but both can be severe and require first aid.

TABLE 23-1 Common Myths About Suicide

Myth	Fact
People who talk about suicide do not die by suicide.	Of every 10 people who die by suicide, 8 have given definite warnings of their suicidal intentions. All suicide threats and attempts must be taken seriously.
Suicide happens without warning.	Studies reveal that the person contemplating suicide gives many clues and warnings about suicidal intentions. Being alert to these cries for help may prevent suicidal behavior.
People who contemplate or attempt suicide are fully intent on dying.	Most people who contemplate suicide are undecided about living or dying, and they gamble with death, leaving it to others to save them. Almost no one dies by suicide without letting others know how they are feeling. Often this cry for help is given in code. Decoding these distress signals can save lives.
Once a person attempts suicide, they are suicidal forever.	Fortunately, people who want to kill themselves are suicidal only for a limited time. If they are saved from self-destruction, they can lead meaningful lives.
Improvement following a suicidal crisis means that the suicidal risk is over.	Most suicides occur within 3 months after the beginning of improvement, when the person has the energy to put morbid thoughts and feelings into effect. Relatives and physicians should be especially vigilant during this period.
Suicide strikes more often among the rich; or, conversely, it occurs more frequently among the poor.	Suicide strikes all socioeconomic groups and is represented proportionately at all levels of society.
Suicide is inherited or runs in a family (ie, is genetically determined).	Suicide risk is not inherited. It is an individual decision and can be prevented.
All people who attempt or die by suicide have a mental illness.	Studies of hundreds of genuine suicide notes indicate that although a person who attempts or dies by suicide is extremely unhappy, they do not necessarily have a mental illness. The overpowering unhappiness may result from a temporary emotional upset, a long and painful illness, or a complete loss of hope.

Data from US Department of Health and Human Services.

However, improvisation is often needed, just as it is in splinting a fracture. Whatever the situation, you will have your own emotional reactions toward the person. These reactions are important; they can enhance or hinder your ability to help the person. Especially when you are tired or worried, you may easily become impatient with the person who seems to be "making a mountain out of a molehill." You may feel resentful toward the person for being a burden. Be on guard against becoming impatient, intolerant, or resentful. People who can see the first aid provider's calmness, confidence, and competence will be reassured.

On the other hand, do not be overly sympathetic or overly concerned. Excessive sympathy for an incapacitated person can be as harmful as negative feelings. The person needs solid help but does not need to be overwhelmed with pity.

What to Look For	What to Do
▪ Aggressive, hostile, or violent behavior, which may be a response to illness or may be a way of coping with feelings of helplessness ▪ Person standing or sitting in a threatening position (eg, clenched fists) ▪ Presence of lethal object ▪ Yelling or verbal threats of harm to others	**1.** Size up the situation before you do anything. An angry, violent person is ready to fight with anyone who approaches and may be difficult to control. If the scene appears unsafe, **DO NOT** enter. If necessary, contact law enforcement. **2.** Avoid responding with anger. Many angry or violent people can be calmed by someone who is trained and who appears confident that the person will behave well. **3.** Encourage the person to speak directly about the cause of their anger. A statement like, "I am not sure I understand why you are angry," often brings results. Reassure the person that you are there to help. **4.** Notify the police if you are unable to communicate with a person who is dangerous to themselves or to others. **5.** Confronting a person who is experiencing a psychological emergency can be a trying and frustrating experience. Use these guidelines if you must try to calm a person who is upset: ▪ Acknowledge that the person seems upset, and reiterate that you are there to help. ▪ Maintain a comfortable distance. ▪ Encourage the person to state what is troubling them. ▪ **DO NOT** make quick moves. ▪ Respond honestly to the person's questions. ▪ **DO NOT** threaten, challenge, or argue with a disturbed person. ▪ Tell the truth—**DO NOT** lie. ▪ **DO NOT** play along with any of a disturbed person's visual or auditory disturbances. ▪ Involve trusted family members or friends. ▪ Be prepared to stay with the person for an extended period of time. ▪ Never leave the person alone. ▪ Avoid unnecessary physical contact. ▪ Maintain eye contact.

TABLE 23-2 Psychological First Aid for Reactions to Emergency Situations

Reaction	Symptoms	Do . . .	Do Not . . .
Normal	■ Trembling ■ Muscle tension ■ Perspiration ■ Nausea ■ Mild diarrhea ■ Urinary frequency ■ Pounding heart ■ Rapid breathing ■ Anxiety	■ Give reassurance. ■ Encourage the person. ■ Talk with the person. ■ Observe to see that the person is gaining composure, not losing it.	■ Show resentment. ■ Overdo sympathy.
Individual panic (flight reaction)	■ Unreasoning attempt to flee ■ Loss of judgment ■ Uncontrolled weeping ■ Wildly running about	■ Try kind firmness. ■ Get help to isolate the person from others, if necessary. ■ Be empathetic. ■ Encourage the person to talk. ■ Be aware of your own limitations.	■ Use forceful physical restraint. ■ Strike the person physically. ■ Douse the person with water. ■ Give sedatives.
Depression (underactive reactions)	■ Stands or sits without moving or talking ■ Vacant expression ■ Lack of emotional display	■ Make contact gently. ■ Secure a rapport. ■ Get the person to tell you what happened. ■ Be empathetic. ■ Recognize feelings of resentment in the person and yourself. ■ Give the person a simple, routine task to complete.	■ Tell the person to "snap out of it." ■ Overdo sympathy. ■ Give sedatives. ■ Argue with the person.
Overactive	■ Argumentative ■ Talks rapidly ■ Jokes inappropriately ■ Makes endless suggestions ■ Jumps from one activity to another	■ Let the person talk about the situation. ■ Find the person a job that requires physical effort. ■ Supervision is necessary. ■ Be aware of your own feelings.	■ Suggest that the person is acting abnormally. ■ Give sedatives. ■ Argue with the person.
Physical (conversion disorder [a mental disorder in which psychological conflict manifests itself as physical symptoms])	■ Severe nausea and vomiting ■ Cannot use some part of the body	■ Show interest in the person. ■ Find a small job for the person to distract and occupy their thoughts. ■ Make the person comfortable. ■ Get professional medical care as soon as possible.	■ Tell the person that there is nothing wrong with them. ■ Place blame. ■ Ridicule the person. ■ Ignore the disability.

Data from M51-400-603-1, Department of Nonresident Instruction, Medical Field Service School, Brooke Army Medical Center, Fort Sam, Houston, Texas.

Abuse

Abuse includes situations that involve mistreatment of others, such as sexual assault and rape, child abuse and neglect, domestic violence, and elder abuse.

Sexual Assault and Rape

The definitions of rape and sexual assault vary widely. Rape is generally defined as the criminal act of penetrating another person without their consent. Categories of rape include the following:

- *Acquaintance rape*, which involves people who knew each other before the rape; includes relatives, neighbors, or friends.
- *Date rape*, which takes place within a relationship but without the consent of one person and may involve harm or the threat of harm by the other person or the use of drugs slipped into a drink.
- *Marital rape*, which occurs when the person and the offender are married to each other.
- *Stranger rape*, which occurs when the person and the offender have no relation to each other.

The person may hesitate to report a rape for various reasons, such as shame, guilt, fear of retaliation, or reluctance to deal with law enforcement officials or the judicial system. The person may even begin to doubt whether a "real" rape occurred. Rape is a traumatic crisis that disrupts the physical, psychological, social, and sexual aspects of the person's life. The most common physical injuries are bruises, black eyes, and cuts.

As a first aid provider, you must be tactful and sensitive with the person. The person may find it extremely difficult to discuss what happened and may feel fear or hostility toward a first aid provider who is the same sex as the attacker. Every effort should be made to understand the person's feelings and to respond with kindness and reassurance. The emotional trauma of rape is usually more prolonged and severe than the physical trauma. The attitude shown toward the person during their initial care can have a substantial influence—for good or ill—on future psychological and physical recovery. Convince the person to seek counseling through community resources such as a rape crisis center and to report the crime to the police. Ask the person not to change clothes or to bathe because doing so can alter legal evidence. For the same reason, suggest that the person not urinate, douche, defecate, or wash before being examined by a physician. Care for any injuries incurred during the attack. For more information, see Chapter 22, *Childbirth and Gynecologic Emergencies*.

Child Abuse and Neglect

Because child abuse usually occurs in the privacy of the home, no one knows exactly how many children are affected. **Child abuse** is doing or failing to do something that results in physical or emotional injury to a minor, and **neglect** is a caregiver's failure to provide necessities. Of reported cases, 75% involve neglect, 17% involve physical abuse, and 8% involve sexual abuse. In addition, 7% of these cases involve other forms of maltreatment, such as emotional abuse, threats, exposure to drugs and alcohol, or lack of supervision. Child abuse and neglect can cause permanent damage to a child's physical, emotional, and mental development. The physical effects can include damage to the brain, vital organs, eyes, ears, arms, and legs, which, in turn, can result in mental retardation, blindness, deafness, or loss of a limb. At its most serious, abuse or neglect can result in a child's death.

Child abuse and neglect are usually divided into four major categories: physical abuse, neglect, sexual abuse, and emotional maltreatment. Each has recognizable characteristics, and all may be encountered by a first aid provider. Still, children who have been mistreated are often afraid to tell anyone because they think they will be blamed or that no one will believe them. Other parents or adults also tend to overlook symptoms because they do not want to face the truth. The longer a child continues to be abused or is left to deal with the situation on their own, the less likely they are to make a full recovery.

The National Center on Child Abuse and Neglect has set forth physical and behavioral indicators of child abuse and neglect. The list is not intended to be exhaustive; many more indicators exist than can be included. The presence of a single indicator does not necessarily prove that child abuse or neglect has occurred **TABLE 23-3**.

However, the repeated occurrence of an indicator, the presence of several indicators in combination, or the appearance of serious injury should alert you to the possibility of child abuse **FIGURE 23-1**.

TABLE 23-3 Physical and Behavioral Indicators of Child Abuse and Neglect

Type of Child Abuse or Neglect	Physical Indicators	Behavioral Indicators
Physical abuse	■ Unexplained bruises and welts on face, lips, mouth, torso, back, buttocks, and/or thighs in various stages of healing as indicated by different colors ■ Clustered injuries on several different surface areas; formed by regular patterns reflecting the shape of the articles used to inflict the injury (electric cord, belt buckle) ■ Regularly appearing injuries after an absence, weekend, or vacation, especially about the trunk and buttocks ■ Old bruises in addition to fresh ones ■ Unexplained burns (such as those from a cigar or cigarette) especially on soles, palms, back, or buttocks ■ Immersion burns (sock-like, glove-like, doughnut-shaped on buttocks or genitalia) ■ Pattern burns, as from an electric burner or iron, for example ■ Rope burns on arms, legs, neck, or torso ■ Unexplained fractures (particularly if multiple) to skull, nose, and/or facial structures in various stages of healing ■ Multiple or spiral fractures ■ Unexplained lacerations or abrasions to mouth, lips, gums, eyes, and/or external genitalia	■ Wary of adult contacts ■ Apprehensive when other children cry ■ Behavioral extremes: aggressiveness or withdrawal ■ Frightened of parents, caregivers, or siblings ■ Afraid to go home ■ Reports injury by parents ■ Acts apathetic and does not cry despite injuries ■ Has been seen by emergency personnel for related complaints ■ Was injured several days before medical attention was sought
Physical neglect	■ Consistent hunger, poor hygiene, inappropriate dress ■ Consistent lack of supervision, especially in dangerous activities or for extended periods of time ■ Unattended physical conditions or medical needs ■ Abandonment	■ Begs, steals food ■ Extended stays at school (early arrival and late departure) ■ Constant fatigue, listlessness, or falling asleep in class ■ Alcohol or drug abuse ■ Delinquency (eg, thefts) ■ States there is no caretaker

Type of Child Abuse or Neglect	Physical Indicators	Behavioral Indicators
Sexual abuse	■ Difficulty walking or sitting ■ Torn, stained, or bloody underclothing ■ Pain or itching in genital area ■ Bruises or bleeding in external genitalia or vaginal or anal areas ■ Sexually transmitted disease, especially in preteens ■ Pregnancy	■ Unwillingness to change for gym or participate in physical education class ■ Withdrawal, fantasizing, or infantile behavior ■ Bizarre, sophisticated, or unusual sexual behavior or knowledge ■ Poor peer relationships ■ Delinquency or truancy ■ Reports sexual assault by caretaker
Emotional maltreatment	■ Speech disorders ■ Lags in physical development ■ Failure to thrive	■ Habit disorders (sucking, biting, rocking) ■ Conduct disorders (antisocial, destructive) ■ Neurotic traits (sleep disorders, inhibition of play) ■ Psychoneurotic reactions (hysteria, obsession, compulsion, phobias, hypochondria) ■ Behavior extremes (compliant, passive-aggressive, demanding) ■ Overly adaptive behavior (inappropriately adult, inappropriately infantile) ■ Developmental lags (mental, emotional) ■ Attempted suicide

Data from National Center on Child Abuse and Neglect.

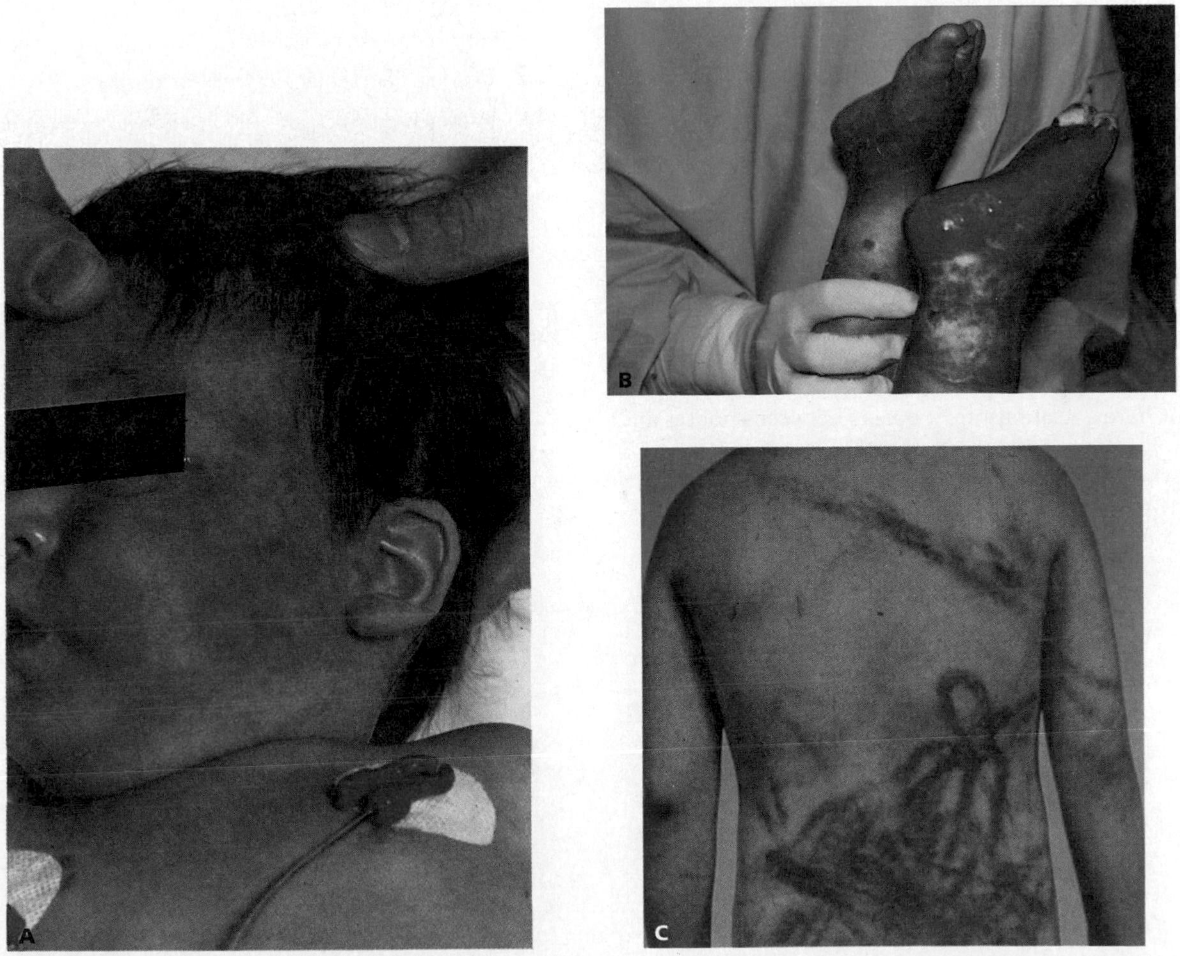

FIGURE 23-1 **A**. The face is a common target for physical abuse. **B**. Stocking/glove burns of the feet/hands are almost always inflicted injuries. **C**. Rope or cord bruises are a commonly inflicted injury.

What to Look For	What to Do

The best way to check for signs of abuse is to be alert to any unexplainable changes in a child's body or behavior.
▪ Physical abuse:
  ▪ Any injury (bruise, burn, fracture, abdominal or head injury) that cannot be explained
▪ Sexual abuse:
  ▪ Fearful behavior (nightmares, depression, unusual fears, attempts to run away)
  ▪ Abdominal pain, bedwetting, urinary tract infection, genital pain or bleeding, sexually transmitted disease
  ▪ Extreme sexual behavior that seems inappropriate for the child's age
▪ Emotional abuse:
  ▪ Sudden change in self-confidence
  ▪ Headaches or stomach aches with no medical cause
  ▪ Abnormal fears, increased nightmares
  ▪ Attempts to run away
▪ Emotional neglect:
  ▪ Failure to gain weight (especially in infants)
  ▪ Desperately affectionate behavior
  ▪ Large appetite and stealing of food
	1. Care for the neglected infant or child. Give appropriate first aid for injuries.
	2. **DO NOT** accuse parents or caregivers, especially at the scene, since you have no idea who the perpetrator of the crime might be.
	3. Report any suspected abuse to the local welfare and social service agency responsible for investigating the issue. Follow the laws for reporting in your state. Be sure to report what you saw and heard, not what you think.

Domestic Violence

Domestic violence, also known as partner abuse, spouse abuse, or battering, occurs when one person inflicts injury—either emotional or physical—upon another person with whom they had or have a relationship. It occurs between spouses and partners, parents and children, children and grandparents, and brothers and sisters. Domestic violence may be the single most common source of serious injury to women.

What to Look For	What to Do
▪ Bruises or injuries on the head, neck, or chest ▪ Type or extent of an injury that is inconsistent with the person's explanation ▪ Substantial delay between when the injury occurred and when the person sought help ▪ Injuries during pregnancy ▪ Evidence of alcohol or drug abuse ▪ Needs medical care as a result of a suicide attempt or rape	1. If you are not aware of immediate danger, but you suspect abuse, check with welfare and social service agencies. Most cities and counties, according to state law, will investigate and protect vulnerable adults. The issue cannot be remedied until it is reported. 2. Call the police if a person is in imminent danger. 3. Treat any injuries.

Elder Abuse

Elder abuse ranges from passive neglect to active assault and includes emotional abuse. Some physically abused older people report having had something thrown at them; some are pushed, grabbed, or shoved; others are slapped, bitten, or kicked. Elder abuse occurs most often in women older than 75 years. Signs of abuse may be quite obvious or subtle. Burns are a common form of elder abuse. Another form of elder abuse is financial abuse. If you suspect this is happening, report it to the police.

FYI

Are You Being Abused?

Just one "yes" answer to these questions means you are involved in an abusive relationship. If so, you are not alone and you have choices. No one deserves to be abused. Does your partner:

- Threaten to hurt you or your children?
- Say it is your fault if they hit you; then promise it will not happen again (but it does)?
- Put you down in public?
- Keep you from contacting family or friends?
- Throw you down or push, hit, choke, kick, or slap you?
- Force you to have sex when you do not want to?

Data from American College of Obstetricians and Gynecologists, www.acog.org.

What to Look For	What to Do

▪ Physical injury:
  ▪ Bruises, cuts, burn or rope marks, and broken bones that cannot be explained
  ▪ Comments about being battered
  ▪ The refusal of the caregiver to allow you to visit the older person alone
▪ Lack of physical care:
  ▪ Dehydration, malnourishment, weight loss, and poor hygiene
  ▪ Bed sores, soiled bedding
  ▪ Unmet medical needs
  ▪ Comments about being mistreated
▪ Unusual behaviors:
  ▪ Agitation, withdrawal, fear or anxiety, apathy
  ▪ Reports of being treated improperly
	1. If you are not aware of immediate danger, but you suspect abuse, check with welfare and social service agencies. Most cities and counties, according to state law, will investigate and protect vulnerable adults. The issue cannot be remedied until it is reported.
	2. If you suspect elder abuse in an institutional setting, such as a nursing home, report your concerns to your state long-term care ombudsman. Each state has a long-term care ombudsman to investigate and address nursing home complaints.
	3. Call the police if a person is in imminent danger.
	4. First aid includes calling 9-1-1 when needed and treating any injuries.

PREP KIT

Ready for Review

- When emotions lead to violence or other inappropriate activities, it is known as a psychological emergency.
- Depression is one of the most common and treatable of all mental illnesses.
- Suicide in the United States is increasingly an issue for adolescents, college-age students, and older people. The National Suicide Prevention Lifeline, at 1-800-273-8255, is a 24-hour service that is available to anyone in suicidal crisis or emotional distress. (By July 2022, 9-8-8 will be the nationwide number.)
- First aid for an emotional injury means being supportive of people with emotional injuries, whether the injuries are a result of physical injury or excessive or unbearable strain on the person's emotions.
- Because child abuse and neglect usually occur in the privacy of the home, no one knows exactly how many children are affected.
- Domestic violence may be the single most common source of serious injury to women.
- The types of physical abuse of older people vary from passive neglect to active assault.

Vital Vocabulary

child abuse Doing something or failing to do something that can result in physical or emotional injury or neglect of a child.

depression A persistent mood of sadness, despair, and discouragement.

domestic violence Injury (emotional or physical) that a person inflicts upon another person with whom they had or have a relationship.

elder abuse Any action on the part of an older person's family member, caregiver, or other associated person that takes advantage of the older person, their property, or emotional state.

neglect Refusal or failure on the part of the caregiver to provide life necessities.

psychological emergency Any situation in which a person is experiencing extreme distress, is unable to cope with everyday life, or is in danger of hurting themselves or others.

suicide Any willful act that ends one's own life.

Assessment in Action

Your good friend has been married for about 3 years. He is normally a quiet, reserved person who cares deeply for others. Lately, you have seen him change; he has been argumentative, jokes inappropriately, and appears to have a hard time concentrating. He no longer engages in several of his hobbies and does little else when not at work. You then find out that he separated from his wife about 1 month ago.

Directions: Circle Yes if you agree with the statement; circle No if you disagree.

1. Your friend is exhibiting an overactive reaction to his situation.
   YES NO
2. You should avoid being too argumentative with your friend.
   YES NO
3. You should not give sedatives to calm him down.
   YES NO
4. Supervision and perhaps even some type of professional therapy may be helpful for your friend.
   YES NO
5. Letting him talk to you about his situation will make things worse.
   YES NO

Check Your Knowledge

Directions: Circle Yes if you agree with the statement; circle No if you disagree.

1. Abnormal behavior may be due to a psychological condition or a physical condition.
   YES NO
2. Low blood glucose in a person with diabetes can affect behavior.
   YES NO

PREP KIT continued

3. Depression cannot be treated.

YES **NO**

4. The rate of suicide for men is higher than the rate for women.

YES **NO**

5. Most people who talk about suicide are not serious.

YES **NO**

6. The only way for you to react to an aggressive person is with anger.

YES **NO**

7. A failure to gain weight may be a sign of emotional neglect in an infant.

YES **NO**

8. Women are rarely subjected to domestic violence.

YES **NO**

9. Burns are a common form of elder abuse.

YES **NO**

10. Feeling shaky during an emergency is not normal.

YES **NO**

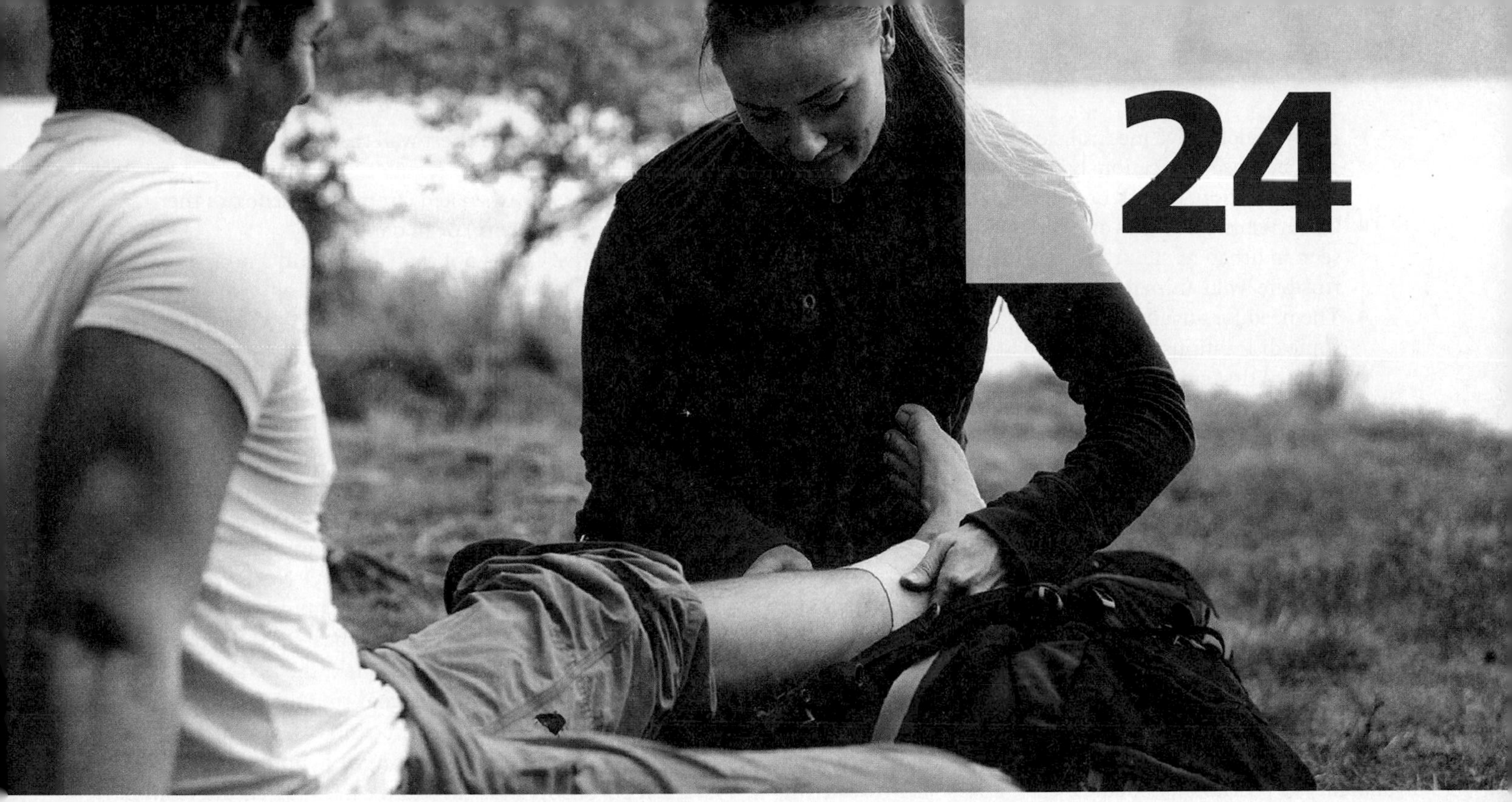

24

Wilderness First Aid

CHAPTER AT A GLANCE

- Wilderness First Aid
- Cardiac Arrest
- Dislocations
- Spinal Injury
- Splinting Femur Fractures
- Avalanche Burial
- Altitude Illness
- Lightning
- Wild Animal Attacks
- Wilderness Evacuation
- Signaling for Help

Wilderness First Aid

At some time, anyone living, working, traveling, or recreating in remote locations will probably encounter dangers unfamiliar to most people. Regardless of precautions, injuries and illnesses happen.

The term **wilderness**, as defined by the Wilderness Medical Society (WMS), is a remote geographic location more than 1 hour from definitive medical care. According to that definition, wilderness could describe a variety of situations, including the following:

- Recreation (eg, fishing, camping, hiking, hunting)
- Occupations in remote areas (such as farming, forestry, fishing)
- Urban areas with overwhelmed emergency medical services (EMS) after a natural or manmade disaster
- Residences in remote communities (such as farms, ranches, vacation homes)
- Developing countries

The millions of people in these wildernesses should be as medically prepared as possible to manage a condition for others and for themselves. First aid with a wilderness focus seems indispensable in the following situations:

- Occurrence of injuries and illnesses in the outdoors, where adverse environmental conditions such as heat, cold, altitude, darkness, rain, or snow may be a major concern

- Delay of definitive medical care for hours or days because of location, bad weather, lack of transportation, or lack of communication
- Occurrence of injuries and illnesses not commonly seen in urban or suburban areas (eg, altitude illness, frostbite, wild animal encounters)
- The need for advanced medical care (eg, reduction of some dislocations, wound cleansing)
- Limited first aid supplies and equipment
- Need to make difficult decisions (cardiopulmonary resuscitation [CPR], evacuation) in a remote setting

Most first aid texts and training courses describe situations in which EMS response is expected within 10 to 20 minutes. In these cases, the first aid provider usually helps for only a few minutes before an ambulance arrives. They report what they found and what they did. When the injured person is transported to a medical facility, the first aid provider's job is finished.

Wilderness first aid is similar to that needed in urban situations, except that extra or extended skills are sometimes needed. Consideration must be given to time, distance, and availability of professional medical care. A first aid provider in the wilderness may have to remain many hours or days with a sick or injured person.

Cardiac Arrest

Because heart activity must be restored within a short time (which may require defibrillation and medications) for a person with cardiac arrest to survive, CPR has limited use in a wilderness or remote setting, especially if severe trauma such as massive head or chest injury, severe blood loss, or a severed spinal cord accompanies the cardiac arrest. In addition, CPR is difficult to continue during a wilderness evacuation.

The WMS recommends *stopping* CPR in the following situations:

- The person revives.
- The rescuers are exhausted.
- The rescuers are in danger.
- The person is turned over to higher-level trained personnel.
- The person does not respond to prolonged resuscitation efforts.

The State of Alaska Cold Injuries Guidelines, the WMS, and the National Association of EMS Physicians (NAEMSP) say that, in the following situations, CPR should not be started:

- The person has been submerged in cold water for more than 1 hour.
- The person has a core temperature of less than 50°F (10°C).
- The person has obvious signs of death or fatal injuries (eg, rigor mortis, decapitation, decomposition).
- The person is frozen (eg, ice formation in the airway).
- The person has a chest wall that is so stiff that compressions are impossible.
- Rescuers are exhausted (from the rescue or other strenuous activity) or in danger.
- Definitive care is not available within 3 hours.

CPR for People with Hypothermia

The person with severe hypothermia must be handled very gently. The cold heart is very prone to spontaneous ventricular fibrillation due to movement. Even cautious movement of the person may induce ventricular fibrillation.

It is difficult to assess breathing in an unresponsive person with hypothermia. If the person is unresponsive and not breathing, check the carotid pulse for 1 minute. If there is no pulse rate after 1 minute, start CPR. **DO NOT** wait to check the person's temperature. **DO NOT** wait until the person is rewarmed to start CPR. Prevent further heat loss by removing the person's wet clothes; insulate and shield the person from wind and additional cold exposure. Avoid rough handling and activate the EMS system as soon as possible. Continue CPR until EMS arrives. In a person with severe hypothermia, CPR can be delayed ("scoop and run") and can be given intermittently during evacuation if it is not possible or safe to perform continuous CPR. CPR can be given for several hours, if necessary. Deliver chest compressions at 100 to 120 beats per minute.

CPR for People in an Avalanche

Avalanche-related deaths are on the rise in North America due to winter recreational activities (eg, backcountry skiing and snowboarding, helicopter and snowcat skiing, snowmobiling, out-of-bounds skiing, ice climbing, mountaineering, and snowshoeing). The most common causes of avalanche-related death are suffocation (hypoxia), injury, hypothermia, or a combination of these three. If the person is unresponsive and is not breathing, begin CPR. Use an automated external defibrillator (AED) as soon as it becomes available. If a person has an airway obstructed by snow or ice and has been buried for 35 minutes or longer, resuscitation should not be attempted. However, if there is no airway obstruction, resuscitation is possible and should be attempted.

CPR for Drowning

First aid providers should give CPR as soon as an unresponsive submersed person is removed from the water. If you are alone, give five sets (about 2 minutes) of CPR before leaving the person to activate the EMS system and get an AED. If you are not alone, send someone to activate the EMS system and get an AED while you continue giving CPR. An AED should be used as soon as it becomes available.

People with only respiratory arrest usually respond after a few rescue breaths. Rescue breathing can be started once the person is in shallow water; however, chest compressions are not recommended in water and may not be effective. There is no need to attempt to clear the airway of water because only a small amount of water is aspirated by most drowning people and is absorbed by the body. **DO NOT** try to remove water by performing abdominal thrusts. If abdominal thrusts are needed, get the patient out of the water to a firm surface as quickly as possible and then begin compressions.

If vomiting occurs during CPR, turn the person to the side and remove the vomitus using a finger or a cloth. If a spinal injury is suspected, the person should be turned as a unit with no twisting. A suggestion is to keep the person's nose and navel pointed in the same direction as they are turned.

CPR for People Struck by Lightning

The National Weather Service estimates an average of 49 deaths occur from lightning strikes in the United States each year. The main cause of death in these people is cardiac arrest. When multiple people are struck at the same time by lightning, rescuers should give the highest priority to people who are unresponsive and not breathing by beginning CPR. An AED should be used as soon as it becomes available.

Dislocations

In a wilderness situation, reducing (a technical term that means aligning) some dislocated joints is recommended. The WMS gives the following reasons for reducing a joint dislocation quickly after it happens:

1. Reduction is easier immediately after the injury, before swelling develops.
2. It is easier to transport a person after reduction.
3. Reduction dramatically relieves pain.
4. The joint can be stabilized and better protected.
5. Reduction lessens the possibility of jeopardizing circulation in the extremity. (If the blood supply is cut off, gangrene could develop, which could result in amputation.)
6. Several simple dislocations can be reduced using simple and safe techniques.

A dislocation is considered simple if it involves the anterior (front) part of the shoulder, a finger, or the patella (the kneecap, not the knee itself). **DO NOT** attempt to reduce a dislocated elbow or hip. Elbow and hip dislocations resemble fractures; reduction techniques for those joints are painful and can cause further injury.

Shoulder Dislocation

Anterior (frontal) shoulder joint dislocations account for more than 90% of shoulder dislocations **FIGURE 24-1**.

There are several methods for reducing a shoulder dislocation; two of the easiest methods are discussed here. With either method, stop if pain increases or resistance is met. **DO NOT** try pulling on the person's arm with your foot in the person's armpit. Check the circulation, sensation, and movement of the hand before and after reducing the dislocation.

What to Look For	What to Do
▪ The person is in extreme pain. ▪ Because the problem often reoccurs, the person can identify the dislocation if it has happened before. ▪ The upper arm is held away from the body in various positions and cannot be brought next to the body into a sling-type position. ▪ The person is unable to touch the uninjured shoulder with the hand of the injured extremity. ▪ Compare the injured shoulder with the uninjured one. The shoulder joint will appear squared off or flattened and a prominence may be seen or felt in the front of the shoulder. ▪ Numbness or paralysis in the arm from pressure, pinching blood vessels, or nerves.	*Simple hanging traction method:* 1. Lay the person facedown on a surface high enough so that the injured arm can hang over the side. Place some cushioning (a folded towel or clothing) under the armpit, between the arm and the surface **FIGURE 24-2**. 2. Attach a 5- to 10-lb (2- to 5-kg) weight to the person's lower arm, between the elbow and the wrist. Cushion and strap the weight, being careful not to impede circulation. Keep the person's palm facing inward. 3. It may take up to 60 minutes to stretch and tire the muscles, allowing the joint to pop back in. 4. After successful reduction, stabilize the arm with a sling and swathe. Secure a sling and swathe (binder) using the method shown in Chapter 16, *Splinting Extremities*.
	5. The patient will need a radiograph to ensure there was no fracture. 6. After successful reduction, stabilize the arm with a sling and secure the sling with a swathe (binder) **FIGURE 24-3**. *Note:* This method should be used to reduce a shoulder dislocation when professional medical are is more than 1 hour away. There are several other methods that can be used to reduce a shoulder dislocation, such as the Mulch technique, which may be taught in a wilderness first aid course.

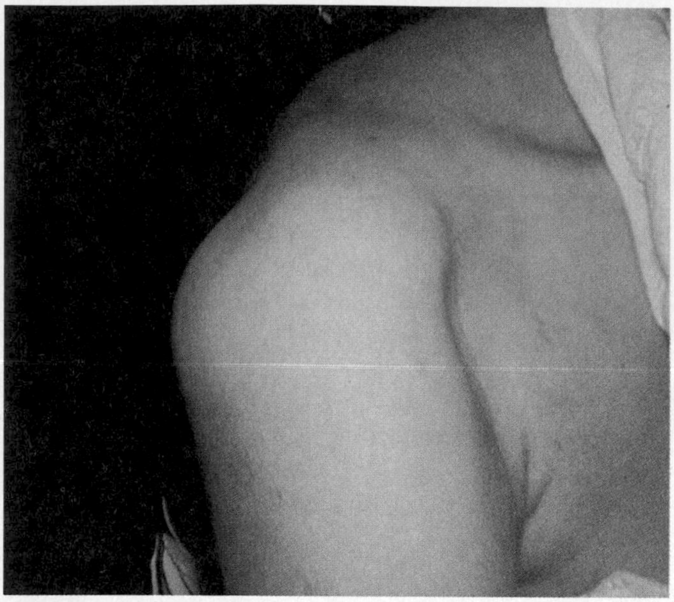

FIGURE 24-1 The shoulder almost always dislocates anteriorly. Note the absence of the normal rounded appearance of the shoulder.

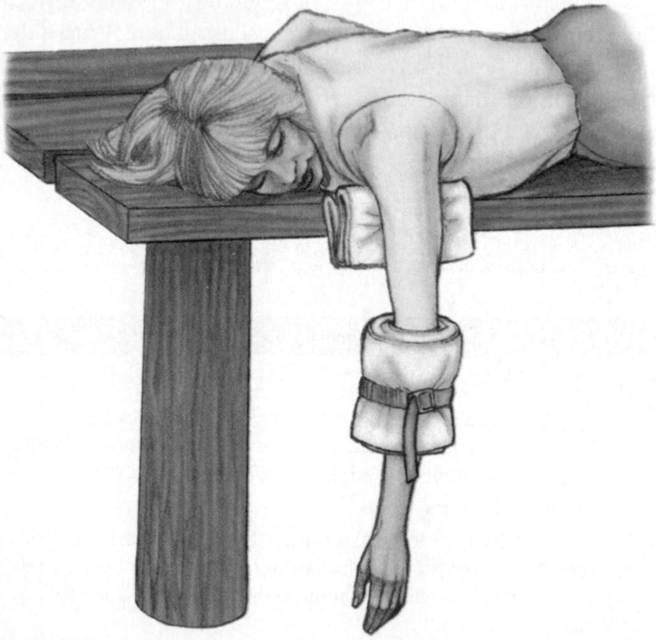

FIGURE 24-2 Simple hanging traction to reduce an anterior shoulder dislocation.

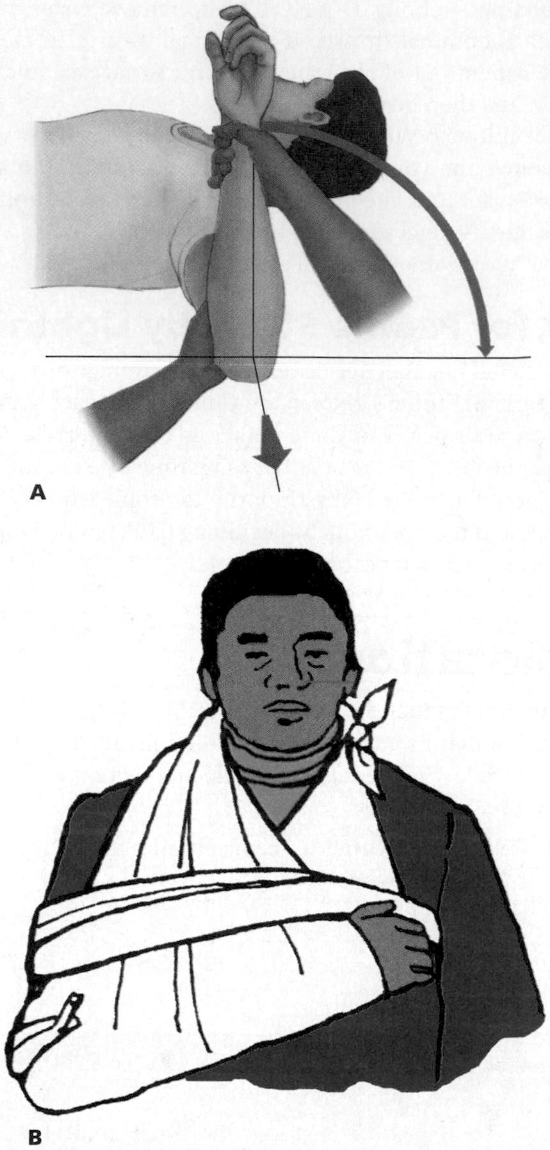

FIGURE 24-3 Sling and swathe (binder).

Finger Dislocation

The fingers are injured easily, and even a minor injury may cause a dislocation **FIGURE 24-4**.

Often, people with this injury can reduce the finger dislocation themselves. In a remote location, you should try to reduce a finger dislocation only once. **DO NOT** attempt to reduce a dislocation at the base of the index finger or at the base of the thumb—those areas may require surgery for reduction.

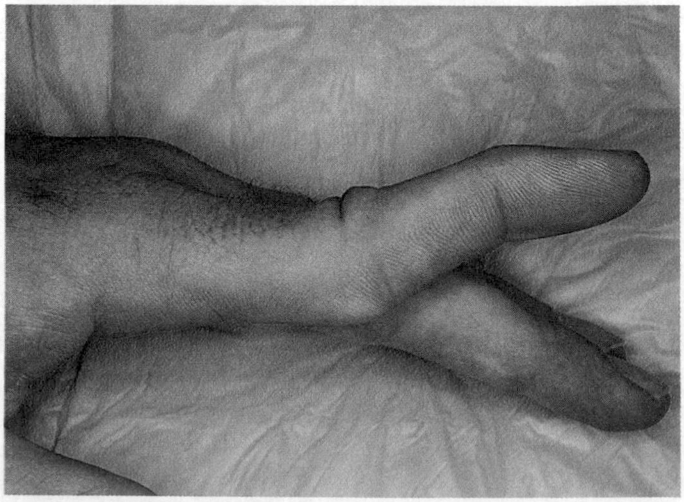

FIGURE 24-4 Dislocation of the finger joint. Do not be tempted to try to "pop" the joint back into place.

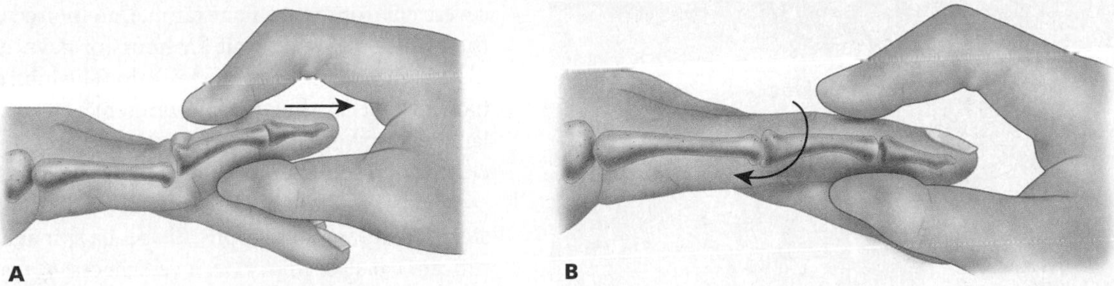

A B

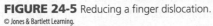

FIGURE 24-5 Reducing a finger dislocation.

What to Look For	What to Do
▪ Deformity and inability to use or bend the finger ▪ Pain and swelling ▪ An abnormal position of the two adjoining bones; looks like a lump at the joint	To reduce a finger dislocation, use one of two methods. *Method 1*: **1.** Hold the end of the finger with one hand and the rest of the finger in the other. **2.** Gently hyperextend the dislocated joint (bend it backwards). **3.** Pull gentle traction. **4.** Push the dislocated bone into place. **5.** Unbend the finger. **6.** Buddy tape it to the next finger. **7.** Splint the finger in the position of function (fingers and hand in a cupping shape, as though holding a baseball).
	Method 2 **FIGURE 24-5**: **1.** Wrap the finger with a piece of cloth to prevent slippage. Hold the end of the finger with one hand and the rest of the finger in the other. **2.** Pull the end of the finger first in the direction it is pointing, then, while maintaining traction, gently swing it back into the normal anatomic position. *Regardless of whether the reduction is successful:* **1.** Stabilize the joint in the position of function (fingers and hand in a cupping shape, as though holding a baseball) by the buddy-taping method—using adhesive tape to secure the injured finger to an adjacent uninjured finger.

Kneecap Dislocation

For most dislocated kneecaps (patella), you should only apply an ice pack and use a splint to stabilize the leg in place as you found it. For remote locations, however, always consider reducing a dislocated kneecap by using the method described in the following table. All dislocations, whether successfully reduced in the field or not, should be seen by a physician.

What to Look For	What to Do
▪ Some people have recurrent dislocations of the patella (kneecap) and can tell you what is wrong. ▪ The patella has moved to the outside of the knee joint (large bulge under the skin) with the leg bent **FIGURE 24-6**. ▪ The person is in pain. ▪ Compare the injured portion with the patella on the other leg.	**1.** Slowly straighten the knee as you gently push the kneecap back into its normal position. Straightening alone may replace the kneecap. **2.** Stabilize the leg straight. The person usually can walk on the injured leg. **3.** With the knee extended (straight) and stabilized, the person may be able to walk well enough for self-evacuation. Because of the heavy physical demands and usually higher altitudes in the backcountry, carrying a person can take 8 to 16 rescuers rotating the task. In the wilderness, a ski pole or a tree branch makes a good walking aid. Helicopter evacuation usually is not justified for a kneecap dislocation. **4.** Seek follow-up care from a physician.

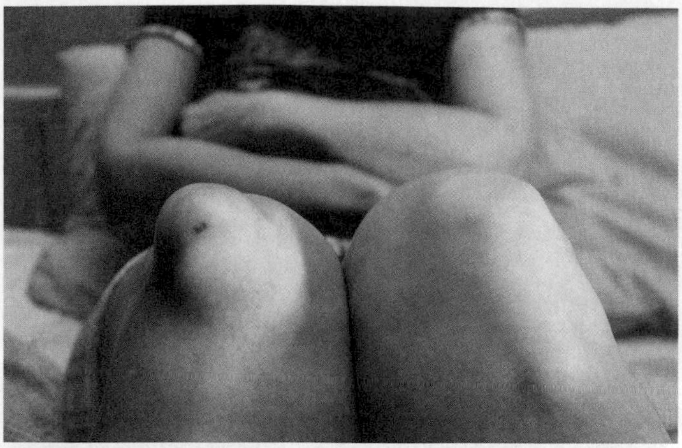

FIGURE 24-6 A dislocated patella typically will appear with the patella displaced lateral to the knee and with the knee moderately flexed.

Spinal Injury

The necessity of restricting spinal motion after trauma is well known. A person with a cervical spinal injury who is moved may become quadriplegic or die. In urban settings, first aid providers should have the person remain as still as possible and wait for EMS to arrive. **DO NOT** apply a cervical collar.

In the wilderness, spinal stabilization may not always be necessary—such a procedure can be difficult, impractical, impossible, or even dangerous during prolonged evacuation in severe environments. For example, an injured climber far above the timberline could wait for hours or days, depending on the distance someone has to go for help. The injured climber would have to wait in a hostile environment and risk death from avalanche, rockfall, or hypothermia. However, if the person were cleared of a spinal injury, they could self-evacuate.

Spinal fractures can be difficult to determine, even by physicians reading radiographs. Suspect a spinal injury when a significant cause of injury (ie, a vehicle crash involving ejection, a rollover, or high speed; a head injury causing unresponsiveness; penetrating wounds of the neck or trunk; diving into shallow water; fall from a height; collisions involving recreational vehicles or bicycles) has occurred.

To clear a spinal injury in the wilderness, determine if the person is reliable or unreliable. A reliable person meets the following criteria:

- Alert (knows name, day of week and where they are)
- Not intoxicated by drugs or alcohol
- Calm, cooperative
- Has no painful, distracting injury

An unreliable person has one or more of the following criteria:

- Altered mental status
- Intoxicated by drugs or alcohol
- Combative, confused
- Has a painful, distracting injury

What to Look For	What to Do
A reliable person with: ▪ Back pain and leg numbness and tingling ▪ Tenderness/pain when you run fingers all the way down the spine (if possible); press each bump of vertebrae and on the depressions produced on each side when you touch or push on the bones.	When a spinal injury is suspected: **1.** Send for medical help. **DO NOT** attempt to evacuate the person. Wait for trained rescuers with proper equipment. **2.** Leave the person on the ground. Cover to prevent heat loss by log rolling the person, keeping the nose and navel pointing in the same direction, and place insulating materials under and over the person.
A reliable person who fails the following tests for sensation and movement (test all four extremities): ▪ Pinch several fingers/toes with the person's eyes closed and ask, "Can you feel this? Where am I touching you?" ▪ Ask, "Can you wiggle your fingers/toes?" ▪ Ask, "Can you squeeze my hands?/ Can you push and pull your feet simultaneously against my hands?"	**1.** Restrict the person against movement. Improvised cervical collars (ie, blanket, SAM splint) alone are inadequate. ▪ Use rolled up blankets on both sides of the person's head. **2.** Tell the person to remain as still as possible and wait for medical help.
A reliable person who is injured and: ▪ Is alert, not intoxicated, and has no distracting injuries. ▪ Does not report neck pain or neurologic symptoms (ie, tingling, numbness). ▪ Has no neck tenderness when felt, no loss of sensation when fingers and toes are pinched, can move the fingers and toes, and can squeeze your hands and push and pull their feet against your hands. ▪ Can rotate their neck 30° left and right when requested.	**1.** Suspect no spinal injury. **2.** Treat other injuries (ie, wounds, bruises, fractures).
An unreliable person with: ▪ A significant cause of injury	**1.** Assume that a spinal injury exists. **2.** Restrict the person against movement. **3.** Tell the person remain as still as possible and wait for professional medical help.

Splinting Femur Fractures

A person with a femur fracture can easily experience 2 quarts (about 2 L) of blood loss in the thigh and develop massive swelling. Because EMS personnel have the training, experience, and equipment, it is best to let them apply traction splints, if possible. However, you can use first aid methods to stabilize a femur fracture. These methods are detailed in Chapter 16, *Splinting Extremities*.

Q&A

Do improvised traction splints work?

Although the advantages of stabilizing a broken femur by applying a traction splint are cited in various manuals, there are dissenting opinions about the effectiveness of improvised traction splints. For example, the Outward Bound organization says, "Improvised traction splints for field use employing ski poles, canoe paddles, and other pieces of equipment are usually more architecturally interesting than medically useful. The simplest, safest, and most universal splint is firm immobilization on a long board or litter without traction." The WMS suggests stabilizing the fractured extremity to the uninjured leg with adequate padding and placing padding behind the knee to create a slight bend, which is more comfortable than being straight.

Avalanche Burial

Avalanches are sliding masses of snow that may also contain rocks, soil, or ice. Since the early 1970s, the number of deaths caused by avalanches has increased rapidly as a result of the tremendous growth in backcountry winter mountain travel (eg, skiing, mountaineering, snowmobiling).

Snow sets up solid after an avalanche. It is almost impossible for people to dig themselves out, even if they are buried under less than a foot of snow. The pressure of several feet of snow sometimes is so great that people are unable to expand their chests to breathe. A completely buried person has a poor chance of survival. During the first 15 minutes, more people are found alive than dead. Between 16 and 30 minutes after an avalanche, an equal number are found dead and alive (50% chance of survival). After 30 minutes, more are found dead than alive.

Most people buried by an avalanche die of suffocation; therefore, in the absence of fatal injuries, speed of extrication from the avalanche and existence of an air pocket are the main factors that determine survival of a buried person. There are no documented reports of anyone surviving a burial of 7 feet (2 m) or more.

FYI

Avalanche Rescue

If you survive an avalanche, follow these steps to find other people:

1. Send a person to notify the ski patrol immediately if you are near a ski area and there are several rescuers. If you are the only rescuer, do a fast surface search for clues before leaving to notify the ski patrol. In remote backcountry, all survivors should remain and search until they cannot or should not continue.
2. With a piece of equipment, clothing, or tree branch, mark the spot where a person was last seen.
3. Search the area below the last-seen point for any clues of the person. Make probes into likely burial spots with a ski, ski pole, or tree limb.
4. If beacons were being used, all survivors must immediately switch their units to receive mode and listen for a beeping sound from buried beacons.
5. If a second avalanche is possible, place one person in a safe location to shout a warning so rescuers can flee to safety.

Rescue transceivers or beacons are an efficient way of locating people. Organized probe lines have found more people than any other method, but because of the time involved, most of the people were dead. Trained search dogs can locate buried people quickly, but they often are brought to the scene only after long periods of burial. One trained dog can search more effectively than 30 searchers.

What to Look For	What to Do
Avalanches kill and injure in two ways: ▪ From the serious injury the person acquires while tumbling down an avalanche path. Trees, rocks, cliffs, and the wrenching action of snow are hazards. About one-third of all deaths are related to trauma, especially trauma to the head and neck. ▪ Snow burial, which causes suffocation in the other two-thirds of avalanche deaths. Inhaled snow clogs the mouth and nose, and people can suffocate quickly if they are buried with the airway already blocked.	After you have first checked for further avalanche danger and then found a person, follow these steps: 1. Quickly free the person's head, chest, and stomach. 2. Send for help. 3. Clear the person's airway and check breathing. 4. If not breathing, begin CPR. 5. Check for severe bleeding. 6. Examine for and restrict spinal movement. 7. Treat for hypothermia, if suspected.

TABLE 24-1 Characteristics of Altitude Illnesses

	AMS	HAPE	HACE
Elevation	Above 8,000 ft (2,438 m)	Usually above 10,000 ft (3,048 m)	Above 12,000 ft (3,658 m)
Time after ascent	Within several hours, up to 2 days later	3 to 4 days, possibly later	Within 24 hours, up to 7 days or later
Cause and symptoms	Symptoms of hypoxia: headache, sleep disturbance, fatigue, shortness of breath, dizziness, loss of appetite, vomiting	Symptoms of fluid in the lungs: shortness of breath, dry cough, mild chest pain, weakness, insomnia, rapid pulse, cyanosis, crackles (formerly known as rales), or gurgling sounds	Symptoms of increased fluid and pressure in the brain: severe headache (unrelieved), vomiting, Cheyne-Stokes breathing (irregular breathing pattern that includes periods of apnea [no breathing]), ataxia (irregular gait or lack of coordination), unconsciousness
First aid	■ Stop ascending or return to a lower altitude. ■ Drink fluids. ■ Rest. ■ Take aspirin or ibuprofen according to package directions. ■ Take acetazolamide. ■ If you are trained, give high-flow supplemental oxygen, if available.	■ Descend at least 2,000 ft (610 m). ■ Seek professional medical attention. ■ **DO NOT** go down alone. ■ **DO NOT** delay descent. ■ If immediate descent is not possible: • Give high-flow supplemental oxygen, if available and you are trained. • Use a portable hyperbaric chamber, if available and you are trained.	■ Descend 4,000 ft (1,219 m). ■ Seek professional medical attention. ■ **DO NOT** go down alone. ■ **DO NOT** delay descent. ■ Give high-flow supplemental oxygen, if available and you are trained. ■ Use a portable hyperbaric chamber, if available and you are trained.

Altitude Illness

If you live in or visit mountainous regions, you need to know about altitude illness. Altitude illness is not simply an exotic affliction of mountaineers—it is a common environmental risk to which millions of people are exposed, often without adequate knowledge.

Altitude illnesses actually are a spectrum of a single problem, **hypoxia**. Hypoxia occurs when the body's tissues do not have enough oxygen. Altitude illnesses include **acute mountain sickness (AMS)**, **high-altitude pulmonary edema (HAPE)**, and **high-altitude cerebral edema (HACE)** TABLE 24-1.

The least serious altitude illness is AMS, which includes symptoms such as dizziness, nausea, headache, and shortness of breath and is the result of the high altitude. It affects about one in four people from lower elevations who visit areas that are 6,000 to 12,000 feet (1,829 to 3,658 m) above sea level. Such elevations are common at ski resorts and on mountain hiking trails.

The actual incidence of altitude illness varies with rate of ascent and altitude attained. A study published in the *Annals of Emergency Medicine* cited about 67% of climbers on Mt. Rainier in Washington have at least mild AMS because of rapid ascent to a moderately higher altitude. The incidence of AMS in a study of Colorado skiers at lower altitudes (usually one day's ascent from Denver or lower) was only 15% to 40%.

Although anyone can get altitude illness, certain factors increase the risk. Under similar conditions, different people sometimes respond quite differently to altitude. For most people, at least four factors determine whether they will be sick or well at a higher altitude: (1) the speed of ascent (the slower the climb, the fewer the symptoms); (2) the altitude reached (the higher one goes, the more likely one will become ill); (3) health at the time (malnutrition, dehydration, fatigue, and any of several illnesses increase the risk); and (4) individual differences and genetic influences.

Altitude illness occurs because oxygen levels decrease as elevation increases, and it takes a few days to adapt to the thinner air. At 11,500 feet (3,505 m), the amount of oxygen in the air is about 65% the amount at sea level, so the body struggles to maintain normal levels of oxygen. As the person breathes more deeply, they "blow off" more carbon dioxide than normal, creating a more alkaline (less acidic) condition in the body, which in turn causes altitude illnesses.

It is important to recognize the symptoms of altitude illness and take steps to treat it. In a small number of people, acute altitude illnesses such as HAPE, in which fluid builds up in the lungs, or HACE, in which fluid collects in the brain, can occur. HAPE and HACE occur when reduced oxygen causes capillary leakage and swelling of body tissues. Although they are uncommon, both conditions can be fatal in less than 12 hours.

At 18,000 feet (5,486 m), humans reach their ceiling and cannot stay for more than a few weeks. Any person at sea level who is quickly taken to 20,000 feet (6,096 m) will be almost incapacitated in less than one-half hour and death will occur soon thereafter.

What to Look For	What to Do
The following symptoms (often mistaken for a cold, flu, or hangover) typically occur during the first 12 hours: ▪ Headache (most common symptom) ▪ Loss of appetite	1. Seek professional medical help if any of the following more serious symptoms appear: ▪ Persistent cough ▪ Shortness of breath while resting ▪ Noisy breathing ▪ Loss of balance

What to Look For	What to Do
▪ Nausea ▪ Insomnia ▪ Fatigue ▪ Shortness of breath with exertion Three-fourths of all people who travel from sea level to above 8,000 feet (2,438 m) have at least one symptom (usually a headache), and the rest have two or more symptoms.	▪ Confusion ▪ Vomiting 2. Have the person rest and let the body acclimatize for a few days. 3. If the person recently ascended to above 6,000 feet (1,829 m) and does not feel better in 1 to 2 days, they should see a physician. 4. If it is not possible for the person to see a physician and symptoms continue, the person should descend 2,000 to 3,000 feet (610 to 914 m), rest, and drink plenty of fluids. Aspirin or a similar pain reliever can be taken according the package directions for a mild headache. 5. If rest and over-the-counter (OTC) medications do not provide relief, consult a physician, who might administer oxygen or prescribe medication. 6. If HACE or HAPE is suspected, early descent is required, because these conditions are serious. The next best step after descent is to breathe additional oxygen so that the inspired oxygen pressure equals that at sea level. This will relieve the headache and make breathing easier. Ibuprofen may also be given if headache is not relieved.

FYI

Preventing Altitude Illness

You can take several measures to lower your risk of getting altitude sickness. Start slowly and avoid overexerting yourself. If possible, gain altitude slowly to allow your body to adjust. By going easy, you allow your body to acclimatize; that is, adjust to different conditions. Simply put, your body becomes more efficient at using oxygen. Unfortunately, the effects of acclimatization do not last after you return to your normal altitude. You must repeat the process whenever you return to higher elevations.

If you cannot or will not take the time, protective medications are available by prescription. Acetazolamide (Diamox) has been effectively used to prevent AMS for more than 30 years. Acetazolamide also seems to prevent HAPE and HACE, although that is almost impossible to prove because HAPE and HACE are rare.

Side effects of acetazolamide include increased urination and tingling or numbness in the fingers and toes. If you are allergic to sulfa drugs, you may be allergic to acetazolamide. Also, you should wear a sunscreen with a sun protection factor (SPF) of at least 15 while taking the drug, since it may increase the risk of sunburn.

Acetazolamide is effective for most lowlanders going to moderate altitudes and perhaps for high-altitude residents returning after a short stay at low altitude. It has been called an artificial acclimatizer. Just how much acetazolamide to take and when to take it are debated. Follow the prescribed dosage; for adults, it is 125 mg twice per day, starting as early as 2 days prior to ascent.

Because dehydration can be a factor at high altitudes, drink plenty of fluids such as water and juice. Mountain air is drier than air at lower elevations. You are drinking enough fluid when your urine is clear. Tea, coffee, and alcohol cause more frequent urination and may lead to dehydration. Eat foods that are easy to digest for a few days.

Avoid taking sleeping pills because they tend to cause shallow breathing while you sleep, which can make it difficult for your body to get enough oxygen. Likewise, do not smoke because it increases carbon monoxide levels in the blood, which diminish the body's ability to use oxygen.

Other Altitude-Related Illnesses

Other altitude-related illnesses include the following:

- *Pharyngitis and bronchitis.* Because of dry air, a sore throat and coughing may develop. Care involves drinking fluids, applying an OTC antibiotic ointment in the nostrils, and sucking on hard candy or throat lozenges.
- *Peripheral edema.* The hands, ankles, and/or face (around the eyes) may swell at high altitude. If possible, raise the affected arms and/or legs. After descending or with acclimatization to higher altitudes, the swelling diminishes. Descend if signs of more serious altitude illness appear.

FYI

Altitude Increases Sunburn Risk

Skiers, hikers, and others who enjoy outdoor activities in the mountains have long believed that it takes less time to sunburn in the mountains than at lower levels. Research confirms that the higher the altitude, the quicker a person will develop sunburn. Ultraviolet (UV) light energy readings were taken at solar noon in direct sunlight on cloudless days at Vail, Colorado; Orlando, Florida; and New York, New York. The high-altitude regions in the United States include areas with some of the fastest population growth, and it is vital that people living or visiting these regions recognize the increase in UV exposure at higher altitudes and take precautions to prevent sunburn.

Data from Rigel DS, Rigel EG, Rigel AC. Effects of altitude and latitude on ambient UVB radiation. *J Am Acad Dermatol.* 1999;40:114–116.

Lightning

Lightning is awesome and frightening **FIGURE 24-7**. The National Oceanic and Atmospheric Administration reports about 10% of lightning strikes to humans result in death. Lightning is one of the leading environmental causes of death in the United

States, according to the Centers for Disease Control and Prevention **FIGURE 24-8**.

In the past, farmers, sailors, and other outdoor workers in isolated areas tended to be the people the most frequently injured by lightning. Today, a larger proportion of people injured by lightning are hikers, campers, golfers, and others who are outdoors for recreational purposes.

Lightning deaths occur more often during daytime hours when people are active and outdoors. Most occur during the months of June through September, when thunderstorms are most frequent. There are more thunderstorm days in the South than in any other region of the United States. Thunderstorms occur frequently over high mountains. People are better protected in urban areas where high buildings have metal frames and lightning devices.

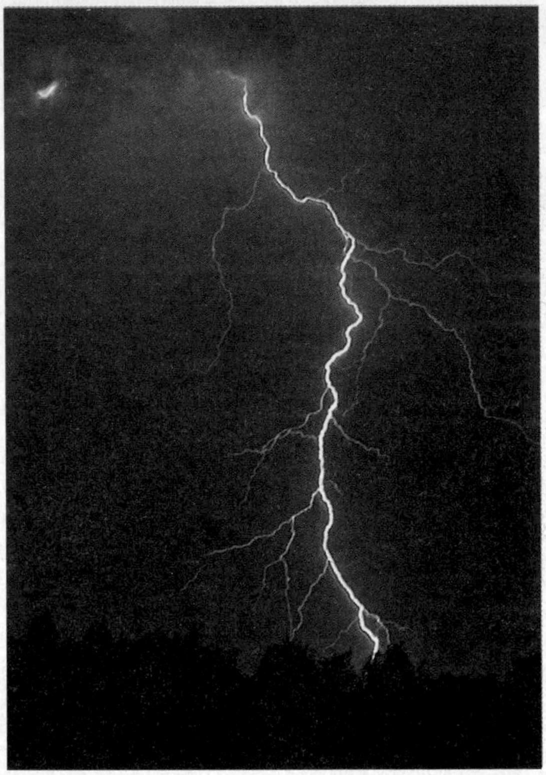

FIGURE 24-7 Lightning strike.

How Lightning Injures

Lightning injures in five ways. A *direct strike* is actually being struck by lightning. Lightning is most likely to hit a person in the open who has been unable to find shelter. Any conductor of electricity that the person carries, especially if it is metal and carried above the shoulder level (eg, an open umbrella or a bag of golf clubs slung over the shoulder), increases the chances of a direct hit.

FYI

Myths About Lightning

- **Lightning strikes are always fatal.** Actually, studies report that lightning strikes kill only 10% of those struck. Generally, only people who sustain immediate cardiac arrest die.
- **A person who has been struck by lightning retains the charge—is "electrified"—and is dangerous to touch.** This false idea has led to a delay of resuscitation efforts and probably to some unnecessary deaths.
- **Lightning strike injuries allow a long resuscitation effort.** Although rescue breathing (when the person has a pulse) can effectively sustain life for long periods, CPR is usually ineffective after 30 minutes for people in cardiac arrest.
- **Lightning never strikes twice in the same place.** In fact, certain places are prone to lightning due to height, location, or material. The Willis Tower (Chicago) and the Empire State Building (New York) are hit hundreds of times per year, as are mountaintops and radio and television antennas.
- **A person inside a building is safe from lightning injury.** Electrical current can travel along plumbing fixtures, telephone wires, and other appliances attached to the outside of the house by metal conductors.

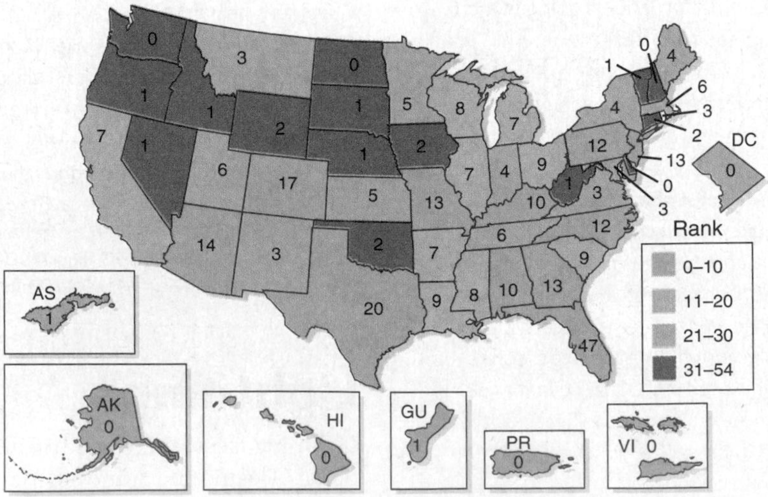

FIGURE 24-8 Lightning fatalities by state, 2007–2016.

Data from National Weather Service, compiled by Vaisala, Inc.

A more frequent cause of injury is a *splash,* which occurs when lightning strikes a tree, building, or other tall object and splashes onto a person seeking shelter nearby. The electrical current seeks the path of least resistance and may jump to the person because bodies have less resistance than trees or other objects. Frequently, a splash can kill groups of animals as they stand near a fence or seek shelter under trees.

Contact injury occurs when a person is holding an object that is directly hit or splashed by lightning.

Ground current is produced when lightning hits the ground or a nearby object. The current spreads like a wave in a pond. Although ground current is less likely to produce fatalities than direct hits or splashes, it often injures multiple people and creates multiple injuries. Large groups have been injured on baseball fields and hiking paths and during military maneuvers.

Finally, people can be injured by the explosive force of the *shock wave* produced as lightning strikes nearby. People actually can be thrown by this blast effect.

Differences Between Generated High-Voltage Electricity Injuries and Lightning Injuries

Lightning contact with the body is instantaneous, leading to flashover, where the current flashes over the body and goes through it. With flashover, the person seldom has burns of any magnitude. Lightning injuries disrupt electrical activity in the heart and nervous system. Exposure to household electricity tends to be much more prolonged because the person freezes to the circuit. The electrical energy surges through the tissues with little resistance to flow, causing thermal injury with severe tissue damage that can result in the loss of the damaged extremity. Electric current can also disrupt the body's electrical activity, as does lightning.

What to Look For	What to Do

▪ No breathing
▪ Seizures, paralysis, and loss of responsiveness (resulting if the central nervous system is damaged)
▪ Minor burns. Most people believe that a person struck by lightning will be severely burned. However, owing to the flashover effect, most people have only the following types of minor burns:
  ▪ Punctate burns (small, circular injuries resembling cigarette burns)
  ▪ Feathering or ferning burns **FIGURE 24-9**
  ▪ Linear burns
  ▪ Burns from ignited clothing and heated metal
	1. If more than one person has been struck by lightning at the same time, go to the quiet and motionless person first, check for breathing and, if absent, begin CPR.
	2. If the person is unresponsive but breathing, place the person on their side in the recovery position.
	3. Check for and treat injuries (fractures, dislocations, burns, spinal injuries).
	4. Evacuate all people to professional medical care.

FYI

Flash-to-Bang: How Close

Be aware of how close lightning is occurring. The flash-to-bang method is the easiest and most convenient way to estimate how far away lightning is occurring. Thunder always accompanies lightning even though its audible range can be diminished due to background noise in the immediate environment and its distance from you. To use the flash-to-bang method, count the seconds from the time the lightning is sighted to when the clap of the thunder is heard. Divide this number by five to obtain how far away (in miles) the lightning is occurring. For example, if you count 15 seconds between seeing the flash and hearing the bang, you divide 15 by 5 to get 3. Therefore, the lightning is about 3 miles (5 km) away.

FYI

30/30 Rule: When to Find Shelter

The 30/30 rule states that people should seek shelter if the flash-to-bang delay (length of time in seconds between a lightning flash and its subsequent thunder) is 30 seconds or less, and that they remain under cover until 30 minutes after the final clap of thunder.

A 30-second lead time is necessary prior to a storm's arrival because of the possibility of distant strikes. A 30-minute wait after the last thunderclap is heard is necessary because the trailing storm clouds still carry a lingering charge. This charge can—and does—occasionally produce lightning on the back edge of a storm, several minutes after the rain has ended.

Studies have shown most people struck by lightning are struck not at the height of a thunderstorm, but before and after the storm has peaked. **DO NOT** wait for the rain to start before seeking shelter, and do not leave shelter just because the rain has ended. One-half of all lightning deaths occur after a storm passes.

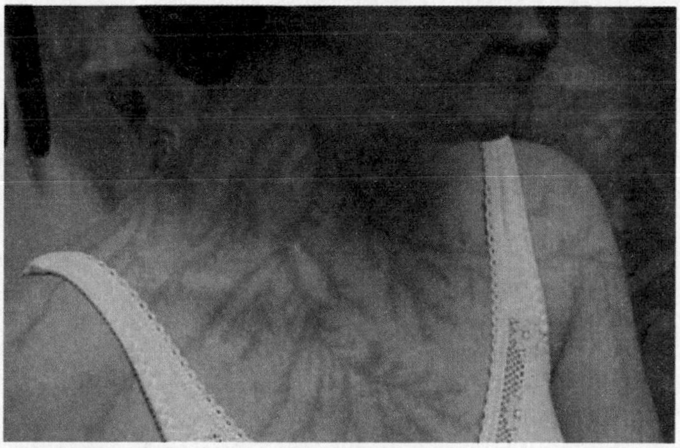

FIGURE 24-9 A feathering burn from a lightning strike can last for hours to days.

FYI

Avoid Lightning Injury

- Be alert about weather conditions and predictions before going outdoors.
- **DO NOT** stand under a natural lightning rod such as a tall, isolated tree in an open area.
- Avoid projecting above the surrounding landscape, as you would do if you were standing on a hilltop, in an open field, on the beach, or fishing from a boat on the open water.
- Get out of and away from open water.
- Get away from tractors and other metal farm equipment.
- Get off and away from motorcycles, scooters, golf carts, and bicycles. Lay down golf clubs.
- Stay away from wire fences, clotheslines, metal pipes, rails, and other metallic paths that could carry lightning to you from some distance away.
- Avoid standing in small, isolated sheds or other small structures in open areas.
- In a forest, seek shelter in a low area under a thick growth of small trees.
- In open areas, go to a low place such as a ravine or valley.
- If you are hopelessly isolated in a level field or prairie and you feel tingling or your hair stand on end—indicating lightning is about to strike—drop to a baseball catcher's crouching position or stance and put your hands over both ears to help avoid an eardrum rupture. **DO NOT** lie flat on the ground. You want as small an area of your body as possible touching the ground to minimize the possibility of your body acting as a conductor.
- If you are indoors during a thunderstorm, avoid open doors and windows, fireplaces, and metal objects such as pipes, sinks, and plug-in electrical appliances. Avoid using the telephone.
- If you are in a motor vehicle (without a cloth top), stay in it. The vehicle will diffuse the current around you to the ground. It is a myth that the rubber tires will provide insulation, but it is true that the metal body affords protection.
- If a group of people is exposed, they should spread out and stay at least 7 yards (20 feet) apart, if possible. That way, should a strike hit, the smallest number will be seriously injured.

Wild Animal Attacks

Despite the fact that few large wild animals (eg, bears, bison, cougars, alligators) remain in the United States, attacks on humans still occur **FIGURE 24-10**. Wild animal attacks outside the United States are more common. Attacks, especially fatal attacks, are often reported and sensationalized in the media.

The incidence of injuries from wild animal attacks is not known **TABLE 24-2**. Reporting is not mandatory, and many attacks are not recorded. Perhaps one or two deaths occur each year in the United States, though deaths from wild animals seem to be increasing as our environments collide.

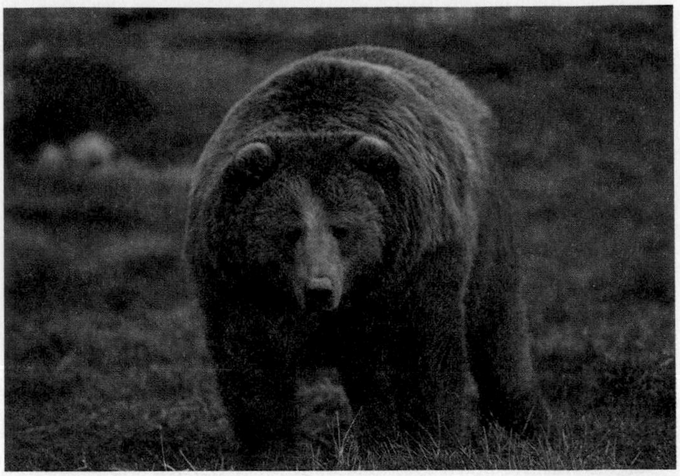

FIGURE 24-10 Large animals do not always retreat from humans and may attack rescuers.

Wild animal attacks occur most often in rural or wilderness settings, a long distance from professional medical care. Preventing wild animal attacks is largely common sense and awareness. An increasing number of parks and wilderness areas are posting warning signs. Recreationalists should be aware of and knowledgeable about the animal habitats through which they travel and take precautions in food handling so as not to attract animals.

Generally, if you encounter a large wild animal, try to remove yourself from the scene quietly and slowly. Running will elicit a predatory response. Never get between an adult animal and its offspring. In most cases, a general rule is to fight back if you are attacked. Vigorous physical resistance, including striking the attacking animal with fists, a weapon, or any other object, has been effective in repelling attacks by cougars, lions, tigers, brown and black bears, and even crocodiles. Exceptions to this recommendation are the grizzly bear and a mother black bear with cubs. In these cases, you should lie down and play dead.

What to Look For	What to Do
Not all injuries are bites; severe injuries result from people being thrown in the air, gored by an antler, butted, or trampled on the ground. Injuries may include the following: ▪ Puncture wounds ▪ Bites ▪ Lacerations ▪ Bruises ▪ Fractures ▪ Rupture of internal organs ▪ Evisceration	1. Stop any bleeding, and bandage and care for wounds as you would any similar injury. See Chapter 8, *Bleeding*, Chapter 9, *Wounds*, and Chapter 10, *Bandaging Wounds*, for specifics regarding bleeding and wound care. 2. Depending on the severity of the injury, either evacuate the person to professional medical care or contact local authorities for evacuation.

TABLE 24-2 Human Deaths from Animal Attacks

Species	Estimated Deaths Annually	Estimated Attacks Annually	Predominant Area	Notes
Humans	200,000	—	Worldwide	Murders only
Wolves	1–5	20–50	Worldwide (mostly Eurasia)	
Hyenas	10–50	Hundreds	Africa	
Domestic dogs	20–50	4.7 million	United States	
Other canines	1–5	200–250	Australia	
Tigers	800	800	India	Frequently maneaters
Leopards	30–100	400	Africa and India	Frequently maneaters
Lions	300–500	—	Africa and India	Frequently maneaters
Cougars	<1	<1	United States	125 attacks, 27 of which were fatal, during the last century
African buffalos	20–100	—	Africa	
Elephants	600	—	Worldwide	
Black rhinoceros	1	—	Africa	
Hippopotami	200–300	—	Africa	Unpredictable
American bison	3	56	United States	
Moose	3	368 injuries	British Columbia, Canada	Auto crashes only
Deer	50	1.3 million incidents	United States	Auto crashes only
Domestic herbivores	20–25	50,000–100,000 injuries	United States and Australia	
Snakes	100,000	—	Worldwide	
Crocodiles	2,000	—	Africa	
Alligators	1–2	—	United States	
Ostrich	1–2	—	Australia	
Kangaroos	1–2	100–200 incidents	Australia	Auto incidents only

Reproduced from Paul Auerbach. *Wilderness Medicine*, 7th Edition. Philadelphia: Mosby, 2017. Reprinted by permission of Elsevier.

Wilderness Evacuation

Determining the best way to evacuate a person (helicopter evacuation versus walking the person out versus carrying the person on a litter) must be based on several factors. The following list is adapted from the WMS Practice Guidelines and suggests factors for determining the level of evacuation:

- Severity of the illness or injury
- Rescue and medical skills of the rescuers
- Physical and psychological condition of the rescuers and the ill or injured people
- Availability of equipment and aid for the rescue
- The estimated time it would take to evacuate the person by other means as determined by distance, terrain, weather, and other conditions
- Cost

When requesting outside assistance, you must consider the safety of incoming rescuers, their time commitment, and the cost of the rescue.

As a general rule, you should delay travel plans or start evacuating a person from the wilderness for any of the following reasons:

- The person's condition is not improving.
- The person is experiencing debilitating pain.
- The person is unable to travel at a reasonable pace owing to a medical problem.
- The person is passing blood via the mouth or rectum (not from an obviously minor source).
- The person has signs and symptoms of serious altitude illness.
- The person has infections that are not improving.
- The person is experiencing chest pain that is not caused by a rib cage injury.
- The person's wounds are severe enough to require professional medical care.
- The person's dysfunctional psychological status is impairing the safety of others.

When to Evacuate

Use the following guidelines to decide whether a person should be evacuated.

Immediate Evacuations

Rapidly evacuate the following injuries, where professional medical care is needed in 30 to 60 minutes or less:

- Open fractures
- Extremity injuries with deformity
- Extremity injuries in which circulation is absent
- Spinal injuries with no sensation in the fingers or toes or inability of the person to move fingers or toes
- Severe altitude illness (signs of HACE or HAPE)
- Decreased level of consciousness
- Signs of shock
- Severe bleeding
- Deep (severe) frostbite

In the wilderness, all bleeding should be controlled. Wounds should be cleaned and irrigated under pressure. The standard rule is not to remove blood-soaked dressings; locate the bleeding vessels and reapply pressure directly over the bleeding vessels. Never attempt to clamp or tie a blood vessel—more damage can result. Do not close a wound with adhesive strips, butterfly bandages, staples, or sutures.

Delayed Evacuations

Professional medical care should be obtained within 6 to 24 hours of injury for the following:

- Limb injuries with deformity, severe pain, or inability to walk
- Superficial frostbite
- Open wounds: Evacuate a wounded person so that a physician can suture a wound within 6 hours for hand or foot injuries and within 24 hours for head or trunk injuries. (If necessary, wounds can be closed by a physician up to about 4 days after injury).
- Hypothermia: It is not necessary to evacuate a person with mild hypothermia if the person has normal mental status and is shivering. Evacuate people who have severe hypothermia (shivering has stopped but the person is still cold and has altered mental status). It is impossible to rewarm a person with severe hypothermia in a wilderness or remote location. See Chapter 20, *Cold-Related Emergencies*, for more information.

Guidelines for Ground Evacuation

If the person is walking out, at least two people should accompany the person. If the person is being carried out, one or two people should be sent to notify authorities that assistance is needed and to give them specifics about the problem.

During a litter evacuation, there should be at least four, and preferably six, litter-bearers at all times. Over rough terrain, eight carriers (six over a smooth trail) should carry the litter 100 yards (91 m) and then rest or rotate with eight other carriers. It is very demanding to carry a loaded litter for more than 15 minutes without a break. The person being carried should be covered to avoid heat loss and secured safely to the litter.

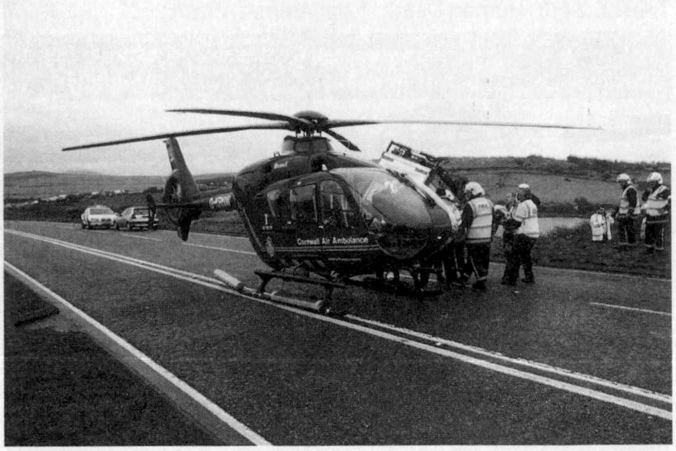

FIGURE 24-11 An EMS helicopter.
Courtesy of Mark Woolcock.

FYI

Hiking: How to Protect One's Health on the Trail

The popularity of backpacking and day hiking has greatly increased, but so have related injuries. A survey of 224 backpackers who hiked the entire 2,100-mile (3,380-km) mountainous Appalachian Trail showed that 82% had injuries (mostly muscle sprains, strains, and stress fractures) and illnesses (mostly diarrhea, skin irritations, foot blisters, and colds). Medical help was needed in 25% of the incidents. Hikers lost an average of 5 days of hiking because of these problems. Because these problems are common, hikers should carry supplies such as water purification equipment, OTC pain medicine, antibiotic ointment, and bandages.

Data from Crouse BJ, Josephs D. Health care needs of Appalachian Trail hikers. *J Fam Pract.* 1993;36:521–525.

Guidelines for Helicopter Evacuation

Helicopters can reduce the time the person has to wait to receive professional medical care. Evacuate by helicopter only if the following conditions apply **FIGURE 24-11**:

- The person's life will be saved or person will have a significantly better chance for full recovery.
- The pilot believes conditions are safe enough for helicopter evacuation.
- Ground evacuation would be unusually dangerous or excessively prolonged or not enough rescuers are available for ground evacuation.

In general, helicopters are not beneficial if ground transport can get the person to the hospital within 30 to 60 minutes.

Refer to **FLOWCHART 24-1** for additional information on evacuating.

Flowchart 24-1 How to Evacuate

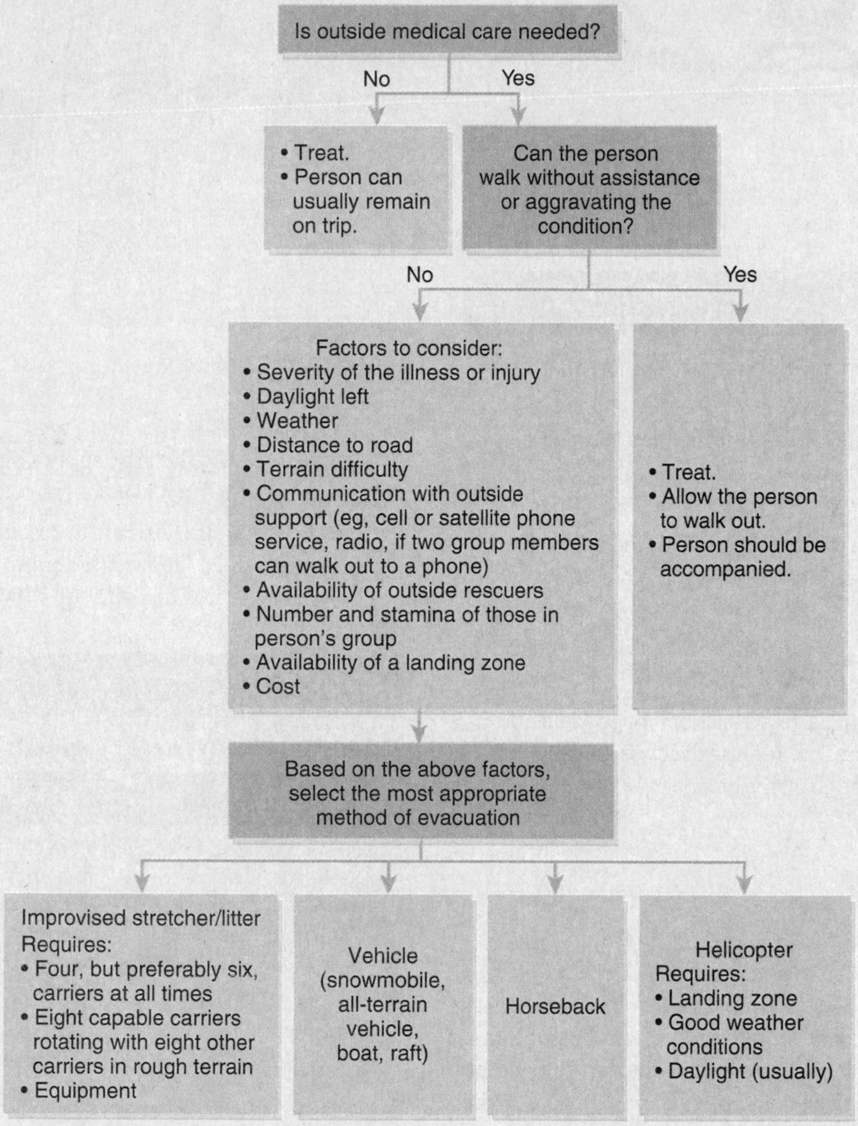
Is outside medical care needed?
No
Yes
• Treat.
• Person can usually remain on trip.
Can the person walk without assistance or aggravating the condition?
No
Yes
Factors to consider:
• Severity of the illness or injury
• Daylight left
• Weather
• Distance to road
• Terrain difficulty
• Communication with outside support (eg, cell or satellite phone service, radio, if two group members can walk out to a phone)
• Availability of outside rescuers
• Number and stamina of those in person's group
• Availability of a landing zone
• Cost
• Treat.
• Allow the person to walk out.
• Person should be accompanied.
Based on the above factors, select the most appropriate method of evacuation
Improvised stretcher/litter
Requires:
• Four, but preferably six, carriers at all times
• Eight capable carriers rotating with eight other carriers in rough terrain
• Equipment
Vehicle (snowmobile, all-terrain vehicle, boat, raft)
Horseback
Helicopter
Requires:
• Landing zone
• Good weather conditions
• Daylight (usually)

Signaling for Help

Many emergency conditions require a search for people in distress. Under such circumstances, it is always better if the people being sought know how to make their presence and their location conspicuous.

Signaling Aircraft

When creating a ground signal that people in an aircraft can see, remember that few straight lines or right angles exist in nature and that things are a lot smaller when viewed from the air. Bigger is almost always better. For ground signals, make a large V for immediate assistance or an X if medical assistance is needed. Make the lines of these signals as large as you can. Construct your signal so that each line is six times as long as it is wide, such as a V with each side 12 feet (4 m) long and 2 feet (1 m) wide. Contrast is another key to ground signals. Examples of materials to use include toilet paper, strips of plastic tarp, strips of tent material, tree branches, logs, and light-colored rocks. In snow and on open ground or sandy shores, signals may be tramped or dug into the surface using shadows to make the signals stand out.

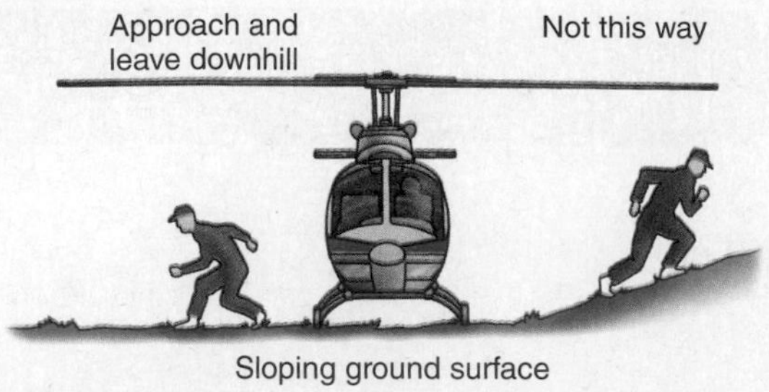

FIGURE 24-12 Helicopter safety.

CAUTION

DO NOT approach a helicopter until one of the aircraft personnel signals it is safe for you to approach.

DO NOT approach a helicopter from the rear, where the fast-spinning tail rotor is invisible and dangerous. Many people walk into spinning rotors each year.

DO NOT forget to protect against wind chill from the rotor blades in the winter and to protect your eyes against flying dirt and debris.

DO NOT approach from the uphill side. The rotor is closer to the ground on the uphill side **FIGURE 24-12**.

DO NOT stand up when approaching a helicopter. Keep as low as possible in a crouched position. Because the blade is flexible, it may dip as low as 4 feet (1 m) off the ground.

Other Signals

A series of three of almost anything indicates "Help." Examples include three shouts, three shots, three blasts from a whistle, or three flashes from a light. Use smoke by day and bright flame by night if other signaling devices are not available. Add engine oil, rags soaked in oil, or pieces of rubber to your fire to make black smoke (best against a light background). Keep plenty of spare fuel on hand. If you are tending a fire as you wait for help, keep fuel handy and throw it on the fire when you hear an aircraft; do not wait, because it takes time for smoke to form and rise. Make sure to start the fire away from combustibles such as grass or trees.

A mirror is an effective means of sending a distress signal. On hazy days, aircraft pilots can see the flash of a mirror before survivors can see the aircraft, so it is wise to flash the mirror in the direction of a plane when you hear it, even when you cannot see it. Mirror flashes have been spotted by rescue aircraft more than 20 miles (32 km) away.

To use a mirror, follow this procedure:

1. Hold the mirror up to the sun with one hand, and stretch your other hand out in front of you. Use your finger or thumb to block your view of your target.
2. Hit your extended finger or thumb with a reflection of the sun from the mirror.

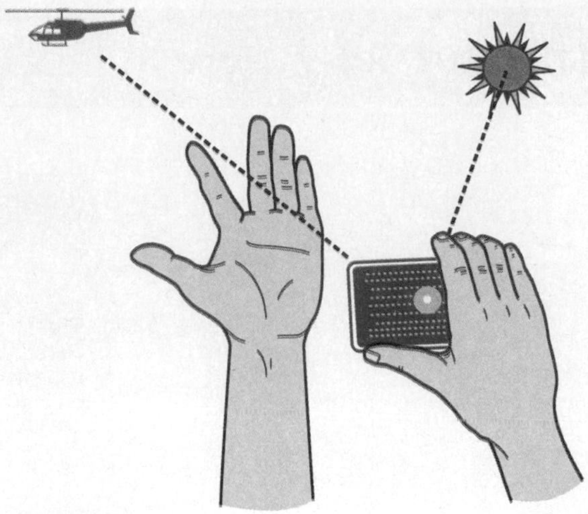

FIGURE 24-13 Signaling.

3. Repeatedly flick the spot of light from the mirror across the finger or thumb and the target.
4. Try to hit the aircraft or rescuers with a flash as much as possible. Do not attempt to do series of three flashes—it is too difficult **FIGURE 24-13**.

FYI

Survival Kit: The Bare Essentials

Minimal items	Purpose
One or two large plastic trash bags or an emergency blanket (space blanket) made of Mylar	Protects against weather (wind, rain, snow). Wear one trash bag by cutting a hole in the bottom of the bag for your head; use the second bag to cover your legs.
Whistle (Fox 40 Mini or Windstorm)	Signal for help.
Signal mirror	Signal for help.
Metal match with striker (magnesium)	Start a fire.
Waterproof match case containing windproof and waterproof matches	Start a fire.
Waterproof match case or empty film canister containing several cotton balls smeared with petroleum jelly (such as Vaseline) or commercial tinder tabs	Petroleum jelly is flammable. Make tinder using cotton balls smeared with petroleum jelly. When using, open a cotton ball up to catch sparks from metal match.
Knife (multitool) and/or wire blade survival saw	Cutting.
Food (such as energy bars and MREs [US military surplus meals-ready-to-eat])	Provides calories and a psychological boost.

PREP KIT

Ready for Review

- Be as medically prepared as possible to manage a problem for others and for yourself.
- Prolonged CPR has little use in a wilderness or remote setting. Once started, CPR should be continued for at least 30 minutes.
- In a wilderness situation, reducing some dislocated joints is recommended.
- Always stabilize an unresponsive person.
- People with a femur fracture can have 2 quarts (about 2 L) of blood loss in the thigh and develop massive swelling. These injuries should be splinted.
- Since the early 1970s, the number of deaths caused by avalanches has increased rapidly.
- Altitude illnesses actually are a spectrum of a single problem: hypoxia.
- Determining the best way to evacuate a person must be based on several factors.
- Many emergency conditions require a search for people in distress.

Vital Vocabulary

acute mountain sickness (AMS) A condition that effects people in high altitudes; symptoms include dizziness, nausea, headache, and shortness of breath.

high-altitude cerebral edema (HACE) A medical condition where high altitude causes the brain to swell with fluid.

high-altitude pulmonary edema (HAPE) When lung vessels constrict and increase pressure causing fluid to leak into the lung tissues and eventually the air sacs.

hypoxia A low oxygen content in the blood; lack of oxygen in inspired air.

wilderness A remote geographic location more than 1 hour from definitive medical care.

Assessment in Action

You have been enjoying a 5-day backpack trip in the high mountains of Colorado. Being from sea level, you knew the high altitude would take some getting used to, but your group is doing very well. On day 4, you must ascend a 1,000-foot (305-m) pass to get to your final campsite. After an hour of never-ending switchbacks, you arrive at the highest point of the trip: 13,500 feet (4,115 m) above sea level. At this elevation, several members in your group report a severe headache and fatigue. Two members cannot seem to catch their breath.

Directions: Circle Yes if you agree with the statement; circle No if you disagree.

1. Because you are above 12,000 feet (3,658 m), you suspect they are suffering from HAPE or HACE.

YES NO

2. Plenty of fluids should be given to the people.

YES NO

3. You should stay at this elevation until they feel well enough to hike down the other side of the pass.

YES NO

4. After descent to your final campsite (3,000 feet [914 m] below the pass), if the people's conditions do not improve, you should seek professional medical care.

YES NO

PREP KIT continued

Check Your Knowledge

Directions: Circle Yes if you agree with the statement; circle No if you disagree.

1. Injuries in the wilderness rarely happen.
   YES **NO**
2. CPR in the wilderness should be stopped if the person does not respond after 30 minutes.
   YES **NO**
3. Reduction of a dislocation dramatically relieves pain.
   YES **NO**
4. When it comes to spinal stabilization, never improvise!
   YES **NO**
5. After an avalanche, it is easy for people to dig themselves out.
   YES **NO**
6. Speed of ascent can affect altitude illness.
   YES **NO**
7. Headache is a common symptom of altitude illness.
   YES **NO**
8. A person with altitude illness should keep moving.
   YES **NO**
9. Most lightning deaths occur during the night.
   YES **NO**
10. Most people struck by lightning will have only minor burns.
    YES **NO**

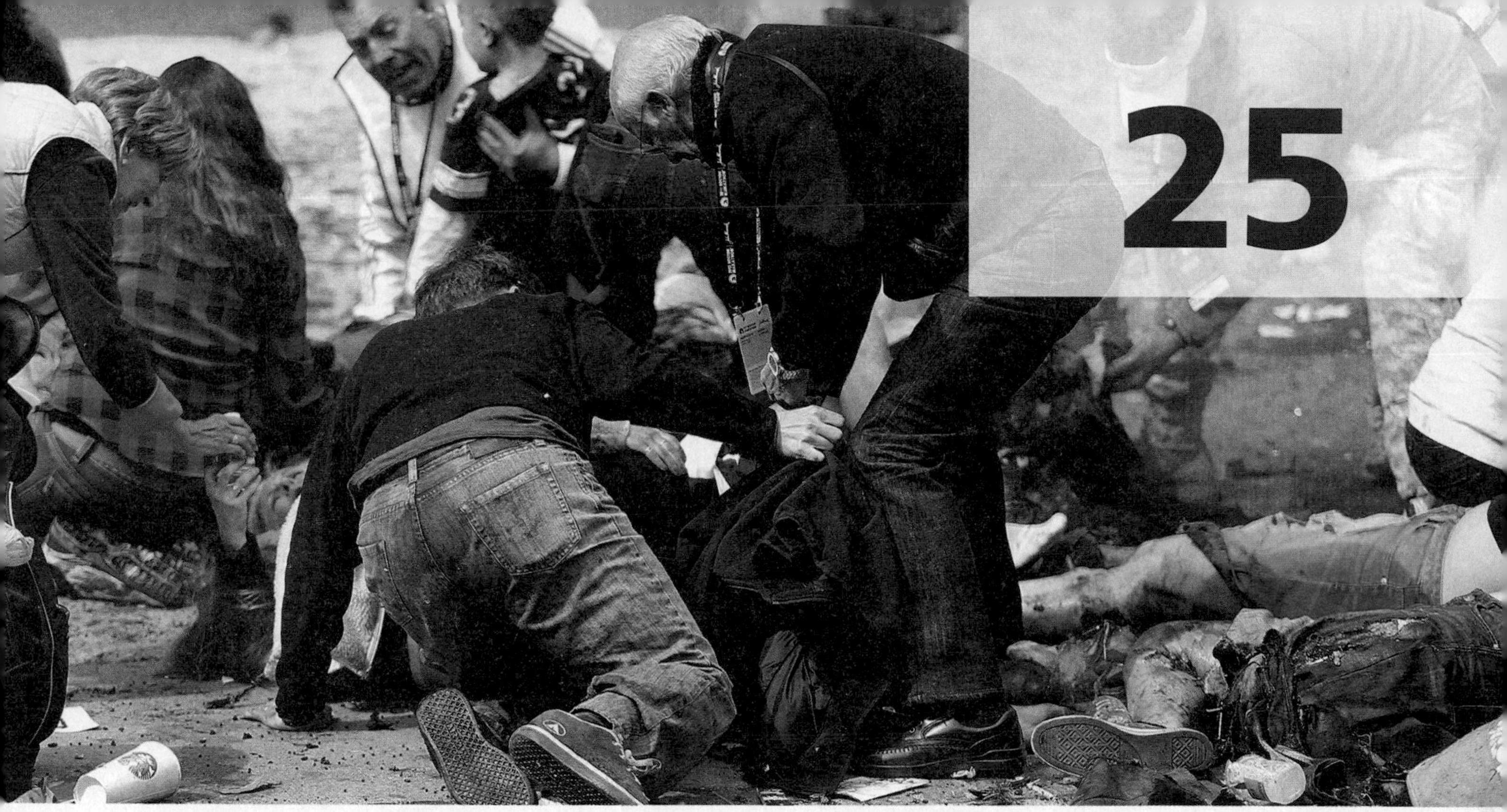

25

Rescuing and Moving Injured People

CHAPTER AT A GLANCE

- Rescue
- Triage: Prioritizing Multiple Injured People
- Moving People

Rescue

Water Rescue

Reach-throw-row-go identifies the sequence for attempting a water rescue. The first and simplest rescue technique is to reach for the person. Reaching requires a lightweight pole, ladder, long stick, or any object that can be extended to the person. Once you have your "reacher," secure your footing and have a bystander grab your belt or pants for stability. Secure yourself before reaching for the person.

You can throw anything that floats: an empty picnic jug, an empty fuel or paint can, a life jacket, a floating cushion, a piece of wood, or an inflated spare tire—whatever is available **TABLE 25-1**. If there is a rope handy, tie it to the object to be thrown so you can pull the person in, or, if you miss, you can retrieve the object and throw it again. The average untrained rescuer has a throwing range of about 50 feet (15 m).

If the person is out of throwing range and there is a rowboat, canoe, motorboat, or boogie board nearby, you can try to row to the person. Maneuvering these craft requires skill learned through practice. Wear a personal flotation device (PFD) for your own safety. To avoid capsizing, never pull the person in over the side of a boat; instead, pull the person in over the stern (rear end) or tow the person to safety.

TABLE 25-1 Effect of Flotation Devices on Survival Times

Situation (50°F [10°C] water)	Predicted Survival Time (hours)
No Flotation Device	
Drownproofing	1.5
Treading water	2.0
With Flotation Device	
Swimming	2.0
Holding still	2.7
HELP (heat escape lessening position)	4.0
Huddle position	4.0

Data from Collis ML. Survival behavior in cold water immersion. In: *Proceedings of the Cold Water Symposium*. Toronto: Royal Life-Saving Society of Canada; 1976.

FYI

Advanced First Aid

While this text provides a solid foundation and overview of advanced first aid procedures, there are a number of rescue disciplines. Additional training can be beneficial in becoming proficient in these disciplines.

CAUTION

DO NOT swim to and grasp a drowning person unless you are trained in lifesaving procedures.

If reach, throw, and row are impossible and you are a capable swimmer trained in water lifesaving procedures, you can go to the drowning person by swimming. Entering even calm water makes a swimming rescue difficult and hazardous. All too often, a would-be rescuer drowns as well.

Drowning

According to the World Health Organization, **drowning** is the process of experiencing respiratory impairment from submersion/immersion in liquid. For drowning to occur, usually at least the person's face (mouth and nose) must be immersed, or covered, in water. During submersion, the entire body, including the face, is under water. Behaviors of a drowning person are found in **TABLE 25-2**.

Care for Drowning Person

1. Survey the scene (see Chapter 2, *Action at an Emergency*), then carry out a water rescue **FIGURE 25-1**.
2. If the person was diving (or it is unknown whether they were diving), suspect a possible spinal injury. Support the person on the surface of the water so that they are floating faceup with the head and spine in a straight line until properly trained rescuers arrive with a backboard.
3. Check breathing and treat accordingly. Any nonbreathing person who has been submerged in cold water should be resuscitated unless submerged for more than 60 minutes.
4. If no spinal injury is suspected, after the person has been resuscitated, place the person on their side to allow fluids to drain from the airway.

FYI

American Academy of Pediatrics Recommendations for Preventing Childhood Drowning (by Age Group)

4 Years and Younger

- Never leave children alone in bathtubs, spas, or wading pools or near water-filled buckets, toilets, irrigation ditches, or other standing water.
- Recognize that swimming lessons do not "drownproof" children.
- Fence the entire pool so that it is separated from the house. Pool covers are not a substitute for fences.
- Learn cardiopulmonary resuscitation (CPR) and keep a telephone and emergency equipment, such as life preservers and a shepherd's crook, poolside.

5 to 12 Years

- Provide children with swimming lessons that include safety rules.
- Never let the children swim alone or without adult supervision.
- Make sure children wear approved flotation devices when playing in or near a body of water.
- Teach children the dangers of jumping or diving into water and of being on thin ice.

13 to 19 Years

- In addition to relaying the preceding safety tips, counsel about the dangers of substance abuse combined with swimming, diving, or boating.
- Teach adolescents how to perform CPR.

Data from American Academy of Pediatrics Committee on Injury, Violence, and Poison Prevention. Prevention of drowning. *Pediatrics* 2019;143(5):2–5.

Cold-Water Immersion

Immersion in cold water is a potential hazard for anyone who participates in activities in the oceans, lakes, and streams of all but the tropical regions of the world. The US Coast Guard defines cold water as water with a temperature of less than 70°F (21°C). However, water does not need to be that cold for a person to become hypothermic. A person can become hypothermic in water that is 77°F (25°C). Most North American lakes, rivers, and coasts are colder than that year-round. The

TABLE 25-2 Behaviors of a Distressed Swimmer and Drowning Person

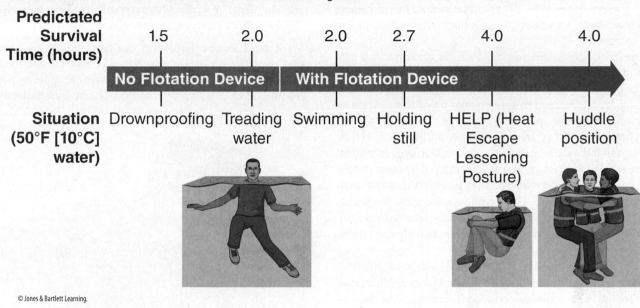

Predictated Survival Time (hours)	1.5	2.0	2.0	2.7	4.0	4.0
	No Flotation Device		With Flotation Device			
Situation (50°F [10°C] water)	Drownproofing	Treading water	Swimming	Holding still	HELP (Heat Escape Lessening Posture)	Huddle position

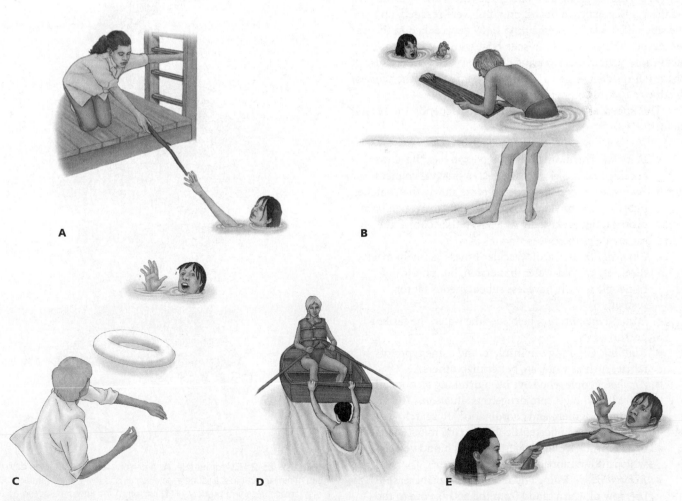

FIGURE 25-1 Water rescue. **A**. Reach for the person with a lightweight pole, ladder, long stick, or other object. **B**. Secure your footing before reaching for the person. **C**. Throw anything that floats. **D**. Row to the person if the person is out of throwing range. **E**. Go to the person if reach, throw, and row are impossible and you are trained in water lifesaving procedures.

risk of immersion hypothermia in North America is nearly universal most of the year. A person immersed in cold water experiences heat loss about 25 times faster than someone exposed to cold air.

The US Coast Guard and other rescue organizations recommend that survivors get as much of their bodies out of the water as possible to minimize cooling rate and maximize survival time. A widespread misunderstanding of the concept of wind chill often causes people to conclude that survivors have higher heat losses if they are exposed to wind, especially if they are wet, than if they are immersed in water. During recreational activities at beaches, lakes, and swimming pools, most people have experienced feeling colder after leaving the water than they do while swimming. That reinforces the misunderstanding, which has sometimes led people to abandon a safe position atop a capsized vessel and reenter the water, usually with tragic results.

Cold-water immersion is associated with two potential medical emergencies: drowning and hypothermia. Numerous case histories and statistical evidence document the prominence of cold-water immersion as a cause of drowning and hypothermia. Perhaps the most famous occurrence of cold-water immersion was the sinking of the ocean liner *Titanic* on April 14, 1912. After striking an iceberg, the ship sank in calm seas. Of the 2,201 people on board, only 712 were rescued, all from the ship's lifeboats. The remaining 1,489 people died in the water, despite the arrival of a rescue boat within 2 hours. Nearly all of those people were wearing life preservers, yet the cause of death was officially listed as drowning. More likely, the cause of death was immersion hypothermia.

The speed at which a person cools depends on several factors:

- *Body fat.* The more body fat a person has, the slower cooling occurs. More fat increases survival chances.
- *Body type.* Bigger people cool more slowly than smaller people. Children cool faster than adults. Women have more fat but are usually smaller, so they cool at the same rate as men.
- *Physical fitness.* Cardiovascular fitness can help meet the stress of cold-water immersion, but physically fit people usually have less subcutaneous fat for insulation.
- *Water temperature.* The colder the water, the faster a person cools.
- *Clothing.* Clothing can insulate, and some types of fabric, such as wool, are better than others.
- *Alcohol.* People who have been drinking alcohol are more likely to get into dangerous situations. Alcohol impairs judgment and coordination. Research studies have implicated alcohol in 10% to 50% of all drownings. Alcohol dilates the skin's blood vessels, which allows more body heat to escape.
- *Behavior.* Swimming and treading water increase the flow of warm blood from the body's core to the muscles, increasing the cooling rate. Thus, swimmers often die first because they are more likely to try to tread water or swim rather than float. Likewise, so-called drownproofing, a technique of bobbing in the water (like a jellyfish), markedly increases heat loss as water circulates around the head.

A **heat escape lessening position (HELP)** has been devised, in which the person draws the knees up close to the chest, presses the arms to the sides, and remains as quiet as possible **FIGURE 25-2**. For two or more people, huddling quietly and

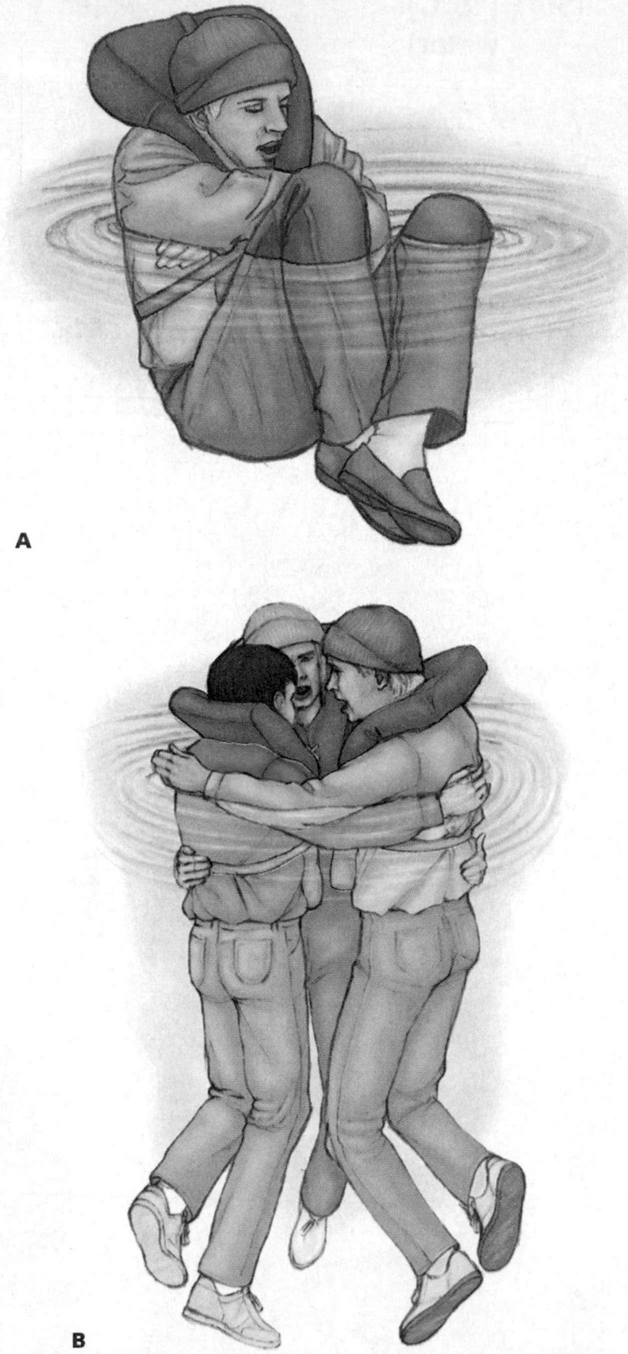

A

B

FIGURE 25-2 HELP or huddle. **A**. A person wearing a flotation device can minimize heat loss and increase chances of survival by assuming the heat escape lessening position (HELP) in which the knees are pulled up to the chest and the arms crossed. **B**. Groups of two or more can conserve heat by wrapping their arms around one another and pulling into a tight circle or huddle.

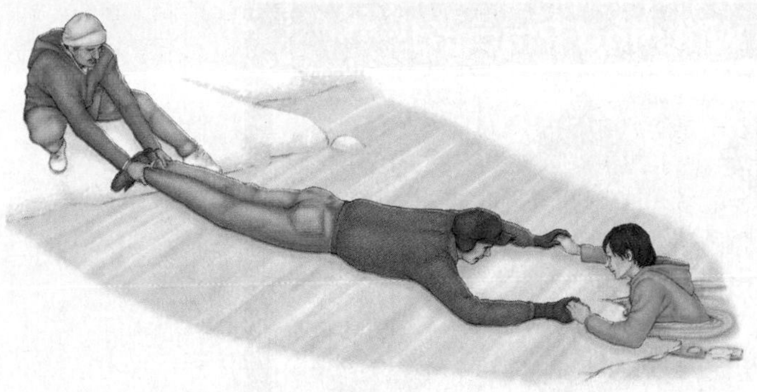

FIGURE 25-3 Ice rescue: Lie flat to distribute the weight over a larger surface area.

closely together (huddle position) will decrease heat loss from the groin and the front of the body. Both of these positions require life jackets, also called PFDs.

Surviving long periods of submersion has been explained by the diving reflex found in all mammals, including humans. The diving reflex, sometimes called the mammalian diving reflex, is the body's natural response to submersion in water and includes limiting oxygen to specific parts of the body in order to conserve energy for survival. The diving reflex is what allows free divers to remain underwater for minutes at a time.

Ice Rescue

If a person has fallen through the ice near the shore, extend a pole or throw a line with a floatable object attached to it. When the person has hold of the object, pull them toward the shore or the edge of the ice.

If the person has fallen through the ice away from the shore and you cannot reach them with a pole or a throwing line, lie flat and push a ladder, plank, or similar object ahead of you **FIGURE 25-3**. You can also tie a rope to a spare tire and the other end to an anchor point on the shore, lie flat, and push the tire ahead of you. Pull the person ashore or to the edge of the ice.

CAUTION

DO NOT go near broken ice without support.

Electrical Emergency Rescue

Electrical injuries can be devastating. Just a mild shock can cause serious internal injuries. A current of 1,000 V or more is considered high voltage, but even the 110 V of household current can be deadly.

When a person receives an electrical shock, electricity enters the body at the point of contact and travels along the path of least resistance (nerves and blood vessels). The current travels rapidly, generating heat and causing destruction.

Most indoor electrocutions are caused by faulty electrical equipment or the careless use of electrical appliances. Before you touch the person, turn off the electricity at the circuit breaker, fuse box, or outside switch box or unplug the appliance if the plug is undamaged.

If the electrocution involves high-voltage power lines, the power must be turned off before anyone approaches the person. If you approach a person and feel a tingling sensation in your legs and lower body, stop. You are on energized ground, and an electric current is entering one foot, passing through your lower body, and leaving through the other foot. You should raise one foot off the ground, turn around, and hop to a safe place. Wait for trained personnel with the proper equipment to cut the wires or disconnect them. If a power line falls over a car, tell the driver and passengers to stay in the car. If a person must get out of the car because of fire or imminent explosion, they should jump out so that the ground and car or wires are not touched at the same time.

CAUTION

DO NOT touch an appliance or the person until the current is off.

DO NOT try to move downed wires.

DO NOT use any object, even dry wood (broomstick, tools, chair, stool), to separate the person from the live electrical source.

Hazardous Materials Incidents

Almost any highway crash scene involves the potential danger of hazardous materials. Clues that indicate the presence of hazardous materials include the following:

- Look for warning signs on the vehicle (eg, "explosive," "flammable," "corrosive"). If you are unable to read the placard or labels, **DO NOT** move closer and risk exposure. If you are able to read the placard with the naked eye, you may be too close and should consider moving farther away. **FIGURE 25-4** shows a chart illustrating the hazardous materials warning placards found on vehicles travelling the roads, and **FIGURE 25-5** shows a chart illustrating warning labels found on packages being shipped.
- Watch for a leak or spill from a tank, container, truck, or railroad car with or without hazardous material placards or labels.
- A strong, noxious odor can denote a hazardous material.
- A cloud or strange-looking smoke from the escaping substance suggests you should stay away.

Stay well away and upwind from the area. Only people who are specially trained in handling hazardous materials and who have the proper equipment should be in the area. Notify the police and fire departments right away if you suspect an incident involving hazardous materials.

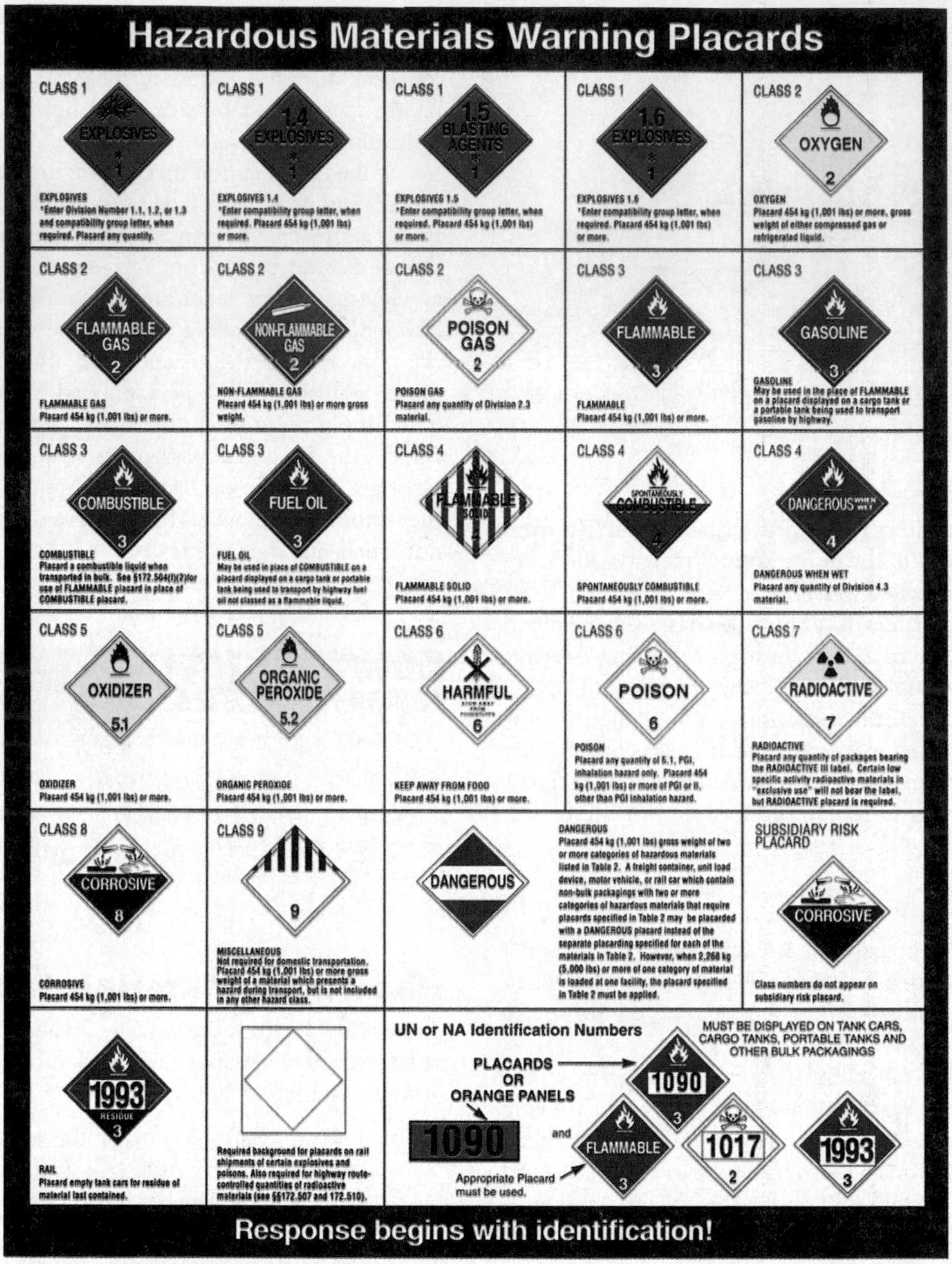

FIGURE 25-4 Hazardous materials warning placards.
Courtesy of U.S. Department of Transportation.

Confined Spaces

A confined space is any area not intended for human occupancy that may have or develop a dangerous atmosphere. They have limited openings for entrance and exit. There are three types of confined spaces: below ground, ground level, and above ground. Below-ground confined spaces include manholes, below-ground utility vaults and storage tanks, old mines, cisterns, and wells. Ground-level confined spaces include industrial tanks and farm storage silos. Above-ground confined spaces include water towers and legged storage tanks.

An incident in a confined space demands immediate action. If someone enters a confined space and signals for help or becomes unresponsive, follow these steps:

1. Call 9-1-1 for immediate assistance.
2. **DO NOT** rush in to help. If you do, you risk needing rescue as well.
3. When help arrives, try to rescue the person without entering the space.
4. If rescue cannot be accomplished from the outside, only trained and properly equipped (respiratory protection plus safety harnesses or lifelines) rescuers should enter the space to remove the person.
5. Once the person is removed, provide care. Additional training is required for first aid providers who are on-call for helping to rescue people in a confined space.

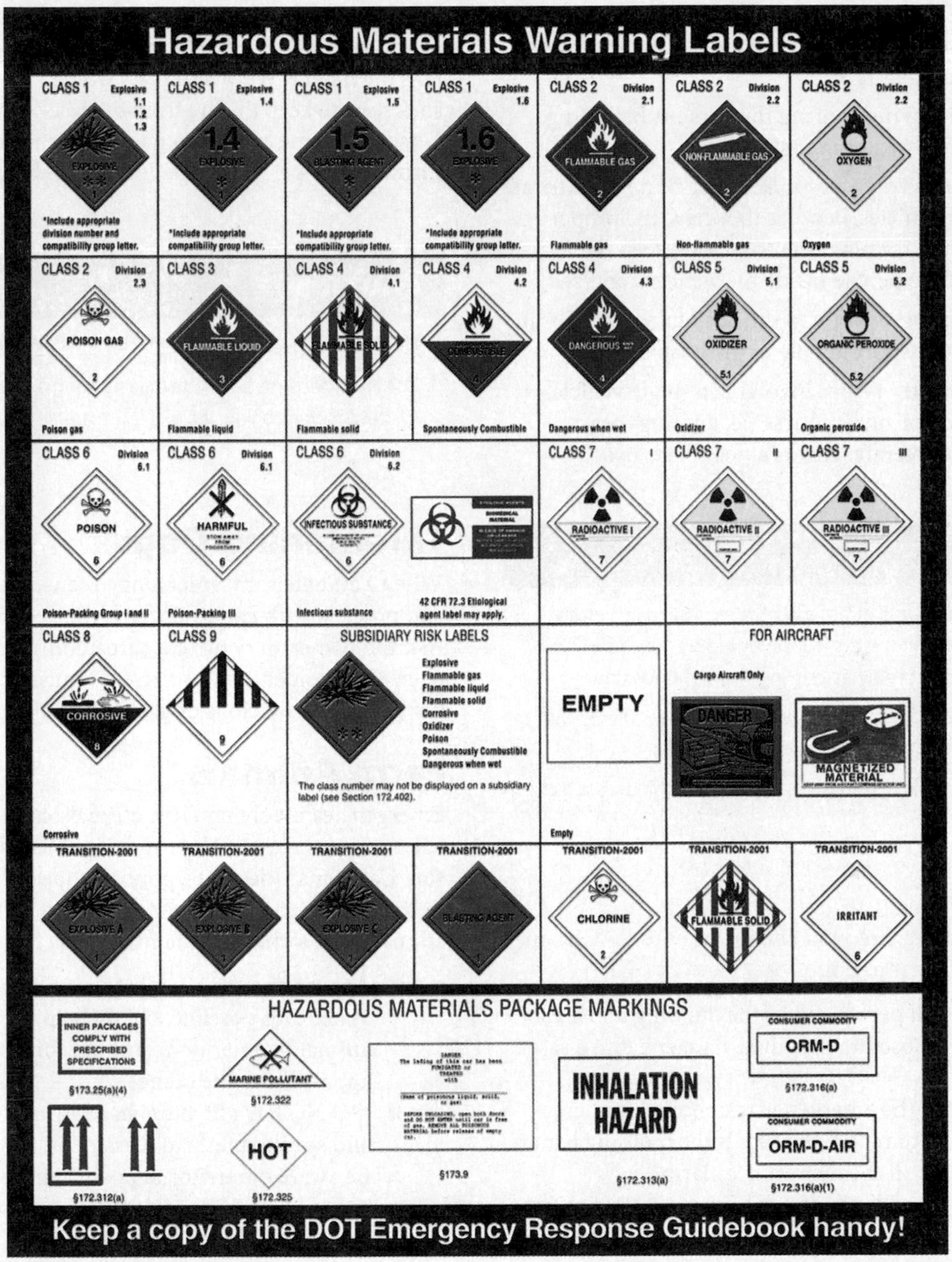

FIGURE 25-5 Hazardous materials warning labels.
Courtesy of U.S. Department of Transportation.

Motor Vehicle Crashes

In most states, you are legally obligated to stop and give help when you are involved in a motor vehicle crash. If you arrive at a crash shortly after it happens, the law does not require you to stop, although it might be argued that you have a moral responsibility to provide any aid that you can.

1. Stop and park your vehicle well off the highway or road and out of active traffic lanes. Park at least five car lengths from the crash. If the police have taken charge, **DO NOT** stop unless you are asked to do so. If the police or other emergency vehicles have not arrived, call or send someone to call 9-1-1 as soon as possible. Ways to call include the following:
   - Using a mobile phone
   - Using a phone at a nearby house or business
   - Finding a pay phone or roadside emergency phone
2. Turn on your vehicle's emergency hazard flashers.
3. Make sure everyone on the scene is safe.
   - Ask the driver to turn off the ignition or turn it off yourself and put the vehicle in park.
   - Ask bystanders to stand well off the roadway.
   - Place flares or reflectors 250 to 500 feet (76 to 152 m) behind the crash scene to warn oncoming drivers of the crash. **DO NOT** ignite flares around leaking gasoline or diesel fuel.

4. If the driver or passenger is unresponsive or might have spinal injuries, use your hands to stabilize the person's head and neck.
5. Check and keep monitoring the person's breathing. Treat any life-threatening injuries.
6. Whenever possible, wait for EMS personnel to extricate people from vehicles, because they have the proper equipment and training. In most cases, keep the condition of the people inside the vehicle stabilized.
7. Do not transport anyone to the hospital yourself, wait for EMS to transport people to the hospital.
8. In motor vehicle crashes involving a single vehicle, consider sudden-onset illness (ie, fainting, heart attack, hypoglycemia, etc) as a possible cause.

CAUTION

DO NOT rush to get people out of a car that has been in a crash. Contrary to "television wrecks," most vehicle crashes do not involve a fire, and most vehicles stay in an upright position.

DO NOT move people or allow people to move unless there is an immediate danger such as fire or oncoming traffic.

DO NOT transport people in your car or any other bystander's vehicle.

Fires

Should you encounter a fire, you should use the RACE mnemonic to remember what to do:

R = *Rescue.* Get all people out of the building and area quickly. Help those in immediate danger get to a safe place.
A = *Activate.* Call the emergency telephone number (usually 9-1-1) to report the fire. If the building has an alarm system, pull the nearest fire alarm.
C = *Confine.* If it can be done safely, prevent the fire from spreading by closing doors and windows. **DO NOT** lock doors and windows.
E = *Extinguish.* If it is safe to do so and you are competent in its use, retrieve and use the nearest fire extinguisher.

You should only fight the fire yourself with a fire extinguisher if the fire is small and if your own escape route is clear. You may be able to put out the fire or at least hold damage to a minimum. Because a fire can spread quickly, efforts to contain it within the first 5 minutes of a blaze can make a substantial difference in the eventual outcome.

To operate a fire extinguisher, use the PASS technique:

P = *Pull* the extinguisher's lock pin.
A = *Aim* the nozzle at the base of the fire.
S = *Squeeze* the handles together.
S = *Sweep* from side to side at the base of the flames.

Extinguishers expel their contents quickly; it takes only 8 to 25 seconds for most home models containing dry chemicals to empty.

If clothing catches fire, tear the article off, in a motion away from the face. Keep the person from running, because running fans the flames. Wrap a rug or a woolen blanket around the person's neck to keep the fire from the face or throw a blanket on the person. In some cases, you may be able to smother the flames by throwing the person to the floor and rolling them in a rug.

CAUTION

DO NOT let people run if their clothing is on fire.

DO NOT become trapped while fighting a fire. Always keep a door behind you so you can exit if the fire gets too big.

Threatening Dogs

When you enter any emergency scene, look for signs of a dog and proceed with caution even if the animal is not threatening. Ask the owner to control a threatening dog. If you cannot be delayed, consider using a fire extinguisher, water hose, or pepper spray. For a vicious dog, call the police for assistance.

Farm Animals

Emergencies involving farm animals can be dangerous to rescuers. Horses kick and bite and, if panicked, may trample a person. Cattle may kick, bite, gore, or squeeze people against a pen or barn. Pigs can deliver severe bites. In a situation that involves animals, you should do the following:

- Approach a situation involving animals with caution. Whenever possible, obtain help from an experienced animal handler or an animal control officer before approaching the scene.
- **DO NOT** frighten or chase an animal. Move slowly and speak quietly to reassure it.
- Be aware of territorial posturing by male livestock, such as bulls, rams, stallions, ganders, or roosters. Avoid making eye contact or facing the animal fully, as this may be interpreted as aggression. If the animal seems to be preparing to charge, back away slowly, as running may provoke it.
- If possible, close gates or fences between you and livestock before assisting injured people.
- **DO NOT** attempt to capture a loose or panicking animal. If food is available, use it to lure the animal away from the injured person. Placing food in a bucket and shaking it may be enough to attract and calm the animal, enabling the rescuer to lead it into an enclosure.

Triage: Prioritizing Multiple Injured People

Situations requiring first aid usually involve only one person. Rarely will you encounter a large-scale event involving more than one person who needs care. Such events may seem

TABLE 25-3 Examples of Disasters Involving Two or More People

Natural Disasters	Human-Caused Disasters
Earthquakes	Highway crashes
Tornadoes	Air crashes
Hurricanes	Train derailments
Floods	Terrorist attacks
Lightning strikes	Riots
Winter storms	Mass shootings
Heat waves	Explosions

commonplace because, when they do occur, they are frequently reported in the mass media **TABLE 25-3**.

When many people are injured, use a process called **triage** (a French word meaning "to sort") to distinguish among the following:

- Those needing immediate care for one of the "killers"—closed airway and severe bleeding (immediate care)
- Those who can wait for care until after others have been triaged (delayed care)
- Those who are deceased (dead/deceased)

The intent of triage is to provide the greatest good for the greatest number of people. Some people have a greater need for emergency care than others. Someone has to go last. Triage is especially effective in situations in which there are more injured people than first aid providers and rescuers present, and in situations where time is critical.

Q & A

What is the origin of the word triage?

Triage is a French word meaning to sort, separate, or select. It refers to the procedure of prioritizing people's care based on the severity of their condition. Several triage methods exist, varying among countries (even within a country) and the type of care provider (eg, paramedic, nurse, first aid provider) involved. The idea originated in World War I with French physicians treating the battlefield wounded at aid stations behind the front lines of battle.

Triage Categories

During triage, evaluate and sort every injured person into one of three categories **TABLE 25-4**.

While EMS personnel may have ribbons, cards, or tags to place on people to identify their category, you will rarely have these items. You can, however, improvise (eg, write on a piece of tape placed on the person's forehead or around the wrist). After triage, take injured people, according to their category,

TABLE 25-4 Triage Categories

Category	Description
Immediate	Person has life-threatening injuries (airway closed or severe bleeding) demanding immediate action to save their life.
Delayed	Person's life is not threatened. They may need care, but it can be delayed while other people are triaged.
Dead/deceased	Person is not breathing after their airway has been opened. There may be no time or people to perform CPR when others need immediate help. A volunteer from the walking-wounded group might be able to perform compression-only CPR or, if trained, CPR. An exception to bypassing the dead to treat the moderately or severely injured occurs when a lightning strike involves multiple people; in this event, CPR should be given to those who are motionless and appear to be dead *before* aiding people in other categories. (See Chapter 24, *Wilderness First Aid*, for more information.)

Abbreviation: CPR, cardiopulmonary resuscitation

to a medical facility, if available, or to an area designated for medical treatment.

Conducting Triage

Step 1: Conduct a voice triage by calling out, "If you can walk, come to me." People who can get up and walk rarely have life-threatening injuries. **DO NOT** force a person to move if they complain of pain. People who can walk can be placed in the "delayed" category. Direct them to a designated safe area; have them sit down and stay together. If you need more assistance, you can ask for volunteers from this group to help.

Step 2: Start surveying each person who did not get up and walk. Begin with the person closest to where you are standing. Quickly get to each person and sort each by their need for care. Tag everyone as "immediate," "delayed," or "dead." **DO NOT** stop to treat anyone during triage except to quickly open the airway and control severe bleeding.

When performing triage, take the following steps **FLOWCHART 25-1**:

- If a person fails one of the tests (or checks), tag them as immediate.
- If a person passes all of the tests (or checks), tag as delayed.
- Give every person a tag.

Reassess people regularly for changes in their condition. Only after people with immediate life-threatening conditions receive care should people with less serious conditions be given care. You may have to care for multiple people without adequate help until more highly trained emergency personnel arrive, at which point you may be asked to provide first aid, help move people, or help with ambulance or helicopter transportation.

Flowchart 25-1 Prioritizing Multiple Injured People

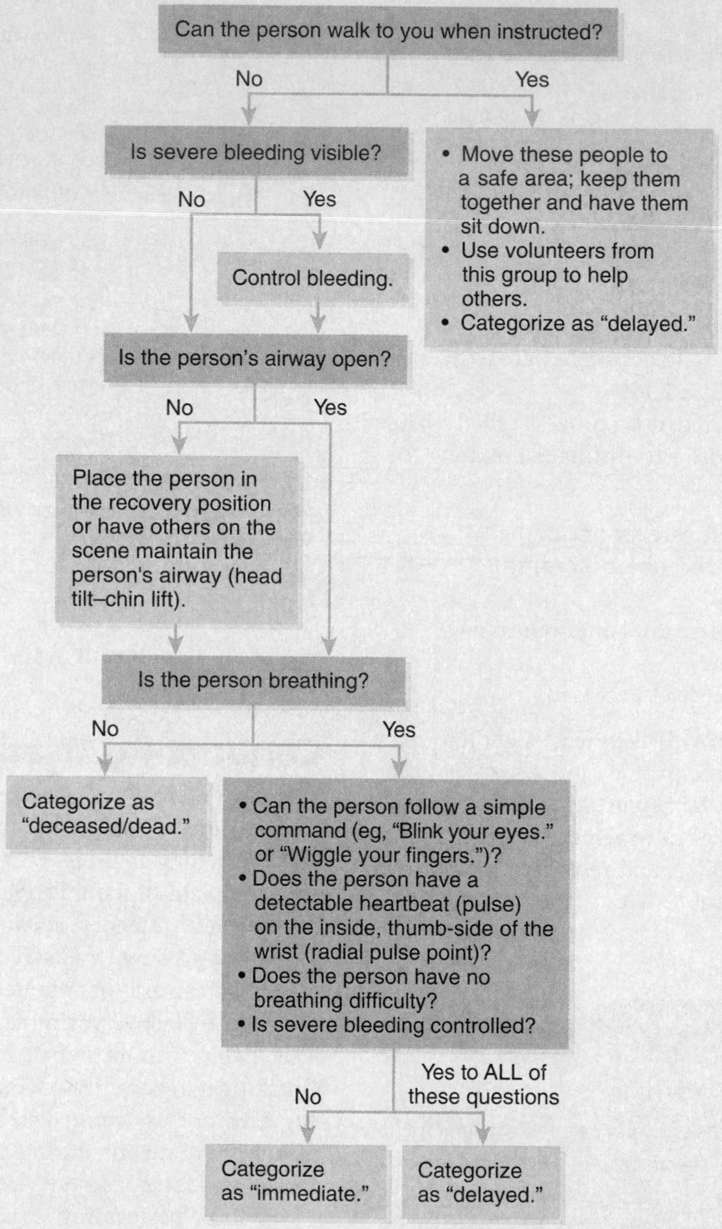

Can the person walk to you when instructed?
No
Yes
Is severe bleeding visible?
• Move these people to a safe area; keep them together and have them sit down.
• Use volunteers from this group to help others.
• Categorize as "delayed."
No
Yes
Control bleeding.
Is the person's airway open?
No
Yes
Place the person in the recovery position or have others on the scene maintain the person's airway (head tilt–chin lift).
Is the person breathing?
No
Yes
Categorize as "deceased/dead."
• Can the person follow a simple command (eg, "Blink your eyes." or "Wiggle your fingers.")?
• Does the person have a detectable heartbeat (pulse) on the inside, thumb-side of the wrist (radial pulse point)?
• Does the person have no breathing difficulty?
• Is severe bleeding controlled?
No
Yes to ALL of these questions
Categorize as "immediate."
Categorize as "delayed."

Moving People

A person should not be moved until they are ready for transportation to a hospital, if required. All necessary first aid should be provided before moving a person. A person should be moved only if there is an immediate danger, such as the following:

- There is a fire or danger of a fire.
- Explosives or other hazardous materials are involved.
- It is impossible to protect the scene from hazards.
- It is impossible to gain access to other people in the situation who need life-saving care (such as in a motor vehicle crash).

A person with cardiac arrest is usually moved unless they are already on the ground or floor because CPR must be performed on a firm, level surface.

Emergency Moves

The major danger in moving a person quickly is the possibility of aggravating a spinal injury. In an emergency, every effort should be made to pull the person in the direction of the long axis of the body to provide as much protection to the spinal cord as possible. If the person is on the floor or ground, you can move them away from the scene by using the various techniques **TABLE 25-5**. Refer to **FLOWCHART 25-2** for additional information regarding emergency rescue moves.

TABLE 25-5 Emergency Rescue Moves

Moves for Three to Six First Aid Providers	When to Use
Hammock carry **FIGURE 25-6**	Used when no equipment is available and the person cannot walk and cannot use the arms to hang onto the two first aid providers, or if the person is unresponsive
Moves for Two First Aid Providers	**When to Use**
Two-person assist **FIGURE 25-7**	Used when the person has a leg injury
Two-handed seat carry **FIGURE 25-8**	Used when no equipment is available and the person cannot walk but can use the arms to hang onto the two first aid providers
Extremity carry **FIGURE 25-9**	Used when no equipment is available and the person cannot walk and cannot use the arms to hang onto the two first aid providers
Chair carry **FIGURE 25-10**	Used for narrow passage or up or down stairs when a chair is available
Moves for One First Aid Provider	**When to Use**
Human crutch **FIGURE 25-11**	Used when person has a leg injury
Cradle carry **FIGURE 25-12**	Used for children and lightweight adults who cannot walk
Pack-strap carry **FIGURE 25-13**	Used for long distances when injuries make carrying the person over the first aid provider's shoulder unsafe
Piggyback carry **FIGURE 25-14**	Used when the person cannot walk but can use the arms to hang onto the first aid provider
Firefighter's carry **FIGURE 25-15**	Used for long distances when the person can be carried over the first aid provider's shoulder
Shoulder drag **FIGURE 25-16**	Used for short distances over a rough surface
Ankle drag **FIGURE 25-17**	Used for short distances over a smooth surface
Blanket drag **FIGURE 25-18**	Used for short distances

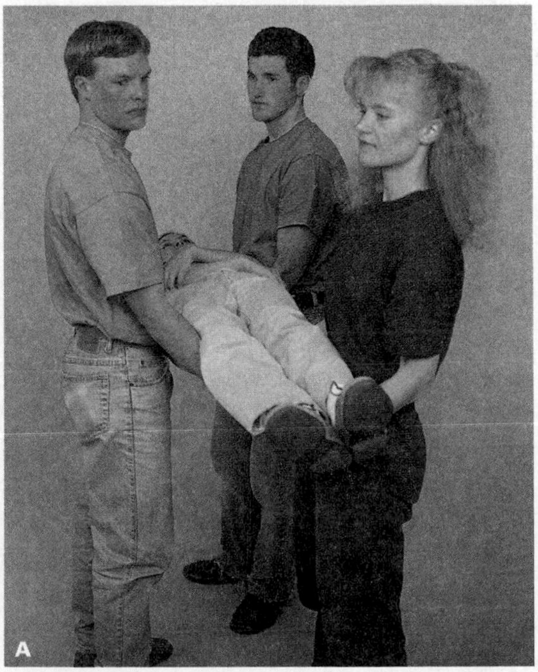

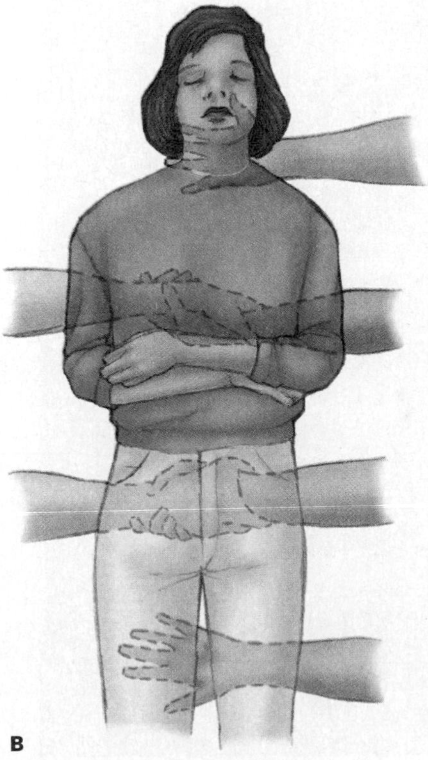

FIGURE 25-6 **A**. Hammock carry. **B**. Three to six people stand on alternate sides of the injured person and link hands beneath the person.

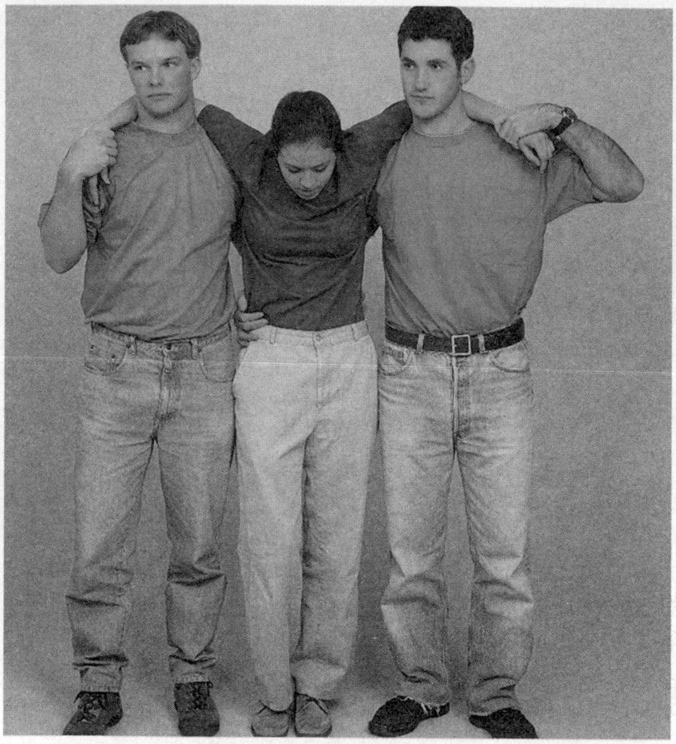

FIGURE 25-7 Two-person assist. This method is similar to the human crutch.

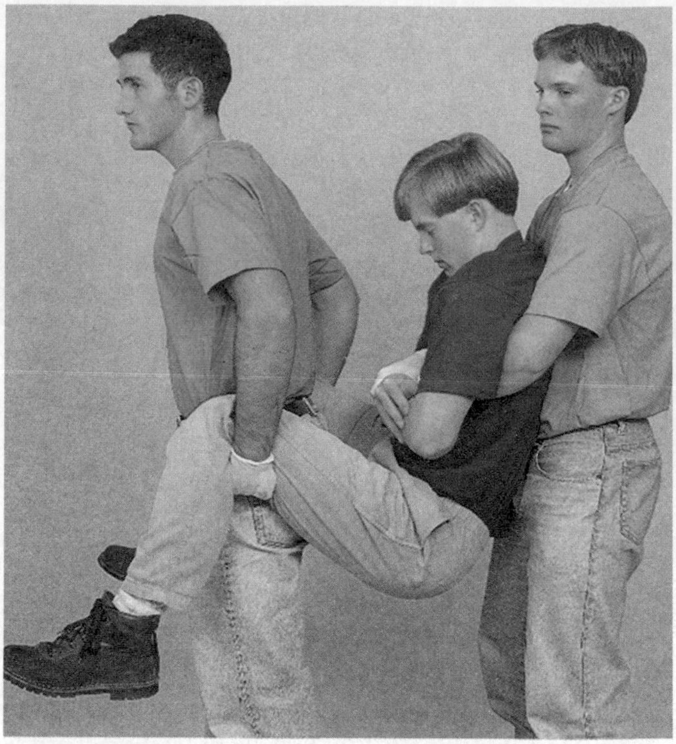

FIGURE 25-9 Extremity carry.

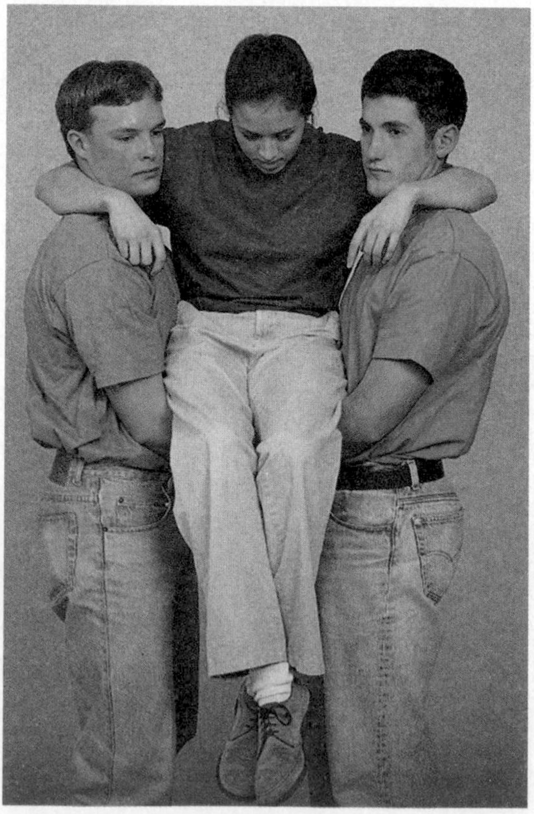

FIGURE 25-8 Two-handed seat carry.

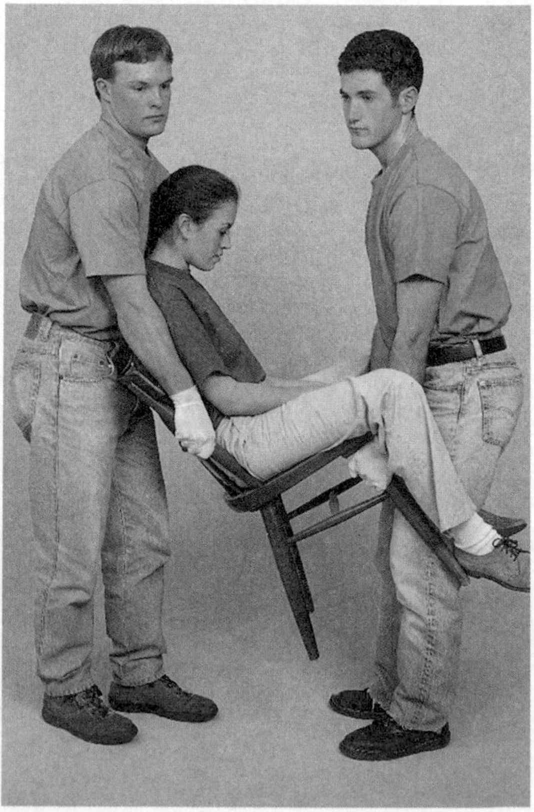

FIGURE 25-10 Chair carry. This method is useful for a narrow passage or up or down stairs. Use a sturdy chair that can take the person's weight.

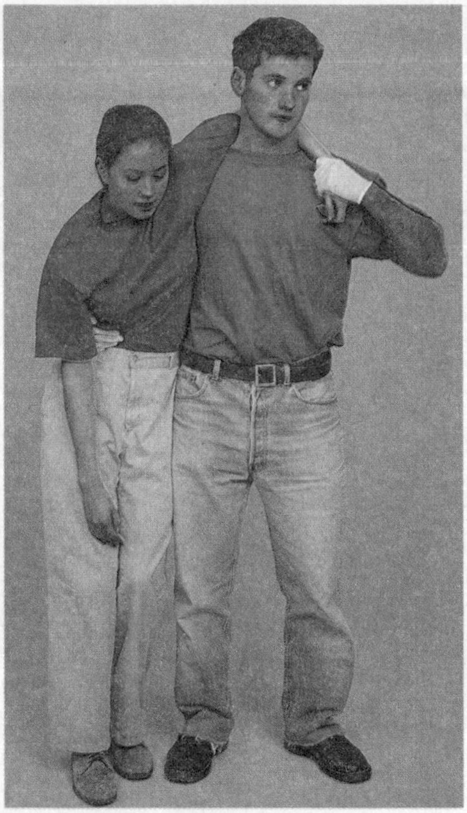

FIGURE 25-11 Human crutch (one person helps the person to walk). If one leg is injured, help the person to walk on the good leg while you support the injured side.

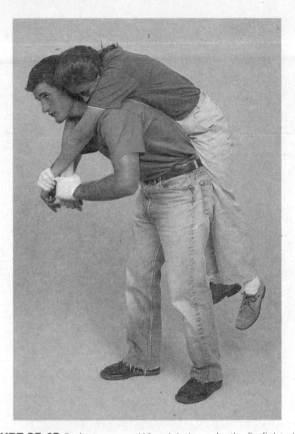

FIGURE 25-13 Pack-strap carry. When injuries make the firefighter's carry unsafe, this method is better for longer distances.

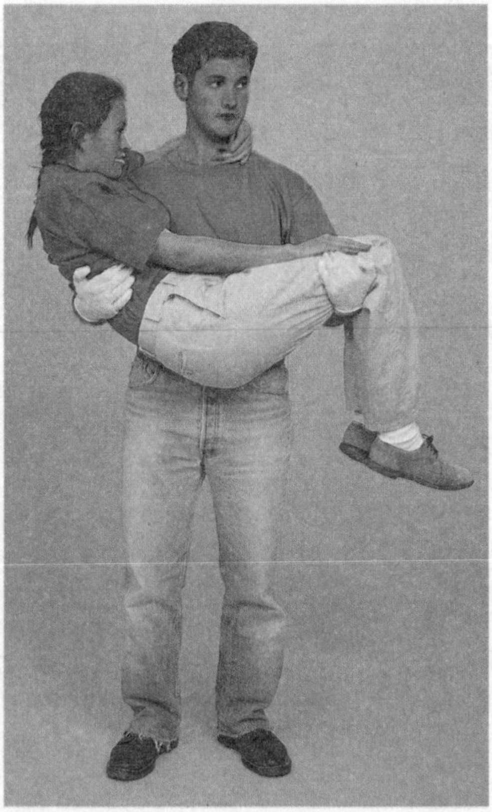

FIGURE 25-12 Cradle carry. Use this method for children and lightweight adults who cannot walk.

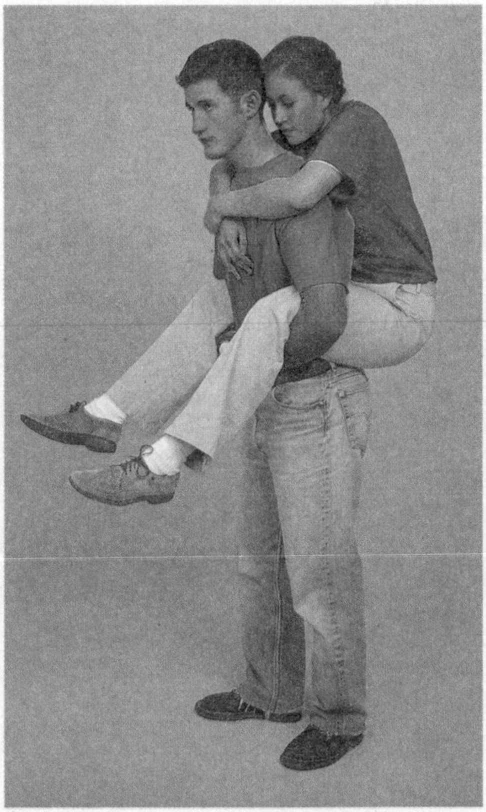

FIGURE 25-14 Piggyback carry. Use this method when the person cannot walk but can use the arms to hang onto the rescuer.

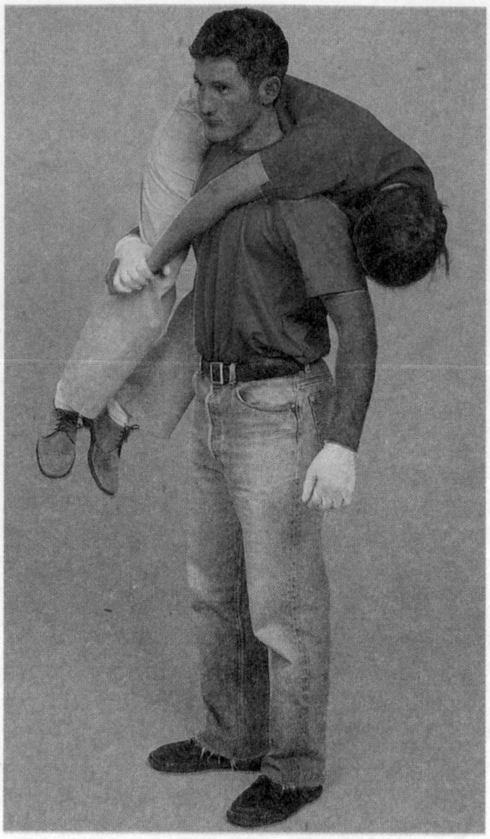

FIGURE 25-15 Firefighter's carry. If the person's injuries permit, you can travel longer distances if you carry the person over your shoulder.

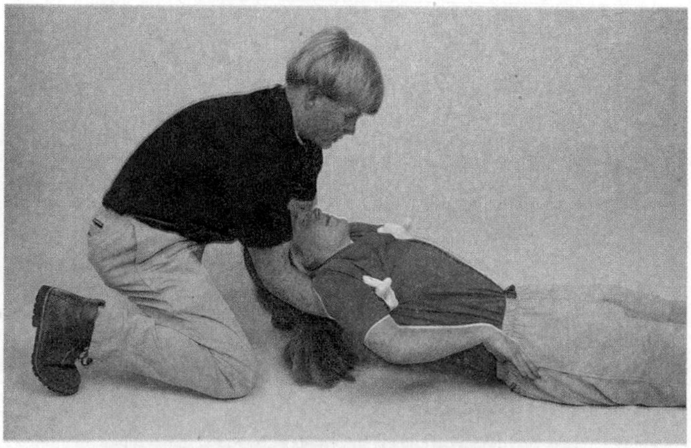

FIGURE 25-16 Shoulder drag. Use for short distances over a rough surface; stabilize the person's head with your forearms.

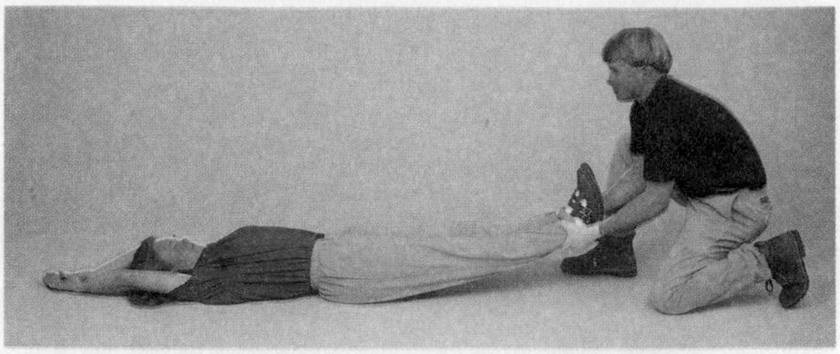

FIGURE 25-17 Ankle drag. This is the fastest method for a short distance on a smooth surface.

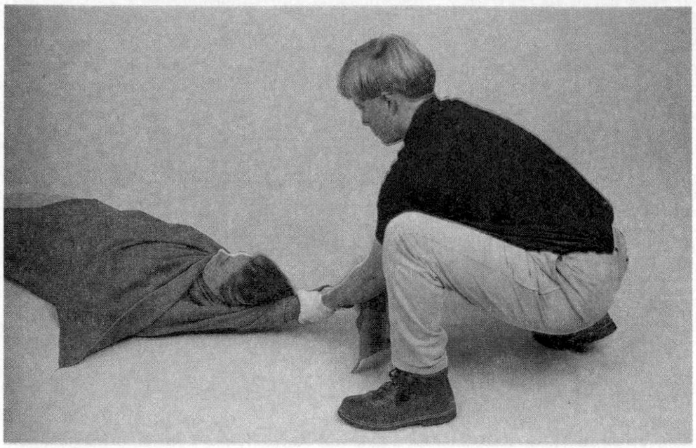

FIGURE 25-18 Blanket drag. Roll the person onto a blanket, and pull from behind the person's head.

FYI

Principles of Lifting and Carrying

- Know your capabilities. **DO NOT** try to handle a load that is too heavy or awkward; seek help.
- Use a safe, nonslip grip. Use as much of your palms as possible.
- Keep your back straight **FIGURE 25-19**. Tighten the muscles of your buttocks and abdomen.
- Bend your knees to use the strong muscles of the thighs and buttocks.
- Keep your arms close to your body and your elbows flexed.
- Position your feet shoulder width apart for balance, one in front of the other.
- When lifting, keep and lift the person close to your body.
- While lifting, **DO NOT** twist your back; pivot with your feet.
- Lift and carry slowly, smoothly, and in unison with the other lifters.
- Before you move a person, explain to them what you are doing.

Flowchart 25-2 Emergency Rescue Moves

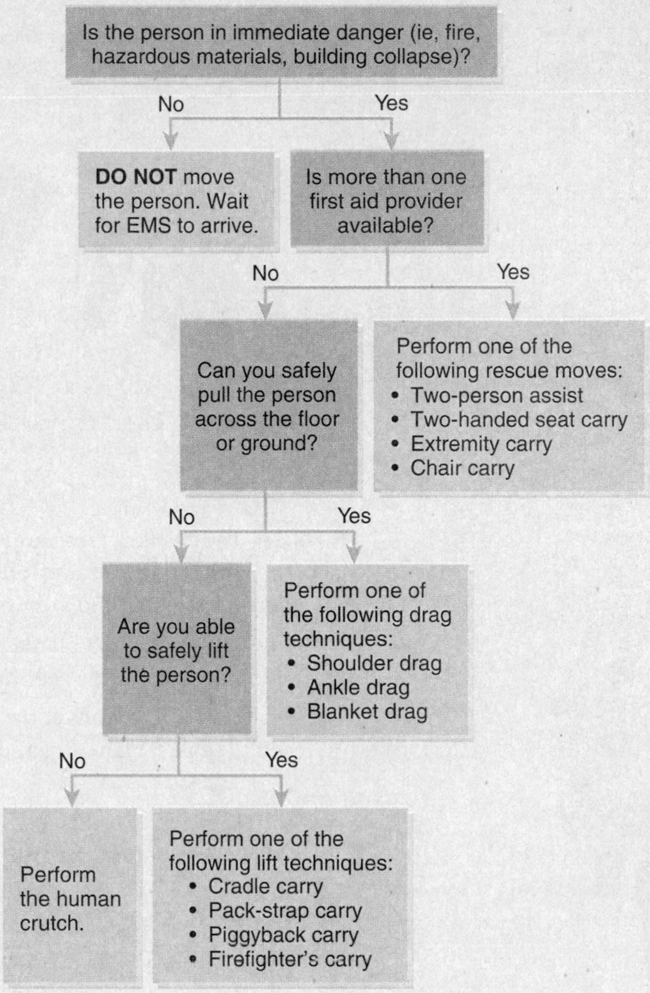

Nonemergency Moves

All injured parts should be stabilized before and during moving. If rapid transportation is not needed, it is helpful to practice on another person about the same size as the injured person.

Stretcher or Litter

The safest way to carry an injured person without a spinal injury is on a stretcher or litter, which can be improvised. Before using an improvised stretcher, test it by lifting a rescuer about the same size as the injured person.

Important cautions regarding improvised stretcher use include the following:

- Test improvised stretchers before use by lifting a rescuer who is about the same size as the person.
- Improvised stretchers do not give sufficient support of a suspected spinal injury.
- Improvised stretchers should be used only when the person is able to stand some sagging, bending, or twisting without serious consequences.

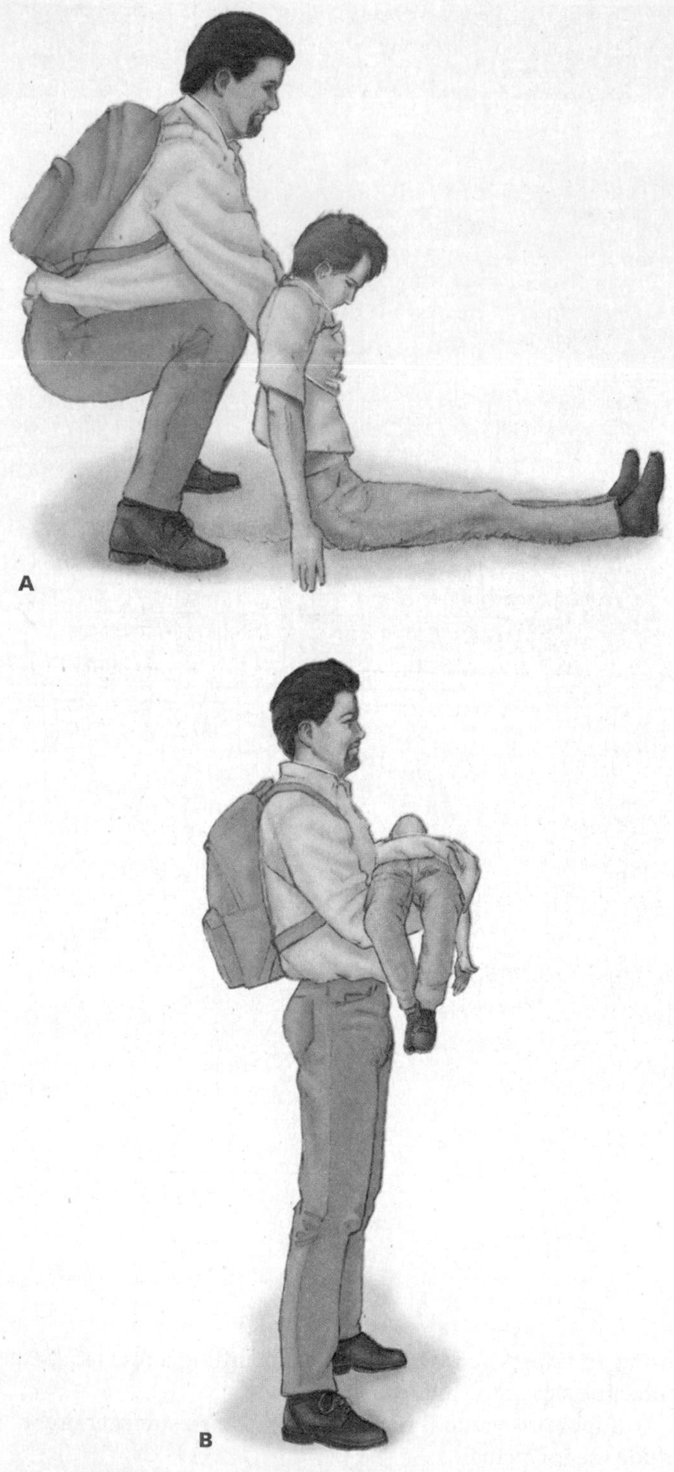

FIGURE 25-19 When lifting and carrying a person, keep your back straight and bend your knees. Keep the person close to your body.

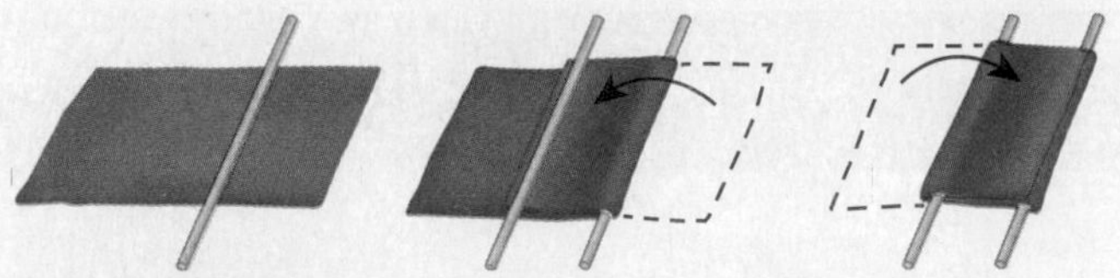

FIGURE 25-20 Blanket-and-pole improvised stretcher.

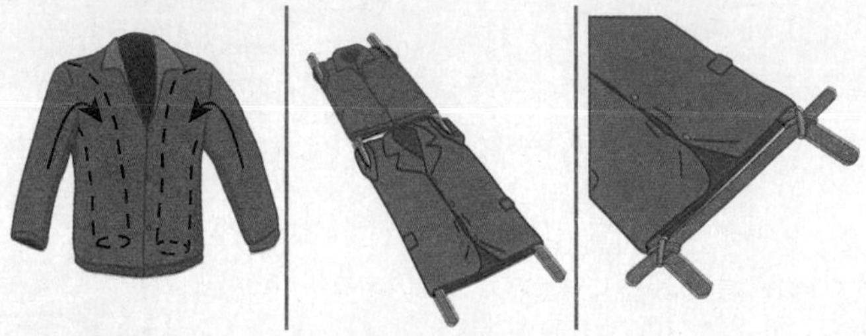

FIGURE 25-21 Jacket-and-pole improvised stretcher.

Blanket-and-Pole Stretcher

A blanket, tarp, tent fly, or other material may be used for a blanket-and-pole improvised stretcher **FIGURE 25-20**. Two sturdy poles may be used from such objects as strong tree limbs, skis, 2 × 4–inch wood boards, etc. The poles should be long enough to reach beyond the ends of the blanket in order that the carriers may get a firm grip on the poles. The person's weight will keep the blanket from unwinding if it is properly wrapped. To build a blanket-and-pole improvised stretcher, reference Figure 25-20 and the following steps:

1. Spread out a blanket and lay a pole one-third of the distance between the edges.
2. Fold the blanket over the pole and place the second pole 6 inches from the edge on top of the folded-over part.
3. Fold the 6-inch part over the second pole and fold the longer part over the same pole and body of stretcher.

Jacket-and-Pole Stretcher

Two or three jackets are required to construct a jacket-and-pole improvised stretcher for adults **FIGURE 25-21**. The sleeves are turned inside out (for greater strength). The poles are passed through the sleeves of the jackets. Button or zip up the jackets. Follow these steps to build a jacket-and-pole stretcher:

1. Turn the sleeves of two or three jackets inside out (inverted).
2. Thread the poles through the jacket sleeves inside the jacket and button or zip up the jackets.
3. Attach a cross-brace (eg, tree limb) to the ends of the poles for added stability.

Blanket-Lift-and-Carry

Where no poles are available, a stretcher can be made by placing the person in the middle of a blanket **FIGURE 25-22**. A minimum of two people are needed to perform this move, but three people on each side is better. To perform the blanket-lift-and-carry, follow these steps:

1. Kneel and roll the edges of the blanket toward the person until the edges are tightly rolled (about 2 inches from the body) and are large enough grasp securely.

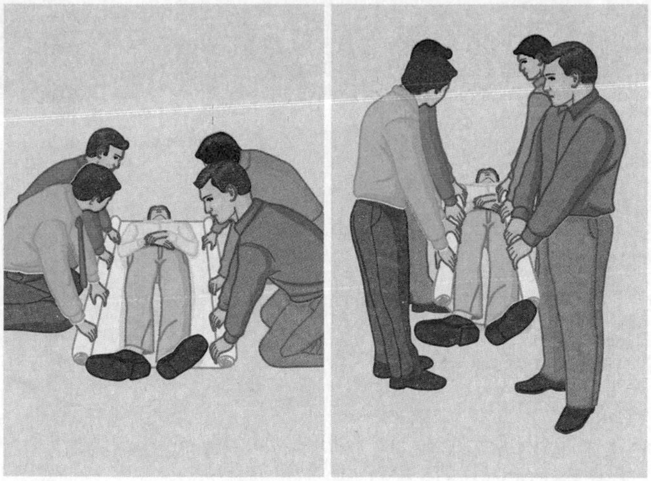

FIGURE 25-22 Blanket-lift-and-carry when no poles are available. Tightly role the edges of the blanket and use to grasp and lift.

2. Slowly pull outward to remove any slack that could jar the person on lifting.
3. After the slack has been removed, the person can be lifted and carried.

Improvised Board Stretcher

An improvised board stretcher is sturdier than a blanket-and-pole stretcher but is also heavier and less comfortable. Secure the person to the board. Skis, pack frames, and sleds can also be used to make stretchers. Pad stretchers well, using sleeping bags, clothing, or sleeping pads. Commercial stretchers are seldom available except with rescue groups.

If the person is being carried out, be sure to do the following:

- Call or send someone to notify authorities that help is needed.
- At least four, preferably six, bearers should carry the stretcher (litter) at all times.
- Over rough terrain, eight carriers (six over smooth trail) should carry the litter for 15 minutes and then rest or rotate with other carries.

CAUTION

DO NOT move a person unless absolutely necessary, such as if the person is in immediate danger or must be moved to shelter while waiting for EMS personnel to arrive.

DO NOT make the injury worse by moving the person.

DO NOT move a person who could have a spinal injury unless absolutely necessary due to other threats to life, such as fire.

DO NOT move a person without splinting the injured part.

DO NOT move a person unless you know where you are going.

DO NOT leave an unresponsive person alone except for taking a short time to call 9-1-1.

DO NOT move a person when you can send someone for help. Wait with the person.

DO NOT try to move a person by yourself if other people are available to help.

DO NOT enter certain hazardous areas (eg, a confined space filled with gas or vapors) unless you have the proper training and equipment.

PREP KIT

Ready for Review

- *Reach-throw-row-go* identifies the sequence for attempting a water rescue.
- If a person has fallen through the ice near the shore, extend a pole or throw a line with a floatable object attached to it.
- Electrical injuries can be devastating.
- Almost any highway crash scene involves the potential danger of hazardous chemicals.
- A confined space is any area not intended for human occupancy that may have or develop a dangerous atmosphere.
- In most states, you are legally obligated to stop and give help when you are involved in a motor vehicle crash.
- Should you encounter a fire, you should:
  - Get all people out fast.
  - Call 9-1-1.
- When you enter any emergency scene, look for signs of an animal and proceed with caution if the animal is not threatening.
- Emergencies involving farm animals can be dangerous to rescuers.
- The goal of triage is to do the greatest good for the greatest number of people.
- A variety of systems are used to identify care and transportation priorities.
- A person should not be moved until they are ready for transportation to a hospital, if required.
- The major danger in moving a person quickly is the possibility of aggravating a spinal injury.
- All injured parts should be stabilized before and during moving.

Vital Vocabulary

drowning The process of experiencing respiratory impairment from submersion/immersion in liquid.

heat escape lessening position (HELP) The recommended position (knees pulled up, arms crossed) for a person who is in cold water and wearing a flotation device; meant to minimize heat loss and increase chances of survival.

triage A system used for sorting people to determine the order in which they will receive medical attention.

Assessment in Action

You are fishing at the nearby lake. Several swimmers and others in canoes are also enjoying the lake. One swimmer decides to swim to the other side but begins to struggle about 30 feet (9 m) from shore.

Directions: Circle Yes if you agree with the statement; circle No if you disagree.

1. This type of drowning situation is called distressed nonswimmer.

   YES **NO**

2. You are a very strong swimmer so you should immediately jump in the lake to rescue the person.

   YES **NO**

3. You could try throwing a floating object to the person.

   YES **NO**

4. The best option in this situation would be to use a canoe to rescue the person.

   YES **NO**

Check Your Knowledge

Directions: Circle Yes if you agree with the statement; circle No if you disagree.

1. You should attempt to move downed power lines away from a person by using a broom or other wooden object.

   YES **NO**

2. Strong, unusual odors or clouds of vapor are possible indications of the presence of hazardous materials.

   YES **NO**

3. To keep from becoming trapped while attempting to extinguish a fire, you should always keep a door behind you for rapid exit.

   YES **NO**

4. In a situation involving several people, those with breathing difficulties need immediate attention.

   YES **NO**

PREP KIT continued

5. A major concern in moving a person quickly is the possibility of aggravating a spinal injury.

   YES **NO**

6. Row-throw-reach-go represents the safe order for executing a water rescue.

   YES **NO**

7. In most states, you are legally obligated to stop and give help when you see a motor vehicle crash.

   YES **NO**

8. The first thing to do in case of a fire is to use a fire extinguisher and try to put out the fire.

   YES **NO**

9. When using a fire extinguisher, aim it at the base of the flames.

   YES **NO**

10. When several people are injured, those crying or screaming should receive your attention first.

    YES **NO**

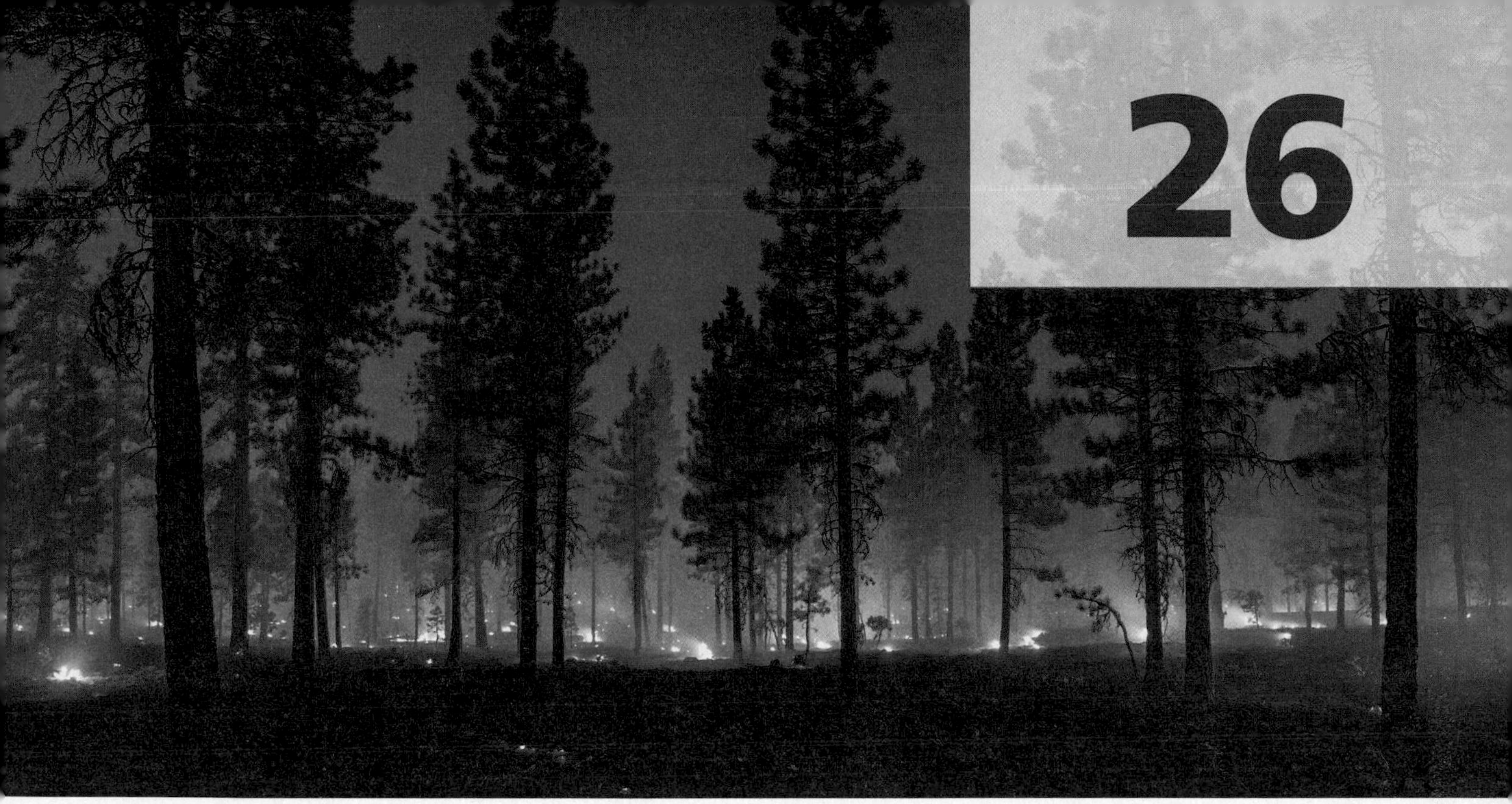

26

Disaster Preparedness

CHAPTER AT A GLANCE

Disaster Preparedness

Disasters are a fact of life. Each year, thousands of disasters, large and small, natural and caused by humans, strike somewhere in the world. Many people have survived disasters, thanks to good luck and willpower, but that is not enough. Training about disasters needs to be modified from "nice to know" to "must know." Every American will likely experience or witness at least one disaster during their lifetime. The tragedy is that each citizen could be better prepared than they are now for that disaster. When a disaster strikes, you must be ready to act.

Valuable information about disasters is discussed in this chapter. This information is adapted from US government documents provided by the Federal Emergency Management Agency (FEMA), the US Department of Homeland Security, the National Weather Service, the US Department of Labor, and the US Geological Survey.

Natural Disasters

Natural disasters such as earthquakes, floods, hurricanes, and tornados claim many lives each year. Becoming informed about the dangers of natural disasters and steps you can take to protect yourself and others can help minimize injuries and deaths.

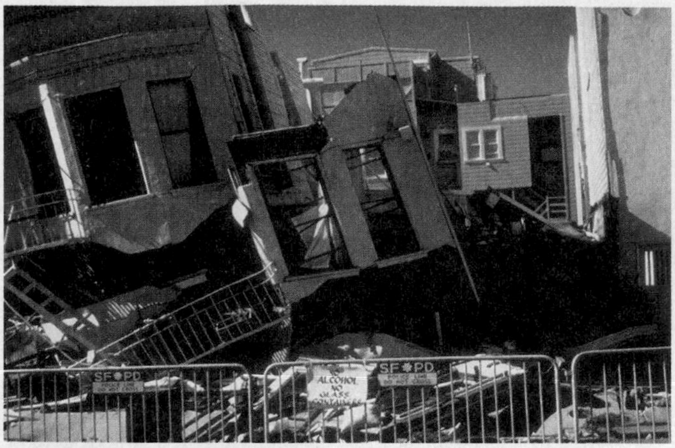

FIGURE 26-1 Devastation resulting from the California earthquake that crippled San Francisco in 1989.
Courtesy of D. Perkins/USGS.

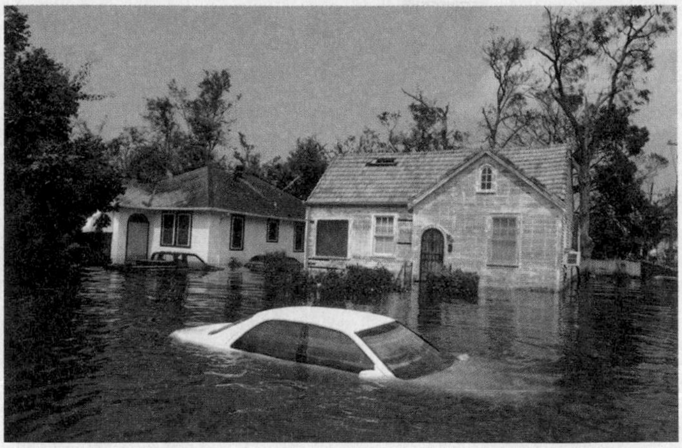

FIGURE 26-2 Hurricane Katrina (2005) caused massive floods in New Orleans.
Courtesy of Jocelyn Augustino/FEMA.

Earthquake

An earthquake is a sudden, rapid shaking of the earth caused by the breaking and shifting of rock deep beneath the earth's surface. This shaking can cause buildings and bridges to collapse; disrupt gas, electric, and phone service; and sometimes trigger landslides, avalanches, flash floods, fires, and huge, destructive ocean waves known as tsunamis. Earthquakes can occur at any time of the year **FIGURE 26-1**.

What to Do During an Earthquake

Follow these safety guidelines if you experience an earthquake:

- If you are indoors, take cover under a sturdy desk, table, or bench or against an inside wall. If the earthquake is severe, crouch next to a large, sturdy object such as a refrigerator or file cabinet. Should the ceiling collapse, a triangle of space next to the object will provide a safe place. Stay away from glass, windows, outside doors, walls, and anything that could fall. If there is no table or desk nearby, cover your face and head with your arms and crouch down; a door frame may offer some protection.
- Stay inside until the shaking has stopped and you are sure exiting is safe. It is dangerous to try to leave a building during an earthquake because objects can fall on you. Beware of aftershocks, and if they occur, follow the same precautions for an earthquake.
- If you are in bed, stay there, and protect your head with a pillow, unless you are under a heavy light or fan fixture that could fall. If the earthquake is severe, move to the floor next to, but not under, the bed. This will also provide a safe space if the ceiling collapses.
- If you are in a high-rise building, expect the fire alarms and sprinklers to go off during an earthquake. **DO NOT** use the elevators; use the stairs.
- If you are outdoors, find a clear spot away from buildings, trees, streetlights, and power lines. Drop to the ground and stay there until the shaking stops.
- If you are in a vehicle, pull over and stay there with your seat belt fastened until the shaking has stopped. If the earthquake is severe and you are under a highway overpass, exit your car and lie next to, but not underneath, your vehicle. The falling debris may crush the roof of the car, but beside the car will be a safe place for you to stay until help arrives.
- If you are trapped in debris, do not panic. Move carefully.
  - **DO NOT** use a flame for light because of possible gas leaks.
  - **DO NOT** move about or kick up dust.
  - Cover your mouth with a handkerchief or clothing.
  - Tap on a pipe or wall so rescuers can locate you.
- Learn how to turn off your gas supply where it enters the house. Turn off the gas if you smell gas or have to evacuate.
  - If you smell gas, **DO NOT** use light switches or any other devices that can spark.

Flood

With the exception of fire, floods are the most common and widespread of all natural disasters. Most communities have experienced some type of flooding after heavy storms or winter snow thaws **FIGURE 26-2**. Pay attention to flash flood warnings in your area even if skies are clear, because runoff can occur from storms that occur miles away. Be especially aware of storms in hills above you. Flash floods occur when heavy rain causes runoff into channels and low-lying areas. The flood can be very fast and can occur miles from the rain, often catching people off guard.

What to Do During a Flood

Follow these safety guidelines if conditions exist that could cause a flood:

- Be aware of the likelihood of flooding in your area. If there is any possibility of a flood or flash flood, move immediately to higher ground. Be aware of streams, drainage channels, canyons, and other areas prone to flooding quickly and suddenly.

- Listen to your local radio or television stations or check social media outlets for information.
- If local authorities issue a flood watch, prepare to evacuate.
- Secure your home, if you have time. Move essential items to upper floors.
- If instructed, turn off utilities at the main switches or valves. Disconnect electrical appliances. **DO NOT** touch electrical equipment if you are wet or standing in water.
- If you are not evacuating, you still need to prepare for the worst. If you do not have access to adequate bottled water, you can fill the bathtub with water in case water becomes contaminated or services are cut off. Before filling the tub, sterilize it with a diluted bleach solution (1 part bleach to 10 parts water).
- **DO NOT** walk through moving water. Six inches (15 cm) of moving water can knock you off your feet. Use a stick or pole to check the firmness of the ground and water depth in front of you.
- **DO NOT** drive into flooded areas. A foot of water can float a vehicle. Two feet (61 cm) of water can carry away most vehicles, including sport utility vehicles and pickup trucks.
- If flood water rises around your car and you cannot drive out, abandon the car and move to higher ground, but only if you can safely do so.

Heat Wave

In extreme heat and high humidity, cooling of the body by evaporation is slowed, and it is difficult for the body to maintain normal temperature **FIGURE 26-3**. People living in urban areas may be at greater risk from the effects of a prolonged heat wave than those living in rural areas. Asphalt and concrete store heat longer and gradually release heat at night. A devastating heat wave struck Europe in 2003, resulting in over 35,000 injuries and deaths.

What to Do During a Heat Wave

Follow these safety guidelines if you experience a heat-wave emergency:

- Stay in the coolest available location. Stay indoors as much as possible. If air-conditioning is not available, stay on the lowest floor out of the sunshine. Circulate the air with a fan, and use cool, wet cloths to help keep your body temperature down.
- Drink plenty of water regularly, even if you do not feel thirsty.
- Avoid drinking alcoholic beverages, because they cause further dehydration.
- Never leave children or pets alone in vehicles.
- Dress in loose-fitting clothes. Lightweight, light-colored clothing reflects heat and sunlight and helps maintain normal body temperature.
- Protect your face and head outdoors by wearing a wide-brimmed hat.
- Avoid too much sunshine. Sunburn slows the skin's ability to cool itself.
- Avoid strenuous work during the warmest part of the day (usually at 10:00 to 15:00 hours).
- Spend at least 2 hours of the day in an air-conditioned place. If your home is not air-conditioned, consider spending the warmest part of the day in public buildings (eg, libraries, movie theaters, shopping malls).
- Check on family, friends, and neighbors who do not have air-conditioning and who spend much of their time alone. Refer to Chapter 21, *Heat-Related Emergencies*, for first aid procedures for heat-related emergencies (eg, heatstroke, heat exhaustion, heat cramps).

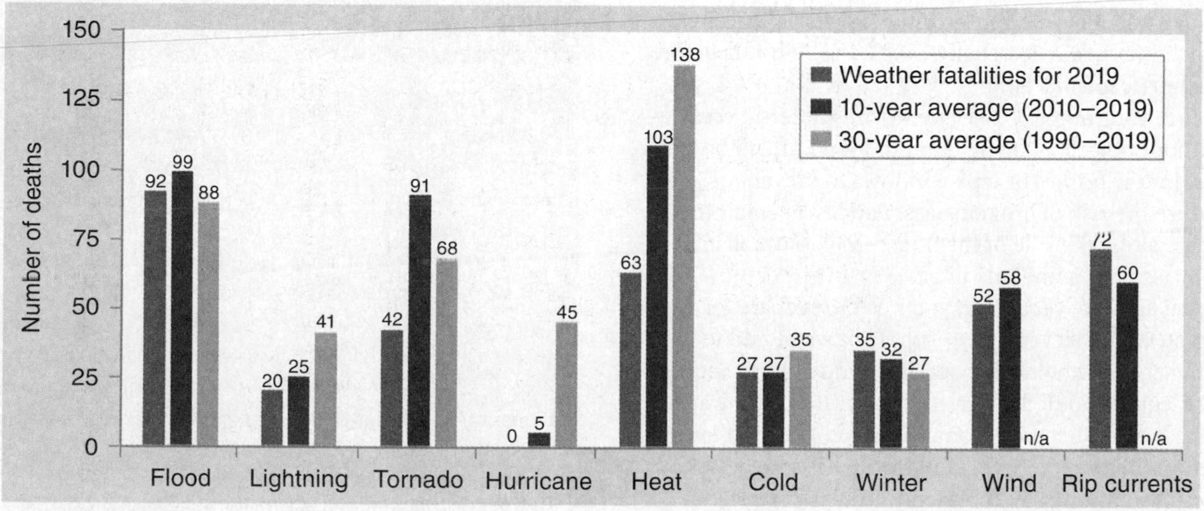

FIGURE 26-3 Deaths caused by weather events.
Data from NOAA's National Weather Service Office of Climate, Water, and Weather Services (http://www.weather.gov/om/hazstats.shtml).

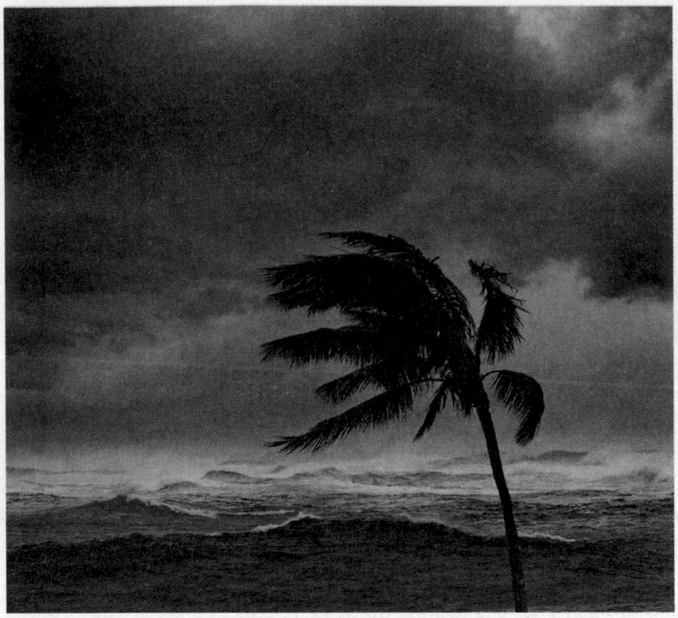

FIGURE 26-4 Hurricanes are among the most costly and dangerous disasters.

Hurricane

A **hurricane** is a tropical storm with winds that have reached a constant speed of at least 74 miles per hour (119 kph). As a hurricane nears land, it can bring torrential rains, high winds, and flooding from the ocean, called storm surges. All Atlantic and Gulf of Mexico coastal areas are subject to hurricanes or tropical storms. August and September are the peak months of hurricane activity during the storm season, which lasts from June to November **FIGURE 26-4**. In the Pacific Ocean, these storms are called typhoons.

What to Do During a Hurricane

Follow these safety guidelines if you experience the threat of a hurricane:

- Listen to your local radio or television stations or check social media outlets for information. If a hurricane watch is issued, you usually have 24 to 36 hours before the hurricane hits land.
- Secure your home. Close any storm shutters. Secure outdoor objects or bring them indoors. Attach boards to window frames or tape windows to prevent or reduce the risk of broken glass. Park cars remaining at home along the side of the house. Make sure that all vehicles have a full tank of gas.
- If you are not evacuating, you need to prepare for the worst. Gather several days' supply of water and food for each household member. If you do not have access to adequate bottled water, fill the bathtub with water in case water becomes contaminated or services are cut off. Before filling the tub, sterilize it with a diluted bleach solution (1 part bleach to 10 parts water).
- If you are evacuating, prepare backpacks to take your disaster supplies with you to the shelter. Be sure to include essential medications and mobile phone chargers.
- When preparing to evacuate, fuel your vehicle and review evacuation routes. If instructed, turn off utilities at the main valves or switches before departing your residence.
- Evacuate to an inland location early in the following situations:
  - Local authorities announce an evacuation and you live in an evacuation zone.
  - You live in a mobile home near the path of the hurricane.
  - You live in a high-rise building near the path of the hurricane.
  - You live on the coast, on a flood plain near a river, or near an inland waterway.
  - You think you are in danger.
- Leave immediately if local authorities order an evacuation. Follow evacuation routes; stay away from coastal areas, riverbanks, and streams; and tell others where you are going.
- If you are not required to evacuate or are unable to evacuate, stay indoors and away from windows and glass doors during the hurricane. Keep pets and necessary supplies such as food close by.
- To protect yourself against the strong winds:
  - Take refuge in a small interior room, closet, or hallway.
  - Close all interior doors; secure and brace exterior doors.
  - In a multistory building, go to the first or second floor and stay in interior rooms away from the windows.
  - Lie on the floor under a table or other sturdy object if a hurricane or any associated tornado approaches.
- Phone lines are likely to be busy with emergency traffic. Avoid using the phone except for serious emergencies.

Q&A

What part does first aid play in disasters?

The value of first aid training for laypeople has increased during natural and man-made disasters. When a sudden disaster strikes, survivors often constitute the only source of initial help because medical help takes time to mobilize or is insufficient.

Reports from bombings in New York and London state that first aid by bystanders saved lives. In the Madrid bombings, 67% of the injured people arrived at the hospital in nonambulance vehicles. Transport by bystanders occurs in many mass casualty disasters if ambulance transport is lacking. Officials interviewed after disasters strongly agree that first aid training for laypeople decreases death tolls.

Data from Van de Velde S, et al. Effectiveness of nonresuscitative first aid training in laypeople: a systematic review. *Ann Emerg Med.* 2009;54(3):447–457.

Landslides

Landslides occur in almost every US state when masses of rock, earth, or debris move down a slope. They may be small or large and can move at slow or high speeds. They are usually associated with periods of heavy rainfall or rapid snowmelt.

What to Do During a Landslide

Follow these safety guidelines if conditions exist that could cause a landslide:

- Stay alert. Many landslides occur when people are sleeping.
- If you are in an area that is susceptible to landslides, consider evacuating if it is safe to do so.
- Listen for unusual sounds that might indicate moving debris, such as trees cracking, boulders knocking together, or rumbling.
- If you are near a stream or channel, be alert for any sudden increase or decrease in water flow and for a change from clear to muddy water. Such changes may indicate landslide activity upstream, so be prepared to move quickly.
- Be alert when driving. Embankments along roadsides are susceptible to landslides. Watch the road for collapsed pavement, mud, fallen rocks, and other indications of possible debris flow.
- If you remain at home, move to a second level if possible to distance yourself from the direct path of landslide debris.

Tornado

A tornado is a violent windstorm characterized by a twisting, funnel-shaped cloud. It is spawned by a thunderstorm (or sometimes as a result of a hurricane). Tornado season is generally March through August, although tornadoes can occur at any time of the year. Every state is at some risk from this hazard, but tornados are most frequently reported east of the Rocky Mountains **FIGURE 26-5**.

What to Do During a Tornado

Follow these safety guidelines if you experience a tornado. If you are at home:

- Go immediately to a windowless interior room, storm cellar, basement, or the lowest level of the building. If there is no basement, go to an inner hallway or a smaller inner room with no windows, such as a bathroom or closet.
- Get under a piece of sturdy furniture (such as a heavy table or desk) and hold on to it.

If you are outdoors:

- If possible, get inside a building.
- If shelter is not available or there is no time to get indoors, lie in a ditch or low-lying area or crouch near a strong building.

If you are at work or school:

- Avoid places with wide-span roofs such as auditoriums, cafeterias, large hallways, and shopping malls.
- Go to a predetermined shelter area (signs are usually posted).
- Get under a piece of sturdy furniture (such as a heavy table, desk, or workbench).

If you are in a vehicle:

- **DO NOT** try to outrun a tornado.
- Get out of the vehicle immediately and take shelter in a nearby building. If there is no time to get indoors, get out of the car and lie in a ditch or low-lying area away from the vehicle.

Tsunami

A **tsunami** (pronounced soo-NAHM-ee) is a series of waves generated by an undersea disturbance (eg, an earthquake). From the area of disturbance, the waves travel outward in all directions, much like the ripples caused by throwing a rock into a pond. Tsunamis reaching heights of more than

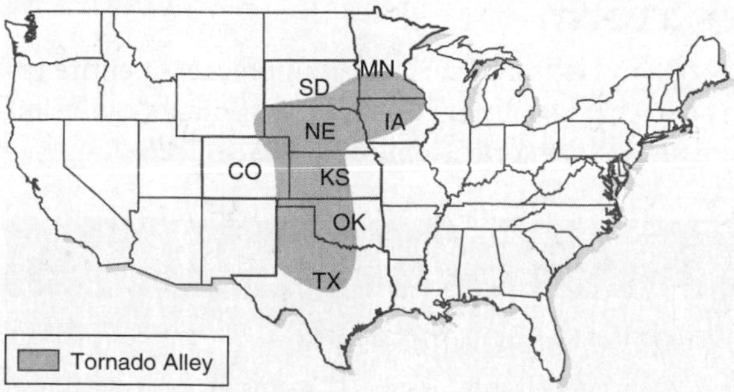

A

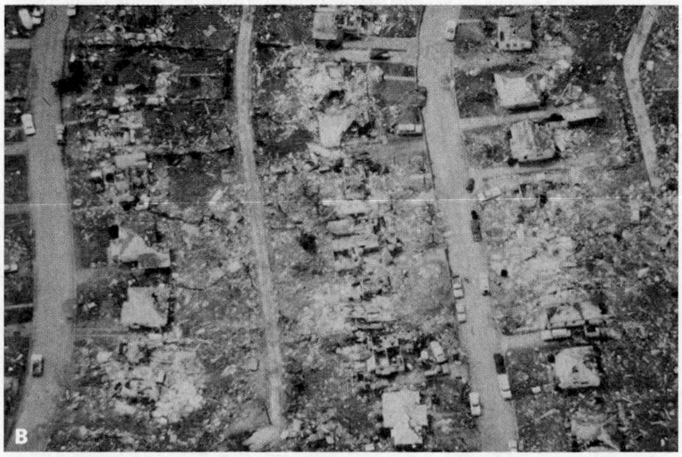

FIGURE 26-5 **A**. Tornados are most frequently reported east of the Rocky Mountains. **B**. The tornado in Wichita Falls, Texas, in 1979 was one of the worst tornadoes in US history.

100 feet (30 m) have been recorded near coastlines, although most waves are less than 18 feet (5 m) high. Areas of greatest risk are less than 50 feet (15 m) above sea level and within 1 mile (2 km) of the shoreline. Drowning is the most common cause of death due to a tsunami.

What to Do During a Tsunami

Follow these safety guidelines if conditions exist that could cause a tsunami:

- Listen to your local radio or television stations or check social media outlets for information. If you are advised to evacuate, do so immediately.
- Stay away from the area until local authorities say it is safe to return.
- **DO NOT** go to the shoreline to watch for a tsunami. If you can see the wave, you are too close to escape it. Because a tsunami is a series of waves, do not assume that the danger is over after one wave.

Volcano Eruption

A volcano is a mountain that opens downward to a reservoir of molten rock below the earth's surface. When the pressure from gases and molten rock becomes strong enough to cause an explosion, eruptions occur. Gases and rock shoot up through the opening and spill over the mountainsides and/or spew into the air. Most injuries and deaths are due to ash, falling rocks, landslides, and floods, rather than hot flowing lava.

What to Do During a Volcano Eruption

Follow these safety guidelines if a volcano erupts:

- Follow the evacuation order issued by local authorities. Avoid areas downwind from the volcano.

If caught indoors:

- Close all windows, doors, and chimney and stove dampers.

If caught outdoors:

- Seek shelter indoors.
- Avoid low-lying areas where poisonous gases can collect and flash floods and lava and mudflows can be dangerous.
- Put all machinery inside a garage or barn.

Protect yourself:

- Wear long-sleeved shirts and pants.
- Use goggles to protect your eyes.
- Use a dust mask or hold a damp cloth over your face to keep from breathing in the hot ash or gases.
- Stay out of the area around the erupting volcano. Trying to watch an erupting volcano can be deadly.

Wildfire

Forest, brush, and grass fires can occur at any time of the year, but mostly during long, dry hot spells. The majority of these fires are caused by human carelessness or ignorance (for example, fireworks, campfires, railroad sparks, and downed power lines can all cause wildfires if not properly cared for) **FIGURE 26-6**.

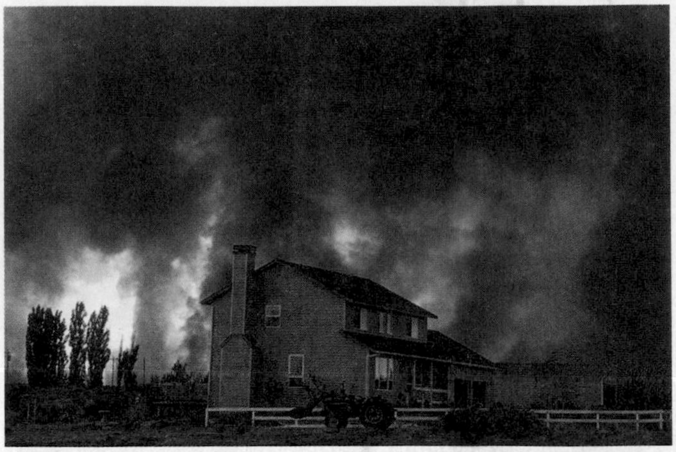

FIGURE 26-6 Wildfires can move quickly, threatening lives and homes.
Courtesy of John Hutmacher/USFS.

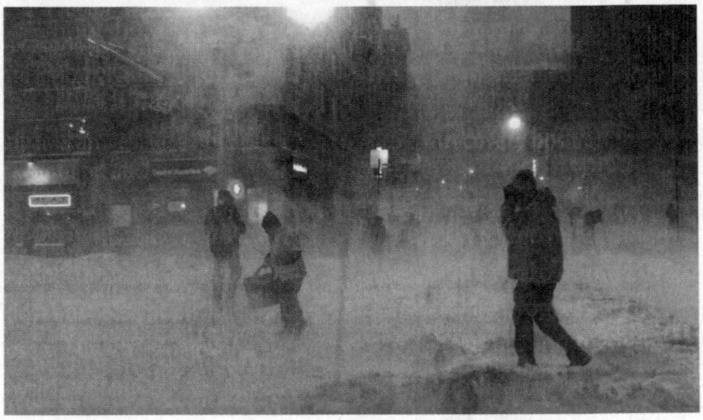

FIGURE 26-7 Major winter snowstorms can tie up a city.
© Ipedan/Shutterstock.

What to Do During a Wildfire

Follow these safety guidelines if a wildfire occurs:

- Listen to your local radio or television stations or check social media outlets for information.
- If advised to evacuate, do so immediately. Choose a route away from the fire hazard. Watch for changes in the speed and direction of fire and smoke. **DO NOT** block firefighting entrance routes.

Winter Storm

Heavy snowfall and extreme cold can immobilize an entire region. Even areas that usually experience mild winters can be hit with a major snowstorm or extreme cold **FIGURE 26-7**.

FYI

Storm Watch Versus Storm Warning

Government agencies such as the National Weather Service issue alerts when threats arise. A watch, such as a tornado watch, is issued when conditions are ripe for the development of that threat. A warning is issued if the threat is actually occurring or has been detected.

What to Do During a Winter Storm

Follow these safety guidelines if a winter storm occurs. If indoors:

- Listen to your local radio or television stations, social media outlets, or the National Oceanic and Atmospheric Administration (NOAA) weather radio for weather reports and emergency information.
- Conserve fuel by lowering the thermostat to 65°F (18.3°C) during the day and 55°F (12.8°C) at night. Close off unused rooms.
- Eat regularly and drink ample fluids, but avoid caffeine and alcohol.
- If using kerosene heaters, maintain ventilation, refuel the heater outside, and keep heaters at least 3 feet (1 m) from flammable objects.
- Never use heat sources or generators designed for outside use in an enclosed space. If you are using these sources outside, be aware of where the smoke or exhaust is going.

If outdoors:

- Dress warmly (ie, several layers of loose-fitting clothing, a hat, gloves, boots, and a scarf to cover your mouth and protect your lungs).
- Avoid overexertion (eg, shoveling snow or pushing a car), which can bring on a heart attack.
- Be aware of signs of frostbite and hypothermia.
- Keep dry by changing wet clothing, which does not insulate well.

If trapped in a vehicle during a winter storm:

- Pull off the highway. Turn on the vehicle's hazard lights. Hang a distress flag from the window or radio antenna.
- Stay inside the vehicle. Rescuers are more likely to find you. **DO NOT** set out on foot unless you can see a building close by where you know you can take shelter.
- Run the engine and heater about 10 minutes each hour to keep warm. When the engine is running, open a window slightly for ventilation, and clear snow from the exhaust pipe to prevent carbon monoxide poisoning.
- Exercise (eg, clap your hands and move your arms and legs occasionally) to maintain body heat, but avoid overexertion.
- In extreme cold, use floor mats, seat covers, road maps, newspapers, and other available resources for insulation. Huddle with other passengers.
- Take turns sleeping. One person should be awake at all times to look for rescue crews.
- Drink fluids to avoid dehydration.
- Watch for signs of frostbite and hypothermia.
- Be careful not to waste battery power.
- At night, turn on the inside light so work crews or rescuers can see you.
- Once the winter storm passes, you may need to leave the car and proceed on foot.

FYI

Winter Travel Supplies

When traveling during the winter, carry disaster supplies in the vehicle. The kit should include the following:

- Shovel
- Windshield scraper
- Flashlight
- Extra batteries
- Battery-powered radio
- Water
- Snack food
- Gloves and mittens
- Hat
- Blankets
- Tow chain or rope
- Tire chains
- Bag of road salt or sand
- Fluorescent distress flag
- Jumper or booster cables
- Road maps
- Emergency flares
- Cell phone, portable battery pack, and charging cables
- Emergency heating candles and container

Technological Hazards

Hazardous Materials Incidents

Chemicals are found everywhere. They can become hazardous during their production, storage, transportation, and disposal. It is not always possible to identify a situation as one involving hazardous materials, but clues such as a leaking cargo trailer, color-coded placards (signs) on abandoned drums, and unusual odors can be good indicators **FIGURE 26-8**.

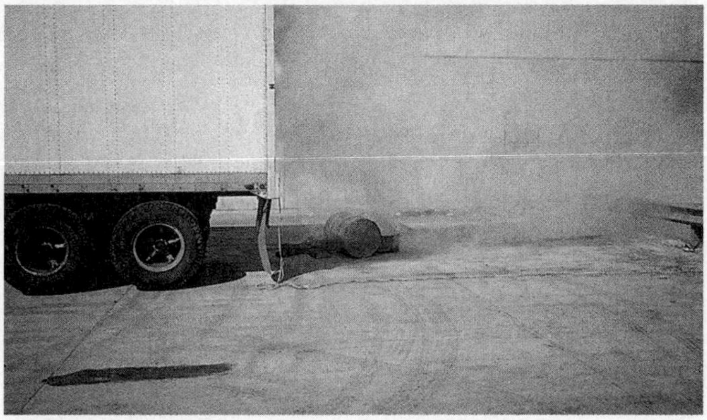

FIGURE 26-8 Fumes leaking from a cargo truck could be an indication of a hazardous materials incident.

What to Do During a Hazardous Materials Incident

Follow these safety guidelines if a hazardous materials incident occurs:

- If you witness an incident that you believe to be a hazardous materials incident, call 9-1-1.
- Stay away from the incident site.
- If caught outside, remember that gases and mists are usually heavier than air. Try to stay upstream, uphill, and upwind. Try to go at least one-half mile from the danger area.
- If in a vehicle, stop and seek shelter in a permanent building, if possible. If you must remain in the vehicle, keep the windows and vents closed and shut off the air conditioner and heater.
- If asked to evacuate your home, do so immediately.
- If requested to stay indoors rather than evacuate:
  - Follow all instructions and close all exterior doors, windows, vents, and fireplace dampers.
  - Turn off air conditioners and ventilation systems.
  - Go into an above-ground room with the fewest openings to the outside; close the doors and windows; tape around the sides, bottom, and top of the door; and cover each window and vent in the room with a single piece of plastic sheeting.
  - Listen to local emergency broadcasts.
  - When advised that it is safe to leave your shelter, open all doors and windows and turn on air-conditioning and ventilation systems to flush out any chemicals that infiltrated the building.

Nuclear Power Plants

Nuclear power plants operate in most states and produce about 20% of the nation's power. Millions of Americans live within 10 miles (16 km) of a nuclear power plant, according to the Natural Resources Defense Council. Although these plants are closely monitored and regulated, unintentional radiation exposures are possible. Local and state governments, federal agencies, and electric utility companies have emergency response plans for nuclear power plant incidents.

FYI

Disaster Myths

Myth	Reality
Myth: Disasters are truly exceptional events.	Reality: They are a normal part of daily life and in many cases are recurring events.
Myth: Disasters kill people without respect for socioeconomic status.	Reality: The poor and marginalized are more at risk of death than are rich people or the middle classes.
Myth: People can survive for many days when trapped under the rubble of a collapsed building.	Reality: The vast majority of people brought out alive from the rubble are saved within 24 or perhaps even 12 hours of impact.
Myth: When disaster strikes, panic is a common reaction.	Reality: Most people behave rationally in a disaster. While panic is not to be ruled out entirely, it is of such limited importance that some leading disaster sociologists regard it as insignificant or unlikely.
Myth: After disaster has struck, survivors tend to be dazed and apathetic.	Reality: Survivors rapidly start reconstruction. Activism is much more common than fatalism (this is the so-called therapeutic community). Even in the worst scenarios, only 15% to 30% of people show passive or dazed reactions.
Myth: Looting is a common and serious issue after disasters.	Reality: Looting is rare and limited in scope. It mainly occurs when there are strong preconditions, as when a community is already deeply divided.
Myth: Disease epidemics are an almost inevitable result of the disruption and poor health caused by major disasters.	Reality: Generally, the level of epidemiologic surveillance and health care in the disaster area is sufficient to stop any possible disease epidemic from occurring. However, the rate of diagnosis of diseases may increase as a result of improved health care.
Myth: In order to manage a disaster well, it is necessary to accept all forms of aid that are offered.	Reality: It is better to limit acceptance of donations to goods and services that are actually needed in the disaster area.
Myth: Unburied dead bodies constitute a health hazard.	Reality: Not even advanced decomposition causes a significant health hazard. Hasty burial demoralizes survivors and upsets arrangements for death certification, funeral rites, and, where needed, autopsy.
Myth: One should donate used clothes to people affected by disasters.	Reality: This often leads to accumulations of huge quantities of useless garments that people cannot or will not wear.

Myth	Reality
Myth: Companies, corporations, associations, and governments are always very generous when invited to send aid and relief to disaster areas.	Reality: This may be true sometimes, but in the past, disaster areas have been used as dumping grounds for outdated medicines, obsolete equipment, and unusable goods, all under the cloak of apparent generosity.
Myth: There is usually a shortage of resources when disaster occurs, and this prevents disasters from being managed effectively.	Reality: The shortage, if it occurs, is almost always temporary. There is more of an issue in deploying resources well and using them efficiently than in acquiring them. Often, there is also an issue of coping with a superabundance of certain types of resources.

Data from: Alexander DE. Misconception as a barrier to teaching about disasters. *Prehosp Disaster Med.* 2007;22(2):95–103.

What to Do During a Nuclear Power Plant Emergency

Follow these safety guidelines in a nuclear power plant emergency:

- Stay tuned to local radio and television stations. Local authorities will provide specific information and instructions.
- Evacuate if you are advised to do so.
- If told not to evacuate, remain indoors. Close the doors and windows and turn off the air conditioner, ventilation fans, furnace, and other air intakes. Go to a basement or other underground area if possible. Keep a battery-powered radio with you at all times.
- Do not use the telephone unless absolutely necessary. Lines will be needed for emergency calls.
- If you suspect exposure, take a thorough shower. Change clothes and shoes. Put all exposed clothing in a plastic bag. Seal the bag and place it out of the way.
- Seek professional medical care for any symptoms, such as nausea, that may be related to radiation exposure.

National Security Emergencies

Terrorism

Terrorism is the unlawful use of force or violence against people or property for purposes of intimidation, coercion, or ransom. Acts of terrorism range from threats of terrorism, assassinations, kidnappings, hijackings, bomb scares and bombings, and cyberattacks to the use of chemical, biologic, and nuclear weapons **FIGURE 26-9**.

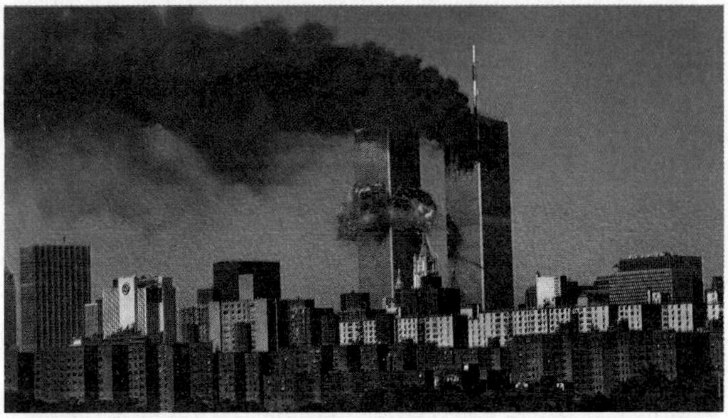

FIGURE 26-9 The September 11, 2001 terrorist attacks on the World Trade Center in New York City.

The Homeland Security Advisory System is designed to provide quick, comprehensive information about the potential threat of terrorist attacks or threat levels. Threat conditions can apply nationally, regionally, by industry, or by specific target. You should be aware of the current Homeland Security threat level at all times **TABLE 26-1**.

TABLE 26-1 Homeland Security Advisory System

Threat Level	Protective Measures You Should Take
Severe	■ Avoid high-risk areas such as public gatherings. ■ Listen attentively to news for advisories and instructions. ■ Contact employers to determine work status.
High	Review evacuation and sheltering measures for different types of attacks (chemical, biologic, or radiologic).
Elevated	Watch and report any suspicious activity. Contact schools to determine their emergency procedures.
Guarded	■ Review home disaster plan and update supplies. ■ Meet with your family to discuss what to do, where to go, and how to communicate if an attack occurs.
Low	Develop a home disaster plan and disaster supply kit.

Chemical and Biologic Agents

Chemical warfare agents are poisonous vapors, aerosols, liquids, or solids that have toxic effects on people, animals, or plants. They can be released by bombs; sprayed from aircraft, boats, or vehicles; or used in liquid form to create a hazard to people and the environment. Some chemical agents may be odorless and tasteless. They can have an immediate effect (a few seconds to a few minutes) or a delayed effect (several hours to several days). Although potentially lethal, chemical agents are difficult to deliver in lethal concentrations. Outdoors, the agents often dissipate rapidly.

Biologic agents are organisms or toxins that can kill or incapacitate people, livestock, and crops. The three basic groups of biologic agents likely to be used as weapons are bacteria, viruses, and toxins.

What to Do During a Chemical or Biologic Attack

If a chemical or biologic weapon attack occurs near you, authorities will instruct you on the best course of action, which may be to evacuate the area immediately, seek shelter at a designated location, or take immediate shelter where you are and seal the premises. The best way to protect yourself is to take emergency preparedness measures ahead of time and get medical attention as soon as possible, if needed.

Follow these additional safety guidelines if a chemical or biologic attack occurs:

- Listen to your local radio or television stations or check social media outlets for instructions from authorities, such as whether to remain inside or to evacuate.
- If instructed to remain in your home, office building, or other shelter during a chemical or biologic attack:
  - Turn off all ventilation, including furnaces, air conditioners, vents, and fans.
  - Seek shelter in an internal room, preferably one without windows. Seal the room with duct tape and plastic sheeting.
  - Avoid the furnace or utility room.
  - **DO NOT** use any major appliances (eg, furnace, oven or range, clothes dryer, washing machine).
- Remain in protected areas where toxic vapors are reduced or eliminated, and take a battery-operated radio with you.
- If caught in an unprotected area, try to get upwind of the contaminated area, try to find shelter inside a building as quickly as possible, and listen to your local radio or television stations or check social media outlets for official instructions.

Nuclear and Radiologic Weapons

Nuclear explosions can cause deadly effects such as blinding light, intense heat (thermal radiation), initial nuclear radiation, blast fires started by the heat pulse, and secondary fires caused by the destruction. Surface-level explosions also produce radioactive particles called fallout that can be carried by wind for hundreds of miles.

Terrorist use of a radiologic dispersion device, often called a dirty bomb, is considered far more likely than use of a nuclear device. These radiologic weapons are a combination of conventional explosives and radioactive material designed to scatter dangerous and sublethal amounts of radioactive material over a general area. There is no way of knowing how much warning time there would be before an attack by a terrorist using a nuclear or radiologic weapon.

What to Do During a Nuclear or Radiologic Attack

Follow these safety guidelines if a nuclear or radiologic attack occurs:

- Avoid looking at the flash or fireball; it can blind you.
- If you hear an attack warning:
- Take cover as quickly as you can, below ground if possible, and stay there until instructed to do otherwise.
- If caught outside and unable to get inside immediately, take cover behind anything that might offer protection. Lie flat on the ground and cover your head.
- If the explosion is some distance away, it could take 30 seconds or more for the blast wave to hit. Be aware of a second, returning blast wave.
- Protect yourself from radioactive fallout by taking shelter, even if you are many miles from the source of the explosion.
- Keep a battery-powered radio with you, and listen for official information. Follow the instructions given. Local instructions should always take precedence; officials in your area know the local situation best.

FYI

Disaster Preparedness

The US Department of Homeland Security offers these general guidelines for food and water needs for survival during emergency situations.

Water

- One gallon (4 L) of water per person per day, for drinking and sanitation.
- Keep at least a 3-day supply of water per person.
- Children, nursing mothers, and people who are ill may need more water.
- If you live in a warm-weather climate, more water may be necessary.

Food

- Store at least a 3-day supply of nonperishable food.
- Select foods that require no refrigeration, preparation, or cooking and little or no water.
- Pack a manual can opener and eating utensils.
- Choose foods your family will eat:
  - Ready-to-eat canned meats, fruits, and vegetables
  - Protein or fruit bars
  - Dry cereal or granola
  - Peanut butter
  - Dried fruit
  - Nuts
  - Crackers
  - Canned juices
  - Nonperishable pasteurized milk
  - High-energy foods
  - Vitamins
  - Food for infants
  - Comfort foods

First Aid Kit

- Maintain a well-stocked first aid kit. See Appendix A and Appendix D for suggestions for your first aid kit.

PREP KIT

Ready for Review

- Disasters are a fact of life, and you need to be prepared.
- Natural disasters such as earthquakes, floods, hurricanes, and tornados claim many lives each year.
- Chemicals are found everywhere; they can be hazardous during their production, storage, transportation, and disposal.
- Terrorism is the unlawful use of force or violence against people or property for purposes of intimidation, coercion, or ransom.
- When disaster strikes, you must be ready to act.

Vital Vocabulary

biologic agents Organisms or toxins that can kill or incapacitate people, livestock, and crops.

chemical warfare agents Poisonous vapors, aerosols, liquids, or solids that have toxic effects.

hurricane A tropical storm with winds that have reached a constant speed of at least 74 miles per hour (119 kph). Those in the Pacific Ocean are called typhoons and those in the Indian Ocean are known as cyclones.

terrorism The unlawful use of force or violence against people or property for purposes of intimidation, coercion, or ransom.

tsunami A series of waves generated by an undersea disturbance.

Assessment in Action

Seismologists have been predicting a large earthquake for your region of the country within the next 10 years. While at work on the top floor of your three-story office building, the predictions come true. Sudden shaking begins, and you feel the building move. Wall hangings and items on shelves begin to fall to the ground.

Directions: Circle Yes if you agree with the statement; circle No if you disagree.

1. This is most likely not the "big one," so you can continue your work as normal.
   YES **NO**
2. You should take cover under your desk.
   YES **NO**
3. You should call 9-1-1 to report the emergency.
   YES **NO**
4. You should know all the exit routes from your building.
   YES **NO**
5. If you smell gas, you should not delay your evacuation from the building.
   YES **NO**

Check Your Knowledge

Directions: Circle Yes if you agree with the statement; circle No if you disagree.

1. Earthquakes most often occur in the winter.
   YES **NO**
2. Never walk through moving water.
   YES **NO**
3. People in urban areas may be at greater risk from the effects of a prolonged heat wave than those in rural areas.
   YES **NO**
4. Hurricane season is from April until August.
   YES **NO**
5. Hide in a room with open windows if you are in the path of a tornado.
   YES **NO**
6. Never go near the shoreline to watch for a tsunami.
   YES **NO**
7. If you are trapped inside your car during a winter storm, run the engine and heater 10 minutes each hour to keep warm.
   YES **NO**

PREP KIT continued

8. If you witness a hazardous materials incident, get up close to find out the name of the hazardous material before calling 9-1-1.

YES **NO**

9. You should be aware of the Homeland Security threat level at all times.

YES **NO**

10. All chemical agents have a smell or taste.

YES **NO**

Appendix A

First Aid Supplies

Many injuries and sudden illnesses can be cared for without medical attention. For these situations and for situations requiring medical attention later, it is a good idea to have useful supplies on hand for emergencies.

Supplies in a first aid kit should be customized to include those items likely to be used on a regular basis. For example, a first aid kit for the home may be different from one at a workplace or one found on a boat.

The list in **TABLE A-1** includes nonprescription (over-the-counter [OTC]) medications. Some drug products lose their potency over time, especially after they have been opened. Therefore, buying a large, family size of a product that you use infrequently may not be economical. Note the expiration date on every medication.

TABLE A-1 Sample Items for a First Aid Kit

Items for Bleeding Control	
Disposable medical exam gloves (nonlatex)	Protects against potentially infected blood, body fluids, or contaminated items
Hemostatic wound dressing	Use only when direct pressure fails to control bleeding.
Tourniquet (manufactured, ie, CAT preferred)	Use only when direct pressure fails to control extremity bleeding.
Items for Wound Care	
Alcohol hand sanitizer (medium bottle)	Cleans hands and the area around the wound (not inside wound)
Antibiotic ointment (Polysporin, Neosporin, Bacitracin, or triple-antibiotic ointment) single-use packets	Reduces healing time and reduces the risk of skin infections that are associated with shallow wounds and small second-degree burns
Surgical tape (Micropore paper tape) (1 and 2 in. [3 and 5 cm])	Covers blisters
Elastic tape (Elastikon) (2 and 4 in. [5 and 10 cm])	Covers wounds and blisters
Blister pad (Spenco 2nd Skin) (1 and 3 in. [3 and 7 cm])	Covers wounds and blisters
Adhesive bandages (1 × 3 in [3 × 7 cm] and other sizes) **FIGURE A-1**	Covers minor wounds
Sterile gauze pads (3 × 3 in. and 4 × 4 in. [7 × 7 cm and 10 × 10 cm]; individually wrapped) **FIGURE A-2**	Covers wounds
Nonstick pads (3 × 4 in. [7 × 10 cm])	Covers burns, blisters, and scrapes
Self-adhering roller gauze bandage (ie, Kling/Kerlix conforming bandages) (2, 3, and 4 in. [5, 7, and 10 cm] wide) **FIGURE A-3**	Holds dressings in place
Sterile trauma pad (5 × 9 in., 8 × 10 in. [13 × 23 cm, 20 × 25 cm]) **FIGURE A-4**	Covers large wounds
Triangular bandages (about 40 × 40 × 56 in. [102 × 102 × 142 cm])	When folded (known as a cravat bandage), it can hold dressings and splints in place or it can be applied as a swathe (binder) for an arm sling.
Sterile eye pads	Cover both eyes to prevent both eyes from moving, even if only one is injured.
Items for Bone, Joint, and Muscle Care	
Cold pack (instant and disposable)	Use on sprains, dislocations, fractures, and insect stings when ice is not available.
Splint (padded and malleable, ie, SAM Splint)	Stabilizes broken bones and dislocations
Elastic bandage (ie, ACE bandage) (3 in. [7 cm] wide) **FIGURE A-5**	Provides compression to reduce the swelling of joint injuries
Plastic bags (sealable)	Holds ice to apply on insect stings and bone, joint, and muscle injuries; contains embedded tick after its removal
Nonprescription (OTC) Medications *Keep all medications out of the reach of children and use child-resistant containers. For schools and worksites, giving oral medications is often prohibited; check the local policies.*	
Glucose tablets	Treats hypoglycemia (low blood sugar)
Acetaminophen (Tylenol)	Treats pain and fever

Continues

TABLE A-1 Sample Items for a First Aid Kit (*Continued*)

Ibuprofen (Advil)	Treats pain, fever, and inflammation
Aspirin (Excedrin, preferably chewable)	Treats pain, fever, and inflammation; may be used for suspected heart attack. **DO NOT** give aspirin to children.
Antihistamine (Benadryl) *Warning*: First aid kits at workplaces, schools, and public places should not contain products known to cause drowsiness.	Relieves allergy symptoms; treats poison ivy or oak itching and rash; reduces nausea and motion sickness; causes drowsiness and induces sleep
Hydrocortisone cream, 1%	Relieves itchiness and skin-related reactions, including rashes associated with insect bites and stings, poison ivy and oak, and other allergic skin rashes. It may be too weak for some conditions.
Aloe vera gel (100% gel) **FIGURE A-6**	Soothes sunburn or superficial frostbite
Sports drink packets (eg, Gatorade, Powerade)	Treats heat stress, dehydration, and water intoxication when too much water has been consumed and sodium has been depleted from the body.
Antacids tablets (eg, Tums, Rolaids)	Treats heartburn and acid indigestion (upset stomach)
Antidiarrheal tablets (eg, Pepto-Bismol and Imodium A-D)	Treats diarrhea
Anticonstipation/laxative tablets (eg, Metamucil)	Treats constipation
Equipment	
CPR breathing barrier device (with one-way valve)	Protects against potential infection during CPR
Face masks for public health	Protects against respiratory droplets carrying infectious viruses, such as COVID-19
Scissors (various types available) **FIGURE A-7**	Cuts dressings, bandages, and clothing
Thermometer	Monitors temperature for possible fever or hypothermia
Tweezers (angled tip)	Removes splinters and ticks
Safety pins (2 in. [5 cm] long) **FIGURE A-8**	Creates sling from shirttail or sleeve, secures dressings, and drains blisters
Emergency blanket (eg, state highway department trash bags; household polyethylene trash bags; space blanket made of Mylar, although it may tear in wind)	Protects against body heat loss and weather (wind, rain, and snow)
First Aid, CPR, and AED Guide (first aid booklet from Jones & Bartlett Learning)	Provides quick reference during an emergency and for review of first aid procedures

Abbreviations: COVID-19, coronavirus disease 2019; CPR, cardiopulmonary resuscitation; OTC, over the counter

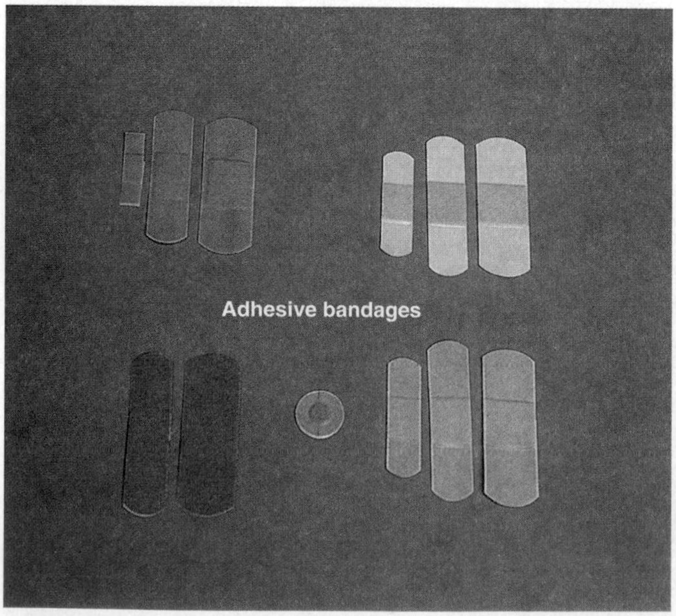

FIGURE A-1 Adhesive bandages.

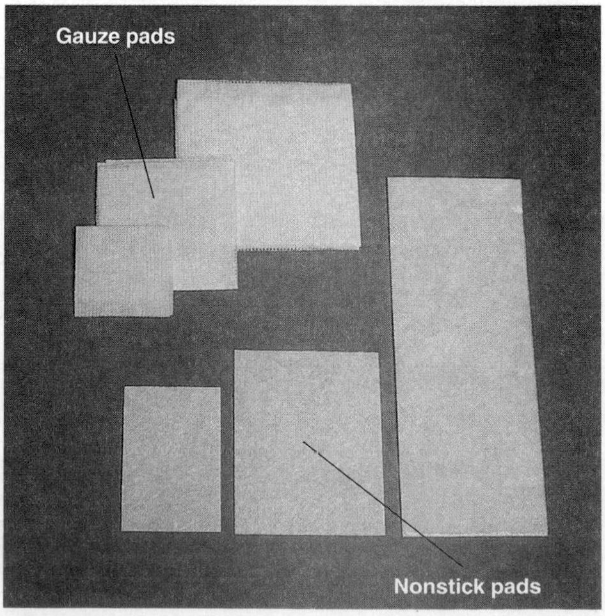

FIGURE A-2 Gauze pads and nonstick pads.

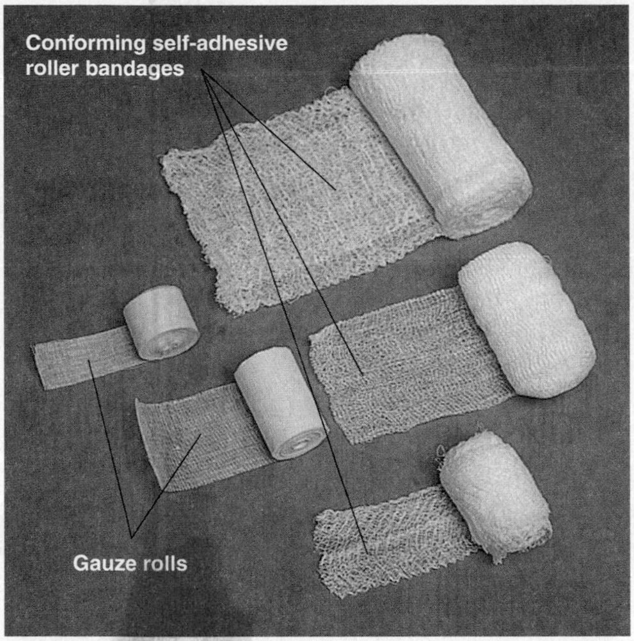

FIGURE A-3 Gauze rolls and self-adhering roller bandages.

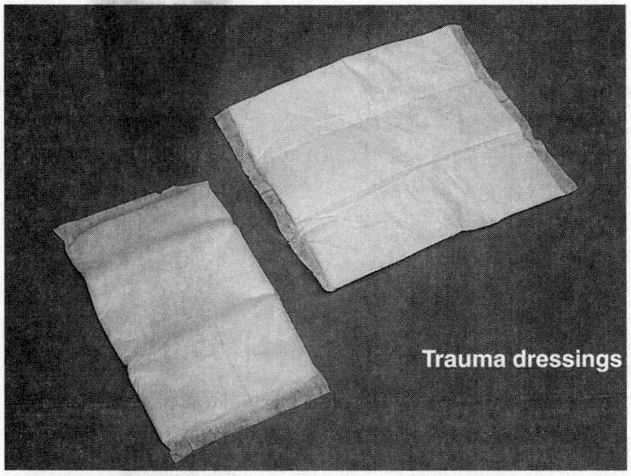

FIGURE A-4 Trauma pads.

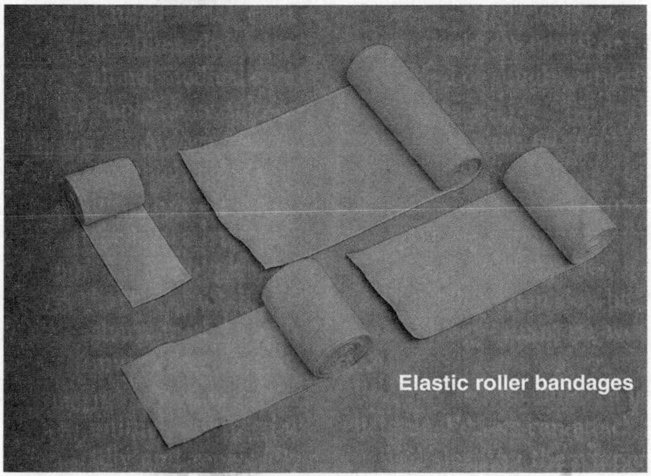

FIGURE A-5 Elastic roller bandages.

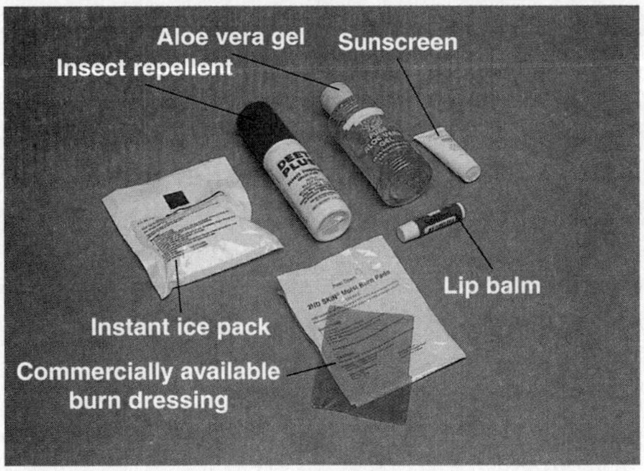

FIGURE A-6 Aloe vera gel, instant ice pack, burn dressing, and optional first aid kit items (insect repellent, sunscreen, and lip balm).

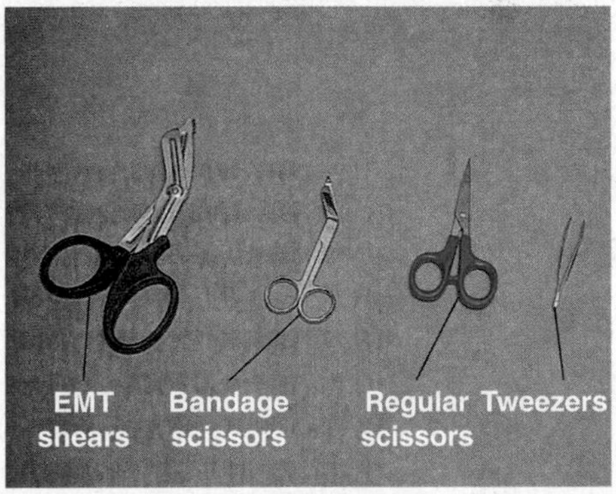

FIGURE A-7 Trauma shears, bandage scissors, regular scissors, and tweezers.

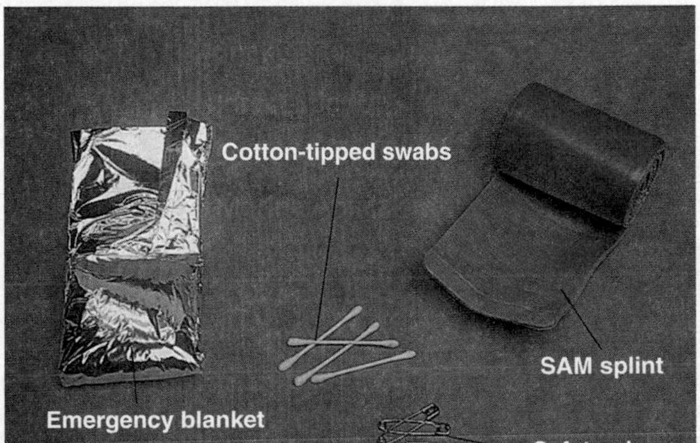

FIGURE A-8 Emergency blanket, cotton-tipped swabs, safety pins, and SAM splint.

Keep all medicines out of reach of children. Read and follow all directions for properly using medications. Consider keeping your first aid supplies in either a fishing tackle box or a tool box.

Workplace First Aid Kit Contents

In the absence of a medical facility in close proximity to a workplace, the Occupational Safety and Health Administration (OSHA) requires that the workplace have adequate supplies readily available and a person or people at the workplace who is adequately trained to render first aid to all injured employees. Neither OSHA's general industry standard 1910.151 nor its construction standard 1926.50 require specific contents be included in the workplace first aid kit.

OSHA refers to the *American National Standard (ANSI) Z308.1, Minimum Requirements for Workplace First Aid Kits.* The recommended supplies and their quantities and size/volume are found in **TABLE A-2**.

Two classes of first aid kits are identified as Class A and Class B. Class A kits contain supplies for the most common workplace injuries (eg, minor wounds, burns, sprains). Class B kits contain supplies for injuries in large employee workplaces with a complex or high-risk environment (eg, factories, warehouses, outdoor areas).

To comply with the ANSI/ISEA Z308.1 standards that OSHA uses, neither workers nor employers can subtract from the minimum requirements listed in Table A-2, but they may add to it. OSHA recommends employers also consider the availability of an automated external defibrillator (AED) in the workplace.

TABLE A-2 Recommended Minimum Items for a Workplace First Aid Kit

Equipment	Class A Minimum Quantity	Class B Minimum Quantity
Adhesive bandages (1 × 3 in. [2.5 × 7.5 cm])	16	50
Adhesive tape (1 in. [3 cm] width, 2.5 yards [2.3 m] length) **FIGURE A-9**	1 roll	2 rolls
Antibiotic ointment	10 packets	25 packets
Antiseptic towelette/swab **FIGURE A-10**	10 packets	50 packets
Breathing barrier (face mask with one-way valve) **FIGURE A-11**	1	1
Burn dressing (gel-soaked; 4 × 4 in. [10 × 10 cm])	1 packet	2 packets
Burn treatment (1/32 oz. [1 g])	10 packets	25 packets
Cold pack (instant, disposable; 4 × 5 in. [10 × 12.5 cm])	1	2
Eye covering (with means of attachment, 3 in.^{2} and 7.5 cm^2)	2	2
Eye/skin wash	1-oz (30-mL) bottle	4-oz (118-mL) bottle
First Aid, CPR, and AED Guide (booklet from Jones & Bartlett Learning)	1	1
Hand sanitizer (60% alcohol)	6 packets or 1 small bottle	10 packets or 2 small bottles
Medical exam gloves (nonlatex [Nitrile recommended]; size large) **FIGURE A-12**	2 pairs	4 pairs
Roller gauze bandage (2 in. [5 cm] width, 4 yards total length)	1	2
Roller gauze bandage (4 in. [10 cm] width, 4 yards total length)	0	1
Scissors	1	1
Splint (eg, SAM splint, 4 × 24 in. [10 × 61 cm])	0	1
Sterile gauze pads (3 × 3 in. [7.5 × 7.5 cm])	2	4
Sterile trauma pads (5 × 9 in. [13 × 23 cm])	2	4
Tourniquet (1 in. [2.5 cm] wide)	0	1
Triangular bandage (40 × 40 × 56 in. [102 × 102 × 142 cm])	1	2

Note: Nonprescription (over-the-counter [OTC]) medications can be put in first aid kits if packaged in single dose, tamper-evident packaging and labeled as required by FDA regulations. Nonprescription (OTC) drug products should not contain ingredients known to cause drowsiness. Please read all labels and only use as directed.

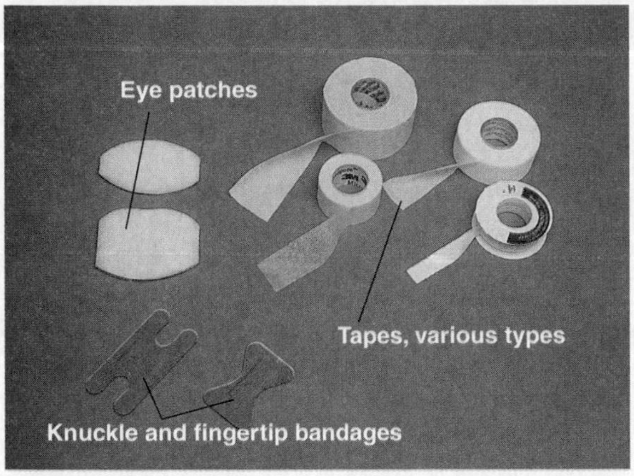

FIGURE A-9 Eye patches, knuckle and fingertip bandages, and tape.

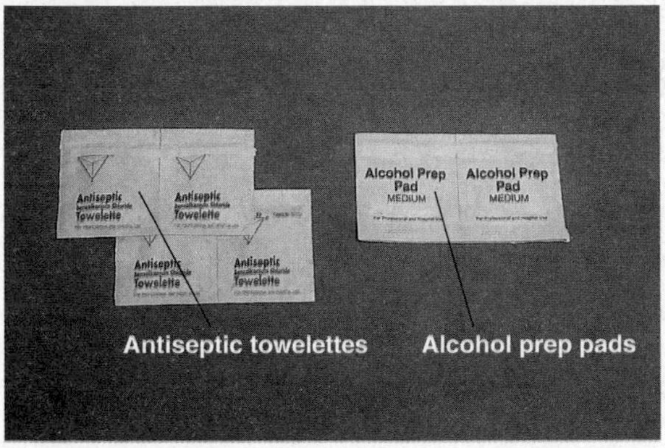

FIGURE A-10 Antiseptic towelettes and alcohol prep pads.

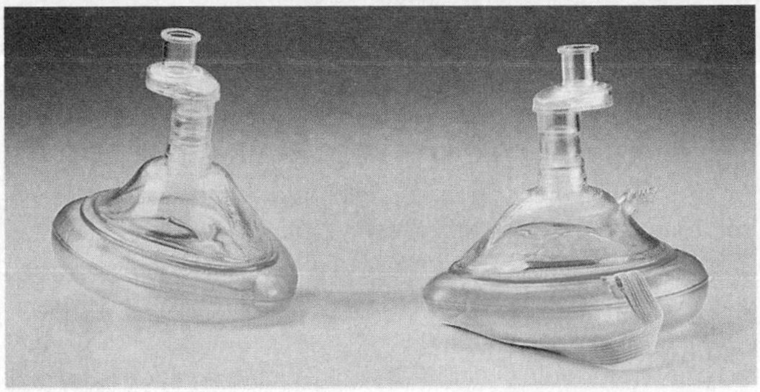

FIGURE A-11 Face masks.

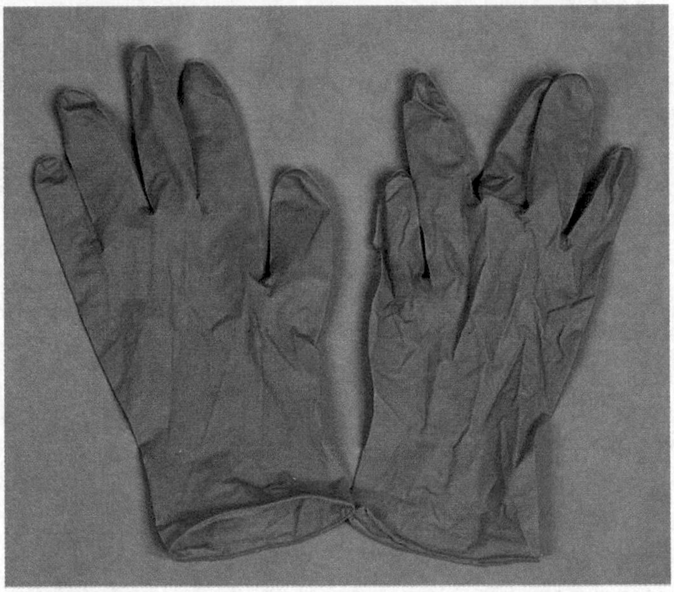

FIGURE A-12 Medical exam gloves.

Appendix B

Medication Information

As a first aid provider, you might be in a situation that requires you to give a person certain medications (or to assist a person in taking their own medication). Never give a medication that is expired, that was prescribed to someone else, or to someone with a known allergy to that medication. A knowledgeable first aid provider should be familiar with the following medications:

- Over-the-counter pain relievers:
  - Acetaminophen
  - Aspirin
  - Ibuprofen
  - Naproxen
- Physician-prescribed medications:
  - Metered-dose inhaler
  - Nitroglycerin
  - Epinephrine
- Over-the-counter medications carried in a first aid kit or available from the person:
  - Oral glucose
- Naloxone

Pros and Cons of Popular Pain Relievers

Acetaminophen

BRAND NAME: Tylenol®

ADVANTAGES: Relieves pain and fever, does not irritate stomach

DISADVANTAGES: Can damage liver with heavy or prolonged use

Aspirin

BRAND NAMES: Bufferin®, Anacin®, Bayer®

ADVANTAGES: Relieves pain, fever, inflammation; useful for heart attacks and their prevention

DISADVANTAGES: Interferes with blood clotting; might trigger stomach bleeding; can cause Reye syndrome in children with viral infections

Ibuprofen

BRAND NAMES: Advil®, Nuprin®, Motrin®

ADVANTAGES: Relieves pain, fever, and inflammation

DISADVANTAGES: Interferes with clotting; can cause stomach bleeding, ulcers, irritation; heavy or prolonged use can damage liver and kidneys

Naproxen

BRAND NAME: Aleve®

ADVANTAGES: Relieves pain, fever, and inflammation; one dose lasts 8 to 12 hours

DISADVANTAGES: Can cause stomach bleeding, ulcers, irritation; prolonged use can harm kidneys

---

Nitroglycerin

Give a person nitroglycerin (Nitrostat®) if the following conditions exist:

- The person is an adult.
- The person has chest pain.
- The person has physician-prescribed sublingual tablets or spray.

DO NOT give a person nitroglycerin if any of the following conditions applies:

- The person has a head injury.
- The person is an infant or a child.
- The person has already taken three doses.
- The person has hypotension.
- The person has taken erectile disfunction medication such as Viagra.

Medication Forms

Tablet (about one-tenth the size of an aspirin), sublingual spray, and patch.

Dosage

One dose

Procedure

Once you have decided to administer nitroglycerin, follow these steps:

1. Check the expiration date of the nitroglycerin.
2. Ask the person about the previous dose taken (time and amount taken).

3. Ask the person to lift their tongue. Place the tablet or spray dose under the tongue or have the person do so. Do not touch the tablet; wear gloves because your skin can absorb nitroglycerin, which could drop your blood pressure.
4. Have the person keep their mouth closed (if doing so will not interfere with easy breathing) with the tablet under the tongue (without swallowing) until the tablet dissolves and is absorbed.

Actions

Nitroglycerin takes the following actions:

- Relaxes (dilates) blood vessels
- Reduces the workload of the heart

Side Effects

Side effects of nitroglycerin include the following:

- Lower blood pressure (person should sit or lie down)
- Headache
- Heart rate changes

Epinephrine Auto-Injector

Give a person epinephrine (Adrenalin, EpiPen®) if both of the following conditions exist:

- The person exhibits signs of a severe allergic reaction (including breathing distress or shock).
- The person has physician-prescribed medication.

Medication Form

Liquid from automatic needle-and-syringe injection system

Dosage

- Adult: One adult auto-injector (0.3 mg) **FIGURE B-1**
- Child/infant: One infant/child auto-injector (0.15 mg)

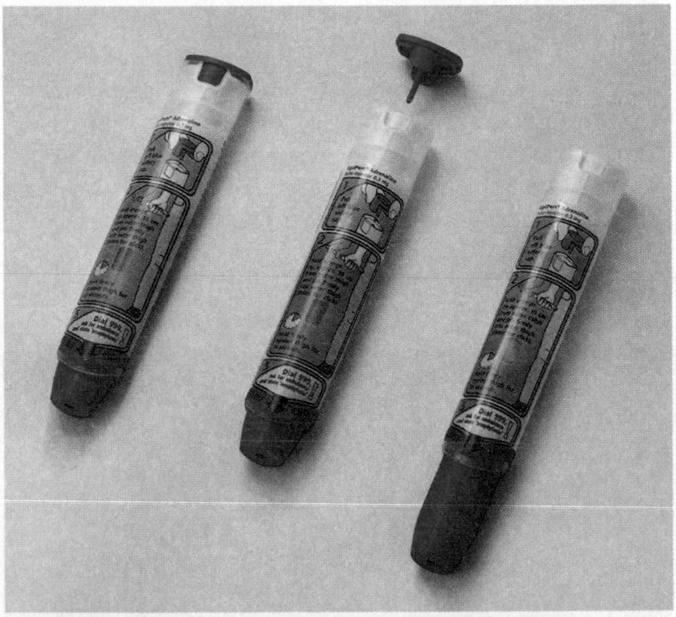

FIGURE B-1 Epinephrine auto-injectors.

Procedure

Use these steps when administering epinephrine:

1. Obtain the person's physician-prescribed auto-injector.
2. Remove the safety cap.
3. Place the tip of the auto-injector against the person's thigh.
4. Push the injector firmly against the thigh until you hear it click to inject medication.
5. Hold the injector in place for 3 seconds.
6. When a person with anaphylaxis does not respond to the first dose and the arrival of emergency medical services will exceed 5 to 10 minutes, a second dose may be considered if a second device is available.
7. Call 9-1-1.

Actions

Epinephrine takes the following actions:

- Dilates the bronchioles (small tubes in lungs)
- Constricts blood vessels

Side Effects

Epinephrine has the following side effects:

- Increased heart rate
- Dizziness
- Headache
- Chest pain
- Nausea
- Vomiting
- Anxiety

Metered-Dose Inhaler

Give a person a metered-dose inhaler (Albuterol®, Proventil®, Ventolin®) if the person is experiencing asthma, or difficulty breathing with wheezing. The person may have asthma or COPD.

Dosage

Adult/child: one to two inhalations

Procedure

Use these steps when administering a metered-dose inhaler **FIGURE B-2**:

1. Take the cap off the inhaler and inspect the mouthpiece to ensure that it is clean.
2. Shake the inhaler several times and apply the spacer, if available.
3. Holding the inhaler upright, tell the person to place their lips around the inhaler or spacer.
4. For greater benefit, the person can take a breath and then exhale fully. Then, while the person breathes in slowly and deeply, depress the inhaler to release the medication.
5. Tell the person to hold their breath for 5 to 10 seconds and to breathe out slowly.
6. A second dose may be given in 30 to 60 seconds.

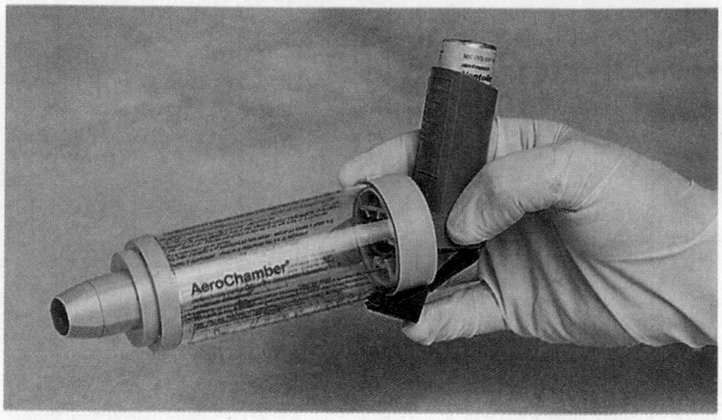

FIGURE B-2 Metered-dose inhaler with a spacer attached.

Actions

A metered-dose inhaler takes the following actions:

- Causes bronchodilation
- Stimulates the nervous system

Side Effects

A metered-dose inhaler has the following side effects:

- Hypertension
- Increased heart rate
- Anxiety
- Restlessness

Oral Glucose

Give a person oral glucose if all of the following conditions exist:

- The person has low blood glucose (hypoglycemia, insulin reaction).
- The person is able to swallow.
- The person is alert and able to follow instructions.

Dosage

Adult: one tube of gel or three tablets

Procedure

Use these steps when administering oral glucose:

1. If the person has a blood glucose monitor, allow them to check their blood glucose.
2. Use the Rule of 15 when:
   - Testing is not possible
   - Testing shows a low blood glucose level
   - Profuse sweating or shaking occurs in a person with diabetes

   The Rule of 15 works as follows:

- Have the person eat 15 grams of sugar (ie, 3 to 5 glucose tablets, 3 to 5 teaspoons [15 mL to 25 mL] of table sugar, or 4 ounces [118 mL] of orange juice or regular soft drink [not diet]) **FIGURE B-3**.
- Wait 15 minutes for the sugar to get into the blood.
- Recheck the blood glucose level. If it is still low or no testing is available, give the person 15 more grams of sugar to consume.

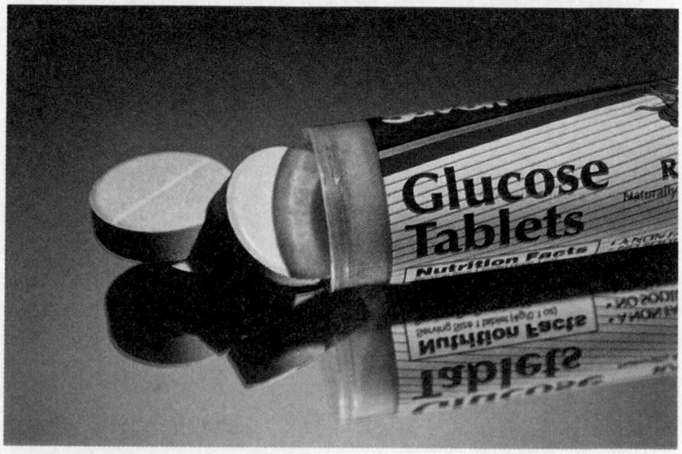

FIGURE B-3 Glucose tablets.

If the person experiences a decline in responsiveness or there is no improvement in the person after 15 minutes, repeat the dose, and if the condition remains the same after another 15 minutes, call 9-1-1.

Actions

When oral glucose is absorbed by the body, it provides glucose for cell use.

Side Effects

Oral glucose has the following side effects.

- Nausea
- Vomiting

Naloxone

Naloxone is available in a prefilled, single-dose *nasal spray* (Narcan) that cannot be reused and a prefilled, single-dose *auto-injector* (Evzio) that cannot be reused.

Dosage

One dose to start; more if needed and if available (the effects of opioids often outlast the effects of naloxone)

Procedure

Once you have decided to administer Naloxone, follow these steps for a single-dose nasal spray (Narcan):

1. Place the person flat on their back, with the head tilted back.
2. Administer the spray into one nostril.
3. If there is no recovery within 2 to 3 minutes and another nasal spray device is available, repeat the dose in the other nostril.

Follow these steps for a single-dose auto-injector (Evzio):

1. Pull the device out of the case.
2. Once activated, the device provides voice directions (similar to automated defibrillators).
3. Inject into the person's outer thigh (similar to an epinephrine auto-injector). It can be given through clothing (eg, pants, jeans) if necessary. If the electronic voice directions do not work, the device can still deliver the naloxone dose.
4. If there is no recovery within 2–3 minutes and there is another auto-injector available, repeat the dose.

Actions

Naloxone takes the following actions:

- Reverses the effect of opioids

Side Effects

Side effects of naloxone include the following:

- Opioid withdrawal symptoms, such as:
  - Body aches
  - Fever
  - Sweating
  - Runny nose
  - Sneezing
  - Goose bumps
  - Yawning
  - Weakness
  - Shivering or trembling
  - Nervousness
  - Restlessness or irritability
  - Diarrhea, nausea, or vomiting
  - Stomach cramps
  - Fast heartbeat
  - Increased blood pressure

Appendix C

Health Care Provider Basic Life Support Review

Examples of health care providers include physicians, dentists, nurses, emergency medical technicians (EMTs), advanced emergency medical technicians (AEMTs), paramedics, fire fighters, and athletic trainers. Health care providers work in a variety of settings such as emergency medical services, hospitals, medical and dental clinics, and athletic facilities. These professionals perform basic life support techniques, such as cardiopulmonary resuscitation (CPR), differently than laypeople.

One-Rescuer Adult CPR

If you find a collapsed, motionless person, make a quick check for dangerous hazards and other clues as to what happened. Refer to **SKILL SHEET C-1** for the appropriate steps and techniques for one-rescuer adult cardiopulmonary resuscitation (CPR).

SKILL SHEET C-1 One-Rescuer Adult CPR

Note: Always use a mouth-to-barrier device to prevent disease transmission. Remember to observe for scene safety as you approach the person.

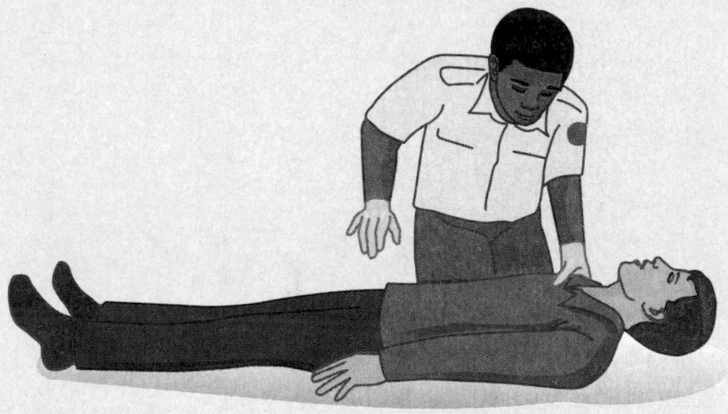

1 Check responsiveness. Tap the person on the shoulder and shout, "Are you okay?"

If the person responds:

- **a.** Ask the person about chief complaints.
- **b.** Use the SAMPLE (signs and symptoms, allergies, medications, pertinent past medical history, last oral intake, events leading up to the illness or injury) history questions.
- **c.** Check the person for DOTS (deformities, open wounds, tenderness, and swelling) if an injury is suspected.

If the person does not respond, continue to **Step 2**.

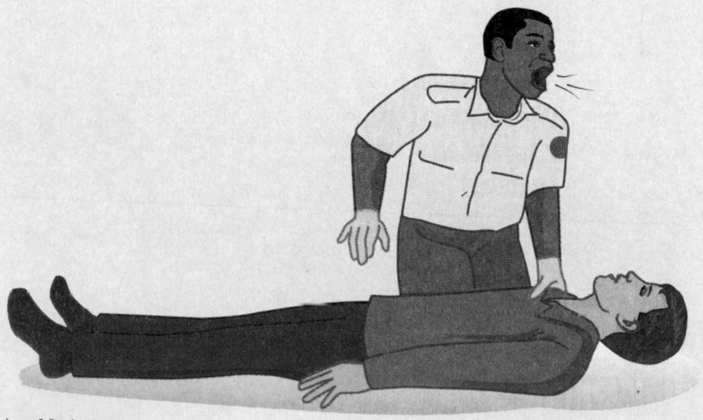

2 Shout for help.

- **a.** If you are alone, leave the person to activate the emergency response system and get an automated external defibrillator (AED) before starting CPR.
- **b.** If another person arrives or is nearby, have them activate the emergency response system and get an AED.

Note: You can either activate the resuscitation team at this time or after checking for breathing and pulse.

SKILL SHEET C-1 One-Rescuer Adult CPR (*Continued*)

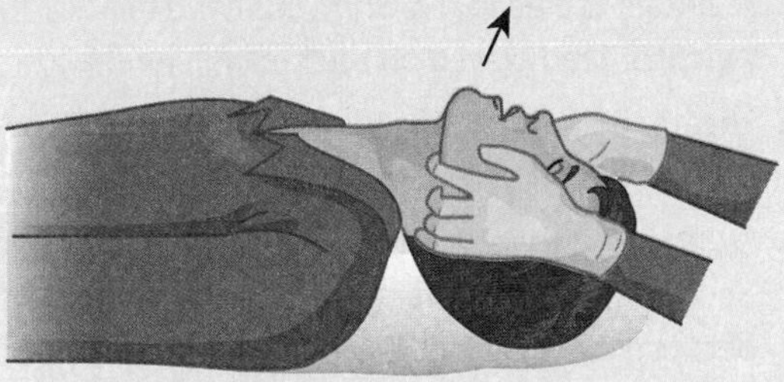

© Jones & Bartlett Learning.

3 Open the person's airway.

a. Take your hand nearest the person's head and place it on their forehead; apply pressure to tilt the head back.

b. Place two fingers of your other hand under the bony part of the person's jaw (near the chin) and lift. Avoid pressing on soft tissues under the jaw.

c. Tilt the head backward.

If you suspect a spinal neck injury, DO NOT move the person's head or neck. Use the jaw-thrust method to open the airway. With both hands, one on each side, place your fingers behind the angles of the jaw and lift upward. Your thumbs can be used to pull down the person's lower jaw to allow breathing through the mouth.

If you see fluid or material in the person's mouth, wear medical exam gloves and use a cloth over your fingers to scoop the liquid out of the person's mouth. If you see a solid object, wear medical exam gloves and remove the object by using a hooking motion. If you see dentures, leave them in place unless they are loose and cannot be kept in place.

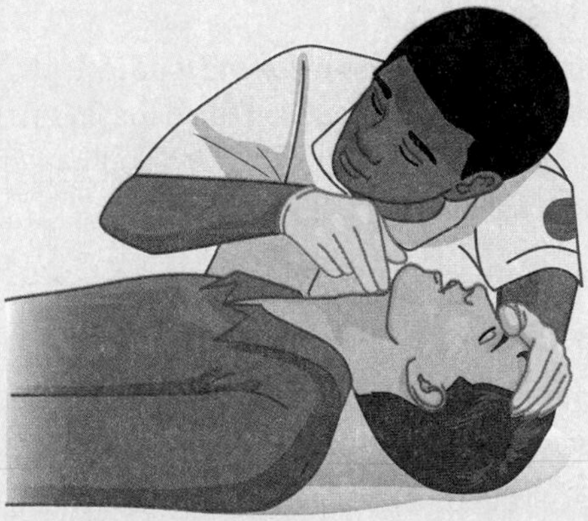

© Jones & Bartlett Learning.

4 Check for breathing.

a. While keeping the airway open, place your ear near the person's mouth and listen and feel for breathing. Observe the person's chest for movement (rise and fall).

b. If the person is not breathing or is only gasping, continue to **Step 5**.

c. If the person is breathing normally, continue to monitor their breathing until emergency responders arrive.

Continues

SKILL SHEET C-1 One-Rescuer Adult CPR (*Continued*)

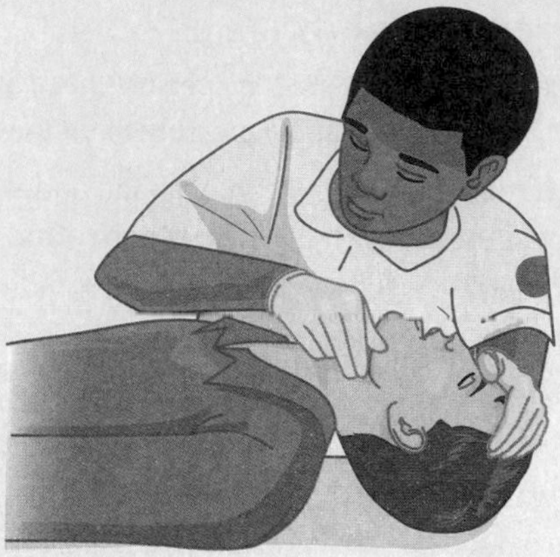

5 Check for pulse. (This step is done simultaneously with Step 4 in at least 5 and no more than 10 seconds.)

a. Maintain the head tilt, with your hand nearest the person's head placed on the person's forehead.

b. Locate the larynx using two fingers of your hand nearest the person's feet.

c. Slide your fingers down into the groove of the person's neck on the side nearest you. DO NOT use your thumb because you may feel your own pulse.

d. Feel for a carotid pulse (take 5 to 10 seconds). The carotid artery is used in adults because it lies close to the heart and is easily accessible.

e. If the person has a pulse and is breathing, keep the airway open and monitor breathing.

f. If the person has a pulse but is not breathing:

- Provide rescue breaths (1 breath every 5 to 6 seconds, or about 10 to 12 breaths per minute).
- After 2 minutes, activate the emergency response system, if not already done.
- Continue providing rescue breaths; check the pulse about every 2 minutes. If the person has no pulse, begin CPR.

g. If the person has no pulse and is not breathing or is only gasping, continue to **Step 6** (begin sets of CPR [30 compressions and 2 breaths] and apply an AED as soon as possible).

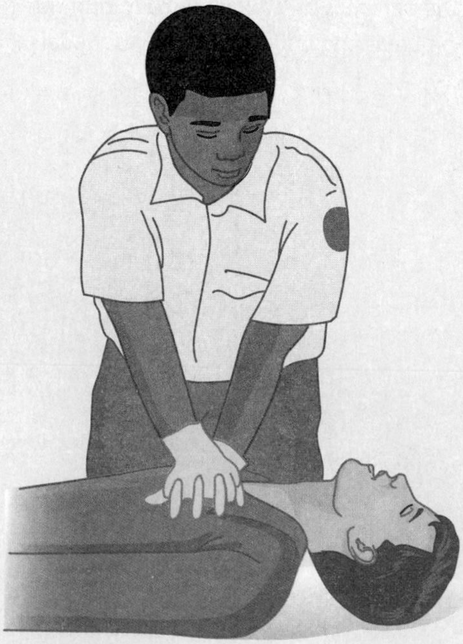

6 Give 30 chest compressions.

a. Place the heel of one of your hands on the center of the person's chest and on the lower half of their sternum.

b. Place your other hand on top of the first one with your fingers interlocked. Hold your fingers off the person's chest and point them directly away from you. DO NOT cross your hands.

c. Keep your arms straight and elbows locked, with your shoulders positioned directly over your hands.

d. Push hard. Press straight down on the sternum, at least 2 to 2.4 inches (5 to 6 cm).

e. Push fast: 100 to 120 compressions per minute. Consider using the beat of the Bee Gees' song "Stayin' Alive" or metronome app on a cell phone.

f. Push smoothly. DO NOT jerk or jab. DO NOT stop at the top or bottom of a compression.

g. Allow the chest to fully recoil after each compression (DO NOT lean on the chest).

SKILL SHEET C-1 One-Rescuer Adult CPR (*Continued*)

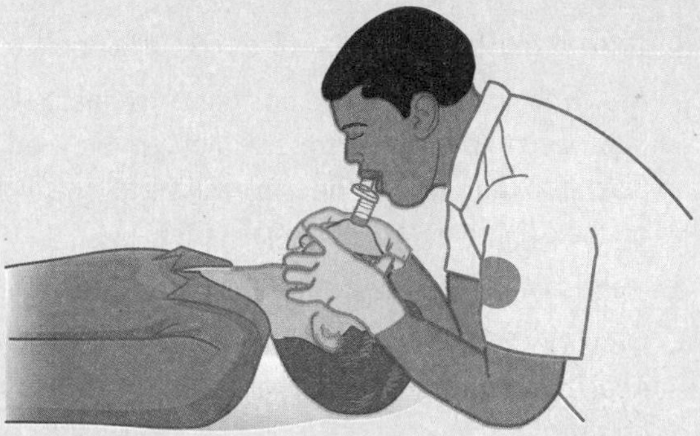

© Jones & Bartlett Learning.

7 Give two breaths.

a. Keep the head tilted back with the head tilt–chin lift method to maintain an open airway.

b. Pinch the person's nose shut.

c. Give two breaths, each lasting 1 second. (Take a normal breath for yourself after each breath.)

d. Watch for chest rise to determine if your breaths go in.

e. Allow for chest deflation after each breath.

f. If you see chest rise after the 2 breaths, give 30 chest compressions.

g. If the first breath does not make the chest rise, retilt the person's head and give a second breath. If the second breath does not make the chest rise, begin CPR (30 compressions and 2 breaths). Each time before giving the first of the two breaths, open the mouth and look for an object; if seen, remove it.

h. If you cannot use the person's mouth (ie, seriously injured mouth, ineffective seal, mouth cannot be opened, person is in water), use the head tilt–chin lift maneuver. Seal your mouth around the person's nose and breathe.

i. If there are two rescuers and a bag-mask device is available, deliver two ventilations, each lasting 1 second. (Note: This is a challenging skill that requires a lot of practice. It may be slower than the mouth-to-mask method.)

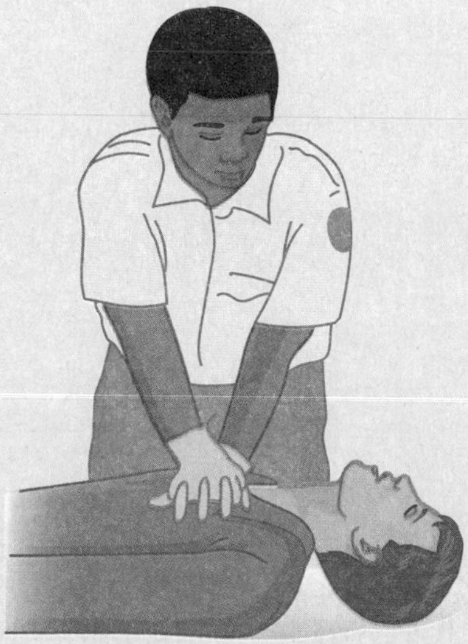

© Jones & Bartlett Learning.

8 Continue sets of 30 chest compressions and 2 breaths until someone with an AED arrives.

Continues

SKILL SHEET C-1 One-Rescuer Adult CPR (*Continued*)

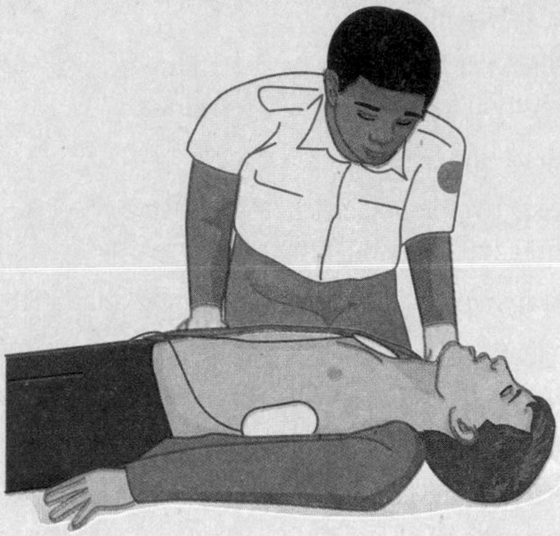

© Jones & Bartlett Learning.

9 When an AED becomes available, apply it as soon as possible.

a. Turn on the AED and follow the voice prompts.

b. Attach the pads to the person's bare, dry chest. (You may need to dry the person's skin or remove medical patches or hair so that the pads will stick.) The diagrams on the pads show where to place them.

c. Make sure no one is touching the person. Say, "Clear!"

d. Allow the AED to analyze the heart rhythm (push the Analyze button, if necessary) and follow the AED's voice prompts.

e. If no shock is advised, immediately resume five sets of 30 chest compressions and 2 breaths (2 minutes).

f. If shock is advised, do not touch the person. Give 1 shock and immediately resume five sets of 30 chest compressions and 2 breaths (2 minutes).

The AED will prompt you to stop CPR every 2 minutes to reanalyze the heart rhythm.

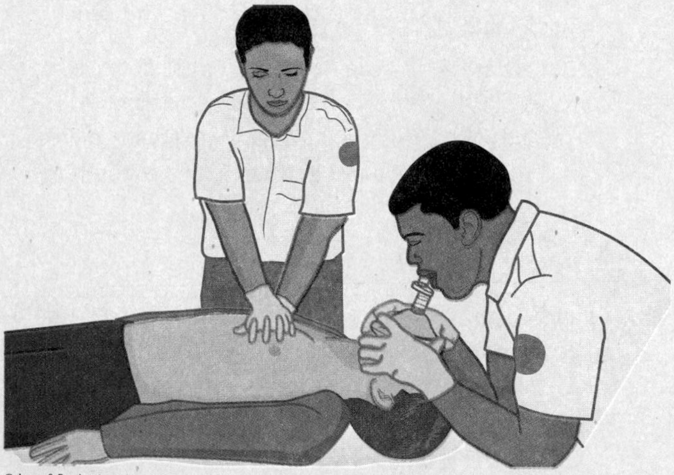

© Jones & Bartlett Learning.

10 When a second rescuer arrives, provide two-person CPR and apply the AED.

Two-Rescuer Adult CPR

Lifeguards and other health care providers are often taught two-rescuer CPR procedures. Having two or more rescuers present has the following advantages:

- One rescuer can activate the emergency response system and obtain an AED
- It is less exhausting for the rescuers. One rescuer can give chest compressions while the other performs rescue breathing. Additionally, the rescuers can switch positions after every five sets of CPR or sooner if the rescuer giving chest compressions becomes fatigued.
- There is less interruption between the compressions and breaths.

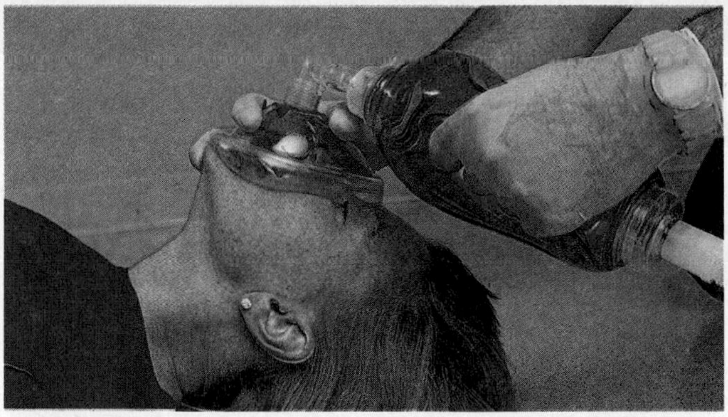

FIGURE C-1 Bag-mask device.

The sequence of steps is the same as for one-rescuer CPR, but the tasks are shared between the two rescuers. The rescuer providing the breaths should be positioned at the person's head on one side while the other rescuer, who is giving chest compressions, should be positioned at the person's side on the other side. Ideally, the rescuers should be on opposite sides of the person to enable a quicker switch of tasks.

Protect against disease transmission by not sharing a mouth-to-barrier device (ie, mask or face shield) or by not giving mouth-to-mouth breaths. One option is for each rescuer to have their own pocket mask or mouth-to-barrier device to use while giving breaths. Another option is to use a bag-mask device **FIGURE C-1**; however, using a bag-mask device properly requires practice.

Appendix D

FEMA Disaster Supplies Checklists

TABLE D-1 First Aid Supplies

Supplies	Home	Vehicle	Work
Adhesive bandages, various sizes			
Sterile dressing (5 × 9 in. [13 × 23 cm])			
Conforming roller gauze bandage			
Triangular bandages			
Sterile gauze pads (3 × 3 in. [8 × 8 cm])			
Sterile gauze pads (4 × 4 in. [10 × 10 cm])			
Roll of cohesive bandage (3 in. [8 cm])			
Germicidal hand wipes or waterless, alcohol-based hand sanitizer			
Antiseptic wipes			
Pairs of large, medical grade, nonlatex gloves			
Tongue depressor blades			
Adhesive tape (2 in. [5 cm] wide)			
Antibacterial ointment			
Cold pack			
Scissors (small, personal)			
Tweezers			
Assorted sizes of safety pins			
Cotton balls			
Thermometer			
Tube of petroleum jelly or other lubricant			
Sunscreen			
CPR (cardiopulmonary resuscitation) breathing barrier, such as a face shield			
First aid manual			

FEMA. (2004). Are You Ready? An In-depth Guide to Citizen Preparedness. Retrieved from https://www.fema.gov/pdf/areyouready/areyouready_full.pdf

TABLE D-2 Nonprescription and Prescription Medicine Kit Supplies

Supplies	Home	Vehicle	Work
Aspirin and nonaspirin pain reliever			
Antidiarrhea medication			
Antacid (for stomach upset)			
Laxative			
Vitamins			
Prescriptions			
Extra eyeglasses/contact lenses			

FEMA. (2004). Are You Ready? An In-depth Guide to Citizen Preparedness. Retrieved from https://www.fema.gov/pdf/areyouready/areyouready_full.pdf

TABLE D-3 Sanitation and Hygiene Supplies

Item
Washcloth and towel
Towelettes, soap, hand sanitizer
Toothpaste, toothbrushes
Shampoo, comb, and brush
Deodorants, sunscreen
Razor, shaving cream
Lip balm, insect repellent
Feminine supplies
Diapers (3-day supply)
Heavy-duty plastic garbage bags and ties for personal sanitation uses and toilet paper
Medium-sized plastic bucket with tight lid (one per person)
Odor control (eg, cat litter)
Disinfectant and household chlorine bleach (When diluted 10 parts water to 1 part bleach, bleach can be used as a disinfectant. Or in an emergency, you can use it to treat water by using 16 drops of regular household liquid bleach per gallon of water. Do not use scented, color safe, or bleaches with added cleaners.)
A small shovel for digging a latrine
Toilet paper
Contact lens solution
Mirror

FEMA. (2004). Are You Ready? An In-depth Guide to Citizen Preparedness. Retrieved from https://www.fema.gov/pdf/areyouready/areyouready_full.pdf

TABLE D-4 Equipment and Tools

Tools	Kitchen Items
Portable, battery-powered radio or television and extra batteries	Manual can opener
National Oceanic and Atmospheric Administration (NOAA) Weather Radio, if appropriate for your area	Mess kits or paper cups, plates, and plastic utensils
Flashlight and extra batteries	All-purpose knife
Signal flare	Household liquid bleach to treat drinking water
Matches in a waterproof container (or waterproof matches)	Sugar, salt, pepper
Shut-off wrench, pliers, shovel, and other tools	Aluminum foil and plastic wrap
Duct tape and scissors	Resealable plastic bags
Plastic sheeting	Small cooking stove and a can of cooking fuel (if food must be cooked)
Whistle	
Small canister, ABC-type fire extinguisher	**Comfort Items**
Tube tent	Games
Compass	Cards
Work gloves	Books
Paper, pens, and pencils	Toys for kids
Needles and thread	Food
Battery-operated travel alarm clock	

Continues

TABLE D-4 Equipment and Tools (*Continued*)

Tools		Kitchen Items	
Zip ties and superglue in a sealed tube			
KN95 or N95 dust mask, to help filter contaminated air and plastic sheeting and duct tape to shelter-in-place			
Portable battery pack and charging cable for cell phone			

FEMA. (2004). Are You Ready? An In-depth Guide to Citizen Preparedness. Retrieved from https://www.fema.gov/pdf/areyouready/areyouready_full.pdf

TABLE D-5 Food and Water

Supplies	Home	Vehicle	Work
Water (1 gallon of water per person per day for at least 3 days, for drinking and sanitation)			
Ready-to-eat meats, fruits, and vegetables (at least a 3-day supply)			
Canned or boxed juices, milk, and soup			
High-energy foods such as peanut butter, jelly, low-sodium crackers, granola bars, and trail mix			
Vitamins			
Special foods for infants or persons on special diets			
Special food for pets			
Cookies, hard candy			
Instant coffee			
Cereals			
Powdered milk			

FEMA. (2004). Are You Ready? An In-depth Guide to Citizen Preparedness. Retrieved from https://www.fema.gov/pdf/areyouready/areyouready_full.pdf

TABLE D-6 Clothes and Bedding Supplies

Item	
Complete change of clothes	
Sturdy shoes or boots	
Rain gear	
Hat and gloves	
Extra socks	
Extra underwear	
Thermal underwear	
Sunglasses	
Blankets/sleeping bags and pillows	

FEMA. (2004). Are You Ready? An In-depth Guide to Citizen Preparedness. Retrieved from https://www.fema.gov/pdf/areyouready/areyouready_full.pdf

TABLE D-7 Documents and Keys

Item	Location Where Stored
Personal identification	
Cash and coins	
Credit cards	
Current list of medications, nutritional supplements and the name and contact information of the doctors who prescribed the medications	
Extra set of house keys and car keys	

Item	Location Where Stored
Copies of the following:	
■ Birth certificate	
■ Marriage certificate	
■ Driver's license	
■ Social Security card	
■ Passport	
■ Will	
■ Deeds	
■ Inventory of household goods	
■ Insurance papers	
■ Immunization records	
■ Bank and credit card account numbers	
■ Stocks and bonds	
■ Emergency contact list and phone numbers	
■ Map of the area and phone numbers of places you could go	

FEMA. (2004). Are You Ready? An In-depth Guide to Citizen Preparedness. Retrieved from https://www.fema.gov/pdf/areyouready/areyouready_full.pdf

Appendix E

Answer Key

Assessment in Action

Chapter 1

1. No; **2.** Yes; **3.** No; **4.** No

Chapter 2

1. Yes; **2.** No; **3.** Yes; **4.** Yes

Chapter 3

1. No; **2.** No; **3.** Yes; **4.** No

Chapter 4

1. No; **2.** Yes; **3.** Yes; **4.** Yes

Chapter 5

1. Yes; **2.** No; **3.** No; **4.** Yes; **5.** Yes; **6.** Yes

Chapter 6

1. Yes; **2.** Yes; **3.** No; **4.** Yes; **5.** No

Chapter 7

1. Yes; **2.** Yes; **3.** No; **4.** No

Chapter 8

1. Yes; **2.** Yes; **3.** No; **4.** Yes

Chapter 9

1. No; **2.** No; **3.** Yes; **4.** No

Chapter 10

1. Yes; **2.** Yes; **3.** Yes; **4.** No; **5.** Yes

Chapter 11

1. No; **2.** No; **3.** Yes; **4.** Yes; **5.** Yes

Chapter 12

1. No; **2.** Yes; **3.** Yes; **4.** No

Chapter 13

1. Yes; **2.** Yes; **3.** No; **4.** Yes; **5.** Yes

Chapter 14

1. Yes; **2.** Yes; **3.** Yes; **4.** No; **5.** Yes

Chapter 15

1. Yes; **2.** Yes; **3.** No; **4.** Yes

Chapter 16

1. Yes; **2.** Yes; **3.** No; **4.** Yes

Chapter 17

1. No; **2.** Yes; **3.** Yes

Chapter 18

1. No; **2.** No; **3.** Yes; **4.** Yes

Chapter 19

1. No; **2.** No; **3.** No; **4.** Yes; **5.** Yes

Chapter 20

1. Yes; **2.** Yes; **3.** No; **4.** Yes; **5.** Yes

Chapter 21

1. No; **2.** Yes; **3.** Yes; **4.** No; **5.** Yes; **6.** Yes

Chapter 22

1. No; **2.** No; **3.** No; **4.** Yes; **5.** Yes

Chapter 23

1. Yes; **2.** Yes; **3.** Yes; **4.** Yes; **5.** No

Chapter 24

1. Yes; **2.** Yes; **3.** No; **4.** Yes

Chapter 25

1. No; **2.** No; **3.** Yes; **4.** Yes

Chapter 26

1. No; **2.** Yes; **3.** No; **4.** Yes; **5.** Yes

Check Your Knowledge

Chapter 1

1. No; **2.** Yes; **3.** No; **4.** No; **5.** Yes; **6.** No; **7.** Yes; **8.** Yes; **9.** Yes; **10.** No

Chapter 2

1. Yes; **2.** No; **3.** Yes; **4.** Yes; **5.** Yes; **6.** Yes; **7.** Yes; **8.** Yes; **9.** Yes; **10.** No

Chapter 3

1. No; **2.** No; **3.** Yes; **4.** Yes; **5.** No; **6.** Yes; **7.** No; **8.** Yes; **9.** Yes; **10.** Yes

Chapter 4

1. Yes; **2.** No; **3.** Yes; **4.** No; **5.** Yes; **6.** No; **7.** Yes

Chapter 5

1. Yes; **2.** Yes; **3.** Yes; **4.** Yes; **5.** No; **6.** Yes; **7.** Yes; **8.** Yes; **9.** No; **10.** Yes

Chapter 6

1. Yes; **2.** Yes; **3.** No; **4.** No; **5.** No; **6.** Yes; **7.** No; **8.** Yes; **9.** Yes; **10.** No

Chapter 7

1. No; **2.** Yes; **3.** No; **4.** No; **5.** Yes; **6.** Yes; **7.** Yes; **8.** Yes; **9.** Yes; **10.** No

Chapter 8

1. No; **2.** No; **3.** Yes; **4.** No; **5.** Yes; **6.** No; **7.** Yes; **8.** Yes; **9.** Yes; **10.** Yes

Chapter 9

1. Yes; **2.** No; **3.** Yes; **4.** Yes; **5.** Yes; **6.** No; **7.** Yes; **8.** No; **9.** No; **10.** Yes

Chapter 10

1. No; **2.** Yes; **3.** Yes; **4.** No; **5.** No; **6.** Yes; **7.** No; **8.** No; **9.** Yes; **10.** Yes

Chapter 11

1. No; **2.** No; **3.** Yes; **4.** No; **5.** Yes; **6.** Yes; **7.** Yes; **8.** No; **9.** Yes; **10.** No

Chapter 12

1. No; **2.** No; **3.** No; **4.** Yes; **5.** No; **6.** Yes; **7.** No; **8.** Yes; **9.** Yes; **10.** Yes

Chapter 13

1. Yes; **2.** No; **3.** No; **4.** No; **5.** Yes; **6.** Yes; **7.** No; **8.** Yes; **9.** No; **10.** Yes

Chapter 14

1. Yes; **2.** Yes; **3.** Yes; **4.** Yes; **5.** No; **6.** No; **7.** No; **8.** Yes; **9.** No; **10.** Yes

Chapter 15

1. Yes; **2.** No; **3.** Yes; **4.** No; **5.** No; **6.** Yes; **7.** Yes; **8.** No; **9.** No; **10.** Yes

Chapter 16

1. Yes; **2.** No; **3.** Yes; **4.** Yes; **5.** No; **6.** Yes; **7.** No; **8.** No; **9.** Yes; **10.** Yes

Chapter 17

1. Yes; **2.** Yes; **3.** Yes; **4.** Yes; **5.** Yes; **6.** No; **7.** Yes; **8.** No; **9.** Yes; **10.** Yes

Chapter 18

1. Yes; **2.** No; **3.** No; **4.** No; **5.** No; **6.** No; **7.** Yes; **8.** Yes; **9.** Yes; **10.** Yes

Chapter 19

1. Yes; **2.** No; **3.** No; **4.** Yes; **5.** Yes; **6.** Yes; **7.** Yes; **8.** No; **9.** No; **10.** Yes

Chapter 20

1. Yes; **2.** No; **3.** Yes; **4.** Yes; **5.** Yes; **6.** No; **7.** No; **8.** Yes; **9.** Yes; **10.** No

Chapter 21

1. Yes; **2.** Yes; **3.** Yes; **4.** Yes; **5.** Yes; **6.** No; **7.** Yes; **8.** No; **9.** Yes; **10.** Yes

Chapter 22

1. Yes; **2.** No; **3.** No; **4.** Yes; **5.** No; **6.** Yes; **7.** Yes; **8.** No; **9.** Yes; **10.** Yes

Chapter 23

1. Yes; **2.** Yes; **3.** No; **4.** Yes; **5.** No; **6.** No; **7.** Yes; **8.** No; **9.** Yes; **10.** No

Chapter 24

1. No; **2.** Yes; **3.** Yes; **4.** No; **5.** No; **6.** Yes; **7.** Yes; **8.** No; **9.** No; **10.** Yes

Chapter 25

1. No; **2.** Yes; **3.** Yes; **4.** Yes; **5.** Yes; **6.** No; **7.** Yes; **8.** No; **9.** Yes; **10.** No

Chapter 26

1. No; **2.** No; **3.** Yes; **4.** No; **5.** No; **6.** Yes; **7.** Yes; **8.** No; **9.** Yes; **10.** No

Glossary

3Es A strategy to produce effective prevention by combining three types of intervention: education, enforcement, and engineering.

abandonment Failure to continue first aid until relieved by someone with an equal or higher level of training.

abdomen The body cavity that contains the major organs of digestion and excretion. It is located below the diaphragm and above the pelvis.

abrasion An injury in which a portion of the skin is removed by rubbing or scraping on a hard, rough surface.

act of commission A breach of duty in which the provider does something that a reasonably prudent person would not do under the same or similar circumstances.

act of omission A breach of duty in which the provider fails to do what a reasonably prudent person with the same or similar training would do in the same or similar circumstances.

acute mountain sickness (AMS) A condition that effects people in high altitudes; symptoms include dizziness, nausea, headache, and shortness of breath.

adhesive bandage A combination of both a sterile dressing and a bandage.

adhesive tape Tape used to secure bandages and dressings; available in rolls and in a variety of widths.

adverse drug interaction An unintended or harmful response to two or more drugs being taken concurrently.

airborne disease An infection transmitted through the air, such as tuberculosis (TB).

airway obstruction A blockage, often the result of a foreign body, in which airflow to the lungs is reduced or completely blocked.

alveoli The air sacs of the lungs in which the exchange of oxygen and carbon dioxide takes place.

amniotic sac A thick, transparent sac that holds the fetus suspended in the amniotic fluid.

amputation An injury in which a body part is completely removed.

anaphylaxis A life-threatening allergic reaction.

angina pectoris A spasmodic pain in the chest, characterized by a sensation of severe constriction or pressure on the anterior chest; associated with insufficient blood supply to the heart, aggravated by exercise or tension, and relieved by rest or medication.

anterior The front surface of the body.

anterior nosebleed Bleeding from the front of the nose.

antivenom An antiserum containing antibodies against reptile or insect venom.

aorta The principal artery leaving the left side of the heart and carrying freshly oxygenated blood to the body.

artery A blood vessel, consisting of three layers of tissue and smooth muscle, that carries blood away from the heart.

arterial bleeding Bleeding from an artery. This type of bleeding initially spurts up to several feet from the wound.

assault A threat or attempt to touch another person without consent.

asthma A condition marked by recurrent attacks of breathing difficulty, often with wheezing, due to spasmodic constriction of the air passages, often as a response to allergens or to mucus plugs in the bronchioles.

automated external defibrillator (AED) A device capable of analyzing the heart rhythm and providing a shock.

avulsion An injury that leaves a piece of skin or other tissue either partially or completely torn away from the body.

bandage A material used to cover a dressing to keep it in place on the wound and to apply pressure to help control bleeding.

barbiturates A group of drugs in the class of drugs known as sedatives.

battery Touching a person or providing first aid without consent.

battle sign A contusion on the mastoid area of either ear; sign of a basilar skull fracture.

biologic agents Organisms or toxins that can kill or incapacitate people, livestock, and crops.

birth canal The vagina and the lower part of the uterus.

blood The fluid that circulates through the heart, arteries, capillaries, and veins, carrying nutrients and oxygen to the body cells and removing waste products such as carbon dioxide and various metabolic products for excretion.

bloodborne disease An infection transmitted through the blood, such as human immunodeficiency virus (HIV) or hepatitis B virus (HBV).

bloody show The bloody mucus plug that is discharged from the vagina when labor begins.

bones The hard form of connective tissue that constitutes most of the skeleton in humans.

brachial artery The artery of the arm that branches at the elbow into the radial and ulnar arteries; used to determine an infant's pulse.

brainstem The area of the brain between the spinal cord and cerebrum, surrounded by the cerebellum; controls automatic functions that are necessary for life, such as respirations.

brain The soft, large mass of nerve tissue that is contained in the cranium.

breach of duty Failure of a first aid provider to deliver the type of care that would be given by a person having the same or similar training.

breech Birth presentation where the baby's buttocks or lower extremities emerge before the head or shoulders.

bronchial tubes The passageways from the trachea to the lungs.

burn An injury in which soft tissue absorbs more energy than it can dissipate from thermal heat, chemicals, or electricity.

capillaries The small blood vessels through whose walls various substances pass into and out of the tissues and on to the cells.

capillary bleeding Bleeding that oozes from a wound steadily but slowly.

carbon monoxide A colorless, odorless, poisonous gas formed by incomplete combustion, such as in fire.

cardiac arrest Stoppage of the heartbeat.

cardiac muscle The heart muscle.

cardiopulmonary resuscitation (CPR) The act of providing chest compressions and rescue breaths for a person in cardiac arrest.

cardiovascular system The arrangement of connected tubes, including the arteries, arterioles, capillaries, venules, and veins, that moves blood, oxygen, nutrients, carbon dioxide, and cellular waste throughout the body.

carotid artery The major arteries that supply blood to the head and brain.

cause of injury The force that causes an injury; sometimes called mechanism of injury or MOI.

cavitation A localized expansion of tissue resulting from the shock wave of a bullet.

central nervous system (CNS) The brain and spinal cord.

cerebellum One of the three major subdivisions of the brain; coordinates voluntary body movements.

cerebrospinal fluid (CSF) A clear, watery solution similar to blood plasma.

cerebrum The largest part of the three subdivisions of the brain, made up of several lobes that control movement, hearing, balance, speech, visual perception, emotions, and personality.

cervix The small opening at the lower end of the uterus through which the baby passes.

chain of survival A concept involving six critical links (recognition and activation of EMS, CPR, defibrillation, advanced care, post-arrest care, recovery) to help improve survival from cardiac arrest.

chemical burn An injury to the skin caused by contact with chemicals.

chemical warfare agents Poisonous vapors, aerosols, liquids, or solids that have toxic effects.

chest compression The act of depressing the chest and allowing it to return to its normal position as part of CPR.

chief complaint The primary symptom a person complains about; also, the person's response to questions such as "What is wrong?" or "What happened?"; the reason EMS or professional medical care was called for in the patient's own words when possible.

chilblain A nonfreezing cold injury that, while painful, causes little or no permanent damage.

child abuse Doing something or failing to do something that can result in physical or emotional injury or neglect of a child.

chronic obstructive pulmonary disease (COPD) A disease that makes it hard for a person to breathe because the normal flow of air into and out of the person's lungs is partially obstructed.

clavicle The collarbone.

clean amputation A clean-cut, complete detachment of an extremity.

closed abdominal injury An injury to the abdomen that occurs as a result of a direct blow from a blunt object. There is no break in the skin.

closed chest injury An injury to the chest in which the skin is not broken; usually due to blunt trauma.

closed fracture A fracture in which there is no wound in the overlying skin.

cold stress An injury that develops when a person has been exposed to a cold environment; can cause shivering, however the person affected will be alert and can move and care for themselves; not to be confused with hypothermia.

communicable disease A disease that can spread from person to person or from animal to person.

concussion A temporary disturbance of brain activity caused by a blow to the head; also known as mild traumatic brain injury.

conduction The process by which heat is directly transmitted from one object to another.

consent An agreement by a person in need of care to accept treatment offered as explained by medical personnel or first aid providers.

contusion A bruise; an injury that causes a hemorrhage in or beneath the skin but does not break the skin.

convection The transfer of heat by the circulation or movement of heated parts of a liquid or gas.

coup-contrecoup Dual impacts of the brain into the skull; coup injury occurs at the site of impact; contrecoup injury occurs on the opposite side of impact, as the brain rebounds.

cramp A painful spasm of a muscle.

cranium The area of the head above the ears and eyes; the part of the skull that contains the brain.

cravat A folded triangular bandage used to hold splints and dressings in place, to apply pressure evenly over a dressing, or as a swathe (binder) for an injured arm in an arm sling.

crepitus A grating sound heard and the sensation felt when the fractured ends of a bone rub together.

crowning The stage of birth when the presenting part of the baby is visible at the vaginal orifice.

crushing amputation An injury in which an extremity separates by being crushed or mashed off.

cyanosis A blue-gray skin color that is caused by a reduced level of oxygen in the blood.

deep Located farther inside the body and away from the skin.

defibrillation The electrical shock administered by an AED to reestablish a normal heart rhythm.

dehydration Loss of water from the tissues of the body.

depressant An agent that produces a depressed or reduced level of stimulation.

depression A persistent mood of sadness, despair, and discouragement.

dermis The inner layer of the skin, containing hair follicles, sweat glands, nerve endings, and blood vessels.

desensitization A process of deconditioning or counterconditioning designed reduce a person's fears and anxieties. The idea is to weaken an undesirable response such as fainting by strengthening an incompatible response.

diabetes A condition that develops when glucose builds up in the blood, overflows into the urine, and passes through the body unused.

diabetic coma A state of unresponsiveness caused by a lack of insulin that goes uncorrected for too long.

diaphragm A muscular dome that forms the undersurface of the thorax, separating the chest from the abdominal cavity. Contraction of the diaphragm brings air into the lungs. Relaxation allows air to be expelled from the lungs.

diffuse axonal Tearing brain injury caused by shaking or strong rotation of the head.

dislocation The displacement of a bone from its normal joint alignment, out of its socket, or out of its normal position.

distal Located away from the center of the body or from the point of attachment, such as the point where the arm or leg attaches to the body.

domestic violence Injury (emotional or physical) that a person inflicts upon another person with whom they had or have a relationship.

dorsalis pedis artery The artery on the anterior (top) surface of the foot between the first and second metatarsals.

DOTS A mnemonic for assessment in which each area of the body is evaluated for deformities, open wounds, tenderness, and swelling.

dressing A sterile gauze pad or clean cloth covering that is placed over an open wound.

drowning The process of experiencing respiratory impairment from submersion/immersion in liquid.

duty to act A person's responsibility to provide care.

ectopic pregnancy A pregnancy that develops outside the uterus, typically in a fallopian tube.

elastic roller bandage A type of bandage used for compression on sprains, strains, and contusions; available in various widths.

elder abuse Any action on the part of an older person's family member, caregiver, or other associated person that takes advantage of the older person, their property, or emotional state.

electrical burn An injury to the skin and the inside of the body caused by contact with electric current.

emergency medical services (EMS) A system that represents the combined efforts of several professionals and agencies to provide emergency medical care.

epidermis The outer layer of the skin, which is made up of cells that are sealed together to form a watertight protective covering for the body.

epiglottis A small flap of tissue that allows air to pass into the trachea but prevents food and liquid from entering.

epinephrine auto-injector A prescribed device used to administer an emergency dose of epinephrine to a person experiencing anaphylaxis.

esophagus A collapsible tube that extends from the pharynx to the stomach. Contractions of the muscle in the wall of the esophagus propel food and liquids through it to the stomach.

evaporation Conversion of water or another fluid from a liquid to a gas.

expressed consent Permission for care that a person gives verbally or with a head nod.

fallopian tubes The tubes that connect each ovary with the uterus.

femoral artery The principal artery of the thigh. It supplies blood to the lower abdominal wall, external genitalia, and leg. There are two, one in each leg. It can be palpated in the groin area.

femur The thigh bone; the longest and one of the strongest bones in the body.

fetus The developing, unborn offspring inside the uterus.

fibula The outer and smaller bone of the two bones of the lower leg.

first aid Immediate care given to an injured or suddenly ill person.

first-degree (superficial) burn A burn affecting only the epidermis; characterized by skin that is red but not blistered or burned through.

flail chest A condition that occurs when several ribs in the same area are broken in more than one place.

floating ribs The 11th and 12th ribs, which do not attach to the sternum.

fontanelles Areas where the infant's skull has not fused together; usually disappear at approximately 18 months of age.

foramen magnum A large opening at the base of the skull through which the brain connects to the spinal cord.

fracture A break or crack in the bone.

frostbite The damage to tissues as a result of prolonged exposure to extreme cold.

frostnip The reversible freezing of superficial skin layers that is usually marked by numbness and yellow to gray skin.

gangrene Permanent damage or death of tissue.

gauze pad A type of sterile dressing used for small wounds; available in separately wrapped packages of various sizes. Some have a special coating to keep them from sticking to the wound.

gauze roller A type of bandage that is cotton and nonelastic, and used to wrap or bind various body parts; available in various widths.

general impression The part of the assessment that helps identify any immediately or potentially life-threatening conditions.

glycogen Main form in which carbohydrate is stored in the liver and then broken down into glucose (sugar) for energy.

Good Samaritan laws Laws that encourage people to voluntarily help an injured or suddenly ill person by minimizing the liability for errors made while rendering emergency care in good faith.

grieving process The emotional process that a person works through after a stressful situation that causes personal pain. People go through several stages of grieving.

Haddon Matrix A strategy for identifying interventions that can be applied to any type of illness or injury. Interventions proceed through three stages: pre-event, event, and post-event.

hallucinogens An agent that produces false perceptions in any one of the five senses.

head tilt–chin lift maneuver A combination of two movements to open the airway by tilting the forehead back and lifting the chin.

heart A hollow, muscular organ that receives blood from the veins and propels it into the arteries.

heart attack A lay term for a condition resulting from blockage of a coronary artery and subsequent death of part of the heart muscle; a myocardial infarction; sometimes called simply "a coronary."

heat cramps A painful muscle cramp resulting from excessive loss of salt and water through sweating.

heat escape lessening position (HELP) The recommended position (knees pulled up, arms crossed) for a person who is in cold water and wearing a flotation device; meant to minimize heat loss and increase chances of survival.

heat exhaustion A prostration caused by excessive loss of water and salt through sweating; characterized by clammy skin and a weak, rapid pulse.

heatstroke An acute and dangerous reaction to heat exposure characterized by high body temperature and altered mental status.

hemorrhage A large amount of bleeding in a short time.

hemostatic gauze dressing A gauze-style dressing that is saturated with an agent that stops bleeding.

hepatitis B virus (HBV) A viral infection of the liver for which a vaccine is available.

hepatitis C virus (HCV) A viral infection of the liver for which no vaccine is currently available.

high-altitude cerebral edema (HACE) A medical condition where high altitude causes the brain to swell with fluid.

high-altitude pulmonary edema (HAPE) When lung vessels constrict and increase pressure causing fluid to leak into the lung tissues and eventually the air sacs.

human immunodeficiency virus (HIV) The virus that can cause acquired immunodeficiency syndrome (AIDS).

humerus The bone of the upper arm.

hurricane A tropical storm with winds that have reached a constant speed of at least 74 miles per hour (119 kph). Those in the Pacific Ocean are called typhoons and those in the Indian Ocean are known as cyclones.

hyperglycemia An abnormally increased concentration of glucose in the blood.

hyperventilation Excessively fast breathing that occurs during emotional distress.

hypoglycemia An abnormally diminished concentration of glucose in the blood.

hyponatremia A condition that occurs when the level of sodium in the body is inadequate.

hypothermia Decreased body temperature; severe hypothermia is life threatening.

hypoxia A low oxygen content in the blood; lack of oxygen in inspired air.

implied consent The legally permissible assumption that an unconscious person in need of emergency life-saving treatment would accept treatment, were they alert and able.

incision A wound that is usually made deliberately in connection with surgery. The edges are cleanly cut as opposed to a laceration.

infectious disease A medical condition caused by the growth of small, harmful organisms within the body.

inferior Located closer to the feet.

inferior vena cava Large vein located between the spine and the abdominal organs.

ingested poisoning Poisoning caused by swallowing a toxic substance.

joint The place where two bones come into contact.

labor The process or period of childbirth; especially, the muscular contraction of the uterus designed to expel the fetus from the mother.

laceration A wound made by the tearing or cutting of body tissues.

larynx The voice box.

lateral Located farther from the middle of the body.

ligament A band of the fibrous tissue that connects bones to bones. It supports and strengthens a joint.

meconium A dark green material in the amniotic fluid that can indicate fetal distress; the infant's first bowel movement.

medial Located closer to the middle of the body.

miscarriage Delivery of the fetus before it is mature enough to survive outside the womb (about 20 weeks), from either natural (spontaneous abortion) or induced causes.

naloxone A medication used to counter the effects of opioids.

narcotics A drug that produces sleep or altered mental status.

nature of illness (NOI) The general type of illness a person is experiencing.

neglect Refusal or failure on the part of the caregiver to provide life necessities.

negligence Deviation from the accepted standard of care that results in further injury to the person.

nematocysts Stinging cells found on certain marine animals.

nervous system The system that controls virtually all activities of the body, both voluntary and involuntary.

neurogenic shock Cardiovascular failure caused by paralysis of the nerves that control the size of the blood vessels, leading to widespread dilation; seen in people with spinal cord injuries.

open abdominal injury An injury to the abdomen in which the skin is broken; can involve a penetrating wound or protruding organs.

open chest injury An injury to the chest in which the chest wall itself is penetrated by an external object such as a bullet or knife.

open fracture A fracture exposed to the exterior; an open wound lies over the fracture.

opiates A drug containing or derived from opium.

opioids A synthetically produced narcotic not derived from opium.

paradoxical movement The movement of the portion of the chest wall that is detached in a flail chest; the movement (in during inhalation, out during exhalation) is the opposite of normal chest wall movement during breathing.

paraplegia Paralysis of the legs caused by damage to the spine.

patella The kneecap; a specialized bone that lies within the tendon of the quadriceps muscle.

perfusion The circulation of oxygenated blood within an organ or tissue in adequate amounts to meet the cells' current needs.

peripheral nervous system A network of nerve cells that originates in the brain and spinal cord and extends to all parts of the body, including the muscles, the surface of the skin, and the special sense organs, such as the eyes and the ears.

personal protective equipment (PPE) Equipment, such as exam gloves, used to block the entry of an organism into the body.

pharynx The throat.

physical exam A part of the secondary assessment process in which a detailed exam is performed, based on the body system of the chief complaint, on people whose conditions cannot be readily identified or when more specific information is needed about a condition.

placenta The vascular organ attached to the uterine wall that supplies oxygen and nutrients to the fetus; also called afterbirth.

plasma A sticky, yellow fluid that carries the blood cells and nutrients and transports cellular waste material to the organs of excretion.

platelets Tiny, disk-shaped elements that are much smaller than cells. They are essential in the initial formation of a blood clot, the mechanism that stops bleeding.

pneumothorax Accumulation of air in the pleural space.

poison Any substance that impairs health or causes death by its chemical action when it enters the body or comes in contact with the skin.

Poison Help A medical facility operated by the National Poison Control Center that provides immediate, free, expert advice any time; can be reached by calling 1-800-222-1222.

posterior nosebleed Bleeding from the back of the nose, which may flow out of the nostrils and into the mouth or throat.

posterior The back surface of the body.

posterior tibial artery The artery just posterior to the medial malleolus; supplies blood to the foot.

posttraumatic stress disorder (PTSD) A delayed stress reaction to a prior emergency event.

primary assessment When a first aid provider checks for life-threatening injuries and gives care for any that are found.

prolapsed cord A condition in which the umbilical cord comes out of the vagina before the infant.

protruding organ injury A severe injury to the abdomen in which the internal organs escape or protrude from the wound; also known as evisceration.

proximal Located closer to the center of the body or to the point of attachment, such as the point where the arm or leg attaches to the body.

psychogenic shock A sudden nervous system reaction that produces a temporary vascular dilation, resulting in fainting, or syncope.

psychological emergency Any situation in which a person is experiencing extreme distress, is unable to cope with everyday life, or is in danger of hurting themselves or others.

pulse The wave of pressure created as the heart contracts and forces blood out of the left ventricle and into the major arteries.

puncture A deep, narrow wound in the skin and underlying organs.

quadrant A section of the abdominal cavity. Imagine a horizontal and a vertical line intersecting at the umbilicus, dividing the abdomen into four equal areas.

quadriplegia Paralysis of the arms and legs caused by damage to the spine.

rabies An acute viral infection of the central nervous system transmitted by the bite of an infected animal.

radial artery A main artery in the forearm. It is palpable at the wrist on the thumb side.

radiation The transfer of heat to colder objects in the environment by radiant energy.

radius The bone on the thumb side of the forearm.

red blood cells Cells that carry oxygen to the body tissues; also called erythrocytes.

respiration The inhalation of cold air that is warmed by the body, leading to heat loss when exhaled.

respiratory system All the structures of the body that contribute to the process of breathing, consisting of the upper and lower airways and their component parts.

roller bandage A type of bandage used to wrap or bind various body parts; available in various widths, lengths, and types of material.

rule of thirds A system that divides each long bone into thirds to determine which section or sections of an injured bone should be splinted.

safety data sheet (SDS) A form, provided by manufacturers and distributors of chemicals, containing information about chemical composition, physical and chemical properties, health and safety hazards, first aid procedures, and handling and storage of a specific chemical.

SAMPLE history A brief history of a person's condition to determine signs and symptoms, allergies, medications, pertinent past medical history, last oral intake, and events leading to the illness/injury.

scapula The shoulder blade.

scene size-up A quick assessment of the scene and the surroundings for safety issues, the cause of injury or nature of illness, and the number of people; it is completed before starting first aid.

second-degree (partial-thickness) burn A burn affecting the epidermis and some portion of the dermis but not the subcutaneous tissue; characterized by blisters and skin that is white to red and moist.

sedatives A class of drugs that act as a central nervous system depressant.

seizure Generalized, uncoordinated muscular activity associated with a loss of responsiveness; a convulsion; an attack of epilepsy.

self-adhering, conforming bandage A type of bandage that bonds to itself as it is wrapped, helping to secure itself in place; available as rolls of slightly elastic, gauzelike material in various widths.

severe acute respiratory syndrome coronavirus 2 (SARS-CoV-2) The virus that causes an infection called coronavirus 2019 (COVID-19), which primarily affects the lungs and can lead to respiratory failure and death.

shock Inadequate tissue perfusion resulting from serious injury or illness.

sign Evidence of an injury or disease that can be seen, heard, or felt; objective findings.

skeletal muscle Muscle that is attached to bones and usually crosses at least one joint. It is striated, or voluntary, muscle.

skeleton The framework that gives us our recognizable form; also designed to allow motion of the body and protection of vital organs.

skull fracture A break or a crack in the cranium (bony case surrounding the brain).

sling A triangular bandage applied around the neck to support an injured upper extremity; any material long enough to suspend an upper extremity by passing the material around the neck; used to support and protect an injury of the arm, shoulder, or clavicle.

smooth muscle Muscle that constitutes the bulk of the gastrointestinal tract and is present in nearly every organ to regulate automatic activity. It is nonstriated, or involuntary, muscle.

spinal cord An extension of the brain, composed of virtually all the nerves carrying messages between the brain and the rest of the body. It lies inside of and is protected by the spinal canal.

splint Any support used to stabilize a fracture or to restrict movement of a part.

sprain A trauma to a joint that injures the ligaments.

stabilize To minimize further injury by holding a body part to prevent movement.

standard of care The level of care legally and ethically required of a provider. To meet the standard of care when providing first aid, a provider must (1) do what is expected of someone with first aid training and experience working under similar conditions, and (2) treat the person to the best of their ability.

standard precautions Protective measures that have traditionally been developed by the Centers for Disease Control and Prevention (CDC) for use in dealing with objects, blood, body fluids, or other potential exposure risks of communicable disease.

status epilepticus The occurrence of two or more seizures without a period of complete consciousness between them or a lengthy seizure lasting more than 5 minutes.

sternum The breast bone.

stimulant An agent that produces an excited state.

strain An injury to a muscle caused by a violent contraction or an excessive, forcible stretching.

strain A tearing of muscle that occurs when the muscle is stretched beyond its normal range of motion.

stroke A brain injury due to bleeding in the brain tissue or to a blockage of blood flow, causing permanent damage.

sucking chest wound A chest wound that allows air to pass into the chest cavity with each breath.

suicide Any willful act that ends one's own life.

superficial Located closer to or on the skin.

superior Located closer to the head.

swathe A cravat tied around the body to decrease movement of a part.

symptom What a person tells a first aid provider about what they feel; subjective findings.

syncope Fainting; a brief period of unresponsiveness.

tendinitis Inflammation of a tendon caused by overuse.

tendons The fibrous connective tissue that attaches muscle to bone.

terrorism The unlawful use of force or violence against people or property for purposes of intimidation, coercion, or ransom.

thermal (heat) burn Damage to the skin caused by contact with hot objects, flammable vapor, steam, hot liquid, or flames.

thermoregulation The body's ability to maintain a normal body temperature despite environmental conditions of heat or cold.

third-degree (full-thickness) burn A burn that affects all skin layers and possibly the subcutaneous layers, muscle, bone, and internal organs, leaving the area dry, leathery, and white, dark brown, or charred.

thorax The chest cavity that contains the heart, lungs, esophagus, and great vessels.

tibia The shin bone; the larger of the two bones of the lower leg.

tourniquet A bleeding control device that is wrapped tightly around an extremity to stop blood flow from a wound.

toxin A poisonous substance produced by bacteria, animals, or plants that acts by changing the normal metabolism of cells or by destroying them.

trachea The windpipe; the main trunk for air passing to and from the lungs.

tranquilizers (benzodiazepines) A group of drugs in the class of drugs known as sedatives.

transient ischemic attack (TIA) A form of stroke that occurs when a part of the brain is deprived of oxygen-rich blood long enough to cause symptoms but not long enough to cause permanent damage; a mini-stroke.

trauma dressing A type of dressing made of large, thick, absorbent, sterile materials.

trench foot A serious nonfreezing cold injury that develops when the skin on the feet is exposed to moisture and cold for prolonged periods (12 hours or longer); also called immersion foot.

triage A system used for sorting people to determine the order in which they will receive medical attention.

triangular bandage A type of bandage available commercially or that can be made from a square piece of preshrunk cotton muslin measuring 36 to 40 inches (230 to 260 cm) along each side of the square.

tsunami A series of waves generated by an undersea disturbance.

tuberculosis (TB) A bacterial disease usually affecting the lungs.

ulna The inner bone of the forearm, on the side opposite the thumb.

umbilical cord The flexible structure that connects the fetus to the placenta.

vasoconstriction The narrowing of the diameter of a blood vessel.

vasovagal syncope A shock-like state due to severe emotional distress; may result in a fainting spell resulting from a transient decrease in blood flow to the brain.

vein Any blood vessel that carries blood from the tissues to the heart.

vena cava syndrome A set of symptoms that occur when blood flow to the inferior vena cava is compressed or blocked.

venous bleeding Bleeding from a vein. This type of bleeding tends to flow steadily.

ventricular fibrillation (VF) A potentially life-threatening electrical condition, in which the heart muscle contracts and relaxes in a disorganized fashion; the lower chambers of the heart quiver and cannot pump blood.

ventricular tachycardia (VT) A potentially life-threatening electrical condition, in which the heart beats too fast to pump blood effectively.

vertebrae The 33 bones that make up the spinal column.

voluntary muscle Muscle that is under direct voluntary control of the brain and can be contracted or relaxed at will; skeletal or striated muscle.

white blood cells Blood cells involved in the body's immune defense mechanisms against infection.

wilderness A remote geographic location more than 1 hour from definitive medical care.

windchill The relationship of wind velocity and temperature in determining the effect of cold on living organisms.

xiphoid process The lowest part of the sternum.

Index

Note: Page numbers followed by *f* or *t* indicate material in figures and tables, respectively.

A

B

C

D

E

F

G

H

L

M

N

T

X

Y